Operative Surgery of the Colon, Rectum and Anus

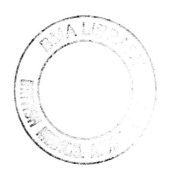

Operative Surgery of the Colon, Rectum and Anus

SIXTH EDITION

Edited by

P Ronan O'Connell MD FRCSI FRCPS(Glas) FRCS(Edin)
Professor of Surgery, University College Dublin;
Consultant Surgeon, St Vincent's University Hospital, Dublin, Ireland

Robert D Madoff MD FACS FASCRS FRCSEd(Hon)
Stanley M. Goldberg MD Professor of Colon and Rectal Surgery;
Chief, Division of Colon and Rectal Surgery,
University of Minnesota, Minneapolis, MN, USA

Michael J Solomon MBBCh(Hons) MSc FRCSI FRACS
Clinical Professor of Surgery, University of Sydney; Academic Head, Department of Colorectal
Surgery and Head, Surgical Outcome Research Centre (SOuRCE); Chairman, Institute of Academic
Surgery at Royal Prince Alfred Hospital and the University of Sydney, Sydney, Australia

Advisory Editor

Sir Norman S Williams MS FRCS FMEDSCI FRCP FRCP(Edin)
FRCA FDS(Hon) FACS(Hon) FRCSI(Hon)
Professor of Surgery; Director of National Centre for Bowel Research and
Surgical Innovation, Barts and the London School of Medicine and Dentistry;
Honorary Consultant Colorectal Surgeon, Barts Health National Centre for
Bowel Research and Surgical Innovation, London, UK

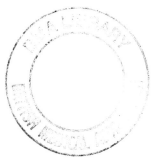

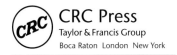
CRC Press
Taylor & Francis Group
Boca Raton London New York

CRC Press is an imprint of the
Taylor & Francis Group, an **informa** business

CRC Press
Taylor & Francis Group
6000 Broken Sound Parkway NW, Suite 300
Boca Raton, FL 33487-2742

© 2015 by Taylor & Francis Group, LLC
CRC Press is an imprint of Taylor & Francis Group, an Informa business

No claim to original U.S. Government works

Printed and bound in India by Replika Press Pvt. Ltd.

Printed on acid-free paper
Version Date: 20150217

International Standard Book Number-13: 978-0-340-99127-5 (Pack – Book and Ebook)

Medical Illustrators: Graeme Chambers, Emily Evans, Brenda L. Bunch, Jennifer C. Darcy, Oxford Designers & Illustrators, Wendy Hiller Gee, Katie Dale, Jennifer Gentry, Elizabeth Nixon Shapiro, Morgan Noonan, Zina Studios, Jeanne Robertson, Bricelyn H. Strauch, Amy D'Camp, Sarah J. Taylor, Jane Fallow

Visit the Taylor & Francis Web site at
http://www.taylorandfrancis.com

and the CRC Press Web site at
http://www.crcpress.com

Contents

Contributors

DF Altomare MD
Associate Professor of Surgery, Department of Emergency and Organ Transplantation, University of Bari, Bari, Italy
8.1, Delorme operation

Kirk KS Austin BSc AFRCSI FRACS
Department of Colorectal Surgery and Surgical Outcomes Research Centre (SOuRCe), University of Sydney, Royal Prince Alfred Hospital, Camperdown, Australia
6.11, Operative technique for pelvic exenteration

Robert W Beart MD
Emeritus Professor, Department of Surgery (Colorectal), University of Southern California, Keck School of Medicine, Los Angeles, CA, USA
1.9, Anastomotic technique – stapled

Chetan Bhan MBBS MSc FRCS (Gen Surg)
Consultant Colorectal Surgeon and Training Programme Director, UCL Partners, Whittington Health, Highgate Hill, London, UK
8.7, The EXPRESS procedure

Rakesh Bhardwaj MD FRCS
Consultant Colorectal Surgeon, Darent Valley Hospital, Dartford, UK
5.14, Colonic stenting

Ian P Bissett MB ChB FRACS MD
Associate Professor and Head, Department of Surgery, University of Auckland, Auckland, New Zealand
1.1, Preparation for colorectal surgery

W Donald Buie MD MSc FRCSC FACS
Associate Professor of Surgery and Oncology, Site Chief, Division of General Surgery, Foothills Hospital; Program Director, Colorectal Surgery Program, Department of Surgery, University of Calgary, Calgary, Alberta, Canada
6.6, Proctocolectomy for inflammatory bowel disease – open

Christopher LH Chan BSc (Hons) PhD FRCS (Eng) FRCS (Gen Surg)
Senior Lecturer in Surgery and Consultant Colorectal Surgeon, Academic Surgical Unit, Barts and the London NHS Trust, Queen Mary University of London, London, UK
9.3, Construction of an electrically stimulated gracilis neoanal sphincter

Pierre H Chapuis DS (Q'ld) FRACS
Clinical Professor, Department of Colorectal Surgery, Concord Hospital, Concord, Australia
2.3, Flexible endoscopy

Hueylan Chern MD
Assistant Professor of Surgery, Section of Colorectal Surgery, University of California, San Francisco, San Francisco, CA, USA
7.2, Martius flap

Hester YS Cheung MD
Consultant Surgeon, Department of Surgery, Pamela Youde Nethersole Eastern Hospital, Hong Kong
6.2, Anterior resection – laparoscopic

Heidi K Chua MD
Assistant Professor of Surgery, Division of Colon and Rectal Surgery, Mayo Clinic, Rochester, MN, USA
1.8, Anastomotic technique – suture

Robert R Cima MD MA
Professor of Surgery and Consultant in Colon and Rectal Surgery, Mayo Clinic College of Medicine, Rochester, MN, USA
5.3, Right colectomy – open

J Calvin Coffey BSc PhD FRCS (Gen Surg)
Professor and Chair, Department of Surgery; Consultant General and Colorectal Surgeon, Graduate Entry Medical School, University of Limerick, University Hospitals Limerick, Limerick, Ireland
4.3, Malrotation

Bard C Cosman MD MPH FASCRS
Staff Physician, Halasz General Surgery Section, VA San Diego Healthcare System; Professor of Clinical Surgery, University of California San Diego School of Medicine, San Diego, CA, USA
2.5, Excision of perianal thrombosis

Michael H Cotton MA FRCS FACS FCS(ECSA)
Consultant Surgeon, Emergency Department, Centre Hospitalier Universitaire Vaudois, Lausanne, Switzerland
2.9, Perianal sepsis

Conor P Delaney MD MCh PhD FRCSI FACS FASCRS
The Jeffrey L. Ponsky Professor of Surgical Education; Chief, Division of Colorectal Surgery; Interim Chair, Department of Surgery; Director, CWRU Center for Skills and Simulation; Surgical Director, Digestive Health Institute, University Hospitals Case Medical Center, Case Western Reserve University, Cleveland, OH, USA
5.4, Right hemicolectomy - laparoscopic

André D'Hoore MD PhD
Department of Abdominal Surgery, University Hospital Leuven, Leuven, Belgium
8.5, Laparoscopic ventral rectopexy

Michael J Earley MCh FRCSI FRCS (Plast)
Consultant Plastic and Reconstructive Surgeon, The Children's
University Hospital and Mater Misericordiae University Hospital;
Associate Clinical Professor, University College Dublin, Dublin,
Ireland
7.3, Local advancement flaps

Yair Edden MD
Clinical Fellow, Department of Colorectal Surgery, Cleveland Clinic
Florida, Weston, FL, USA
1.4, Access to abdominal cavity – laparoscopic

Tim W Eglinton MBChB FRACS
Consultant Colorectal Surgeon, Christchurch Hospital; Senior
Lecturer in Surgery, Department of Surgery, University of Otago,
Christchurch, New Zealand
2.14, Perianal condylomata and anal intraepithelial neoplasia

Khalid A El-Gendy BSc MBBS MRCS
Formerly Colorectal Research Fellow, Academic Surgical Unit,
Centre for Digestive Diseases, Blizard Institute of Cell and
Molecular Science, Barts and the London School of Medicine and
Dentistry, The Royal London Hospital, London, UK
6.18, The APPEAR procedure

Paul J Finan MD FRCS Hon FRCS (Glasg)
Consultant General and Colorectal Surgeon, St James's University
Hospital, Leeds, UK
6.10, Abdominoperineal excision of the rectum and anus

Pascal Frileux MD
Professor of Surgery, Hôpital Foch, Suresnes, France
5.12, Hartmann's procedure

Frank A Frizelle MBChB MMedSc FRACS FACS
Consultant Colorectal Surgeon, Christchurch Hospital; Professor
of Colorectal Surgery, Department of Surgery, University of Otago,
Christchurch, New Zealand
2.14, Perianal condylomata and anal intraepithelial neoplasia

Susan Galandiuk MD
Professor, Department of Surgery; Head, Section of Colon and
Rectal Surgery; Director, Price Institute of Surgical Research,
University of Louisville, KY, USA
5.13, Emergency colectomy

Julio Garcia-Aguilar MD PhD
Professor of Surgery and Chief, Division of Colon and Rectal
Surgery, Memorial Sloan Kettering Cancer Center, New York, NY,
USA
6.4, Anterior resection – robotic

Jean-Claude R Givel MD FACS FRCSEd FRCSEng EBSQcoloproctology
Honorary Professor, Medical Faculty, Cabinet de Chirurgie
Viscérale, Lausanne, Switzerland
2.9, Perinanal sepsis

Marc A Gladman MBBS DRCOG DFFP PhD MRCOG FRCS (Gen Surg) FRACS
Professor of Colorectal Surgery and Head, Colorectal Surgery,
Concord Repatriation General Hospital; Director, Academic
Colorectal Unit, Sydney Medical School – Concord, University of
Sydney, Sydney, Australia
6.19, Vertical reduction rectoplasty for idiopathic megarectum

Stanley M Goldberg MD FACS HonFRACS(Aust) HonFRCS(Eng) HonAFC(Fr)
HonFRCPS(Glasg) HonFRSM(Eng) HonFPCS(Phil) HonFRCS(Edin) Honoris Causa (Lleida)
HonSAS(Spain) HonJSS(Japan)
Clinical Professor of Surgery, Division of Colon and Rectal Surgery,
Department of Surgery, University of Minnesota, Minneapolis,
MN, USA
2.7, Closed hemorrhoidectomy

Katherine Grant MSc FRCS
Resident Surgical Officer, St Mark's Hospital, Harrow, London, UK
3.2, Colostomy

Shashank Gurjar FRCS MSc Dip(MedEd)
Consultant Colorectal Surgeon, Department of Surgery, Luton and
Dunstable Hospital, Luton, UK
2.2, Proctosigmoidoscopy

Toby M Hammond MBChB MD FRCS
General and Colorectal Surgery, Broomfield Hospital, Chelmsford,
UK
2.10, Anal fistula

Alexander Herold MD
Professor, Enddarm-Zentrum, Mannheim, Germany
2.1, Office/outpatient set-up

James Hill MB ChB FRCS ChM
Clinical Professor of Colorectal Surgery, Manchester Academic
Health Science Center; Consultant Colorectal Surgeon,
Manchester Royal Infirmary, Manchester, UK
3.5, Antegrade continence enema procedure in adults

Werner Hohenberger
Professor, Chirurgische Universitätsklinik, Erlangen, Germany
5.9, Colectomy – complete mesocolic excision

Roel Hompes MD
Clinical and Research Fellow, Department of Colorectal Surgery,
Oxford University Hospitals, Oxford, UK
6.15, Transanal endoscopic microsurgery

Tracy L Hull MD
Professor of Surgery, Department of Colon and Rectal Surgery,
Digestive Disease Institute, The Cleveland Clinic Foundation,
Cleveland, OH, USA
2.11, Rectovaginal fistula repair

David Jayne BSc MB BCh FRCS MD
Professor of Surgery, University of Leeds, St James's University
Hospital, Leeds, UK
8.6, STARR

D Brian Jones MD (Melb) FRACP FRCP (Lond)
Clinical Associate Professor, Discipline of Medicine, Sydney
Medical School, The University of Sydney, Concord Hospital,
Concord, Australia
2.3, Flexible endoscopy

Seigo Kitano MD PhD
President of Oita University; Department of Gastroenterological
Surgery, Oita University Faculty of Medicine, Oita, Japan
*1.7, Access to the abdominal cavity: natural orifice transluminal
endoscopic surgery*

Mary R Kwaan MD MPH
Assistant Professor, Division of Colon and Rectal Surgery, Department of Surgery, University of Minnesota Medical School, Minneapolis, MN, USA
5.6, Left colectomy – open

Peter J Lee MBBS BSc(Med) MS FRACS
Colorectal Surgeon, Royal Prince Alfred Hospital, LifeHouse Cancer Centre, Surgical Outcomes Research Centre (SOuRCe), Sydney, Australia
6.12, Pelvic exenteration: radical perineal approaches and sacrectomies

Jérémie H Lefèvre MD
Department of Digestive and General Surgery, Hôpital Saint-Antoine, Assistance Publique–Hôpitaux de Paris, Université Pierre et Marie Curie, Paris, France
6.5, Coloanal anastomosis with intersphincteric resection and colon J-pouch construction; 7.1, VRAM flap

Paul-Antoine Lehur MD PhD
Institut des Maladies de l'Appareil Digestif, University Hospital of Nantes, Nantes, France
9.4, Artificial bowel sphincter

Michael Levitt MD
St John of God Healthcare, Subiaco, Australia
1.2, Safety and positioning in the operating room

Michael KW Li MD
Professor, University College London, London, UK; Honorary Consultant in General Surgery, Hong Kong Sanatorium Hospital, Hong Kong; Director Minimal Access Surgery Training Centre Hong Kong; Consultant Surgeon, Department of Surgery, Pamela Youde Nethersole Eastern Hospital, Hong Kong
6.2, Anterior resection – laparoscopic

Ian Lindsey MB BS FRACS
Department of Colorectal Surgery, Oxford Radcliffe Hospitals, Oxford, UK
2.2, Proctosigmoidoscopy

Ann C Lowry MD
Clinical Professor of Surgery, Division of Colon and Rectal Surgery, University of Minnesota, St Paul, MN, USA
9.1, Surgical repair of the anal sphincters following injury

Kirk A Ludwig MD
The Vernon O. Underwood Professor, Professor of Surgery; Chief, Division of Colorectal Surgery, Department of Surgery, Medical College of Wisconsin, Milwaukee, WI, USA
5.5, Right hemicolectomy - hand-assisted laparoscopic surgery

Peter J Lunniss MS, FRCS
Senior Lecturer, Academic Surgical Unit, Barts and the London School of Medicine and Dentistry; Honorary Consultant Colorectal Surgeon, The Royal London and Homerton Hospitals, London, UK
2.10, Anal fistula

John MacFie MB ChB MD FRCS FRCP
Professor of Surgery and Consultant Colorectal Surgeon, University of Hull and Scarborough Hospital, Scarborough, UK
4.1, Small bowel resection

Anthony R MacLean MD FRCSC FACS
Clinical Associate Professor of Surgery, Program Director General Surgery Residency Program, Department of Surgery, University of Calgary, Calgary, Alberta, Canada
6.6, Proctocolectomy for inflammatory bowel disease – open

Robert D Madoff MD FACS FASCRS FRCSEd (Hon)
Stanley M. Goldberg MD Professor of Colon and Rectal Surgery; Chief, Division of Colon and Rectal Surgery, University of Minnesota, Minneapolis, MN, USA
8.2, Perineal rectosigmoidectomy; 8.3, Abdominal rectopexy – open

Padraig SJ Malone MB MCh FRCSI FRCS FEAPU
Consultant Paediatric Urologist, Department of Paediatric Urology, University Hospitals Southampton Foundation Trust, Southampton General Hospital, Southampton, UK
3.4, Antegrade continence enema procedure in children

Lukas Marti FMH Surgery MD
Consultant Surgeon, EBSQ Coloproctology, District Hospital of St Gallen, St Gallen, Switzerland
8.6, STARR

Klaus E Matzel MD
Chirurgische Klinik mit Poliklinik der Universität Erlangen, Erlangen, Germany
9.2, Sacral nerve stimulation

Clare-Ellen McNaught MB ChB MD FRCS
Consultant Colorectal Surgeon, Scarborough Hospital, Scarborough, UK
4.1, Small bowel resection

Brendan J Moran MCh FRCS FRCSI
Consultant Colorectal Surgeon, Basingstoke and North Hampshire Foundation Trust Hospital, Basingstoke, UK
6.1, Anterior resection of the rectum

Neil Mortensen MA MB ChB MD FRCS
Professor of Surgery, Department of Colorectal Surgery, Oxford University Hospitals, Oxford, UK
6.15, Transanal endoscopic microsurgery

Mark D Muhlmann MBBS (Hons) FRACS
Visiting Medical Officer, Prince of Wales Public Hospital and the Royal Hospital for Women, Randwick, Australia
5.1, Appendicectomy – open

Paul C Neary MD FRCSI (Gen)
Consultant Colorectal Surgeon, Adelaide and Meath Hospital, Dublin, Incorporating the National Children's Hospital, Dublin, Ireland
5.7, Left hemicolectomy – laparoscopic

Graham L Newstead MB BS FRACS FRCS(Eng) FACS Hon FASCRS Hon FRSM Hon FACP (GB&I)
Conjoint Associate Professor, University of New South Wales; Chairman, International Council of Coloproctology, The Bowel Cancer Foundation; Medical Advisory Council and Colorectal Surgery, Prince of Wales Private Hospital, Randwick, Australia
5.1, Appendicectomy – open

R John Nicholls MD FRCS HON FACS
Emeritus Consultant Surgeon, St Mark's Hospital, Harrow; Visiting Professor of Colorectal Surgery, Imperial College, London, UK
6.8, Continent ileostomy (Kock reservoir ileostomy);
6.9, Restorative proctocolectomy with ileal reservoir

John MA Northover MS FRCS
Senior Consultant Surgeon, St Mark's Hospital for Intestinal and Colorectal Disorders; Professor of Intestinal Surgery, Imperial College, London, UK
2.15, Perianal skin and anal cancer

Karen P Nugent MA MS MEd FRCS
Senior Lecturer, Honorary Consultant, Southampton University Hospital Trust, Southampton, UK
2.13, Anoplasty

Per-Olof Nyström MD PhD
Professor of Surgery, Colorectal Surgery, Department of Surgical Gastroenterology, Karolinska University Hospital – Huddinge, Stockholm, Sweden
2.8, Stapled hemorrhoidopexy

P Ronan O'Connell MD FRCSI FRCPS (Glas) FRCS (Edin)
Professor of Surgery, University College Dublin; Consultant Surgeon, St Vincent's University Hospital, Dublin, Ireland
2.6, Open hemorrhoidectomy

MP Pakarinen MD PhD
Associate Professor and Consultant in Paediatric Surgery, Hospital for Children and Adolescents, University of Helsinki, Helsinki, Finland
6.17, Surgery for Hirschsprung's disease

Yann Parc MD PhD
Department of Digestive and General Surgery, Hôpital Saint-Antoine, Assistance Publique-Hôpitaux de Paris, Université Pierre et Marie Curie, Paris, France
6.5, Coloanal anastomosis with intersphincteric resection and colon J-pouch construction

Mike C Parker BSc MS FRCS
Consultant Colorectal Surgeon, Darent Valley Hospital, Dartford, UK
5.14, Colonic stenting

John H Pemberton MD
Professor of Surgery and Consultant in Colon and Rectal Surgery, College of Medicine, Mayo Clinic, Rochester, MN, USA
5.3, Right colectomy – open

Robin KS Phillips MS FRCS
Professor of Colorectal Surgery, St Mark's Hospital, Harrow, UK
3.1, Ileostomy; 3.2, Colostomy

Alessio Pigazzi MD PhD
Associate Professor of Surgery, Division of Colon and Rectal Surgery, University of California Irvine, Orange, CA, USA
6.4, Anterior resection – robotic

Thomas E Read MD FACS FASCRS
Professor of Surgery, Tufts University School of Medicine, Medford; Staff Surgeon, Department of Colon and Rectal Surgery; Program Director, Colon and Rectal Surgery Residency, Lahey Clinic Medical Center, Burlington, MA, USA
1.5, Access to abdominal cavity – hand-assisted laparoscopic surgery; 5.11, Total colectomy – hand-assisted laparoscopic surgery

Feza H Remzi MD FACS FASCRS
Chairman, Department of Colorectal Surgery, Cleveland Clinic Foundation, Cleveland, OH, USA
4.4, Intestinal stricturoplasty

Harry L Reynolds Jr MD FACS FASCRS
Associate Professor of Surgery, Case Western Reserve University; Director, Section of Colon and Rectal Cancer Surgery, University Hospitals Case Medical Center, Cleveland, OH, USA
5.4, Right hemicolectomy - laparoscopic

Matt Rickard MB BS (Hons) MMed (Clin Epi) Dip Paed (NSW) FRACS
Colorectal Surgeon, Concord Hospital, Macquarie University Hospital, Sydney, Australia
2.16, Pilonidal disease

Nicholas A Rieger MBBS MS FRACS
Associate Professor, The Queen Elizabeth Hospital and the University of Adelaide, Woodville, Australia
1.6, Single incision laparoscopic-assisted colectomy

M Rinaldi MD
Senior Lecturer in Surgery, Department of Emergency and Organ Transplantation, University of Bari, Bari, Italy
8.1, Delorme operation

RJ Rintala MD PhD
Professor of Paediatric Surgery, Hospital for Children and Adolescents, University of Helsinki, Helsinki, Finland
6.7, Surgery for Hirschsprung's disease

David A Rothenberger MD
Jay Phillips Professor and Chairman, Department of Surgery, University of Minnesota, Minneapolis, MN, USA
5.6, Left colectomy – open

John H Scholefield MB ChB FRCS ChM (Dist)
Professor, Head of Division of Gastrointestinal Surgery, University Hospital, Nottingham, UK
2.12, Anal fissure

Ruud Schouten MD
Department of Surgery, Erasmus Medical Center, Rotterdam, The Netherlands
6.16, Presacral resections – Kraske

Kieran Sheahan MB BSc FRCPI FRCPath
Clinical Professor, School of Medicine and Medical Science, University College Dublin; Consultant Histopathologist, Histopathology Department, St Vincent's University Hospital, Dublin, Ireland
1.10, Specimen handling

Daniel Shibru MD MPH
Colon and Rectal Surgery, South Sacramento Medical Center, Sacramento, CA, USA
9.1, Surgical repair of the anal sphincters following injury

Conor Shields BSc MD FRCSI
Consultant General and Colorectal Surgeon, Department of Surgery, Mater Misericordiae University Hospital and Dublin Academic Medical Centre, Dublin, Ireland
5.2, Appendicectomy – laparoscopic

Michael J Solomon MBBCh(Hons) MSc FRCSI FRACS
Clinical Professor of Surgery, University of Sydney; Academic Head, Department of Colorectal Surgery and Head, Surgical Outcome Research Centre (SOuRCE); Chairman, Institute of Academic Surgery at Royal Prince Alfred Hospital and the University of Sydney, Sydney, Australia
6.11, Operative technique for pelvic exenteration; 6.12, Pelvic exenteration: radical perineal approaches and sacrectomies

Scott R Steele MD
Clinical Associate Professor of Surgery, University of Washington, Seattle; Chief, Colon and Rectal Surgery, Madigan Army Medical Center, Fort Lewis, WA, USA
6.14, Transanal resection for rectal lesions

Andrew RL Stevenson MBBS FRACS
Head, Colorectal Surgery Unit, Royal Brisbane Hospital; Associate Professor, University of Queensland; Director, Australian Colorectal Endosurgery, Brisbane, Australia
8.4, Abdominal rectopexy – laparoscopic

Russell Stitz MB BS FRACS FRCS Eng FRCS Edin (Hon) FRCST (Hon) FCSHK (Hon) ASDA
Adjunct Professor of Surgery, University of Queensland, Brisbane, Australia
5.10, Total colectomy – laparoscopic

James Sweeney FRACS
Former Head Colorectal Surgery, Flinders Medical Centre, Bedford Park, Australia
3.3, Stoma closure

Paris P Tekkis MD FRCS
Professor of Colorectal Surgery, Imperial College London, The Royal Marsden Hospital, London, UK
6.8, Continent ileostomy (Kock reservoir ileostomy); 6.9, Restorative proctocolectomy with ileal reservoir

Emmanuel Tiret MD
Department of Digestive and General Surgery, Hôpital Saint-Antoine, Assistance Publique-Hôpitaux de Paris, Université Pierre et Marie Curie, Paris, France
7.1, VRAM flap

Judith L Trudel MD MSc MHPE FRCSC FACS
Clinical Professor of Surgery, Division of Colon and Rectal Surgery, University of Minnesota Medical School, Minneapolis, MN, USA
1.3, Access to abdominal cavity – open

H David Vargas MD FACS FASCRS
Staff Surgeon, Department of Colon and Rectal Surgery; Program Director, Colon Rectal Surgery Fellowship, Ochsner Clinic Foundation, New Orleans, LA, USA
5.5, Right hemicolectomy - hand-assisted laparoscopic surgery

Madhulika Varma MD
Associate Professor and Chief, Section of Colorectal Surgery, University of California San Francisco, San Francisco, CA, USA
7.2, Martius flap

Petar Vukasin MD
Department of Surgery (Colorectal), University of Southern California, Keck School of Medicine, Los Angeles, CA, USA
1.9, Anastomotic technique – stapled

Bruce P Waxman OAM FRACS
Associate Professor and Director, Academic Surgical Unit, Monash University, Southern Clinical School; Director of Colorectal Surgery, Monash Health, Victoria, Australia
4.5, Adhesiolysis

Steven D Wexner MD PhD (Hon) FACS FRCS FRCS(ED)
Director, Digestive Disease Center; Chair, Department of Colorectal Surgery; Emeritus Chief of Staff, Cleveland Clinic Florida; Affiliate Professor, Florida Atlantic University College of Medicine; Clinical Professor, Florida International University College of Medicine, Weston, FL, USA
1.4, Access to abdominal cavity – laparoscopic

J Graham Williams MCh FRCS
Consultant Colorectal Surgeon, Royal Wolverhampton Hospitals NHS Trust, New Cross Hospital, Wolverhampton, UK
8.2, Perineal rectosigmoidectomy; 8.3, Abdominal rectopexy – open

Sir Norman S Williams MS FRCS FMedSci FRCP FRCP(Edin) FRCA FDS(Hon) FACS(Hon) FRCSI(Hon)
Professor of Surgery; Director of National Centre for Bowel Research and Surgical Innovation; Co-Clinical Director NIHR Healthcare Technology Cooperative (Enteric); Honorary Consultant Surgeon, Barts Health, Blizard Institute, Barts and the London School of Medicine and Dentistry, National Centre for Bowel Research and Surgical Innovation, London, UK
6.18, The APPEAR procedure; 6.19, Vertical reduction rectoplasty for idiopathic megarectum; 8.7, The EXPRESS procedure; 9.3, Construction of an electrically stimulated gracilis neoanal sphincter

Jonathan M Wilson PhD FRCS
Resident Surgical Officer, St Mark's Hospital, Harrow, UK
3.1, Ileostomy

Desmond C Winter MB FRCSI MD FRCSGlas FRCS(Gen)
Clinical Professor, University College Dublin; Consultant Surgeon, St Vincent's University Hospital, Dublin, Ireland
4.2, Meckel's diverticulum

Bruce G Wolff MD
Chair, Division of Colon and Rectal Surgery, Mayo Clinic, Rochester, MN, USA
1.8, Anastomotic technique – suture

Mark TC Wong MBBS (Sing) FRCS (Edin)
Consultant Colorectal Surgeon, Department of Colorectal Surgery, Singapore General Hospital, Singapore
9.4, Artificial bowel sphincter

Caroline Wright MBBS MS FRACS
Senior Lecturer, Sydney Medical School, The University of Sydney;
Clinical Academic, Royal Prince Alfred Hospital, Camperdown,
Australia
2.4, Treatment of uncomplicated hemorrhoids

Hideaki Yano MD FRCS
Consultant Surgeon, Department of Surgery, National Centre for
Global Health and Medicine, Tokyo, Japan
6.13, Lateral pelvic lymph node dissection in low rectal cancer

Kazuhiro Yasuda MD
Lecturer, Department of Gastroenterological Surgery, Oita
University Faculty of Medicine, Oita, Japan
*1.7, Access to the abdominal cavity: natural orifice transluminal
endoscopic surgery*

Christopher J Young MBBS MS FRACS
Clinical Associate Professor of Surgery, Central Clinical School,
University of Sydney; Director of Surgical Services, Royal Prince
Alfred Hospital, Sydney, Australia
*5.8, Left hemicolectomy – hand-assisted laparoscopic surgery; 6.3,
Anterior resection – hand-assisted laparoscopic surgery*

Tonia M Young-Fadok MD MS FACS FASCRS
Chair, Division of Colon and Rectal Surgery, Mayo Clinic;
Professor of Surgery, Mayo Clinic Foundation, Phoenix, AZ, USA
*6.7, Proctocolectomy for inflammatory bowel disease –
laparoscopic*

Preface

The late Professor Charles Rob and Mr Rodney Smith, later Lord Smith of Marlow, conceived a multi-volume textbook of operative surgery that would encompass the best of modern surgical practice. First published in 1956, *Rob and Smith*, as the work was familiarly known, became the standard reference operative text for surgeons across the English-speaking world, expanding from eight volumes in the first edition to 13 volumes in the fifth edition.

The sixth edition of *Operative Surgery of the Colon, Rectum and Anus* is a comprehensive atlas of contemporary operative surgical practice, presented in 83 chapters in 9 sections. Such have been the changes in surgical practice and techniques since publication of the fifth edition that 39 new chapters are included in the sixth edition, covering all aspects of laparoscopic and minimally invasive surgery, maximally invasive surgery, modern treatment of incontinence and pelvic floor disorders, and perineal reconstruction. The remaining chapters have all been rewritten by acknowledged experts from Europe, North America and Australasia. The familiar halftone illustrations of earlier editions have been replaced by full color illustrations and, where appropriate, intra-operative photographs. The familiar style of previous editions has however been retained, with a focus on illustration of the technique with appropriate but subordinate text. Considerable time and effort have been expended to ensure that the art (both illustrations and photographs) is of the highest and most educational standard to guarantee that this text remains contemporary for decades to come.

As editors we have tried to insure that the techniques illustrated are representative of contemporary practice in coloproctology and that the vision of Charles Rob and Rodney Smith of a comprehensive atlas of surgery of the colon, rectum and anus has been maintained. We recognize that in editing the sixth edition we have relied greatly on the expertise, hard work and patience of our contributing authors and graphic artists. We acknowledge the achievements of past editors, particularly Stanley Goldberg and Peter Fielding, editors of the fifth edition. We are most grateful to our advisory editor Professor Sir Norman Williams for his help in bringing the work to completion.

P Ronan O'Connell
Robert D Madoff
Michael J Solomon
January 2015

1

General principles

Preparation for colorectal surgery

IAN P BISSETT

INTRODUCTION

The relationship between the patient and the surgeon is primarily a human interaction. It begins with a mutual recognition of that humanity and relies on a trust on the part of the patient and a commitment by the surgeon to place the welfare of that patient as paramount. The initial communication between the two must therefore allow that relationship to develop. Although colorectal surgery may be an everyday event for the surgeon, it is impossible to overstate the magnitude of this intervention in the eyes of the patient. Those presenting for colorectal surgery have often just received news of a diagnosis that they had not expected, and face the coming surgery with dread. It is important that the surgeon recognizes this fact and seeks not only to explain the procedure but also to reassure the patient, bringing their expectations into line with the likely sequence of events before, during, and after surgery. Careful preoperative planning and preparation can reduce patient anxiety, prevent complications, and optimize the patient's perioperative course.

Preparation of a patient for colorectal surgery will involve communication, detailed preoperative assessment, optimization of nutrition and hydration, careful management of coagulation, discussion of possible stoma requirements, and antibiotic prophylaxis. Enhanced recovery after surgery is a whole package of interventions including pre-, intra-, and postoperative measures to speed up patient recovery and return to normal function. The preoperative elements are included in this description of patient preparation for surgery.

INFORMED CONSENT

It is the responsibility of the surgeon to ensure that the patient is well enough informed to be able to decide whether to embrace the treatment that is being offered or not. To fulfill this adequately, the surgeon is required to begin with information with which the patient is familiar and bring him or her to a sound understanding of the likely consequences of different treatment options. Time spent listening to the patient is an important starting point in this process. Verbal, diagrammatic, and written information are all helpful.

During this process, the pathophysiology of the condition, the anatomy of the involved area, the likely outcomes and possible complications of the procedure, as well as the consequences of not undergoing the proposed treatment need to be communicated in a way that can be comprehended. It is not sufficient to merely thrust an information sheet into a patient's hands and tell them to read it. It is the author's practice to draw the anatomy for the patient (usually on a preprinted diagram) outlining the abnormalities and the changes proposed by surgery. Where appropriate, a survival curve to illustrate the outcome over time should be drawn (**Figure 1.1.1**). The patient then takes this away along with printed information to consider and to show others prior to the surgery. Decision aids, both in hard copy and web-based, are becoming more commonly used in the cancer consultation, but have yet to be utilized universally in colorectal surgery.

As part of the consent process, patients should also be informed of potential trials in which they could be enrolled. If this occurs at the initial consultation, it is likely to ensure that contentious issues are included in the discussion around consent. It is also valuable to note that patient involvement in cancer research has been shown to be associated with improved outcomes.

Frequently, the expectations of the patient are unrealistic, especially in the setting of surgery for functional disorders. The likelihood of improvement and its longevity are important messages. In addition to the probability of success, the possible complications need to be addressed in a way that provides a realistic idea of the risk associated with these. This would usually take the form of general complications, including deep vein thrombosis (DVT),

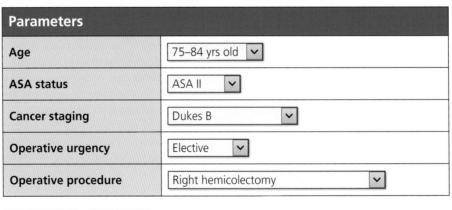

1.1.1 Example of an explanatory diagram drawn for a patient.

be spelt out clearly along with an estimate of the chance of each occurring. The best estimate of complication risk comes from a careful audit of local experience, but this is often absent and one is left with offering the risk as published by others.

Many patients fear that they will die under anesthetic, but fortunately this is extremely rare. Perioperative mortality, however, is more common and an estimate of this is very useful in preoperative decision-making. For patients undergoing surgery for colorectal cancer, an estimate of the predicted risk of 30-day mortality can be obtained from an online risk calculator (**Figure 1.1.2**).[1] Consent can only be considered truly informed when the patient has an understanding of these issues. This process should then be recorded in a manner that does justice to the completeness of the discussion.

In many situations, a second consultation visit is required and this has often been encouraged by consumer groups particularly as research studies have shown less than 50 percent of information imparted in the cancer consultation is remembered by the patient. Patient personalities, such as hypervigilant, buckpassing, and procrastination traits, have been well documented to reflect the patient's desire for information and involvement in the decision-making process. Surgeons should be aware that informed consent is not always the same process for each patient.

MULTIDISCIPLINARY DISCIPLINARY ASSESSMENT

Many different treatment modalities are required to manage colorectal conditions (especially in colorectal cancer, pelvic floor disorders, and inflammatory bowel disease). There is

pneumonia and cardiac events, and specific complications related to the procedure, such as anastomotic leak, wound infection, hemorrhage, pelvic autonomic nerve damage and subsequent adhesions. Each of these complications has significant sequelae for the patient, and these need to

Calculate in ACP score – new model (unpublished)

Choose a value in **each** category that matches your patient from the drop down lists in both the physiological and operative parameters tables below. Defaults values (the commonest national value) are shown for each category.

Parameters	
Age	75–84 yrs old ⌄
ASA status	ASA II ⌄
Cancer staging	Dukes B ⌄
Operative urgency	Elective ⌄
Operative procedure	Right hemicolectomy ⌄

[Calculate risk]   [Reset form]

1.1.2 Thirty-day mortality risk calculator from ACPGBI colorectal cancer model.[1]

mounting evidence, in colorectal cancer particularly, that preoperative discussion in a multidisciplinary forum leads to improved decision-making and outcomes. This approach allows for input from specialists in pathology, radiology, radiation and medical oncology, gastroenterology, genetics, and physiotherapy to be incorporated as necessary. There is an international trend for national bodies to require that cancer patients be assessed in a multidisciplinary forum to ensure that all aspects of the treatment are optimized. In practice, this means that patients will usually need to return for a further discussion with their surgeon following the multidisciplinary meeting. As outlined above, this also has the advantage of giving the patient a further opportunity to ask questions and understand their future management.

ANESTHETIC PREASSESSMENT CLINIC

There is nothing more frustrating for the patient (and the surgeon) than having an operation cancelled at the last minute because of an unrecognized medical condition that requires treatment. The advent of anesthetic preassessment clinics has fortunately made this infrequent. At the preassessment clinic, there is the opportunity to review the patient's medication, check their exercise tolerance, perform respiratory and cardiac studies, and also to reiterate what is involved in the surgery. It is beyond the scope of this chapter to address management of medical problems, such as diabetes, respiratory disorders, and heart disease, which may impact on the perioperative period, but the preadmission clinic allows for the introduction of specialist input where appropriate. Treatment of chronic disease can be optimized prior to surgery and the patient can also be introduced to the ward setting that they will occupy after their surgery. Those likely to require a stoma can meet a stoma therapist and have their skin marked at the appropriate site. Patients can then be safely admitted to hospital on the day of their surgery after sleeping in their own bed, avoiding an unnecessary night in hospital.

NUTRITION

Since the work of Studley in 1936,[2] it has been accepted that severe malnutrition is associated with poorer outcomes after surgery. Preoperative feeding has been shown to reduce complications in those with significant protein depletion or functional impairment associated with weight loss.[3] It is more difficult to prove the benefit of preoperative nutritional supplements in those who are not severely malnourished. A recent meta-analysis has, however, indicated that preoperative feeding with an immune-modulating nutritional supplement (containing arginine, omega-3 fatty acids, and nucleotides) for a minimum of 5 days is associated with reduced infective complications and reduced hospital stay in patients without malnutrition.[4]

Although detailed nutritional assessment is beyond the scope of this discussion, the surgeon should be alert to the patient who has lost weight recently and is physically impaired because of this. A formal nutritional assessment should be obtained if there is concern.

HYDRATION

Conventional surgery has required the patient to take nothing by mouth for 6 hours prior to elective general anesthesia. This has often led to a period of up to 18 hours when there is no fluid intake as patients fast overnight, and may not have surgery until the following afternoon. This has a negative impact on the patient and may lead to dehydration at the time of surgery. It is now accepted that it is safe to consume clear fluids orally up to 2 hours before elective general anesthesia.[5] This should be encouraged, as preoperative fluid intake is associated with an increased feeling of well-being, a reduced thirst and dryness of the mouth, and less anxiety.

ANTICOAGULATION

Patients on preoperative anticoagulation

The perioperative management of patients who have been prescribed antiplatelet or anticoagulation medication warrants discussion. The overriding principle is balancing the risk of bleeding associated with continuing the medication against the risk of a thrombosis and its consequences if the medication is stopped. Three medications will be addressed separately, but clearly discussion with the cardiologist involved and the anesthetist is required to manage these patients' complex conditions.

WARFARIN

The risk associated with stopping warfarin (Coumadin®) depends on the indication for which it is prescribed. Those in whom the condition requires continuous anticoagulation (such as a mechanical heart valve) should stop warfarin 5–6 days prior to surgery, while continuing anticoagulation with therapeutic doses of heparin in the perioperative setting until it is safe to recommence the warfarin postoperatively. There are, however, many patients taking warfarin as prophylaxis in less critical situations (such as in atrial fibrillation), where a brief cessation of anticoagulation over the time of surgery is not associated with major risk. For these patients, stopping warfarin 5–6 days preoperatively allows their INR (international normalized ratio) to decrease to an acceptable level (<1.4) for elective surgery, and the warfarin can be restarted when the patient tolerates oral intake postoperatively. When a patient on warfarin requires emergency surgery, the INR can be corrected over 24 hours by administration of vitamin K, or more quickly by infusion of Prothrombinex and fresh frozen plasma.

ASPIRIN

Traditionally, patients have been advised to stop aspirin treatment 1 week prior to surgery to prevent bleeding complications. More recently, it has become clear that such advice may be ill-founded as the risk of myocardial infarction and cerebrovascular thrombotic events are increased after cessation of aspirin.[6] The increased bleeding associated with aspirin use is likely to be less of a risk to the patient than an associated thrombotic event associated with stopping aspirin. It is now recommended that aspirin is continued unless the risk of bleeding is high, and the consequences of such a bleed are likely to be life-threatening.

THIENOPYRIDINES

Thienopyridines (prasugrel, ticlopidine, clopidogrel) are potent antiplatelet agents, the usage of which is rapidly increasing. The most common indication is in preventing thrombosis associated with coronary artery, peripheral vascular, and cerebrovascular disease. In patients with coronary artery stents, there is a high risk of stent thrombosis, with subsequent sudden death if it is stopped in the early postoperative period (4–6 weeks for bare-metal stents and 12 months for drug-eluting stents).[7] In those with drug-eluting stents, aspirin and thienopyridines should ideally be continued throughout surgery. However, bleeding requiring reoperation is much more common in patients taking thienopyridines even if the patients have stopped taking this 7 days prior to elective surgery. In those with stents in place, consideration should be given to delaying surgery where possible until after the time of greatest risk of stent thrombosis.

Prevention of venous thromboembolism

Major colorectal surgery is associated with a very high incidence of venous thromboembolism (VTE) especially in those with cancer or inflammatory bowel disease. This risk has been reported to be as high as 40 percent for DVT, and 5 percent for pulmonary embolism (PE) in patients without thromboprophylaxis.[8] Patients undergoing major colorectal surgery will benefit from a combination of mechanical and pharmacological VTE prophylaxis. This should consist of a combination of graduated compression stockings and low-dose unfractionated heparin, or a low molecular weight heparin.[9] There is recent evidence to show there is an advantage in continuing this treatment for 4 weeks postoperatively.

BOWEL PREPARATION

Although preoperative mechanical bowel preparation has been recommended prior to colorectal surgery in the past,

there is now a compelling body of evidence that refutes any benefit from this approach. It is clear that in both colonic and rectal surgery there is no difference in any of the important outcomes of anastomotic leak, wound infection, mortality, and postoperative peritonitis (**Figure 1.1.3**).[10] There is an indication for mechanical bowel preparation where concurrent colonoscopy is planned during the surgery, or where the surgery requires the recognition of a small mucosal lesion by palpation of the colon. A further indication in which mechanical bowel preparation may be appropriate is in the setting of a rectal anastomosis with a covering ileostomy constructed to reduce the consequences of an anastomotic leak. Bowel preparation in this situation should avoid the problem of a column of stool proximal to a defunctioned anastomosis. This particular question has not, however, been answered by studies to date.

STOMA EDUCATION

Some operations always result in a stoma and others have the possibility of requiring a stoma. It is essential to discuss this with patients prior to surgery. A few patients respond to the mention of a 'bag' with threats of suicide, and express willingness to take unreasonable risks to avoid it. This provides a major challenge for their surgeon whose patience and communication skills will be severely tested resolving the situation. Most patients, however, are open to discussing the reasons why it may be required and to learn what is involved. The presence of a stoma causes a huge change in a person's body image and what this means in terms of normal daily activities needs to be spelt out. It is useful to have a stoma bag available to demonstrate what it is like and how it is managed. Careful preoperative stoma siting is associated with better stoma function, so this should be addressed in the preassessment clinic. A detailed description of stoma positioning is given in Chapter 3.1.

ANTIBIOTICS

There is robust evidence from multiple randomized controlled trials and systematic reviews that antibiotic prophylaxis is associated with reduced wound infections in patients undergoing colorectal surgery. Antibiotics should be given at the time of induction of anesthesia, and need to provide cover against both aerobic and anaerobic bacteria.[11] There is no advantage in giving more than a single dose of antibiotics. Consideration should be given to the local bacterial resistance patterns and prevention of *Clostridium difficule* when choosing the specific antibiotics.

SUMMARY

The first step in preparing a patient for colorectal surgery is the forming of a relationship in which trust and

Study or sub group	Preparation n/N	No preparation n/N	Peto odds ratio Peto, fixed, 95% CI	Weight	Peto odds ratio Peto, fixed, 95% CI
Brownson 1992	8/67	1/67		4.8%	5.23 [1.36, 20.14]
Bucher 2005	5/78	1/75		3.3%	3.81 [0.75, 19.42]
Burke 1994	3/82	4/87		3.8%	0.79 [0.17, 3.58]
Contant 2007	32/670	37/684		37.2%	0.88 [0.54, 1.42]
Fa-Si-Oen 2005	7/125	6/125		7.0%	1.18 [0.39, 3.58]
Fillmann 1995	2/30	1/30		1.6%	1.99 [0.20, 19.94]
Jung 2007	16/713	17/674		18.3%	0.89 [0.44, 1.77]
Miettinen 2000	5/138	3/129		4.4%	1.56 [0.38, 6.36]
Pena-Soria 2007	4/48	2/49		3.2%	2.06 [0.40, 10.69]
Ram 2005	1/164	2/165		1.7%	0.51 [0.05, 4.98]
Santos 1994	7/72	4/77		5.8%	1.93 [0.57, 6.57]
Tabusso 2002	5/24	0/23		2.6%	8.54 [1.36, 53.51]
Zmora 2003	7/187	4/193		6.1%	1.81 [0.55. 5.99]
Total (95% CI)	**2398**	**2378**		**100.0%**	**1.26 [0.94, 1.69]**

Total events: 102 (preparation), 82 (no preparation)
Hetrogeneity: Chi^2 = 15.77, df = 12 (P = 0.20): I^2 = 24%
Test for overall effect: Z = 1.52 (P = 0.13)

0.1 0.2 0.5 1   2   5   10
Favors preparation   Favors control

1.1.3 Forrest plot showing comparison of mechanical bowel preparation versus no preparation with respect to postoperative anastomotic leak (from Guenaga et al.[10]).

respect are demonstrated. Information relating to the condition, its treatment and possible outcome can then be communicated in a way that the patient understands. Assessment by a multidisciplinary team involving anesthesia, stoma therapists, nurses, and other specialists assists in identifying possible problem areas. Premorbid conditions should be corrected as much as possible, and appropriate measures to prevent complications, such as control of anticoagulation, antibiotic prophylaxis, and correction of nutritional deficits need to be instituted. Careful attention to this preparation will result in a well-informed patient whose perioperative course is optimized.

REFERENCES

1. Smith JJ, Tekkis PP. Risk prediction in surgery. Available from: www.riskprediction.org.uk/index-crc.php.
2. Studley Hiran O. Percentage of weight loss. A basic indicator of surgical risk in patients with chronic pectic ulcer. *Journal of the American Medical Association* 1936; **106**: 458-60.
3. Windsor JA, Hill GL. Weight loss with physiologic impairment. A basic indicator of surgical risk. *Annals of Surgery* 1988; **207**: 290-6.
4. Waitzberg DL, Saito H, Plank LD et al. Postsurgical infections are reduced with specialized nutrition support. *World Journal of Surgery* 2006; **30**: 1592-604.
5. Søreide E, Ljungqvist O. Modern preoperative fasting guidelines: a summary of the present recommendations and remaining questions. *Best Practice and Research. Clinical Anaesthesiology* 2006; **20**: 483-91.
6. Burger W, Chemnitius JM, Kneissl GD, Rücker G. Low-dose aspirin for secondary cardiovascular prevention – cardiovascular risks after its perioperative withdrawal versus bleeding risks with its continuation. Review and meta-analysis. *Journal of Internal Medicine* 2005; **257**: 399-414.
7. American Society of Anesthesiologists Committee on Standards and Practice Parameters. Practice alert for the perioperative management of patients with coronary artery stents: a report by the American Society of Anesthesiologists Committee on Standards and Practice Parameters. *Anesthesiology* 2009; **110**: 22-3.
8. Bergqvist D. Venous thromboembolism: a review of risk and prevention in colorectal surgery patients. *Diseases of the Colon and Rectum* 2006; **49**: 1620-8.
9. Wille-Jørgensen P, Rasmussen MS, Andersen BR, Borly L. Heparins and mechanical methods for thromboprophylaxis in

colorectal surgery. *Cochrane Database of Systematic Reviews* 2001; (3): CD001217.

10. Guenaga KKFG, Matos D, Wille-Jørgensen P. Mechanical bowel preparation for elective colorectal surgery. *Cochrane Database of Systematic Reviews* 2009; (1): CD001544.

11. Nelson RL, Glenny AM, Song F. Antimicrobial prophylaxis for colorectal surgery. *Cochrane Database of Systematic Reviews* 2009; (1): CD001181.

Safety and positioning in the operating room

MICHAEL LEVITT

INTRODUCTION

Notwithstanding the good outcome of the overwhelming proportion of operations performed, surgeons understand only too well what a potentially hazardous place the operating room (OR) can be. The hazards are borne primarily by the patient undergoing the operation, but can extend to every member of the surgical team, as well as to the occasional observer or visitor. The risks include physical injury, inadvertent infection, surgical complications, and even psychological trauma.

In acknowledging these hazards, the surgeon also accepts that it is his or her duty to optimize safety in their OR. As the key decision-maker in the OR, as the person most critically responsible for the safe and correct treatment of the patient, the surgeon sets the standards for both clinical and interpersonal conduct. Where a surgeon demonstrates high regard for the safety – in its broadest interpretation – of their patients and of their colleagues, the OR becomes a safer place for all. Conversely, the surgeon who shows scant regard for these factors will set the scene for any manner of hazard or complication.

The topic of safety in the operating room has numerous aspects and this chapter seeks not to catalog them all in great detail but, rather, to highlight the surgeon's role in overseeing and minimizing each of them. One factor, however, recurs time and again as the root cause of an unsafe OR – haste. Haste is the enemy of safety. A surgeon in a rush will engender an atmosphere that favors the taking of short cuts and that places every member of the surgical team under pressure to put speed ahead of safety and, in turn, that puts them all and, most importantly, their patient at increased risk.

If there is one take-home message about safety in the OR it is to pause and reflect at every opportunity and not to omit the repetitive but necessary cross-checking that demands that the team slows down and focuses precisely on the task at hand. The ultimate responsibility for creating an environment that respects and promotes safe practices through patient and measured conduct rests with the surgeon.

INFORMED CONSENT

Because of the profound impact of litigation, both in financial and psychological terms, there has been intense and sustained focus on the role and importance of informed consent over many years. The surgeon's primary interest is to provide their patient (or their patient's guardian) with sufficient information to participate meaningfully in the decisions surrounding their surgery. Our legal advisors, on the other hand, are equally focused on the surgeon's ability to document that this information has actually been provided.

The end result has been a disproportionate emphasis on the signing of a consent form and upon the precise content of that form. While this remains an important document which offers evidence of the patient's consent to undergo surgery, it does not necessarily mean, let alone prove, that 'informed' consent has been afforded. Likewise, that a patient has been provided with extensive literature dealing with the planned operation and that they might even have signed each page of any relevant document, does not mean that the patient has truly understood what is about to – or what might possibly – happen to them.

The only person who can judge how best to explain the objectives, alternatives, risks, complications, and timeline for recovery of the proposed operation, in terms that the patient can understand and that are relevant to that particular individual, is their surgeon. This cannot be achieved, except in the case of the most minor of procedures, without a commitment on the part of the surgeon to spend the necessary time to do so.

Regrettably, the pressure to attend to large numbers of patients, all demanding of their surgeon's time and expertise, leads to attempts by the surgeon to streamline all manner of procedures including consent. When detailed hand-outs replace direct communication, a valuable opportunity to establish rapport, build trust, and provide truly individualized informed consent is diminished if not lost. When, in addition, even these hand-outs are omitted, consent cannot reasonably be described as informed. Surgeons must also be aware that patients have different personality traits for major decision-making and, as such, demand different levels of communication. Traits such as hypervigilance, buckpassing, and procrastination require and desire different communication levels from clinicians for truly informed consent. The need for multidisciplinary care in areas such as cancer and inflammatory bowel disease also poses challenges for informed consent. Surgeons should be aware also that in cancer consultations, patients rarely remember more than 50 percent of the information discussed by the clinician and that having relatives along to the consultation can help, and the use of second consultations and decision aids (hard copy and web-based) are sometimes helpful.

Ultimately, it is the surgeon who must be satisfied that the necessary information has been provided to – and absorbed by – the patient. This takes time and the preparedness to answer any manner of questions from patients and their relatives and/or friends. It is time-consuming, but the process can still be managed and contained. Supporting this process with a signed form remains important from a medicolegal perspective and offers other members of the surgical team a level of assurance that the nature of their planned surgery has been explained to the patient.

Time, patience, and direct explanation remain the cornerstones of truly informed consent, which should be the goal of the surgeon in every case.

CORRECT PATIENT, CORRECT PROCEDURE, CORRECT SITE

Performing the incorrect procedure on a patient is a fortunately infrequent, but nevertheless, disastrous occurrence. Performing coronary arterial grafts on one patient that were planned for another with the same name; administering a left-sided femoral nerve block for an operation on the right leg; implanting into one patient the intraocular lens intended for another; failing to attend to a concurrent oophorectomy, as agreed prior to surgery, at the time of a colectomy. Numerous scenarios attest to the multitude of opportunities that exist to get things wrong from the time a patient is seen by their surgeon and booked for an operation to the successful completion of the intended procedure. Despite their best intentions, surgeons and their teams can all too easily make fundamental errors at any one – or more – of these opportunities.

Once again, the solution rests with the OR team allowing sufficient time for a series of checks and double-checks to be undertaken. The central elements of ensuring that the correct procedure is performed on the patient about to undergo their surgery are as follows:

- Checking that the patient who is being taken into the OR is the one listed to undergo the surgery and has fasted for an appropriate period of time. This check should occur on several occasions during the patient's journey to the OR – at the hospital or facility reception desk, on admission to the ward, on collection from the ward to be taken to the OR, and on arrival in the OR. On each occasion, the patient should be asked to identify themselves and explain the nature of the operation that they believe they are about to undergo. This should be checked against their details as recorded in the paperwork that accompanies them, especially the consent form, and against the identity band attached to them. It is critical that, wherever there is a disparity between the patient's account of intended events and the documented information, plans for surgery must be put on hold until clarification is obtained. There is absolutely no point in going to the trouble of checking if subsequent inconsistencies in the findings fail to prompt appropriate action.

- Supportive documentation and diagnostic test results must be present and available in the OR. It generally falls to the OR nursing team to double-check that case notes and x-rays are available for viewing before and during the case. In the era of electronic images and test results, this is usually ensured by the availability in the OR of a computer and screen. It remains the absolute responsibility of the surgeon, however, to ensure that the images and test results required for the safe completion of the procedure are at hand before the case commences.

- Marking the body part is an important component of operating on the correct side and at the correct site. The marking should ideally take place well before the patient enters the OR and must be performed by the surgeon performing the procedure. Delegating the marking to anyone other than the operating surgeon is potentially more hazardous than not marking the patient at all. If the patient is not marked, this omission is highlighted upon entry into the OR, drawing the attention of the surgeon and the entire OR team to the omission and permitting them to compensate for that omission. Since the presence of marking sends such a powerful signal to the surgeon about where they should be operating, the presence of an incorrect marking is an especially dangerous mistake. Markings must be clear, useful, and indelible, but they must be made by the operating surgeon.

- Team time-out describes the process whereby the entire OR team stops all activity, after the preparation and draping, but immediately prior to the making of the first incision, to recheck one last time the essential details covered above. It is an obligatory moment to pause, to confirm the identity of the patient, to check for allergies and to reiterate the surgical plan. It is the last chance to avoid a catastrophic mistake or an embarrassing omission, and represents an irreplaceable routine for every case performed in the OR.

Inherent in each of these steps, designed to avoid performing the wrong operation for the patient in question, is the recurrent theme of taking the necessary time to check, document the process and check again that the procedure performed conforms to the plans established well in advance. Haste in the OR – usually as the surgeon or anesthetist drive the OR team to speed up changeover between cases, trying to cover as much ground as possible in the time allotted – is the root cause of these errors. Safety in this regard is as much to do with momentarily halting a seemingly irresistible momentum to press on, as it is to do with performing the checks themselves. A rushed and cursorily performed double-check adds nothing to patient safety, whereas a genuinely reflective pause in otherwise hectic proceedings allows time to identify the simple mistake that had not, to that point, been detected. Haste remains the principal enemy.

MOVING AND POSITIONING THE PATIENT

Handling an unconscious patient places particular responsibility upon the OR team. Spinal and joint injuries are the injuries a patient is most likely to sustain during movement – from operating table to bed, from supine to prone position, or when moving limbs into stirrups. Pressure injury to skin or nerves occurs during prolonged periods of immobility.

Joint and spinal injuries

In practical terms, surgeons are generally just one member of the team that moves patients into position and, later, back on to their bed. In many cases, patient movement is unavoidably undertaken without any assistance from or even oversight by the surgeon. The anesthetist is, however, always in attendance and has primary responsibility for this aspect of the patient's care. Careful planning, gentle handling, and the presence of a sufficient number of staff members to deal with all reasonable contingencies (especially in the case of heavy patients) are the prerequisites for safety during patient movement.

Pressure areas

Positioning the patient and the associated care of potential pressure areas, however, still remain the surgeon's responsibility. Even when positioning is delegated to an assistant (such as when the surgeon is not in the OR at the time), the surgeon remains primarily responsible. Vulnerable pressure areas over the heels in the supine patient, over the head of the fibula and the sacrum when the legs are in stirrups and over the medial humeral epicondyle all require conscious attention from the surgeon, as well as the other members of the OR team. Stretch injury to the brachial plexus due to excessive and prolonged abduction of the arm must be guarded against by both anesthetist and surgeon. Protecting against pressure over the occiput is, by and large, the domain of the anesthetist.

Injuries to staff

All team members involved in moving and positioning the patient also have a duty of care to each other to minimize injury to themselves. Lower back injuries are especially common as a result of poorly judged efforts to move patients in the OR. Surgeons are notorious for self-injury when moving patients, often attempted on their own, when only a few minutes would have seen the arrival of more appropriately able staff members. There is no excuse for injuries sustained as a result of impatience.

Surgical planning

A particularly important aspect of patient positioning relates to the consideration that needs to be given to the possible scenarios that might unfold during the procedure. A good example is a planned left hemicolectomy when access to the anal canal for the purpose of introducing stapling instruments for intestinal reanastomosis is not generally required. This operation can usually be completed in the supine position. Unexpectedly severe sigmoid pathology or certain technical surgical issues might see the resection extended to the upper rectum at which point the surgeon's preference for anastomosis might warrant access to the anal canal.

The patient can always be repositioned during a procedure to ensure that it is completed as safely as possible. However, with a little additional forethought and time at the very outset, the patient might have been positioned differently. The surgeon needs to anticipate the possible scenarios that might unfold during the procedure when positioning the patient at the outset.

THROMBOEMBOLIC PROPHYLAXIS

There is irrefutable evidence that fatality from the thromboembolic complications of surgery can be reduced by the use of lower limb compression devices (both static and dynamic) and low-dose anticoagulation during particular operations (or in particular patients) known to be at increased risk of these complications. Nursing and junior medical staff are generally well briefed on the routine steps required, but surgeons remain primarily responsible for establishing and maintaining awareness within the OR team, as well as on the ward, of the nature of these risks and of the steps required to reduce them. Equally, the surgeon has overall responsibility to ensure that these steps have been implemented in every case in which they are required.

ELECTRICAL SAFETY

While the standard OR houses a myriad of sources of electricity and, hence, potential electrical safety hazards, two mechanisms of electrical injury are of particular importance to the surgeon.

Static electricity

Discharge of static electricity might trigger either fire or explosion or, less likely, induce cardiac arrhythmias. Precautions that are routinely taken in the OR to minimize the risk of there being a discharge of static electricity include:

- avoidance of flammable anesthetic agents;
- avoidance of the use of non-conductive rubber in anesthetic equipment;
- avoidance of woolen/synthetic materials for drapes, sheets, and clothing; cotton and cotton/synthetic materials are advisable;
- use of antistatic flooring materials.

Diathermy equipment

The principal risk associated with the use of diathermy both to the patient and to the surgical team is that of being burnt. In addition, there is the risk associated when the electrical current might 'arc' and provoke either a burn or an explosion in relation to a pool of alcoholic liquid. Key precautions in the OR that minimize these risks include:

- The surgeon should be familiar with the particular settings and mode of operation of the equipment in use; in this context, the surgeon's responsibility is less in the realm of understanding the physics of how the equipment works and very much more in understanding how to use the equipment safely.
- The diathermy plate should be placed as close as possible to the surgical incision.
- Monitoring electrodes (such as electrocardiogram (ECG) electrodes), which might act as alternative earthing pathways, should be placed as far away as possible from the surgical incision.
- Pools of alcoholic skin preparation solutions should be mopped up before the drapes are placed to avoid the risk of arcing or burning.
- A quiver into which the diathermy pencil is returned after use is an important way of avoiding inadvertent burns when the surgeon or an assistant accidentally activates the diathermy when not being used in the operative field.

INFECTION CONTROL

Protecting the patient

Every surgical incision represents a potential point for the entry of infection. Modern OR construction uses laminar air flow to minimize the risk of airborne agents gaining proximity to the surgical site. This is almost entirely beyond the surgeon to both plan and monitor. Likewise, the wearing of masks is more or less mandatory for the operating team and their use generally reflects unequivocal hospital policy. Increasing evidence points to the need for all OR occupants (surgical team, anesthetic, nursing, and observers) to wear masks as a means of minimizing the risk of infection to patients.

There are a number of ways in which the surgeon can more actively reduce the risk of infection to the patient:

- A preoperative wash using chlorhexidine (or other antibacterial) soap has been shown to reduce post-operative wound infection and should be routine prior to all but minor operations.
- Irrefutable evidence dictates that the use of perioperative antibiotics reduces the risk of surgical site infection in operations associated with higher risks of such infection. As a general rule, a single dose of intravenous antibiotics directed at the organisms most likely to be encountered in the operation in question is used. A second dose might be administered during especially long procedures. Although the anesthetist generally administers the antibiotic – and is therefore, almost always familiar with the surgeon's preferences – the surgeon remains primarily responsible for ensuring that the choice of antibiotic is appropriate and for checking that the antibiotic has been administered.
- The greater the amount of human traffic into and out of the OR, the more likely is the laminar air flow to be disrupted and the higher the probability of unwanted organisms being introduced into the OR atmosphere. Limiting the number of people in the OR represents a simple but effective strategy that the surgeon, more than anyone else, can and should oversee.
- Routine hand hygiene involves washing the hands with soap and water or with an alcohol-based hand rub solution. This is standard practice in outpatient clinics and on surgical wards and is performed before and after every episode involving patient contact. Similar standards of care are no less important for all members of OR staff handling patients.
- In addition, the surgeon can ask that that those people intending to pass through the OR do not do so if they are acutely unwell with an infective illness. In this regard, surgeons are, at times, a poor example to their team when they choose to 'battle on' in the face of an acute respiratory or gastroenteric infection. In doing so, they expose their patients (and others) to the risk of the same (usually viral) infection and they also increase the risk of contaminating the surgical site with any superadded (predominantly bacterial) infection. Basic infection control precautions mandate that people who are unwell with acute infections stay away from the OR.
- Finally, increasing evidence suggests that the preparation used for skin cleansing and decontamination immediately

prior to surgery influences the risk of surgical site infection. The use of an alcohol-based agent has been shown to reduce the risk of surgical site infection when compared to agents in which there is no alcohol. The presence of alcohol and other chemicals might, however, be inappropriate where certain body parts are being prepared for surgery – e.g. the genitalia and nipples.

Protecting the surgical team

The entire surgical team is at risk of infection through inadvertent exposure to the patient's body fluids. The use of disposable fabric or other single-use gowns, masks, eye-protection wear and, of course, gloves are all central to minimizing exposure of this sort.

Exposure to the patient's blood through sharps injuries represents an especially grave risk, most notably of acquiring hepatitis B and C and HIV. The safe use and disposal of all sharps – needles, sutures, and scalpels – forms a critical routine in every safely operated OR. Double-gloving, in particular, has been shown to substantially reduce the incidence of skin puncture due to sharps injuries.

The safe handling of sharps consumes extra time and patience, especially towards the end of a long operation when suture handling – and hence the risk of inadvertent sharps injury – is often at its peak. It is the surgical assistant and the scrub nurse who are most at risk of sharps injuries, more so than the surgeon. It is therefore the particular responsibility of the surgeon to maintain and role model safe sharps handling procedures and to commit the time required during the operation to insist upon their use.

ENVIRONMENTAL SAFETY

Temperature

The temperature and humidity in the OR is generally very carefully controlled. With respect to the ambient temperature, a balance needs to be struck between the comfort of the OR team (usually a little cooler) and the best interests of the patient (usually a little warmer.) The use of patient-warming devices generally enables the ambient temperature to be set a little lower, with the comfort of the surgical team in mind, but all members of the OR team must be cognizant of the risks to the patient of even minor degrees of hypothermia prior to the application of the warming device. The surgeon must, then, also be mindful that their patients do not lie exposed in a cool OR for any longer than is absolutely necessary for the correct preparation of the operative field.

Smoke

Smoke generated by diathermy and other electrical devices and the vapors that are generated by high-speed drills and saws are potential contaminants of the OR atmosphere. It has been postulated that the smoke generated by tissue diathermy is carcinogenic, while viral particles contained in the tissue being operated upon might be disseminated as an aerosol and hence pose an infection hazard to members of the OR team.

While these hazards are primarily theoretical, they often generate consternation among members of the surgical team. It is sound practice both from a risk management perspective, as well as with respect to the comfort and happiness of the OR team to take the time to position suckers to evacuate smoke and vapor emanating from the wound during surgery and thereby limit exposure to them.

Radiation and laser

Significant short- and long-term harm can result from exposure to ionizing radiation and laser in the OR. Precautions to protect eyes, gonads, and the thyroid gland, in particular, are readily available and must be used. Surgeons have a duty to their OR teams not only to ensure that the necessary safety equipment is present, but that it is used at all appropriate times. It is essential for the surgeon to demonstrate the safe way for protective equipment and garments to be used.

THE SURGICAL ASSISTANT

The presence of an experienced surgical assistant adds to the safety of surgery in all but genuinely minor procedures. In the case of complex and major surgery, the presence of an independently competent surgeon represents a potentially important step in reducing the danger to the patient associated with surgical misadventure.

In some circumstances, the assistant is provided by the hospital in the form of a surgical trainee or even a member of theater nursing staff. In others, the surgeon engages a colleague, medical or nursing, by private arrangement. Regardless, the surgeon remains primarily responsible for ensuring that the level of surgical assistance is appropriate to their needs and to the needs of the operation in question. No one else is in a position to ascertain the precise skill level required of the surgical assistant; responsibility for ensuring that the surgical assistant is appropriately skilled and experienced rests unequivocally with the surgeon.

THE SURGICAL COUNT

Although most surgeons regard the surgical count as being the domain of the OR nursing team, the surgeon remains ultimately responsible for deciding what to do in the event of an incorrect count. In cases where materials or instruments used in the operation are subsequently found to have been left in the operative field, the ultimate medicolegal responsibility also often falls to the surgeon. For these reasons alone, surgeons must be actively interested in and acutely aware of the counting process and its outcome.

Surgeons must, at all times, handle all surgical equipment – but especially gauze swabs and suture needles – with the consequences of their inadvertent misplacement in mind. Every time a gauze swab is inserted into the operative field, a mental note of its whereabouts must be kept. It is not sufficient to delegate this responsibility entirely to the nursing staff. Likewise, the ease with which a needle can be lost among the surgical drapes or knocked onto the OR floor is well known to every surgeon; conscious care and precision when returning every needle to the scrub nurse is mandatory to minimize this risk.

Perhaps, more than anything else, the surgeon's primary role is to direct and maintain an atmosphere that encourages safe practices within the OR. Rushing to finish a case, usually in the quest of making up valuable time, can place OR staff under immense pressure. A minimum amount of time is required for the completion of the surgical count and the nursing team must be allowed this opportunity to be confident about the count before the surgical wound has been closed. A surgeon pressing his or her OR staff to speed up their work effectively encourages them to take short cuts; the completeness and accuracy of the counting process are often the first to suffer.

Similarly, when an incorrect count is registered, the surgeon is obliged to stop whatever he is doing, calmly establish the nature of the incorrect count and assist the OR team to systematically check the count and, if necessary, look for the missing item. This is not the time for frustrated and angry recriminations; rather, the surgeon might be grateful for the success of the counting process in identifying the error, thus preventing a potentially harmful and professionally damaging oversight.

Again, it is haste that stands in the way of safety in the OR and it is the surgeon who must lead by example, ensuring optimal safety for their patients.

CONDUCT IN THE OPERATING ROOM

The OR can be a scene of considerable stress. While many operations proceed according to plan and sit comfortably within the skill and experience of the surgeon and the surgical team, tense and stressful situations do still regularly arise. Under pressure, all team members – the surgeon no less – are prone to become angry and unreasonable.

Unforeseen technical difficulties and complications of surgery present difficult moments for the surgical team, especially where the consequences are dramatic (e.g. intraoperative hemorrhage). Likewise, operations where there is advanced pathology associated with a clearly poor prognosis, especially in younger patients, create additional pressures for the team in the OR. In these circumstances, tempers can easily become frayed.

However, much of the bad behavior displayed by surgeons in the OR has its origins in more mundane and preventable forces. Easily the most common cause is time pressure. Surgeons generally lead busy working lives and demands upon their surgical services are considerable. As a result, OR lists are often fully booked so that even small delays can see a list overrun, eating into the surgeon's next commitment and delaying the start of the surgeon's next operating session. Faced with these delays – slow changeover between cases, delays in getting the patient to the OR, an unexpectedly difficult or slow case early in the list – some surgeons will become tense, agitated and even aggressive. Rarely does this help speed things up.

Another cause of stress is the lack of availability of familiar equipment or a lack of familiarity with the required equipment. These represent variables that diminish the surgeon's sense of control over the operative environment. Operating with new and unfamiliar equipment introduces additional stress into the surgical equation.

Undoubtedly, personality traits vary widely among surgeons. Ideally, a surgeon will have the capacity to focus entirely on the operation at hand, with primary regard for the safe and correct completion of the operation and with much less regard for the passage of time; doubtless, that is what patients would expect. Accordingly, patience and an even temper are characteristics which are universally respected and admired in a surgeon.

Surgeons who are prone to become stressed and to exhibit angry outbursts in the OR need not be dangerous or ineffective surgeons. However, other members of the OR team are often caught in the angry crossfire, victims of the surgeon's inability to deal more effectively with the pressure of the moment. This can have a debilitating effect upon the affected team member and represents an unacceptable consequence of the surgeon's bad behavior. In time, hospitals can find it difficult to get OR staff to work with surgeons who regularly fail to manage their own emotions during surgery.

The unique culture generated in any surgeon's OR is a direct reflection of the behavior of that surgeon or of the behaviors that the surgeon tolerates or supports in others. The overall standard of conduct in any OR – and the sense of safety felt by other team members working in that OR – remains the primary responsibility of the surgeon. Where the surgeon finds it difficult to control his or her own behavior, they should ensure that as many of the stress-inducing variables as possible are removed; they must ensure that they have an experienced assistant and they must adopt strategies to damp down their more instinctive responses to stress. More than any other factor, however, they must ensure that their operating lists are not overbooked. If time pressure is minimized, stress in the OR is often greatly reduced.

CREDENTIALING AND TECHNICAL COMPETENCE

The vast majority of surgeons have a very clear sense of the boundaries of their clinical skills and competence. Very few surgeons tackle cases for which they have inadequate training and experience. There are, inevitably, difficult cases for which no surgeon has extensive experience and which would extend any surgeon to the limit of his skills and ability.

However, the fact that hospitals have developed such detailed processes for the credentialing of their surgeons reflects the reality that some degree of external control over procedure selection is regarded as necessary. Regrettably, the occasional surgeon may be prone to display poor judgment in selecting cases for surgery, exceeding the limits of his or her training and expertise in the process.

These are matters for individual hospitals to address, but all surgeons can minimize this critical risk to their patients by recognizing circumstances where they have reservations about their own capacity to complete the procedure safely. In this situation, they might choose to involve a colleague in a difficult decision-making process. Even better, where an especially difficult case must be undertaken, the surgeon might obtain the assistance of a suitably experienced peer; operating with another surgeon is a rewarding and comforting experience in technically testing circumstances.

SAFE HOURS

Knowledge gained over decades from the practical experience of surgeons, as well as mounting scientific evidence and the experience of other industries (most notably the airline industry), make a compelling case against extended hours of clinical work for all doctors and especially for surgeons and other proceduralists. Working when fatigued dramatically reduces manual dexterity, adversely affects decision-making and increases the risk of a surgeon making an error. Patient safety is undoubtedly compromised in such circumstances.

That some operations need to be performed at night is an inescapable reality. Likewise, it is unrealistic to expect a contingent of fully rested and suitably qualified surgeons to be available around the clock to deliver the necessary surgical services. Such resources are comfortably beyond the reach of any health-care service.

Inevitably, therefore, surgeons will find themselves obliged to undertake operations when they are tired and when their technical skills might well be suboptimal. The decision to operate when fatigued will be influenced by the urgency of the clinical situation and by the availability of both a surgeon and a properly staffed OR to complete the case. Where the need for surgery is pressing and where the operation has little likelihood of otherwise proceeding in a timely fashion, the decision to operate when potentially fatigued is justified.

However, where the surgeon's fatigue is profound or where the case is entirely elective, the decision to operate when in a fatigued state or late at night, in general, has the potential to compromise patient safety and might be viewed as reckless. The surgeon must, at all times, ensure that his or her physical condition is appropriate to the task at hand.

NEW TECHNOLOGIES

The advance of technology and the steady proliferation of new devices to assist or enhance surgery, driven in part by industry, have created an environment whereby surgeons are continually expected to use new equipment and even new techniques. Many of these new devices have been developed in the era of minimally invasive surgery compounding the confusion associated with having to use new and unfamiliar equipment.

The rate of change, like so many aspects of our technological society, appears to be getting faster and the arrival of new technology is occurring at a pace that stretches human capacity to absorb, analyze, and gain appropriate competence. It is increasingly difficult for surgeons to be expert in the use of so many different techniques and pieces of equipment.

Undeniably, there is pressure upon surgeons to implement new technologies without necessarily having reviewed their scientific foundations or, no better, without having properly prepared themselves from a technical perspective. In this setting, reliance is often placed upon representatives of industry to advise surgeons about the underlying science or to walk surgeons through the use of new technology, sometimes for the first time in the OR. The long-standing basis of the safe practice of surgery – the acquisition of competence through supervision, practice, and analysis of one's performance – can be undermined by a misplaced sense of urgency to implement what is new and 'modern'.

Some of this urgency derives from powerful pressures to conform to the practice of peers who are widely regarded as trendsetters or who are promoted heavily at conferences, especially when the new equipment or technique has been shown to deliver improved outcomes. Surgeons who fail to keep up with the trend might feel that they are being labeled as outdated and their practice as old-fashioned. Notwithstanding the good results they have obtained over time through the sound application of existing equipment and techniques, surgeons often feel obliged to join the bandwagon of progress, attempting things for which their level of training is less than ideal and dramatically affecting patient safety. All surgeons are aware of these pressures and of the discomfort and dangers associated with the premature application of new technologies.

Yet there can be no halting the advance of technology and, to be fair, much of it has the potential to improve patient outcomes. Not all of it, however, has the potential to improve patient safety and there are many examples of improved outcomes for the majority being achieved at the cost of increased rates of complication for the minority. In this respect, surgeons are obliged not only to temper their enthusiasm for the thrill of using (and being seen to use) new technologies, but they have a profound duty to inform their patients about them.

In short, when applying new technologies to surgical practice, surgeons must:

- Dutifully analyze the scientific evidence underpinning the new technology. Every surgeon is familiar with an example of the widespread implementation of a new technology that was based upon the outcome of a single trial from a single center, but which was later shown to be fundamentally flawed and irreproducible at other centers. The caution that is characteristic of the medical profession as a whole has its roots in patient safety. It is altogether better to await the confirmatory results of properly conducted trials of any new technology before implementing them in one's own practice – at the risk of being labeled reactionary – than it is to jump in head first to the often irreversible detriment of our patients.
- Properly practice using the new equipment/technique before applying it independently on a patient. Since so many of these new technologies are subtle variations of what is already in use, it is generally reasonable to trial them live with the input of industry representatives alone. However, when the technology requires a little more in the way of practical application, surgeons are obliged either to assist a colleague already well practiced in the technology or to arrange for such a colleague to assist them when using it initially. Only the surgeon can then be sure whether or not they are comfortable

with the new technology or whether additional supervised practice is required. Finally, when applying a substantially new technology to one's existing practice, the surgeon must ensure that they have undergone the appropriate level of supervised training, obtained meaningful certification of their newly acquired skill and been endorsed to apply this new knowledge by their hospital's credentialing authority.

- Obtain meaningful informed consent from the patient. It is essential that, where any new technology is being applied, patients are advised accordingly. In addition to the usual elements of such informed consent – the objectives, alternatives, risks, complications, and timeline for recovery of the proposed operation – a declaration that the operation involves the use of a new procedure or technique, or one that is new for the surgeon should also form part of the consent process.

Where surgeons have analyzed the data recommending a new technology, have gained appropriate training and supervision in its application, and have advised their patients honestly about their experience, they have attended dutifully to their responsibilities to maintain patient safety; where they have rushed in to use new technology without proper prior analysis and training or where they fail to disclose their inexperience, they substantially raise the risk to their patients.

SUMMARY

There is an almost irresistible worldwide move towards the adoption of the Surgical Safety Checklist (**Figure 1.2.1**) based upon the recommendations of the World Health

Surgical safety checklist (first edition)

Before induction of anaesthesia

SIGN IN

- ☐ Patient has confirmed
  - identity
  - site
  - procedure
  - consent
- ☐ Site marked/not applicable
- ☐ Anaesthesia safety check completed
- ☐ Pulse oximeter on patient and fuctioning

Does patient have a:

Known allergy?
- ☐ No
- ☐ Yes

Difficult airway/aspiration risk?
- ☐ No
- ☐ Yes, and equipment/assistance available

Risk of >500ml blood loss (7ml/kg in children)?
- ☐ No
- ☐ Yes, and adequate intravenous access and fluids planned

Before skin incision

TIME OUT

- ☐ Confirm all team members have introduced themselves by name and role
- ☐ Surgeon, anaesthesia professional and nurse verbally confirm
  - patient
  - site
  - procedure

Anticipated critical events

- ☐ Surgeon reviews: what are the critical or unexpected steps, operative duration, anticipated blood loss?
- ☐ Anaesthesia team reviews: are there any patient-specific concerns?
- ☐ Nursing team reviews: has sterility (including indicator results) been confirmed? are there equipment issues or any concerns?

Has antibiotic prophylaxis been given within the last 60 minutes?
- ☐ Yes
- ☐ Not applicable

Is essential imaging displayed?
- ☐ Yes
- ☐ Not applicable

Before patient leaves operating room

SIGN OUT

Nurse verbally confirms with the team:

- ☐ The name of the procedure recorded
- ☐ That instrument, sponge and needle counts are correct (or not applicable)
- ☐ How the specimen in labelled (including patient name)
- ☐ Whether there are any equipment problems to be addressed
- ☐ Surgeon, anaesthesia professional and nurse review the key concerns for recovery and management of this patient

1.2.1

Organization.[1] The checklist comprises three series of checks – before the induction of anesthesia, immediately prior to the making of the surgical incision, and on completion of the procedure. According to the WHO process, these various points must be signed off for every operation. They encompass many of the safety issues highlighted in this chapter.

A multicenter, multinational study has demonstrated discernible benefits and enhanced safety associated with the use of this checklist. Meticulous and repetitive checking clearly do make for safer surgery; allowing the necessary time to be set aside for this checking to be completed is, perhaps, the surgeon's most important contribution towards enhancing patient safety.

REFERENCE

1. Haynes AB, Weiser TG, Berry WR *et al.* A surgical safety checklist to reduce morbidity and mortality in a global population. *New England Journal of Medicine* 2009; **360**: 491–9.

Access to abdominal cavity – open

JUDITH L TRUDEL

INTRODUCTION

The abdominal incision is the only portion of the surgeon's work which is accessible to the patient for examination. Despite the advent of minimally invasive and natural orifice transluminal endoscopic surgery, the need remains for traditional open access to the abdominal cavity. Patients' demand for smaller incisions for cosmetic purposes is supported by scientific data showing the deleterious impact of large incisions on healing and the immune response. Therefore, the wise selection of patient-appropriate incisions is a crucial surgical decision.

PRINCIPLES FOR CHOOSING AN INCISION

Selecting an incision rests on the following basic principles:

1 The incision must provide ready and direct access to the organ(s) of interest, and provide room for adequate exposure and maneuvering.
2 The incision must be extensible in the direction that may be required should the scope or extent of the procedure be modified during the procedure.
3 The incision should cause minimal interference with abdominal wall function, e.g. minimize injury to motor nerves, division of abdominal wall muscle, etc.
4 The incision should not jeopardize potentially needed future abdominal sites, specifically potential stoma sites.
5 The incision should be amenable to secure closure, leaving the abdominal wall at least as strong as it was before the operation.
6 If at all possible and appropriate, the incision should be cosmetically acceptable to patients.

PATIENT FACTORS INFLUENCING THE CHOICE OF INCISION

For individual patients, the choice of incision for access to the colon or rectum is also predicated on additional factors, including the location and extent of the colonic pathology, the patient's body habitus and internal anatomy (particularly the height of the hepatic and/or splenic flexures), the presence of previous surgical incisions, the potential need (immediate or future) for stomas, and the need for speedy entry into the abdomen in emergency cases.

TYPES OF INCISION

Abdominal incisions are broadly divided into four categories: vertical, oblique, transverse, and special combined incisions. As any of the four types of incision may provide adequate access and exposure to a given colonic pathology, final selection should be guided by the principles listed above.

The name of an incision usually describes the location of the incision or the technique used to gain access to the abdominal cavity. Over the years, many eponyms have become associated with specific incisions. Vertical incisions include midline/median, paramedian, trans-rectus muscle-splitting, and para-rectus (Battle-Kammerer) incisions. Vertical incisions may be supra- or infraumbilical. Oblique incisions include the right subcostal (Kocher) incision, the right lower quadrant gridiron muscle-splitting (McBurney) incision, and the right lower quadrant (Rockey-Davis) incision. Transverse incisions include the transverse suprapubic (Pfannenstiel) incision, and the generic transverse abdominal incision. Special combined incisions include the upper abdominal chevron incision and the thoracoabdominal incision.

Several of the incisions listed above are now mostly of historical interest and will not be described in detail here. In addition to those, a large variety of other little used or obsolete incisions have been described over the course of the centuries. Our goal is to describe the incisions which are nowadays most useful and most frequently used to gain open access to the abdominal cavity for colon and rectal procedures: the vertical midline/median incision, the paramedian incision, the transverse abdominal incision, and the suprapubic Pfannenstiel incision. The right lower quadrant McBurney incision used for access to the appendix will also be described.

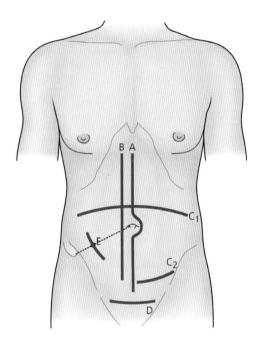

1.3.1 Types of incision: A, midline/median incision; B, paramedian incision (right); C$_1$, upper transverse incision (bilateral); C$_2$, lower transverse incision (left); D, Pfannenstiel incision; E, McBurney's incision.

Vertical versus transverse incisions

A vertical midline/median incision is the open incision of choice for most surgeons operating on colorectal pathologies as it provides optimal exposure to the entire abdomen.

Generally speaking, vertical incisions have the following advantages:

- They are quick and easy to make and easy to close; a vertical midline incision is the incision of choice for emergencies.
- They are technically the easiest to extend if the need arises.
- They destroy few if any important abdominal wall structures, such as nerves or blood vessels.

- They bleed less than transverse incisions as they are made through relatively avascular planes.
- They preserve potential stoma sites which may be needed in the future.
- They avoid division of the rectus abdominis muscles and epigastric arteries, thus preserving the option of a vertical rectus abdominis myocutaneous (VRAM) flap.

The proponents of transverse incisions state the following advantages:

- They parallel Langer's lines of the skin and provide a better final cosmetic result.
- They inflict less tension on suture lines and aponeuroses when the abdominal wall muscles are contracting.
- They run parallel to important abdominal structures, such as nerves and blood vessels, which can then easily be avoided by placing the transverse incision at the appropriate level.

Traditional transverse incisions may be useful for exposure in select cases, at the cost of dividing abdominal wall muscles and possible interference with potential stoma sites. The popularity of the suprapubic Pfannenstiel incision for colorectal pelvic procedures has increased with the use of laparoscopic and hand-assisted laparoscopic approaches.

DESCRIPTION OF THE SURGICAL TECHNIQUE FOR SELECT INCISIONS

For all the procedures described throughout this section, it is assumed that hemostasis will be secured at all stages as the operation proceeds, and that irrigation will be carried out as appropriate during wound closure. These statements will therefore not be repeated in any of the descriptions of the open approaches to the abdomen.

In addition, we will use the term 'ligation' to describe any technically appropriate method of vascular control, including ties, suture ligations, or any approved sealing or hemostatic device used within the range of recommended vessel size for safe use.

Vertical midline/median incision

INDICATIONS FOR USE

The vertical midline/median incision is the open incision of choice for most colorectal pathologies as it provides optimal exposure to the entire abdomen. The supraumbilical or infraumbilical location and the total length of the incision are predicated on the patient factors and principles discussed earlier in this chapter.

TECHNIQUE

At the desired level, a vertical midline incision is made by sharply incising the skin and subcutaneous tissues with either the scalpel or the electrocautery, exposing the shiny white linea alba. If the planned incision extends across the umbilicus, the surgeon should curve around this structure to the left or right, depending on personal preference. The umbilicus should not be excised, unless involved by pathology (an exceptional occurrence).

The linea alba is quite broad and best defined in the supraumbilical portion of the abdomen. Division of the linea alba at that level does not expose the rectus muscle nor does it allow for identification of individual aponeuroses. It is considerably narrower below the umbilicus, and often one of the rectus muscles is exposed while attempting to find the right line. If infraumbilical identification of the linea alba is difficult, a helpful maneuver is to carefully incise the anterior rectus sheath just above the symphysis pubis, exposing the paired pyramidalis muscles anterior to the rectus muscles. The upward direction of the fibers of these paired muscles leads directly to the linea alba. The linea alba proper is avascular.

The linea alba is divided sharply in the midline with either the scalpel or the cautery, exposing well-vascularized extraperitoneal fat of variable thickness. The underlying parietal peritoneum is then grasped with forceps and a small incision is made to confirm entry in the free abdominal cavity. A finger is inserted carefully in the abdomen in order to protect the abdominal viscera while the incision is extended to the required length. At the upper portion of the incision in the epigastric area, the ligamentum teres/falciform ligament of the liver runs just right of the midline. It is best avoided by slipping a finger in the abdomen under the midline, by sweeping the ligamentum teres/falciform ligament to the right and opening the upper portion of the incision under direct manual and visual control. If necessary, the ligamentum teres/falciform ligament can be divided and ligated. Conversely, at the lower portion of a midline incision, care must be taken not to injure the urinary bladder. Gentle blunt finger dissection may be used to push back the bladder out of harm's way prior to dividing the lowermost part of the linea alba, the peritoneum and entering the abdomen.

Once the abdomen is open, complete exploration is performed. Presence of ascites, peritoneal contamination, or carcinomatosis is noted. If present, ascitic fluid is collected and submitted for histopathology to rule out malignancy. Exploration must be performed in a sequential standardized fashion. The exact sequence may vary according to the surgeon's preference. The preoperative findings are confirmed, and additional findings which may alter the surgical plan or the need for extension of the original incision are noted and handled appropriately. Findings directly pertaining to the known pathology and planned procedure must be verified: tumor location, clinical resectability, presence of metastatic disease, local invasion of adjacent organs, adequacy of bowel preparation, adequacy of bowel for primary anastomosis, or any intestinal findings which may impact the surgical plan. Additional non-intestinal findings (aortic aneurysm, gynecological pathology (particularly ovarian), severe vascular disease, etc.) may also alter the original plan.

WOUND CLOSURE

Historically, vertical midline/median incisions were closed in separate layers. Nowadays, most surgeons use a mass closure technique. Options for closure are abundant, and are largely based on the surgeon's preference. The wound may be closed in a continuous or interrupted fashion, using non-absorbable or slowly absorbable suture materials. Staples may be used for the skin.

Vertical paramedian incision

INDICATIONS FOR USE

Paramedian incisions may be made on the right or left side of the abdomen, and may be located in the upper, middle, or lower abdomen. Proponents of this approach argue that they heal more rapidly than midline incisions because of better blood supply compared with the avascular linea alba; and are less prone to herniation because of better buttressing of the suture line by the intact overlying rectus muscle.

TECHNIQUE

At the desired level, a vertical incision parallel to and approximately 2–2.5 cm from the midline of the abdomen is made with either the scalpel or the electrocautery, incising sharply through the skin and subcutaneous tissues. The exposed anterior rectus sheath is cleared of fat and incised vertically approximately 2–2.5 cm from the midline. The medial sheath flap thus created is lifted up, exposing the rectus muscle proper. Using the handle of the scalpel, the medial edge of the rectus muscle is released from its attachment to the midline and to the anterior

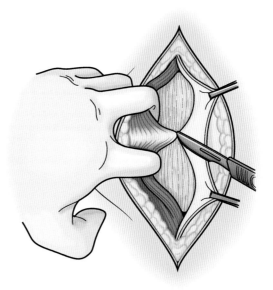

1.3.2 Dissection of rectus muscle tendinous insertions from anterior rectus sheath.

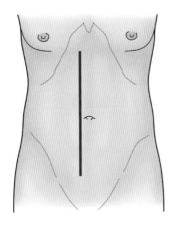

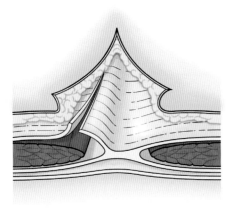

1.3.3 Transverse section paramedian incision on the right (above umbilicus).

rectus sheath itself. The freed muscle is then retracted laterally, protecting the epigastric vessels which run deep to the rectus muscle (**Figure 1.3.2** and **1.3.3**).

The posterior rectus sheath, the transversalis fascia, the properitoneal fat, and the parietal peritoneum are incised carefully approximately 2–2.5 cm from the midline, entering the abdomen. As a reminder, the posterior rectus sheath is absent in the lower abdomen below the level of the semicircular line of Douglas or arcuate line. A finger is inserted carefully in the abdomen in order to protect the abdominal viscera while the incision is extended to the required length. Systematic exploration is then performed, as discussed in the previous section on midline abdominal incisions.

WOUND CLOSURE

The parietal peritoneum, transversalis fascia, and posterior rectus sheath (if present) are closed in a single layer using absorbable suture material. The rectus muscle is allowed to fall back medially in its anatomic position, protecting the underlying suture line. The anterior rectus sheath is closed using interrupted or continuous non-absorbable or slowly absorbable suture material. The subcutaneous tissues and skin are closed according to the surgeon's preference.

Transverse abdominal incision

The lateral abdominal wall muscle compartment extends from the lowermost six ribs superiorly to the anterior portion of the iliac crest inferiorly; medially, its boundary is the lateral edge of the rectus muscle. The relationships between the aponeuroses of the lateral abdominal wall muscles and the anterior and posterior rectus sheaths have already been described.

The most superficial layer is the skin. Immediately under the skin is the subcutaneous layer, consisting mainly of fat with areas of condensation called Camper's (superficial) and Scarpa's (deep) fascia, respectively. The most superficial muscle is the external oblique muscle. Its aponeurosis is well defined medially, while the muscle itself lies more laterally. Its fibers run obliquely in the direction outlined by slipping a hand in a pocket. The internal oblique muscle lies immediately under the external oblique muscle, and its fibers run at 90° with those of the external oblique muscle. The transverse abdominal muscle lies deep to the internal oblique muscle. Its fibers run transversely.

Deep to the muscle layer is the transversalis fascia, followed by a layer of extraperitoneal fat of varying thickness, and finally the parietal peritoneum serving as the innermost layer of the abdominal wall.

INDICATIONS FOR USE

Transverse abdominal incisions may be used to gain access to the upper or lower abdomen. They may be made unilaterally on the right or left side of the abdomen, or extend across the midline at any level of the abdomen. Unilateral or bilateral mid- or lower transverse abdominal incisions are used most frequently to gain open access to the colon and rectum. A transverse mid-abdominal incision is best suited for access to the right, transverse, descending, and sigmoid colon.

TECHNIQUE

At the desired level, a transverse incision is made sharply through the skin and subcutaneous tissues with the scalpel or electrocautery. The length of the incision and its lateral extension are based on the need for exposure and may involve various degrees of the lateral abdominal muscle compartment (**Figure 1.3.4**).

A long incision exposes the anterior rectus sheath and the aponeurosis of the external oblique muscle. Medially, this latter aponeurosis is well defined, but laterally the actual muscle fibers of the external oblique are usually encountered. The anterior rectus sheath is incised transversely, the external oblique aponeurosis is incised in the direction of its fibers and, if the external oblique muscle itself is encountered, its fibers are separated bluntly. The rectus muscle is freed from its attachments to the anterior rectus sheath and a finger is slipped under the lateral border of the rectus toward the midline to guide the surgeon as he/she divides the muscle sharply, usually with

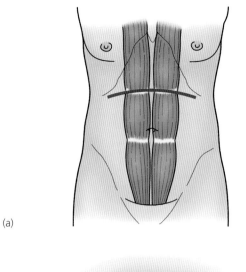

(a)

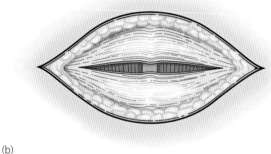

(b)

1.3.4 (a) Transverse abdominal incision; (b) central abdominal wall muscle compartment.

the cautery. As the rectus muscle is divided, the epigastric vessels and any discrete bleeders are ligated. Alternatively, if the lateral extent of the incision is limited and does not involve the lateral abdominal muscle compartment, the freed rectus muscle may be retracted laterally without division. Depending on the level of the incision, either the ninth or the eleventh intercostal nerve can be seen running just anterior to the posterior rectus sheath; it is protected and retracted superiorly. The posterior rectus sheath, the transversalis fascia and the parietal peritoneum are then incised transversely in the midline and the abdomen is entered. Starting at the lateral edge of the rectus, the internal oblique and transverse abdominal muscles are split in the direction of their fibers and retracted superiorly and inferiorly. The transverse incision across the transversalis fascia and parietal peritoneum may be extended as far laterally as needed.

WOUND CLOSURE

The parietal peritoneum, transversalis fascia, and posterior rectus sheath (if present) are closed in a single layer using absorbable suture material. The divided rectus muscle itself is not closed but the anterior rectus sheath is closed using interrupted or continuous non-absorbable or

slowly absorbable suture material. Laterally, the transverse abdominal muscle is usually too attenuated to hold sutures, but both the internal oblique and the external oblique muscles are reapproximated in layers using interrupted non-absorbable or slowly absorbable suture material. The subcutaneous tissues and skin are closed according to the surgeon's preference.

Pfannenstiel incision

INDICATIONS FOR USE

This suprapubic incision provides good open access to the pelvis, but limited room for maneuvering in the mid and upper abdomen. The popularity of the suprapubic Pfannenstiel incision for colorectal pelvic procedures has increased with the use of laparoscopic and hand-assisted laparoscopic approaches, as mobilization and vascular control of mid and upper abdominal structures is achieved before the abdomen is open, decreasing the need for long or high abdominal incisions. It is cosmetically pleasing to the patients, the scar being hidden in the skin folds parallel to Langer's lines of the skin and/or covered by pubic hair.

TECHNIQUE

A slightly curved (smiling) incision is made transversely across the lower abdomen, approximately 5 cm above the symphysis pubis, in the pubic hair-bearing area (**Figure 1.3.5a**). The skin and subcutaneous tissues are incised sharply using the scalpel or the electrocautery, exposing both rectus muscle sheaths. Both rectus muscle sheaths and the linea alba are divided transversely exposing the paired rectus and the apex of the pyramidalis muscles in their sheath (**Figure 1.3.5b**). The upper and lower sheath flaps are grasped with forceps or hemostats and the rectus muscle is then freed superiorly and inferiorly from its attachments to its sheath as far as is possible. The rectus muscles are separated at their junction in the midline and each is retracted laterally. As there is no posterior rectus sheath below the arcuate line or semicircular line of Douglas, the transversalis fascia and parietal peritoneum are directly accessible. They are incised vertically in the midline, taking care not to injure the bladder just above the symphysis pubis as the pelvis is accessed (**Figure 1.3.5c**).

WOUND CLOSURE

The parietal peritoneum and transversalis fascia are closed in a single continuous layer using absorbable suture material. The rectus muscles are allowed to fall back medially in their anatomic position, but do not get sutured. The anterior rectus sheaths and linea alba are closed using interrupted or continuous non-absorbable or slowly absorbable suture material. The subcutaneous tissues and skin are closed according to the surgeon's preference.

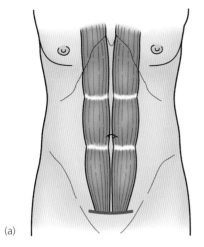

(a)

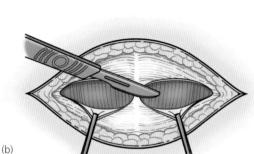

(b)

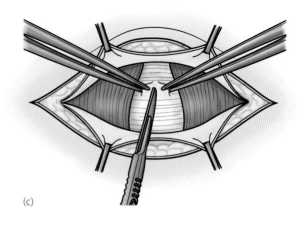

(c)

1.3.5 Pfannenstiel incision.

McBurney's incision

INDICATIONS FOR USE

The McBurney muscle-splitting gridiron incision is the incision of choice for a planned open appendectomy. The exposure is quite limited and does not allow for extensive abdominal exploration. It also does not lend itself to easy extension if the need arises.

The McBurney incision may also be used to access the abdomen when making a cecostomy, an operation with few if any indications nowadays. A mirror image incision may be made in the left abdomen to access the sigmoid colon.

TECHNIQUE

McBurney's point is located two-thirds of the way between the umbilicus and the right anterior iliac spine. The McBurney incision is made approximately 3 cm (two fingerbreadths) above and medially to the right anterior iliac spine, encompassing McBurney's point. Classically, the incision is made in an oblique direction in a line parallel to the directions of the fibers of the underlying external oblique muscle. Depending on the surgeon's preference, the skin incision may be made transversely, and is then called a 'Rockey-Davis incision'. The skin and subcutaneous tissues are incised sharply using the scalpel or the electrocautery, exposing the aponeurosis of the external oblique muscle. The aponeurosis is incised and opened in the direction of its fibers (**Figure 1.3.6**a). Medially, the aponeurosis is well defined, but laterally the actual muscle fibers of the external oblique are usually encountered and separated bluntly. The external oblique muscle is retracted bluntly, exposing the fibers of the internal oblique muscle. Using blunt dissection once again, the internal oblique muscle is separated in the direction of its fibers (**Figure 1.3.6**b), exposing the transverse abdominal muscle, which is also separated bluntly in the direction of its fibers and retracted (**Figure 1.3.6**c). Any adhesions between the transversalis fascia and the transverse abdominal muscle are freed by sweeping the finger under the surface of the muscle. The transversalis fascia and parietal peritoneum are then incised sharply and carefully, making sure that the underlying viscera are not injured (**Figure 1.3.6**d). Limited exploration is carried through this incision.

WOUND CLOSURE

The parietal peritoneum and transversalis fascia are closed in a single continuous layer using absorbable suture material. The split transverse abdominal and internal oblique muscles are approximated loosely with a few interrupted sutures of absorbable suture material. The external oblique muscle is allowed to fall back in its anatomic position and reapproximated in a separate layer with interrupted absorbable suture material. The subcutaneous tissues and skin are closed according to the surgeon's preference.

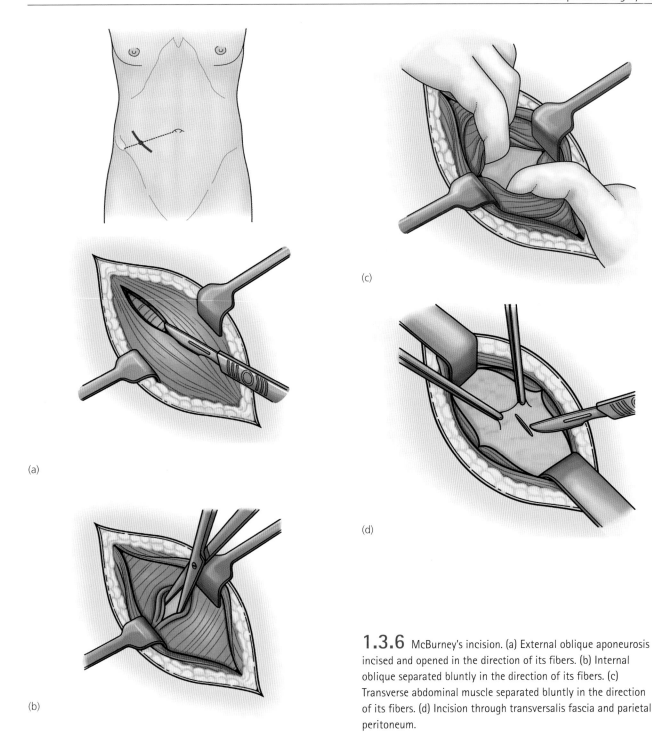

1.3.6 McBurney's incision. (a) External oblique aponeurosis incised and opened in the direction of its fibers. (b) Internal oblique separated bluntly in the direction of its fibers. (c) Transverse abdominal muscle separated bluntly in the direction of its fibers. (d) Incision through transversalis fascia and parietal peritoneum.

REOPERATIVE SURGERY

Access to the previously operated abdomen presents additional challenges and is thus considered separately. The surgeon must first decide whether to enter the previously operated abdomen through a previously used incision or at a relatively new site. The major disadvantage of using a previous incision is the almost universal presence of some adhesions to the innermost abdominal layer and the underside of the wound. Special care and attention must

be taken to avoid damaging or entering the adhered intra-abdominal structures (particularly hollow viscera, such as the small/large bowel or bladder).

Access to the previously operated abdomen at a distance from previous incisions must adhere to all the basic principles outlined at the beginning of the chapter regarding access, extensibility, security of closure, and preservation of potentially needed future sites. Special consideration must be given to the possibility that an additional incision may negatively impact abdominal wall function through cumulative injury to motor nerves or abdominal muscles. General weakening of the abdominal wall may predispose to herniation. All incisions are liable to develop adhesions; consideration should be given to take appropriate measures to minimize additional adhesions.

There is therefore no hard and fast recommendation, and the decision to re-enter the abdomen through a previous or new incision must be individualized.

FURTHER READING

Agur AMR, Dalley AF. *Grant's atlas of anatomy*, 12th edn. Baltimore, MD: Wolters Kluwer, Lippincott Williams & Wilkins, 2008.

McMinn RMH, Hutchings RT. *Color atlas of human anatomy*. Chicago, IL: Year Book Medical Publishers, 1977.

Zuidema GD, Yeo CJ. *Shackelford's surgery of the alimentary tract*, vol. II, 5th edn. Philadelphia, PA: WB Saunders, 2002.

Access to abdominal cavity – laparoscopic

YAIR EDDEN AND STEVEN D WEXNER

INTRODUCTION

The introduction of practical laparoscopic surgery in the early 1980s was initially greeted with reservation and disdain. However, over the last 30 years, the minimally invasive approach has become one of the most significant transformations of its era for both patients and surgeons. Originally used exclusively as a diagnostic tool, laparoscopy has evolved into a commonly accepted approach performed for almost all abdominal operations. The introduction of technical innovations such as high definition cameras, tissue-sealing devices, articulating staplers, and new methods of access and tissue visualization has permitted accomplishment of ever more complicated surgical challenges.

Aside from obvious cosmetic advantages, laparoscopic surgery minimizes immediate and late postoperative complications. Numerous independent, large multicenter studies have proven that laparoscopy shortens hospital stay, causes less operative pain, and is superior to laparotomy.

This chapter addresses the primary step necessary to undertake all laparoscopic procedures: accessing the abdominal cavity and creating a pneumoperitoneum that provides the adequate operating space needed for safe and successful surgery.

PRINCIPLES

In order to perform minimally invasive surgery inside the peritoneal cavity, a working space must be created. This goal is achieved by insufflating the peritoneal cavity with gas, usually CO_2. It is only after this primary step that the laparoscopy camera and the various operative instruments can be safely inserted under direct vision. Since this step is blindly done, it poses a specific challenge to the surgeon. In most reported cases, the complications associated with this step are injury to major blood vessels or to hollow viscera.[1]

OPERATIVE APPROACH, CREATING PNEUMOPERITONEUM

The Veress needle – closed technique

The closed technique to induce pneumoperitoneum is performed by using a Veress insufflating needle (**Figure 1.4.1**). This specifically designed device, introduced in 1932 by Janos Veress, has a hollow needle placed inside a protecting sheath to minimize the risk of damage to adjacent structures.

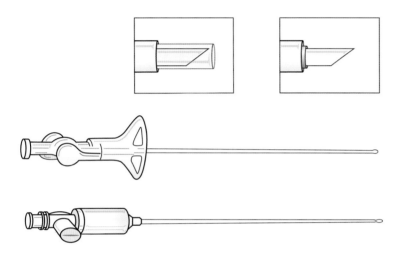

1.4.1 Veress needle: the needle's tip is protected by a retracting sheath that minimizes the risk of damaging intraperitoneal organs.

While pressure is applied against the abdominal wall, the sheath is retracted, exposing the needle tip that is intended to penetrate into the peritoneal cavity (**Figure 1.4.2**). A small skin incision is made over the relevant site and the needle is inserted at a 30° angle with one hand while the abdominal wall is lifted by the other hand with the aid of towel clips. This maneuver facilitates a controlled insertion of the device while elevating the abdominal wall from the underlying structures (**Figure 1.4.2**). After the needle traverses the abdominal wall, the sheath rapidly covers the needle tip to avoid damage to intra-abdominal organs (**Figure 1.4.3**).

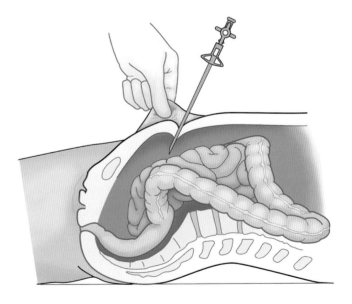

1.4.2 The abdominal wall is lifted to allow safe insertion of the Veress needle into the peritoneal cavity.

In order to ensure the correct intraperitoneal position of the tip, several tests can be performed:

1 Aspiration using a saline-filled syringe. If the needle's tip is inside the peritoneal cavity, air bubbles are expected. The presence of stool or blood in the aspirate indicates an intra-abdominal organ injury.
2 Placing a few drops of normal saline into the needle hub and pulling the abdominal wall upward. If the needle is within the potential space of the peritoneal cavity, the fluid will be drawn inside (**Figure 1.4.3**).
3 Initiate insufflation with CO_2. If the needle tip resides within the peritoneal cavity, there should be no resistance and the gas pressure should be low until the abdomen is distended and the peritoneum is filled with gas.

Although one or more of these methods may be used, the most reliable and accurate test is the CO_2 pressure test.[2] Under normal circumstances with correct needle placement, pressure remains low while the gas flows until the abdomen distends to the optimal pressure of 15 mmHg. If the initial measured pressure is too high, or if high pressure is reached almost immediately without evident distention of the abdominal wall, needle position is presumed to be incorrect and another access attempt should be made.

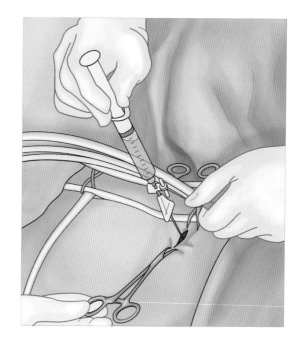

1.4.3 Aspiration on syringe connected to the back of the Veress needle can give indication as for the needle's tip position.

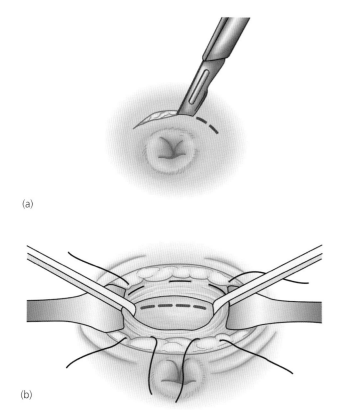

(a)

(b)

The Hasson – open technique

This approach is based on creating a mini-laparotomy.[3] A skin incision 1.5–2 cm is performed and the fascia is exposed by blunt dissection (**Figure 1.4.4**). Once visualized, the fascia is grasped with two Kocher clamps, and a small incision is performed. Anchoring sutures are placed at each edge of the fascia. Traction on these sutures exposes the peritoneum, which is grasped between the two fine clamps and divided with scissors, providing access to the peritoneal cavity.

1.4.4 Hasson technique: skin incision is performed above or below the umbilicus (a) followed by blunt dissection exposing the fascia (b).

A finger or a blunt curved instrument is used to evaluate the presence of adhesions or adherent organs. A Hasson trocar is next inserted into the abdomen and secured to the fascia with the anchoring sutures, which also prevents gas leak after the pneumoperitoneum is created. Gas insufflation is established through this trocar (**Figure 1.4.5**).

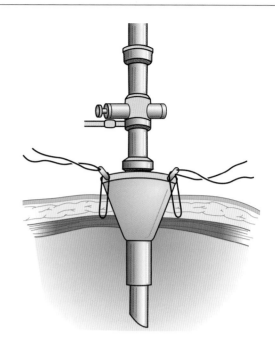

1.4.5 The Hasson trocar is anchored to the fascia with two stitches, helping to maintain adequate intraperitoneal pressure.

Despite the feasibility of laparoscopic surgery in patients who have had prior abdominal surgery, special consideration should be given in these patients. In most patients who have not had previous surgery, the optimal site for placing the first port is over the midline immediately above or below the umbilicus. This location, where only fascia separates the subcutaneous fat and the peritoneum, minimizes the risk of injury to muscle or blood vessels. The presence of a previous scar is a reasonable predictor of possible intra-abdominal adhesions that could complicate the access or make safe entry into the abdomen impossible. Under these circumstances, alternative access points must be considered. Generally speaking, when a midline scar already exists, the access incision should be located adjacent to the umbilicus on the opposite side of the existing scar. In these cases, the open (Hasson) technique is safer than and recommended over the closed (Veress) approach.

Although the Veress technique usually takes less time to perform, after some experience the open technique can be quickly undertaken. In several large studies, no significant difference in complication rates were noted between the two methods.[4,5,6] With lack of evidence-based results, it is a matter of personal surgeon preference that should dictate the method of access. However, the authors of this chapter perform all access using the Hasson technique for all initial and reoperative surgery.

Secondary access

After the first port is placed and pneumoperitoneum is induced, additional ports are inserted under direct vision to prevent injury to intra-abdominal organs. Skin incisions are made according to the port's diameter and the ports are inserted into the abdominal cavity. Originally, the ports had a sharp obturator, but they were later replaced with a covered blade, similar to the Veress needle principle. Lately, several manufacturers have introduced bladeless ports that further reduce the risk of injury during insertion. For the purpose of colorectal surgery, most ports used are either 5 or 10 mm in diameter. Larger and smaller ports are also available for pediatric surgery or in the event that a larger diameter device is required. The number and position of ports placed varies according to the planned procedure, the patient's body habitus, surgeon's preference, and intraoperative requirement.

CONCLUSIONS

Laparoscopic surgery is one of the most important advances during the last several decades. In order to perform safe and successful laparoscopic surgery, a pneumoperitoneum must be created, and the inability to create this space mandates conversion to laparotomy. The two major access methods are the Veress closed technique and the Hasson open technique. To date, there are no compelling data to favor one approach over the other. However, whichever approach is chosen, it must be performed following a standard surgical routine and utilizing sound surgical judgment.

REFERENCES

1. Vilos GA, Ternamian A, Dempster J, Laberge PY, The Society of Obstetricians and Gynaecologists of Canada. Laparoscopic

entry: a review of techniques, technologies, and complications. *Journal of Obstetrics and Gynaecology Canada* 2007; **29**: 433–65.

2. Teoh B, Sen R, Abbott J. An evaluation of four tests used to ascertain Veres needle placement at closed laparoscopy. *Journal of Minimally Invasive Gynecology* 2005; **12**: 153–8.

3. Hasson HM. Open laparoscopy. *Biomedical Bulletin* 1984; **5**: 1–6.

4. Opilka M, Starzewski J, Lorenc Z *et al.* Open versus closed laparoscopy entry – which are the evidences? *Hepatogastroenterology* 2009; **56**: 75–9.

5. Ahmad G, Duffy JM, Phillips K, Watson A. Laparoscopic entry techniques. *Cochrane Database Systematic Reviews* 2008; (**16**): CD006583.

6. Munro MG. Laparoscopic access: complications, technologies, and techniques. *Current Opinion in Obstetrics and Gynecology* 2002; **14**: 365–74.

Access to abdominal cavity – hand-assisted laparoscopic surgery

THOMAS E READ

PRINCIPLES AND JUSTIFICATION

The advantages of laparoscopic approach to colectomy are largely related to a relatively small abdominal incision that reduces wound complications and postoperative pain, and results in modest reductions in the duration of postoperative ileus and improvements in postoperative functional status. Excluding those surgeons who perform transrectal or transvaginal specimen extraction, the majority of surgeons utilize an abdominal incision of 4–8 cm to extract the colectomy specimen. This incision can also be used to perform mesentery division and anastomosis, provided that adequate mobilization of the colon has been accomplished intracorporeally. If such an incision is to be made at some point during the operation, it seems sensible to make it at the start of the procedure and utilize it throughout. The current generation of hand-assist devices allows this concept to be put into practice to facilitate the performance of laparoscopic colectomy. Hand-assist technology allows the novice laparoscopic colectomist to improve tactile sensation and proprioception, and allows the experienced surgeon to approach complex problems laparoscopically and potentially shorten operative times.

Hand-assist devices have evolved since their inception in the 1990s, just as other laparoscopic equipment has evolved. Cumbersome at the outset, with sleeves that prevented easy user exchange, or with bases that limited use of the incision, hand-assist devices now possess most of the qualities necessary for their smooth integration into laparoscopic colorectal procedures. The optimal device includes a stable, sturdy platform base that crosses the abdominal wall and provides circumferential retraction of the wound with a low vertical profile; and a self-sealing membrane that allows for rapid and easy hand exchange, and accommodates trocar placement through the device.

The application of hand-assisted laparoscopic techniques to laparoscopic colectomy may allow the surgeon to solve problems in the operating theater, and allow performance of more complex procedures than straight laparoscopy. The approach to large inflammatory phlegmons or fibrotic masses, such as those associated with diverticulitis or Crohn's disease may be easier using a hand-assisted technique. Similarly, the hostile abdomen with numerous adhesions may be more efficiently sorted out with a hand in the peritoneal cavity. The human hand is an exquisite instrument with five individually functioning digits that all give tactile feedback to the operator. Its use in difficult cases cannot be overstated. Occasionally, however, the placement of a hand in the abdomen may create problems with visualization for the novice surgeon and may force the surgeon to creatively solve ergonomic problems. These difficulties are most often encountered early in the learning curve, and can be abolished completely by withdrawing the hand if so desired, as the current generation of hand-assist devices allows without loss of pneumoperitoneum.

'Peek port' technique

Another benefit of hand-assist technology is that it allows immediate access to the peritoneal cavity via minilaparotomy. Trocars can be placed under direct vision after the hand-assist incision has been made. Thus, trocar-related injuries are minimized and the need for specialized, expensive trocars to establish pneumoperitoneum is eliminated. Additionally, the hand-assisted laparoscopic surgery (HALS) approach allows for the surgeon to assess the peritoneal cavity prior to deciding on whether to proceed with a laparoscopic procedure. The author has used a modification of the hand-assisted technique to minimize the rate of conversion to formal laparotomy, as it is these conversions that generate the most expense, and are often associated with the poorest outcomes. This strategy is associated with a low rate of conversion from laparoscopy to laparotomy.[1]

Patients deemed to be at high risk for conversion (e.g. those with large, inflammatory phlegmons and/or multiple prior laparotomies) are evaluated initially via a small (8 cm) incision placed in the line of the incision which would be used if the case was approached via formal laparotomy. The laparoscopic equipment is kept in the operating theater, but remains unopened. If intraperitoneal conditions are favorable, a hand-assist device is placed through this incision and the procedure performed laparoscopically. If intraperitoneal conditions are unfavorable, the incision is simply extended and the unopened laparoscopic instruments removed from the room.

Adoption of this technique should reduce overall cost by avoiding the use of laparoscopic equipment in patients who ultimately require formal laparotomy, and avoid potential trocar-related complications.

PREOPERATIVE ASSESSMENT AND PREPARATION

Although hand-assisted laparoscopic colectomy can be considered for patients with prior laparotomy and/or complex intra-abdominal pathology, a detailed history should be obtained so as to assess the patient's appropriateness for laparoscopic management of their pathology. Details of prior operative procedures should be obtained, with special attention paid to the difficulty of prior adhesiolysis and whether permanent mesh was placed in the abdominal wall. A thorough assessment of disease pathology should be undertaken and the optimal position of the HALS incision considered. Potential intestinal stoma sites should be marked preoperatively. HALS incisions should not be placed within the anticipated boundaries of the stoma appliance. Comorbid medical conditions should be assessed, and a determination made of the patient's cardiopulmonary status, as prolonged operation and carbon dioxide pneumoperitoneum can be detrimental in some cases. Body mass index also has some influence on the choice of operative technique. Hand-assisted laparoscopic colectomy is easier to perform in the obese patient than straight laparoscopic colectomy, although the super-obese may be better served by laparotomy to perform colectomy.

ANESTHESIA

General endotracheal anesthesia is used for hand-assisted laparoscopic colectomy. Peak airway pressures should be assessed in the extremes of table position prior to draping to ensure that the patient can be adequately ventilated during the case.

OPERATION

Positioning

The patient should be secured to the operating table. My preference is to secure the patient by using a deflatable bean bag. The pads are removed from the thoracoabdominal portion of the table and wide strips of Velcro are placed on the metal of the bed and the posterior aspect of the bean bag. This prevents the bean bag (and the patient) from slipping during the procedure. A large gel pad is placed inside the bean bag and the arms and shoulders padded. The arms are tucked at the sides and the bean bag wrapped around the torso and shoulders to cocoon the patient. The legs are typically placed supine or in split leg position if routine access to the anus is contemplated, such as for endoscopy or passage of a surgical stapling device. The legs are placed in lithotomy for procedures in which greater access to the perineum is required (hand-sewn coloanal or ileoanal anastomosis, resection of the perineum, etc.). The bed is then tested in all the extremes of position to ensure that the patient does not slide and that access to the anus is maintained.

Choice of incision

HALS incisions can either be made proactively, as part of a planned HALS colectomy, or reactively, during straight laparoscopic colectomy in response to complex intra-abdominal situations. The choice of incision is based on where the surgeon feels the incision will maximize safe completion of the procedure. This may be directly over the pathology (phlegmon, fistula, locally advanced tumor) or over the anticipated site of anastomosis. For patients with complex sigmoid diverticular disease or rectosigmoid cancer, these are one and the same.

HALS right colectomy

HALS right colectomy can be accomplished using a variety of incisions. The author's preference is to use an upper midline incision (**Figure 1.5.1**). This allows the case to begin with dissection of the greater omentum from the transverse colon and mesocolon under direct vision. The omentum can be split at the site of anticipated anastomosis, which facilitates retraction. In obese patients, the ability to perform these maneuvers through the incision accelerates performance of the procedure. After the limit of dissection through the incision is reached, an infraumbilical camera port and a working port are placed, and the operation proceeds laparoscopically. The specimen is extracted and the anastomosis performed through the incision. The placement of the incision directly over the mid-transverse colon facilitates anastomosis between ileum and transverse colon.

Other incision sites for HALS right colectomy can be used. For complex colonic disease involving the duodenum, an oblique incision directly over the pathology may be optimal. For ileal Crohn's disease with fistula to the bladder or sigmoid colon, a Pfannenstiel incision can be used. The surgeon should be aware that placement of the incision remote from the anastomotic site will require additional mobilization of the transverse colon, and that placement of an incision on the patient's right side may make insertion of the hand for laparoscopic mobilization of the right colon difficult.

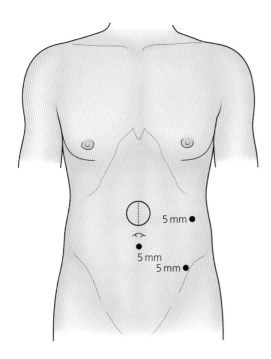

5 mm ●

5 mm
5 mm ●

1.5.1 Hand-assisted laparoscopic surgery (HALS) right colectomy. Schematic of incisions.

HALS left colectomy

The HALS device is typically placed via a Pfannenstiel (**Figure 1.5.2**) or lower midline incision for left colectomy, sigmoid colectomy, and anterior resection of the rectosigmoid. Since the incision is immediately over the pelvic inlet, complex dissection of phlegmons, fistulae, or locally advanced tumors can be performed though the incision. Transection of the rectum and mesorectum, one of the most difficult aspects of laparoscopic proctectomy, can be performed through this incision. Construction of the anastomosis can be performed under direct vision, and any anastomotic problems identified on leak testing can also be repaired directly. In addition, the Pfannenstiel incision is cosmetically appealing to many patients.

Some surgeons utilize a left lower quadrant incision for HALS sigmoid colectomy or anterior resection of the rectosigmoid. Although tolerated well by the patient, such a technique requires closure of the wound and recreation of pneumoperitoneum to perform colorectal anastomosis laparoscopically. Any anastomotic problems must also be addressed laparoscopically.

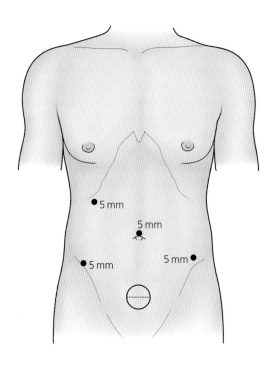

1.5.2 Hand-assisted laparoscopic surgery (HALS) anterior resection. Schematic of incisions.

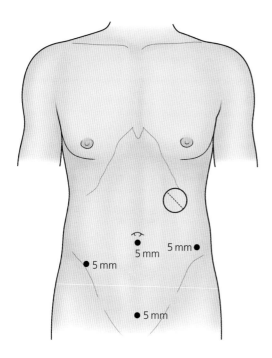

1.5.3 Hand-assisted laparoscopic surgery (HALS) incision for complex left upper quadrant pathology or subtotal colectomy.

There are clinical situations where a left lateral oblique incision (either in the left upper quadrant or left mid abdomen) may be optimal for HALS colectomy. These include patients with complex pathology of the descending colon or splenic flexure, where having the incision directly over the site of disease facilitates safe dissection, and patients requiring subtotal colectomy and ileal-descending colon anastomosis (**Figure 1.5.3**).

HALS total abdominal colectomy and proctocolectomy

HALS total abdominal colectomy or proctocolectomy are most easily performed using a Pfannenstiel or lower midline incision to place the HALS device (**Figure 1.5.4**). Pelvic dissection and anastomosis can be performed under direct vision in many cases.

POSTOPERATIVE CARE

Routine postoperative care is appropriate following HALS colectomy.

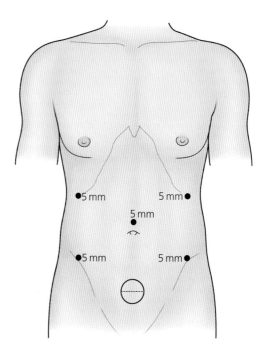

1.5.4 Hand-assisted laparoscopic surgery (HALS) total abdominal colectomy or restorative proctocolectomy incisions. Schematic of incisions.

OUTCOME

A number of well-designed trials have compared results of hand-assisted laparoscopic colectomy versus open colectomy or 'standard' or 'straight' laparoscopic colectomy. In summary, published studies demonstrate that short-term outcomes after hand-assisted laparoscopic colectomy are similar to those following straight laparoscopic colectomy, with similar incision size, similar reduction in duration of ileus when compared to open colectomy, with the advantage of reduced operative times and conversion rates in the hand-assisted groups.[2, 3, 4, 5, 6]

REFERENCES

1. Read TE, Salgado J, Ferraro D *et al.* 'Peek port': a novel approach for avoiding conversion in laparoscopic colectomy. *Surgical Endoscopy* 2009; **23**: 477–81.

2. Kang JC, Chung MH, Chao PC *et al.* Hand-assisted laparoscopic colectomy vs open colectomy: a prospective randomized study. *Surgical Endoscopy* 2004; **18**: 577–81.

3. Marcello PW, Fleshman JW, Milsom JW *et al.* Hand-assisted laparoscopic vs. laparoscopic colorectal surgery: a multicenter, prospective, randomized trial. *Diseases of the Colon and Rectum* 2008; **51**: 818–26; discussion 26–8.

4. Martel G, Boushey RP, Marcello PW. Hand-assisted laparoscopic colorectal surgery: an evidence-based review. *Minerva Chirurgica* 2008; **63**: 373–83.

5. Rivadeneira DE, Marcello PW, Roberts PL *et al.* Benefits of hand-assisted laparoscopic restorative proctocolectomy: a comparative study. *Diseases of the Colon and Rectum* 2004; **47**: 1371–6.

6. Targarona EM, Gracia E, Garriga J *et al.* Prospective randomized trial comparing conventional laparoscopic colectomy with hand-assisted laparoscopic colectomy: applicability, immediate clinical outcome, inflammatory response, and cost. *Surgical Endoscopy* 2002; **16**: 234–9.

Single incision laparoscopic-assisted colectomy

NICHOLAS A RIEGER

HISTORY AND INTRODUCTION

Single incision laparoscopic (SIL)-assisted colectomy is an innovative variant of minimally invasive surgery. The first documented colectomy performed via a single incision was reported in the medical literature in 2008.[1, 2] Standard laparoscopic-assisted surgery for resection of the colon involves multiple trocar sites and an incision to extract the bowel and assist with performing the anastomosis. For SILS, a single incision alone through the abdomen (usually the umbilicus) allows trocar placement, extraction of the mobilized bowel and an extracorporeal anastomosis.

NOMENCLATURE

SILS comes under many guises. This includes single port access (SPA) surgery, laparoendoscopic single site (LESS) surgery, single laparoscopic incision transabdominal (SLIT) surgery, embryonic natural orifice transluminal endoscopic surgery (NOTES), and transumbilical endoscopic surgery (TUES). No doubt there are many more acronyms presently or yet to be devised.

JUSTIFICATION AND ADVANTAGES

SILS has proposed benefits to patient outcomes. These include less postoperative pain, faster recovery and improved cosmesis over standard multiport laparoscopy. None of these factors are proven and there are no large cohorts of patients or comparative studies to justify these claims. There may be other factors to justify SILS. These include fewer port sites from which there may be bleeding, infection, neurapraxia, or development of a hernia. SILS may be considered by some authors as a stepping stone to NOTES. Experience of operating via a single port or site may give experience to operate via a natural orifice.

DISADVANTAGES

SILS has many disadvantages. The site of the wound is generally in the midline. There is a greater risk of subsequent incisional hernia with this wound compared to the laterally placed wounds that are often used in laparoscopic-assisted multiport procedures. During dissection, the procedure is hampered by the clash of instruments and the camera extracorporeally, the loss of triangulation of the tissues intracorporeally and operating with instruments in parallel compared to multiport laparoscopy. This is offset to some degree by specialized instruments that can be angulated (articulated) intracorporeally, an inline camera and the assistance of gravity with high degrees of tilt applied to the operating table. In addition, SILS may only enable the use of three ports, one for the camera and two for instrumentation. This gives one or two fewer ports compared to multiport laparoscopy, further reducing the ability to dissect tissue planes. There is also an increased cost for the procedure compared to multiport laparoscopy. This comes from the use of a specialized port and instruments that are used. The cost–benefit has yet to be justified.

INDICATIONS

All colorectal procedures including resection of the rectum and total colectomy have been reported. SILS is an advanced form of minimally advanced surgery and should not be attempted until a high level of competence has been achieved with standard multiport laparoscopy. It should only be performed in patients who are able to give adequate informed consent, are accepting that conversion to standard laparoscopy or open surgery may be required, and in ideal circumstances where the pathology is of an early stage, size, or site.

CONTRAINDICATIONS

SILS is a developing procedure. It is relatively contraindicated in the obese, patients with potential adhesions from prior surgery, and will be limited by the site, stage and site of pathology. Until more experience is obtained, difficult cases are better performed with multiport laparoscopy or open surgery.

PREOPERATIVE PREPARATION

For tumors of the colon or rectum, the site of the pathology should be accurately sited with careful colonoscopy and the use of a tattoo (carbon ink) to the site to make it easily visible with laparoscopy. Bowel preparation is at the discretion of the surgeon, but can often be avoided. A general anesthetic is required with careful patient positioning on the operating table. This includes arm placement at the side away from the site of surgery. The left arm is placed to the side for right colectomy and the opposite for left colectomy. The patient is appropriately fixed to the operating table to avoid movement of the torso or limbs during the procedure when tilt is applied to the operating table. As for all major colonic procedures, an indwelling urine catheter is placed, intravenous antibiotics are given and deep vein thrombosis (DVT) prophylaxis is used.

INSTRUMENTATION

1 **Operating table**. The operating table should be electric to allow easy tilt to be applied during the procedure.
2 **Ports**. The technology is evolving. SILS may be performed with insertion of standard laparoscopic ports through a single incision. The surgery, however, may be facilitated with devices fixed at the site of the incision to allow passage of laparoscopic instruments. These devices are the SILS™ port (Covidien, Dublin, Ireland), Endocone™ (Storz, Tuttlingen, Germany), X-Cone™ (Storz), Gelport System (Applied Medical, Rancho Santa Margarita, CA, USA), Quad and Triports (Advanced Surgical Concepts, Bray, Ireland; Olympus, Hamburg, Germany) and the Uni-X™ single-port access laparoscopic system (Pnavel Systems, Morganville, NJ, USA).
3 **Camera**. The best system is a long 5 mm camera, 30° with inline camera head and light lead. A camera with a flexible tip may also be used. This helps to prevent instrument clash extracorporeally.
4 **Articulated instruments**. These are 5 mm laparoscopic (graspers and scissors) instruments that once inside the abdomen may be angulated at their head to assist with triangulation of tissues and dissection (**Figure 1.6.1**).

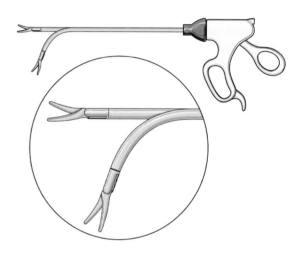

1.6.1 Angulated scissors to enable tissue dissection.

SURGICAL PROCEDURE

Port placement

The individual laparoscopic ports[3] (**Figure 1.6.2**a) or the single port device (**Figure 1.6.2**b) are placed via an open technique through the umbilicus (**Figure 1.6.3**). It is important that the heads of the ports are small and that they are inserted to different depths to avoid them clashing extracorporeally. The port device is replaced or used as a wound protector site and used for specimen extraction. The anastomosis is performed or assisted extracorporeally as for multiport laparoscopic surgery.

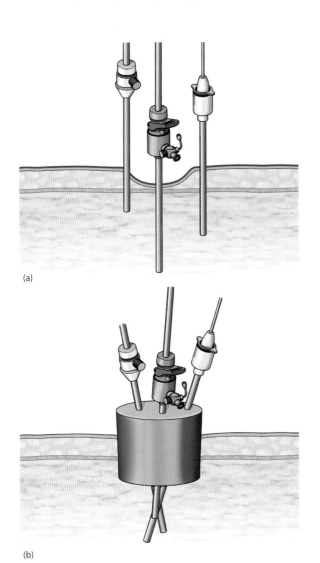

(a)

(b)

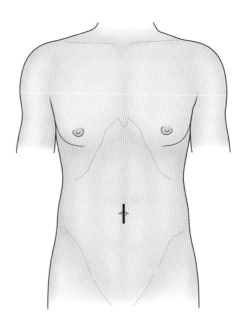

1.6.3 Incision at umbilicus 2.5–3 cm in length vertically.

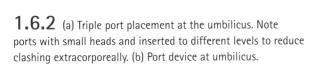

1.6.2 (a) Triple port placement at the umbilicus. Note ports with small heads and inserted to different levels to reduce clashing extracorporeally. (b) Port device at umbilicus.

Dissection and vessel ligation

The operation is assisted by positioning of the operating table to assist retraction of the bowel and adjacent structures. There is no alteration to the operating technique in regard to the tissue planes and mesenteric or vessel division compared to standard multiport laparoscopic surgery.

There are only three ports. One is for the camera, one is for the retracting grasper, and one is for the dissecting device. Five mm articulated scissors are used for the dissection. In combination with an articulated grasper, the instruments can be used without clash and not in parallel to triangulated and dissect tissues. This involves crossing the instruments intracorporeally with the right hand operating from the left intracorporeally and the left hand from the right. The grasping forceps need constant adjustment to expose the planes for dissection.

For a right colectomy, a lateral to medial approach has been used. Initially, the omentum will need to be dissected off the proximal transverse colon and hepatic flexure. The hepatic flexure is mobilized to view the first and second part of the duodenum (**Figure 1.6.4**). The cecum, ascending colon, and small bowel mesentery are mobilized to expose the second and third parts of the duodenum. Its attachments are divided and the cecum is lifted cranially and to the midline to expose the duodenum (**Figure 1.6.5**). After the bowel has been fully mobilized, the cecum can

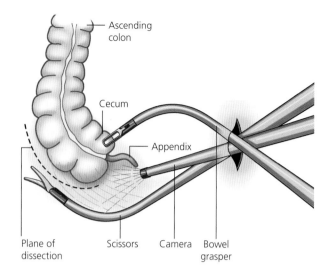

1.6.5 The cecum, ascending colon, and small bowel mesentery are mobilized to expose the second and third parts of the duodenum.

be grasped and put on tension toward the right iliac fossa. This places the ileocolic vessels on stretch. The mesenteric windows above and below the ileocolic vessels are opened to isolate the vessels (**Figure 1.6.6**). The duodenum will be visible through these windows.

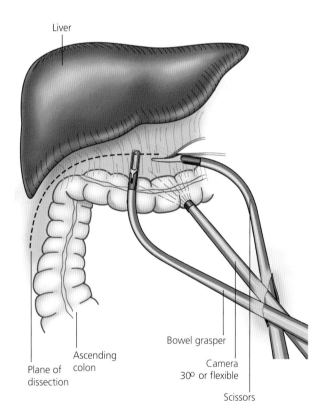

1.6.4 Drawing showing the plane of dissection for a right colectomy.

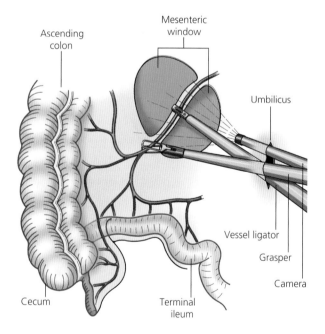

1.6.6 The mesenteric windows above and below the ileocolic vessels are opened to isolate the vessels.

The vessels can be divided with the surgeon's preferred device. This may include an energy source, such as a harmonic scalpel or a coagulation device. Alternatively, vascular staples or clips may be used. The instrument used for the vessel ligation will determine port size (5 or 11 mm) and consideration must be given to whether an instrument with a flexible tip needs to be used. When dividing the vessels, it is wise to leave a short stump of the pedicle. If there is bleeding from the pedicle, an endoloop can be used easily to achieve hemostasis.

Once the bowel has been fully mobilized and the vessels ligated, it can be delivered through the umbilical incision. The pathology is resected and an anastomosis performed (the surgeon's preferred method). Closure of the mesentery is not performed by the author for laparoscopic or open resections.

A left-sided resection is performed in the same manner. A lateral to medial approach has been adopted. The sigmoid and descending colons are mobilized and the splenic flexure taken down (**Figure 1.6.7**). The ureter and gonadal vessels are identified and protected. The bowel is then grasped and held laterally to expose the medial side of the mesentery. This is dissected to the root of the mesentery caudal to the inferior mesenteric artery. The ureter can be seen through the window created, and protected. The window above the artery is exposed and entered, to isolate the inferior mesenteric vascular pedicle. The pedicle can then safely be divided. The mesentery and bowel is divided below the level of the pathology. The proximal divided end of bowel can be delivered through the umbilicus, the pathology resected, and the anvil of a circular stapler inserted. This is then returned to the abdominal cavity, the wound closed and ports reinserted or the port device reinserted and the anastomosis is completed laparoscopically with a circular staple gun inserted through the anus.

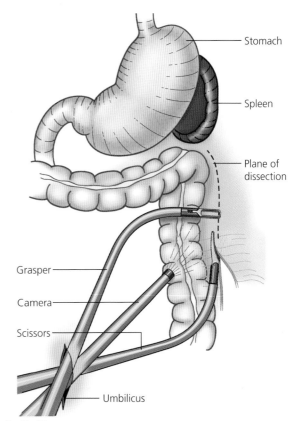

1.6.7 A left-sided resection is performed in the same manner.

theater (luminal bleeding from a stapled right colectomy anastomosis). The mean age was 62 years (range, 30–83 years), mean body mass index (BMI) was 25 (range, 21–33), mean node yield was 14 (range, 6–26), mean incision length was 4 cm (range, 2.5–10 cm), operating time was 87 minutes (range, 65–151 minutes), and mean length of stay was 5 days (range, 3–11 days).

POSTOPERATIVE CARE

Immediately postoperatively, the patient may take oral fluids and analgesia. Early mobilization, introduction of a full diet, removal of the urine catheter, and cessation of intravenous fluid should be strived for to allow for early discharge from hospital and return to normal activity.

OUTCOMES

Two publications relating to outcome are available in the literature,[3, 4] but each only describe seven cases. They demonstrate that SILS is feasible with good operative and patient outcomes. The author's experience is now of 13 cases, with one conversion (bleeding) and one return to

REFERENCES

1. Remzi FH, Kirat HT, Kaouk JH, Geisler DP. Single-port laparoscopy in colorectal surgery. *Colorectal Disease* 2008; **10**: 823–6.
2. Bucher P, Pugin F, Morel P. Single port access laparoscopic right hemicolectomy. *International Journal of Colorectal Disease* 2008; **23**: 1013–16.
3. Chambers W, Bicsak M, Lamparelli M, Dixon A. Single-incision laparoscopic surgery (SILS) in complex colorectal surgery: a technique offering potential and not just cosmesis. *Colorectal Disease* 2011; **13**: 393–8.
4. Rieger NA, Lam FF. Single-incision laparoscopically assisted colectomy using standard laparoscopic instrumentation. *Surgical Endoscopy* 2010; **24**: 888–90.

Access to the abdominal cavity: natural orifice transluminal endoscopic surgery

SEIGO KITANO AND KAZUHIRO YASUDA

HISTORY

Natural orifice transluminal endoscopic surgery (NOTES) is a new, evolving, minimally invasive surgical technique that aims to reduce the impact of surgical access by eliminating abdominal wounds together.[1, 2] In this innovative technique, the abdominal cavity is accessed with a flexible endoscope through a natural body orifice (e.g. the mouth, anus, or vagina) to perform diagnostic and therapeutic procedures. NOTES has potential benefits over conventional laparoscopic surgery that include less pain, quicker recovery, fewer wound complications, fewer adhesions, and better cosmesis. The concept of NOTES has been tested in animal models since 2004, and many experimental studies have shown the potential for application of this technique to various surgical procedures. Recently, human applications of NOTES have been introduced.

PRINCIPLES AND JUSTIFICATION

Clinical application of NOTES in the field of colorectal surgery is mainly for transgastric or transvaginal appendicectomy. However, current human NOTES experience is limited, and the general principles and justification for natural orifice access to the abdominal cavity have not been established. This chapter outlines our technique of transgastric and transvaginal access.

ANESTHESIA

As in standard laparoscopic surgery, general anesthesia is administered and a Foley urethral catheter is inserted. Preoperative single-dose antibiotic prophylaxis is performed to control gastric or vaginal contamination.

OPERATION

Transgastric access

Different techniques for transgastric access to the abdominal cavity, including small linear incision, balloon dilatation after needle-knife puncture, and submucosal tunnel technique, have been described, and a variety of closure techniques for gastric wall incision have also been reported, including endoscopic clips, endoloops, tissue-anchoring systems, and endoscopic suturing. The authors and other investigators have shown that use of a submucosal tunnel with mucosal closure using endoclips is effective for safe transgastric peritoneal access and reliable closure.[3, 4, 5, 6]

The patient is placed in the left lateral decubitus position.

The surgical field, including the oral cavity, is prepared with chlorhexidine gluconate solution and covered with sterile drapes. A clean, disinfected endoscope (XQ 240; Olympus Medical Systems, Tokyo, Japan) with a transparent hood (disposable distal attachment, D-201-10704; Olympus) is inserted perorally into the stomach. To prevent bowel dilatation, carbon dioxide (CO_2) insufflation with an endoscopic CO_2 regulation unit (UCR; Olympus) is used during the procedure instead of air.

A longitudinal narrow submucosal tunnel is created using the endoscopic mucosal resection (ESD) technique. The site for creating the submucosal tunnel is identified on the anterior wall of the stomach by using endoscopy to locate the imprint of the operator's finger pressing on the abdominal wall.

First, normal saline solution is injected into the submucosal layer to create a submucosal cushion for safe cutting (**Figure 1.7.1**).

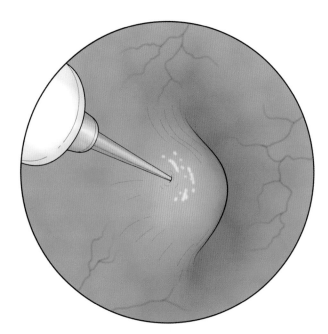

1.7.1

After making a small incision of the mucosa with a Flex knife (KD-630L; Olympus) (**Figure 1.7.2**), the mucosal incision is extended to a length of 2 cm with an insulation-tipped (IT) knife (KD-610L; Olympus) (**Figure 1.7.3**).

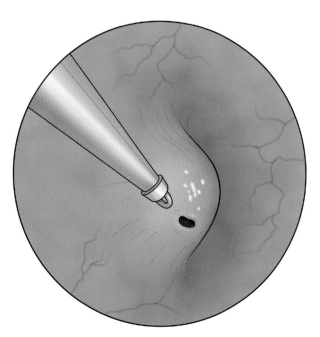

1.7.2

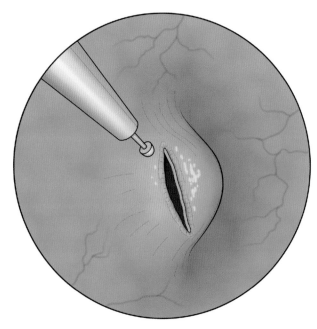

1.7.3

Dissection of the submucosal layer is then performed with the IT knife (**Figure 1.7.4**) to make a 5 cm-long submucosal tunnel (**Figure 1.7.5**).

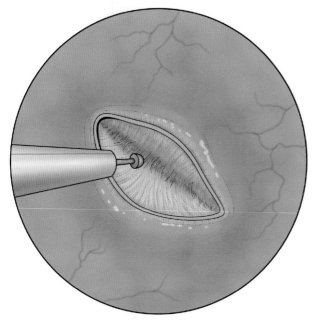

1.7.4

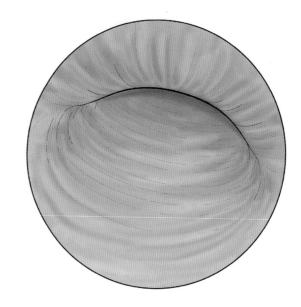

1.7.5

A small incision is made in the seromuscular layer at the end of the submucosal tunnel, and then the opening is enlarged with a 15 mm diameter endoscopic dilation balloon (CRE 5842; Boston Scientific, Natick, MA, USA) (**Figures 1.7.6** and **1.7.7**).

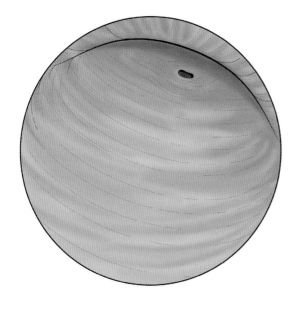

1.7.6

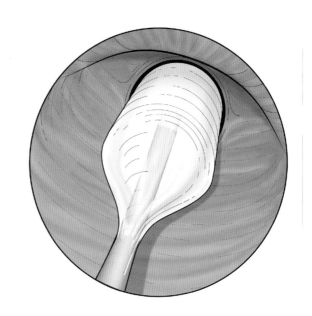

1.7.7

The endoscope is then introduced into the abdominal cavity to perform diagnostic or therapeutic procedures. A pneumoperitoneum is made with an endoscopic CO_2 insufflator (**Figures 1.7.8** and **1.7.9**).

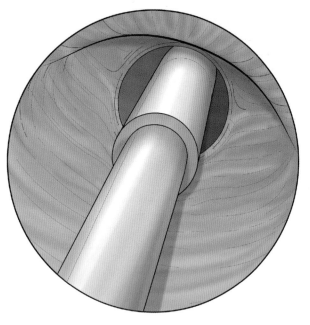

1.7.8

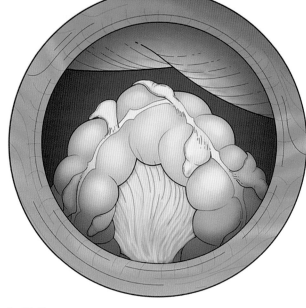

1.7.9

After completing the procedure in the peritoneal cavity, the endoscope is withdrawn back into the stomach, and the mucosal incision site is closed with endoclips (**Figure 1.7.10**).

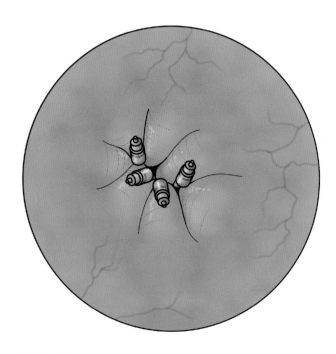

1.7.10

Transvaginal access

The patient is placed in the lithotomy position. The surgical fields, including the anterior abdomen, perineum, and vaginal area are disinfected with povidone iodine and covered with sterile drapes. To prevent injury to the adjacent organs during transvaginal access, hydrotubation and transvaginal ultrasonography are used. A Foley catheter is inserted into the endocervical canal, and normal saline solution is injected. After confirmation of pooling of the normal saline solution in the Douglas pouch, a posterior colpotomy is performed under direct view by use of a vaginal speculum and a grasper to retract the uterus. The ideal diameter of the incision is 2.5 cm. A sterile endoscope (XQ 240; Olympus) with a transparent overtube is carefully inserted into the abdominal cavity through the vaginal incision site under endoscopic observation. The transparent overtube is used for sclerosing any esophageal varices. Intra-abdominal insufflation with CO_2 is achieved with an endoscopic CO_2 regulation unit (UCR; Olympus). After completion of the intra-abdominal procedure, the pneumoperitoneum is aspirated just before removal of the endoscope, and the vaginal wound is closed with interrupted sutures under direct vision.

In the hybrid NOTES technique, a pneumoperitoneum is created first with a 5 mm trocar placed in the umbilicus. Then, transgastric or transvaginal access is performed under laparoscopic view.

Transcolonic access

Transcolonic access appears to have several theoretical advantages over the transgastric approach. It can provide improved endoscope reach and enhanced visualization of the upper abdominal organs by eliminating the need for scope retroflection. The large distensible capacity of the anal orifice may allow passage of larger devices and retrieval of larger specimens. However, most human NOTES procedures have been performed via transgastric and transvaginal approaches to gain abdominal access because of the potential disadvantages of the transcolonic approach, including heavy bacterial load and issues of sterility, and the risk of adjacent organ injury or colonic wall shearing during the procedure. With additional refinements in colonic sterilization and management of the colonic incision site, transcolonic access may be a useful approach for the performance of NOTES procedures.

REFERENCES

1. Rattner D, Kalloo A. ASGE/SAGES Working Group on Natural Orifice Translumenal Endoscopic Surgery, October 2005. *Surgical Endoscopy* 2006; **20**: 329–33.
2. Kitano S, Tajiri H, Yasuda K *et al.* Current status and activity regarding natural orifice translumenal endoscopic surgery (NOTES) in Japan. *Asian Journal of Endoscopic Surgery* 2008; **1**: 7–10.
3. Kitano S, Yasuda K, Shibata K *et al.* Natural orifice translumenal endoscopic surgery for preoperative staging in a pancreatic cancer patient. *Digestive Endoscopy* 2008; **20**: 198–202.
4. Yoshizumi F, Yasuda K, Kawaguchi K *et al.* Submucosal tunneling using endoscopic submucosal dissection for peritoneal access and closure in natural orifice transluminal endoscopic surgery: a porcine survival study. *Endoscopy* 2009; **41**: 707–11.
5. Yasuda K, Kitano S. Lymph node navigation for pancreatic and biliary malignancy by NOTES. *Journal of Hepatobiliary Pancreatic Surgery* 2010; **17**: 617–21.
6. von Delius S, Gillen S, Doundoulakis E *et al.* Comparison of transgastric access techniques for natural orifice transluminal endoscopic surgery. *Gastrointestinal Endoscopy* 2008; **68**: 940–7.

Anastomotic technique – suture

BRUCE G WOLFF AND HEIDI K CHUA

HISTORY

The earliest records of bowel anastomosis date back to ancient Egypt where the oldest suture was found in a mummy's abdomen. Materials used in ancient Egypt included plant fibers, hair, tendon, or wool threads. Since then, significant advances have been made in the types of suture material, allowing surgeons several options for different situations. The addition of stapling devices has provided surgeons with yet another dimension to creating bowel anastomosis, but familiarity with suturing techniques is still required for students learning the art of surgery. The literature shows that there are no statistically significant differences between stapling and hand-sewn anastomoses, except that stapling has had more stricturing and is more expensive.

PATIENT CHARACTERISTICS

Equally important to the selection of suture material and techniques are patient characteristics. Certain medical conditions inhibit wound healing, including smoking, diabetes mellitus, corticosteroids or immunosuppression, malnutrition, and obesity. Optimizing patients for colorectal surgery may involve such things as smoking cessation, strict control of glucose, or institution of parenteral nutrition prior to planning the operation. In some cases, the use of stomas may be necessary if the risk of creating the anastomosis is prohibitive.

FACTORS INFLUENCING ANASTOMOTIC HEALING

The bowel anastomosis heals in phases. The acute inflammatory response occurs in the first few days. The anastomosis has no intrinsic strength at this phase until phase 2, where fibroblasts are incorporated. This is the time for collagen production. The final phase shows collagen maturation to increase the strength of the anastomosis. Failure of any component in these three phases would lead to an anastomotic breakdown.

The purpose of the sutures is to allow for good tissue apposition until collagen is laid down at phase 2. This requires minimal tissue trauma with good blood supply to the tissues involved in creating the anastomosis. Visual inspection of the tissues noting its color and presence of bleeding, palpation of the arterial pulse, Doppler examination, and fluorescein injection are ways to evaluate adequacy of the blood supply to the edges of the bowel. An anastomosis should not be performed when the adequacy of the blood supply is uncertain. A tension-free anastomosis is likewise important. Adequate dissection to ensure adequate length for a tension-free anastomosis is paramount, even if it requires extending the incision or conversion of a laparoscopic case to an open procedure. Meticulous attention to the creation of the anastomosis will minimize the potential of an anastomotic leak.

Anastomotic leaks

An anastomotic leak is one of the most dreaded complications in colorectal surgery. The surgeon should be aware of potential factors that increase the risk of an anastomotic leak. These include both patient factors, such as poor nutritional status, high-dose corticosteroid use, and a history of radiation therapy, and the location of the anastomosis (intra-abdominal versus below the peritoneal reflection). In addition, there are specific operative concerns. The presence of an obstruction distal to the newly created anastomosis, whether it is benign or malignant, will prevent proper healing of the anastomosis. Creation of the anastomosis in the setting of sepsis is also a factor. Severe bleeding with hypotension may result in mesenteric ischemia, altering the blood supply to the bowel edges. Improper techniques in suturing and undue tension on the newly created anastomosis can also compromise the anastomosis.

SUTURING TECHNIQUES

There are currently two techniques used in suturing bowel anastomosis: the single and the two-layered anastomosis. Each technique has its proponents. Various absorbable and non-absorbable sutures are available, but most surgeons use a non-absorbable suture for the single layer anastomosis, while the two-layered anastomosis is created with an absorbable inner layer and non-absorbable outer layer.

Single-layered anastomosis

The single-layered anastomosis is created usually with interrupted non-absorbable sutures. There are several techniques described for single-layered anastomosis: seromuscular stitch (**Figure 1.8.1**a), full thickness vertical stitch (**Figure 1.8.1**b), or horizontal mattress suture (**Figure 1.8.1**c). Since the sutures are placed in an interrupted fashion, proponents of this technique believe there is less risk of interfering with the blood supply. Proponents also feel that interrupted sutures are less likely than continuous ones to compromise the anastomotic lumen.

Two-layered anastomosis

The two-layered anastomosis consists of a seromuscular bite of the bowel wall, incorporating all but the mucosa. This is usually considered the strength layer of the anastomosis and provides apposition of the bowel wall. The inner layer is through the mucosa and submucosa and inverts the mucosa. Some consider this layer the

hemostatic layer. Others question whether the inner layer strangulates the mucosa, leading to bowel ischemia and leaks. However, data from randomized trials do not show a difference in anastomotic leak rates between these two techniques.[1] One needs to avoid excessive tension and advancing the suture too much as this can cause a 'purse-string' effect, drawing the suture line up and reducing the lumen diameter.

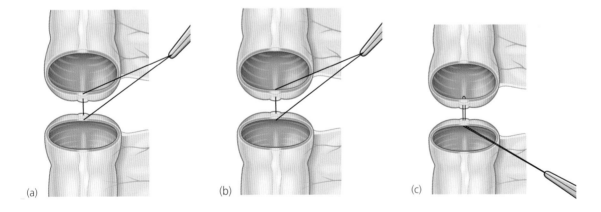

(a)   (b)   (c)

1.8.1

ANASTOMOTIC CONFIGURATIONS

The bowel anastomosis may be created end to end, end to side, side to end, or side to side. Special circumstances include closure of a loop stoma or creation of the ileoanal J pouch or the coloanal anastomosis.

End to end

This anastomosis is applicable anywhere in the gastrointestinal (GI) tract. For the colorectal surgeon, this can be used in the small or large intestine, but a low rectal anastomosis can be challenging. The two-layered anastomosis starts with the divided ends of the bowel held side by side by non-crushing clamps. The clamps are applied lightly to occlude the lumen and not the mesentery. The two ends of the bowel are lined mesentery to mesentery. The anastomosis is begun by placing posterior seromuscular sutures with interrupted silk sutures spaced 3–4 mm apart (**Figure 1.8.2**a). Stay sutures are placed on the mesenteric and antimesenteric side of the bowel. They can be tied at the start or tagged with clamps. The sutures are either tagged individually with clamps or tied sequentially as they are being placed. Sutures that were tagged individually are tied once all the sutures are placed

for the posterior wall. The sutures are then cut with the exception of the two stay sutures on each end of the bowel. The authors use the stay sutures to align the two sections of bowel for ease of doing the anastomosis.

The inner layer is created with a running layer of polyglycolic acid suture and starts at the corner closest to the surgeon (**Figure 1.8.2**b,c). The first stitch runs full thickness on one side of the bowel, runs across through the mucosa of the posterior layer and exits full thickness on the other side of the anastomosis. The knot is tied on the serosal side and the short end of the suture is tagged with a clamp. The suture is then inserted full thickness again to end up on the inside of the bowel. A continuous over-and-over suture technique with mucosa and submucosa is applied to the posterior wall, suturing away from the surgeon, until the opposite side is reached. The stitch is continued over-and-over as the suture transitions to the anterior wall, once again taking only the mucosal layer. A Connell stitch may be used to transition the stitch for ease of the over-and-over technique. Care should be taken to invaginate the mucosa. Tying the suture to the short end tagged with the clamp completes the anterior wall. At this time, the non-crushing clamps can be removed to minimize trauma to the bowel tissue and to minimize ischemia time. The final layer of the anastomosis is placement of the interrupted silk sutures for the outer layer (**Figure 1.8.2**d).

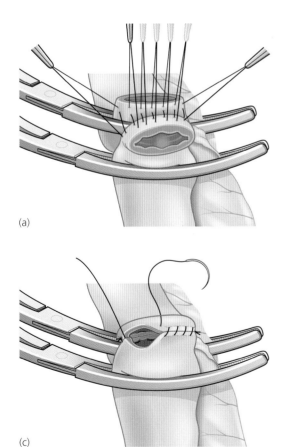

(a)

(c)

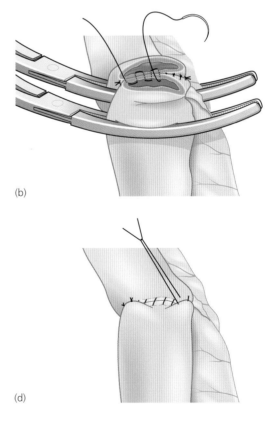

(b)

(d)

1.8.2

As with the posterior outer layer, the sutures are inserted seromuscularly in the manner used on the posterior wall. In the setting of a small bowel anastomosis, when lumen size is narrow, care should be taken not to occlude the lumen. If lumenal size is compromised, an alternate anastomotic configuration should be considered (side to side or end to side). All the sutures can be cut at this time including the two stay sutures. Closure of the mesenteric defect is sometimes done at this time. The entire anastomosis is carefully inspected to assure adequate blood supply, lack of tension, and proper bowel alignment.

Other surgeons prefer placement of the inner layer first (**Figure 1.8.3**a,b). Once completed, the outer layer of sutures is placed. This method requires rotating the anastomosis (**Figure 1.8.3**c) for placement of the posterior layer, which can be problematic for lower colon to rectal anastomoses.

In the single-layered technique, the stay sutures are placed on the mesenteric and antimesenteric borders and they can be tied at the start or tagged with clamps (**Figure 1.8.4**). The posterior row of sutures is placed first at regular intervals (5 mm). The second author prefers the full thickness vertical stitch with silk (**Figure 1.8.4**). The

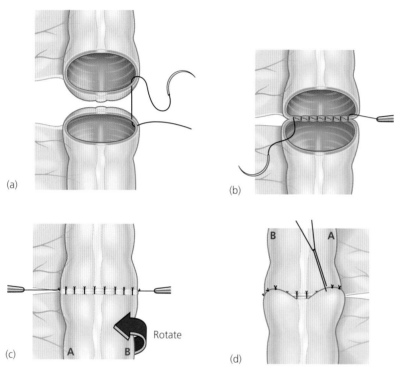

(a)

(b)

(c) Rotate A B

(d)

1.8.3

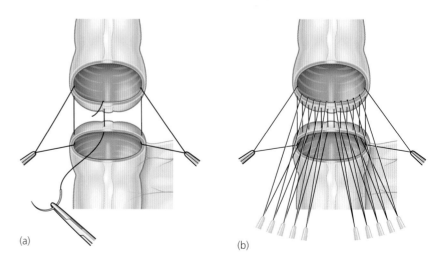

1.8.4 (a) (b)

sutures are tagged with clamps and tied on the mucosal side after the entire row of sutures has been placed. Once the sutures are tied, the anterior row of sutures is placed in the same fashion, taking care to invert the mucosa. For the anterior row, the knots are tied on the outside. This technique comes in handy for low colorectal anastomosis where use of the two-layered technique may be especially difficult. The availability of stapling devices has limited the use of hand-sewn low colorectal anastomosis, but the colorectal surgeon needs to know the option and the technique of creating this challenging anastomosis.

Another option for the single-layered suturing for the low colorectal anastomosis is the placement of three sutures through the full thickness of the bowel wall (**Figure 1.8.5a**). The first two sutures are the mesenteric and antimesenteric sutures and the third is placed in the middle of the posterior row. This middle stitch allows for traction and exposure of the posterior row. The posterior row of sutures should once again be placed through the full thickness of the bowel wall at close intervals (**Figure 1.8.5b**). Once all the posterior sutures are placed, they are tied with the knots on the mucosal side. The same technique of placing a stitch mid-point on the anterior wall will also facilitate placement of the anterior row of sutures (**Figure 1.8.5c–e**). This also ensures that the posterior wall is not incorporated into the anterior wall, closing off the lumen. Care should be taken to completely invert the mucosa.

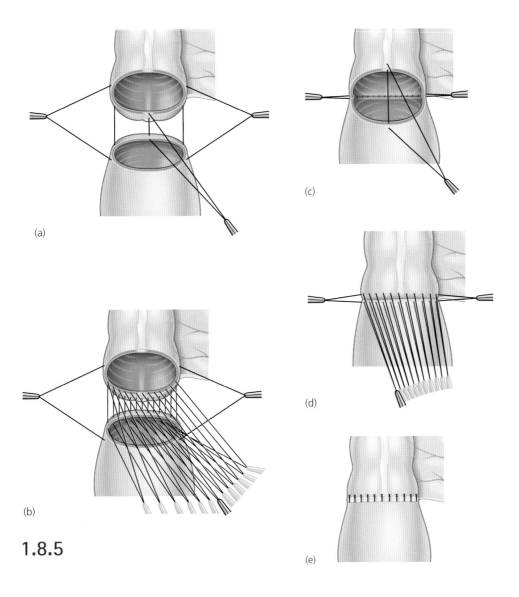

(a)

(b)

1.8.5

(c)

(d)

(e)

The first author prefers a single layer running anastomosis with polydioxanone sutures (PDS). This can also be the inner layer of a two-layered anastomosis. **Figure 1.8.6** illustrates the single-layer anastomosis. The two ends of the bowel are lined up as described above with non-crushing clamps. The bowel ends are oriented in a vertical fashion to facilitate suturing towards the surgeon. The anastomosis is started at the far end with the suture starting on the outside of the bowel wall. The first stitch goes full thickness on one side of the bowel, goes across through the full thickness of the two posterior layers and exits full thickness on the other side of the anastomosis. The knot is tied on the serosal side and the short end of the suture is tagged with a clamp. The suture is then inserted full thickness again to end up on the inside of the bowel (**Figure 1.8.6**a). A continuous over-and-over full thickness suturing technique is applied to the posterior wall, suturing towards the surgeon. Once the suture reaches the near corner, the stitch is placed through the wall of the bowel to end up on the serosal side. The entire anastomosis is rotated 90° clockwise to lie horizontally. The surgeon can then continue the full thickness over-and-over stitch closing the anterior layer of the anastomosis (**Figure 1.8.6**b). Tying the suture to the short end tagged with the clamp completes the anterior wall. This technique allows for a single-layer closure without the need for the Connell transition stitch. Care should be taken not to purse string the anastomosis, which could compromise the lumen diameter.

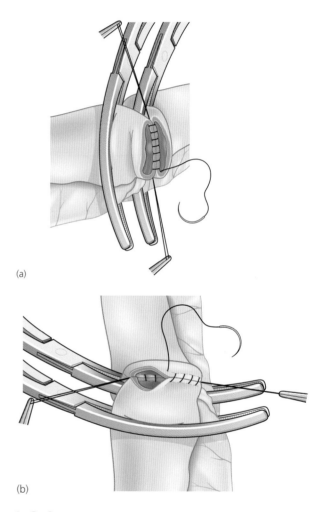

(a)

(b)

1.8.6

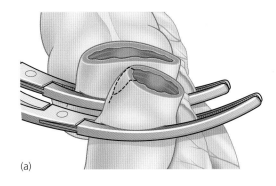

(a)

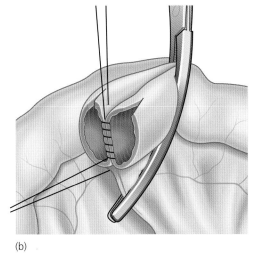

(b)

1.8.7

SIZE DISCREPANCY

In the setting of size discrepancy between the two limbs of bowel, as in the setting of the smaller small bowel to the larger caliber colon, an incision known as the Cheatle slit can be placed along the antimesenteric border of the smaller limb. In some cases, the 'triangle' in **Figure 1.8.7** is excised. The surgeon's preferred anastomosis can then be performed. Another option to address size discrepancy is to create an end-to-side anastomosis.

End to side or side to end

The authors prefer this method to perform an ileorectal anastomosis with the side of the small bowel and the top end of the rectum.

This technique requires that one end of the two limbs has to be closed. A one- or two-layer closure can be used, or the end can be stapled. A non-crushing clamp is used to occlude the lumen and not compromise the blood supply. For the two-layer closure, the first layer is the inner layer of running absorbable suture. The first stitch involves only the mucosal layer, starting at the corner furthest away from the surgeon. An over-and-over suturing technique is used (**Figure 1.8.8**a). Once the other end is reached, the knot is tied on the outside. The outer layer of interrupted absorbable or non-absorbable seromuscular sutures are then placed (**Figure 1.8.8**b). If the single layer closure is used, the same principles of full-thickness stitches and close intervals as described for single layer anastomosis are used.

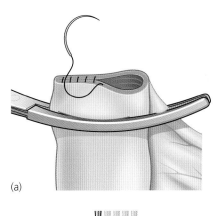

(a)

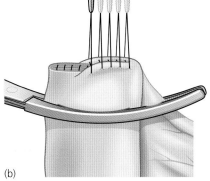

(b)

1.8.8

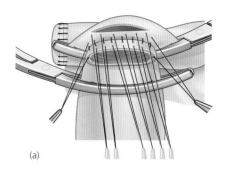

(a)

With the one end closed, the two sections of bowel are ready for the anastomosis. The two-layered anastomosis will be described first. As with the end-to-end anastomosis, a non-crushing clamp is placed on the rectum. The second clamp is placed on the antimesenteric border of the small bowel near the closed end. The author prefers the Foss bowel clamp for this maneuver. The enterotomy is then made to fit the length of the open rectal lumen. Now, both lumens are ready for the anastomosis as described above and illustrated in **Figure 1.8.2**a–d. Other surgeons place the outer posterior layer of non-absorbable sutures prior to making the enterotomy to minimize size discrepancies (**Figure 1.8.9**a–c). There is usually no need to close the mesentery between the two limbs of intestine, but if there is concern about the potential of internal hernia, the mesentery for both limbs can be closed with polyglycolic acid suture.

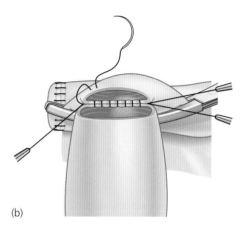

(b)

With the single-layer anastomosis, the enterotomy is created on the side of the small bowel to fit the end of the rectum. Full-thickness interrupted stitches are placed in close intervals with absorbable or non-absorbable sutures starting from the corner furthest away from the surgeon. The sutures can be tagged and tied once all the sutures for the posterior wall are placed. The anterior row of sutures is placed in the same fashion, taking care to not incorporate the posterior wall into the sutures. As with any anastomosis, careful inspection of the entire anastomosis with attention to blood supply, tension, and alignment should also be done.

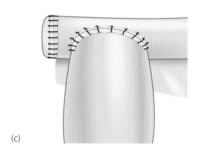

(c)

1.8.9

Side to side

The side-to-side anastomosis is more commonly used in the setting of intestinal bypass where no resection has been done. The technique of the two-layered closure works well in this setting. The anastomosis starts with identifying the two sections of intestine suitable for the anastomosis. This usually means one is proximal and the other distal to the obstructing lesion. The authors once again favor the non-crushing Foss clamps. They are placed on the antimesenteric border of the two limbs of bowel and are away from the mesentery. The anastomosis can be started either by creating the enterotomies/colostomies first to the desired length, or by placing the outer layer of non-absorbable sutures prior to incising the bowel wall (**Figure 1.8.10**).

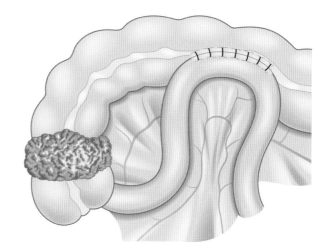

1.8.10

CONCLUSION

Techniques for creating bowel anastomosis have been handed down generation to generation and will continue to be part of each surgical resident's training. The introduction of surgical stapling devices has allowed colorectal surgeons to create easy and safe intra-abdominal anastomoses and has made low pelvic anastomoses a matter of routine. However, there remain many instances where sutured anastomoses are easier than or preferable to stapled ones, and they are frequently necessary to salvage an anastomosis after a stapler mishap. For these reasons, it is incumbent upon all colorectal surgeons to develop and maintain their skills with sutured anastomosis.

REFERENCES

1. Shikata S, Yamagishi H, Taji Y. Single- versus two-layer intestinal anastomosis: a meta-analysis of randomized controlled trials. *BMC Surgery* 2006; **6**: 2.

2. Gouvas N, Tan E, Windsor A *et al*. Fast-track vs standard care in colorectal surgery: a meta-analysis update. *International Journal of Colorectal Disease* 2009; **24**: 1119–31.

FURTHER READING

Brandstrup B, Tonnesen H, Beier-Holgersen R *et al*. Effects of intravenous fluid restriction on postoperative complications: comparison of two perioperative fluid regimens. *Annals of Surgery* 2003; **238**: 641–8.

Guenaga KKFG, Matos D, Wille-Jorgensen P. Mechanical bowel preparation for elective colorectal surgery. *Cochrane Database of Systematic Reviews* 2009; **(3)**: CD001544.

Lobo DN, Bostock KA, Neal KR *et al*. Effect of salt and water balance on recovery of gastrointestinal function after elective colonic resection: a randomized controlled trial. *Lancet* 2002; **359**: 1812–18.

Van't Sant HP, Weidema WF, Hop WCJ *et al*. The influence of mechanical bowel preparation in elective lower colorectal surgery. *Annals of Surgery* 2010; **251**: 59–63.

Anastomotic technique – stapled

PETAR VUKASIN AND ROBERT W BEART

HISTORY

Surgeons continue to be interested in identifying the best way to create an intestinal anastomosis. In 1893, Nicholas pointed out that '… the ideal method of uniting intestinal wounds is yet to be devised'. Through the years, surgeons have devised numerous types of suture material – absorbable, non-absorbable, synthetic, non-synthetic, braided and monofilament – to create intestinal anastomoses. Mechanical stapling devices might be traced to the early work of Denans in Marseilles, whose work preceded the more famous Murphy Button by 66 years. In 1826, he invaginated intestinal ends over two silver rings, and then approximated the bowel with a special pair of forceps. Inversion was accomplished and the entire circumferences of the serosal surfaces were opposed. Stapling devices were developed to overcome inadequacies with traditional suturing methods. Hulti produced a stapling instrument in 1911. It was cumbersome, weighed over 4.5 kg and took hours to assemble. Petz designed an instrument, similar to Payr's crushing clamp, which placed a row of staples along both edges close to the stomach during gastrectomy. Between 1945 and 1950, a group of Russian engineers in Moscow, including Gudov and Androsov, developed methods to staple blood vessels together, prompted by the difficulties with traditional suture techniques experienced during the Second World War. Their developments continued up until the 1970s and included many gastrointestinal stapling instruments.[1]

Since that time, Ravitch and Steiechen should be given the greatest credit for the proliferation of stapling instruments.[2] They initiated numerous publications outlining surgical techniques for the use of staplers to perform pneumonectomy, lobectomy, gastrectomy, end-to-end bowel anastomosis and transaction of multiple vessels. These instruments have now become commonplace and the majority of intestinal anastomoses in the United States are created with these devices. More recently, similar devices have been placed on long handles for use in laparoscopic surgery. The principles, however, remain the same and their use is very similar. Specific changes include articulation of some of the gastrointestinal (GI) staplers and the varying lengths. The technique descriptions in this chapter will generally apply to both sets of instruments. It is appropriate to review the advantages of these instruments, as well as the potential disadvantages, that have been identified since the early 1970s.

When performing colonic surgery with staplers, there are four fundamental techniques which should be mastered: (1) functional end-to-end anastomosis, (2) end-to-side anastomosis, (3) end-to-end anastomosis, and (4) double/triple stapling methods.

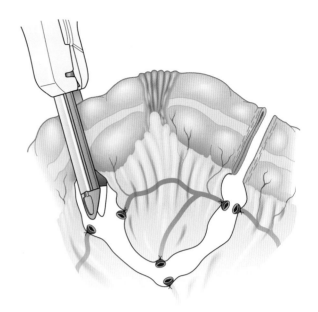

(a)

FUNCTIONAL END-TO-END ANASTOMOSIS

Step 1

In the functional end-to-end method, the bowel is mobilized completely, making sure that all tension has been relieved. The mesentery is dissected to the point where the bowel is to be transected. This can be achieved with a linear stapler which cuts as it divides and seals both ends of the bowel (**Figure 1.9.1**a).

Alternatively, a clamp can be placed on the section to be removed and a stapling device placed across the end to be preserved (**Figure 1.9.1**b).

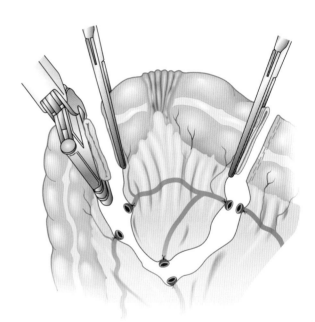

(b)

1.9.1

Step 2

The ends of the small bowel are secured and small enterotomies are made by excising the antimesenteric corners of the staple lines. Orientation of the bowel is important to make sure it is not twisted. Through these enterotomies, the two limbs of the stapler are placed and fired. The length of the anastomosis should not be less than the diameter of the bowel to provide an adequate lumen (**Figure 1.9.2**).

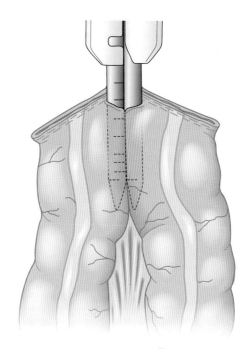

1.9.2

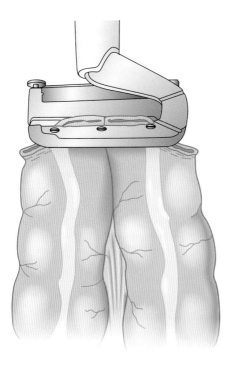

Step 3

This leaves a defect at the site where the limbs of the stapler were inserted, which can be closed with either a mechanical stapler or a traditional hand-sewn technique. The longitudinal staple lines should be offset before the enterotomy site is closed so they do not overlie each other when the anastomosis is complete. This creates a functional end-to-end anastomosis, which has been shown to heal well and function as well as an end-to-end anastomosis (**Figure 1.9.3**).[3]

1.9.3

END-TO-SIDE ANASTOMOSIS

Step 1

An end-to-side anastomosis can be created as an alternative to the functional end-to-end anastomosis. The bowel is similarly mobilized and divided, but the ends of the remaining bowel are not closed with staplers. After sizing the proximal bowel, the appropriate circular stapler anvil is placed into the end of the bowel and the purse-string tied around the shaft of the anvil (**Figure 1.9.4**).

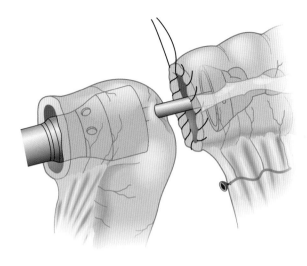

1.9.4

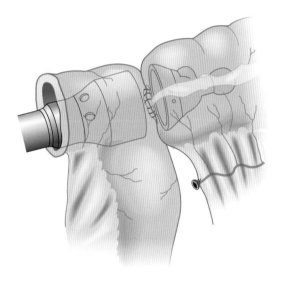

1.9.5

Step 2

The circular staple device[4] is placed through the end of the proximal bowel and the stapler shaft is then extended through its antimesenteric side approximately 5 cm from its cut end (**Figure 1.9.5**).

Step 3

The stapler is reassembled, fired and withdrawn. The end of the proximal bowel is then closed with a linear stapler (**Figure 1.9.6**).

These two anastomotic techniques are used in similar situations. However, the end-to-side anastomosis has a short but real 'blind end', which theoretically may, at a future time, cause problems by the formation of a pulsion diverticulum. In both cases, the mesenteric defect can be closed or not according to the surgeon's preference. Neither anastomotic technique has been shown to be more secure or more rapid than traditional hand-sewn techniques. Therefore, it becomes a matter of personal preference as to which technique a surgeon chooses to use.[5]

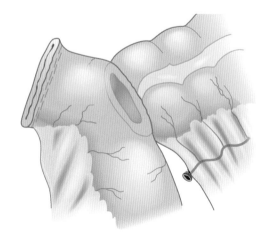

1.9.6

END-TO-END ANASTOMOSIS

The end-to-end anastomosis is most commonly created with the circular stapler. Typically, such an anastomosis will be created in the pelvis where the descending or sigmoid colon is being anastomosed to the rectum. With this technique, the patient must be placed in a modified lithotomy position so that access to the anus is available. The bowel is mobilized and the mesentery ligated and resected to the point where the bowel is to be divided. A clamp is placed across the distal bowel at its margin of transaction, and the distal rectum is irrigated with water or a cytotoxic agent to minimize the presence of any viable cancer cells.

Step 1

A non-crushing bowel clamp can then be placed across the distal bowel, the bowel can be transected and a purse-string suture placed around the open rectum. Proximally, the bowel is transected and a purse-string suture needs to be placed, which can be done with a purse-string clamp. Automatic purse-string devices can be used both proximally and distally, but are quite expensive and probably offer minimal advantage (**Figure 1.9.7**).

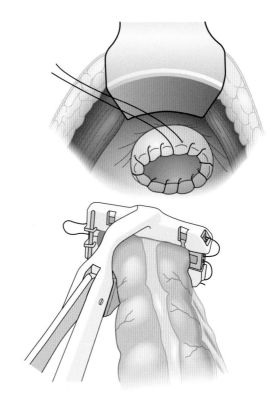

1.9.7

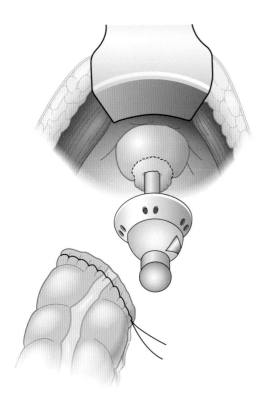

1.9.8

Step 2

Once the purse-strings are placed, the circular stapler is inserted through the anus and advanced through the rectum. As it approaches the rectal purse-string, the assistant opens the stapling device, passing the anvil through the distal purse-string suture. The purse-string is then tied snugly around the shaft and the instrument is opened completely. The anvil can then be completely removed from the stapler to facilitate its insertion into the proximal bowel (**Figure 1.9.8**).

Step 3

The proximal bowel is then placed over the anvil. Placing the bowel over the anvil can be difficult and, before doing this, the edge of the proximal bowel should be grasped with three narrow Allis clamps, one-third of the circumference apart. The bowel can be dilated with ring forceps and glucagon can be given to relax the bowel. The Allis forceps are then used to place the lumen over the posterior aspect of the anvil and, using blunt-tipped forceps, the anterior lip of the bowel is brought over the anvil anteriorly. The proximal purse-string can then be tightened around the shaft of the anvil (**Figure 1.9.9**).

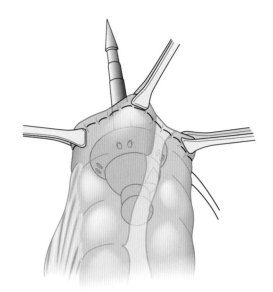

1.9.9

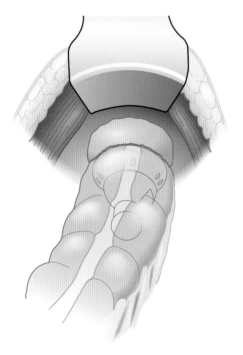

1.9.10

Step 4

Under direct vision and making sure the bowel is not rotated, the anvil is reattached to the stapler's center rod. The stapler can then be tightened and fired. The stapler is then opened two complete times and, using a rotating motion, is withdrawn from the anus. The operating surgeon, working the abdomen, should make an effort to place traction on the rectum to ease the stapler across the anastomosis, because the anastomosis is smaller than the cartridge and removal of the stapler can be somewhat difficult (**Figure 1.9.10**).

At this point, the surgeon must ensure that the anastomosis is not under tension. This is done by making sure that the bowel is lying in the hollow of the sacrum. If there is any 'bow-stringing' across the hollow of the sacrum, the left colon and splenic flexure must be mobilized to remove any evidence of tension. The stapler rings should be inspected. They should be removed from the stapler carefully, maintaining their orientation, and the purse-string sutures should be cut so the rings can be opened fully. Unless the purse-string sutures are cut, small defects in the rings can be hidden. If a defect in the ring is identified, its location in the circumference of the bowel should be noted; this is made possible by having preserved its orientation. The rectum should also be insufflated with air via a proctoscope through the anus to identify any air leaks. If a leak is identified and it can be repaired with sutures, diversion may be unnecessary. If a leak cannot be identified or completely repaired, or if there is any question about the integrity of the anastomosis, a diverting stoma is appropriate.

DOUBLE/TRIPLE STAPLING TECHNIQUES

Step 1

A double or triple staple technique is used in a similar situation to an end-to-end anastomosis. With these techniques, the bowel is similarly mobilized and the mesentery ligated and divided. The distal bowel is transected with a linear stapler. Angulating linear staplers or curved cutting staplers may help transection of the low rectum (**Figure 1.9.11**).[6, 7]

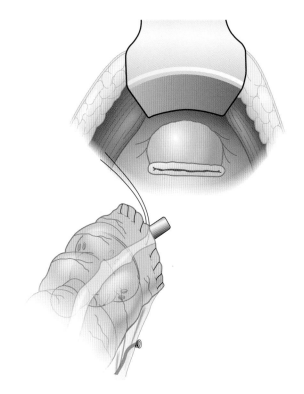

1.9.11

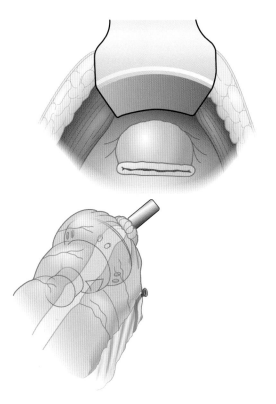

Step 2

In the double stapling method, a purse-string suture is placed in the proximal bowel after its division between clamps, and the detachable anvil inserted proximally with the purse-string suture being tied snugly onto the shaft of the anvil (**Figure 1.9.12**).

1.9.12

Step 3

The circular stapler (without the anvil which has already been placed in the proximal bowel) is then passed through the anus and placed under some pressure against the rectal stump. The shaft of the instrument is then advanced and allowed to perforate the blind stump of the rectum adjacent to the staple line (**Figure 1.9.13**).

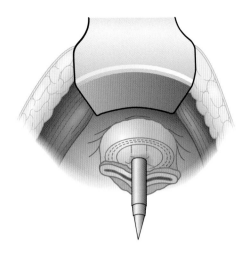

1.9.13

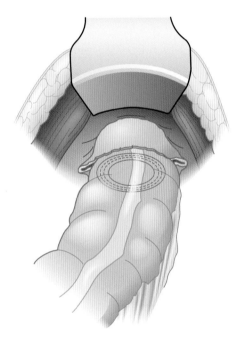

1.9.14

Step 4

The anvil and the stapler are then reunited, making sure that the bowel is not rotated. The stapler is closed, fired, and removed. However, it is vital to ensure that neither the vagina nor other pelvic structures are included in the anastomosis, and after the instrument is closed, all sides of the anastomosis must be carefully inspected before firing the apparatus (**Figure 1.9.14**).

The bowel must not be under tension after the anastomosis has been completed.

Step 5

In the triple stapling technique, an anvil is placed through the open end of the proximal bowel, much like it was done for the end-to-side anastomosis after a right colon resection. The shaft of the anvil can be placed through the antimesenteric border and the end of the bowel can be closed with a linear stapler. A purse-string is generally not necessary around the shaft (**Figure 1.9.15**).

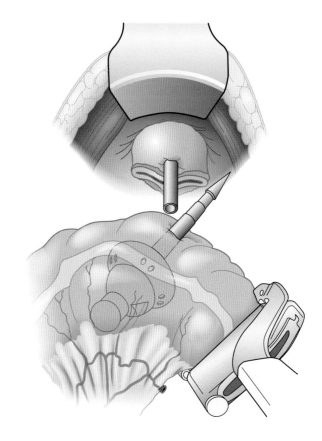

1.9.15

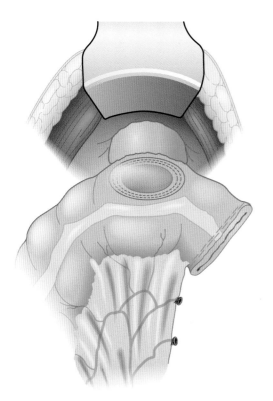

Step 6

The anastomosis is completed as for the double stapling method described above (**Figure 1.9.16**).

1.9.16

STAPLED POUCH PROCEDURES

Stapling devices can be used to construct various types of ileoanal pouches and coloanal pouches.

Step 1

Taking the terminal 45 cm of bowel, two 15 cm limbs are folded upon each other and stapled together with a linear stapler without a knife blade. The bowel is divided along this staple row which opens up the intestine (**Figure 1.9.17**).

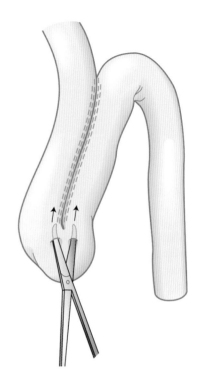

1.9.17

Step 2

The medial edge of the opened pouch is then attached to the other limb of bowel with a linear stapler. Again the bowel is incised along the staple line fully opening the pouch. The outside edges of the pouch can then be stapled together to complete the pouch using a linear stapler (**Figure 1.9.18a,b**).

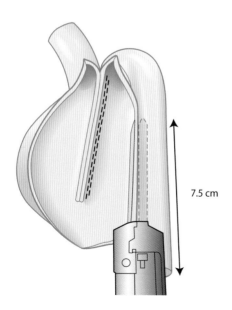

7.5 cm

(a)

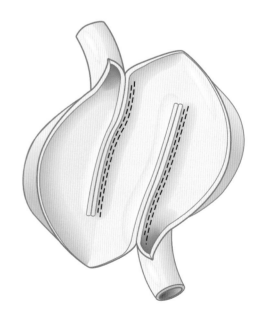

(b)

1.9.18

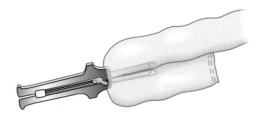

(a)

Step 3

A J-pouch can also be created from the small or large intestine with linear stapling devices. The apex of the pouch is identified and a small enterotomy or colotomy is made. Through this opening, a linear stapler is inserted and fired, taking care to exclude mesentery from the staple line. One or two additional cartridges can be fired as the bowel is 'accordioned' over the stapler. One cartridge is used for colon pouches and two cartridges for a small bowel pouch. The total length of an ileal pouch should be 15–20 cm. In contrast, a colon pouch should be no longer than 5–6 cm due to the risk of emptying difficulties with longer pouches. A circular stapler anvil can then be placed through the enterotomy in the apex of the pouch, pursestringed, and the pouch can be anastomosed to the anus with a circular stapler (**Figure 1.9.19**).

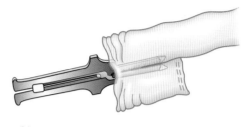

(b)

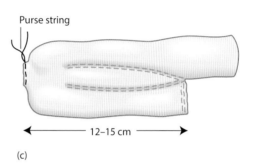

Purse string

◄——— 12–15 cm ———►

(c)

1.9.19

The completed pouch can be stapled to the anus with a circular stapler as described above for colorectal anastomoses (**Figure 1.9.20**). The pouch cannot be stapled to the anus inside the anal canal as this risks damaging the sphincter muscle.

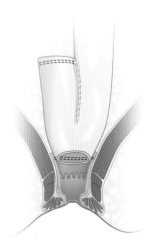

1.9.20

ADVANTAGES AND DISADVANTAGES OF STAPLERS

Staplers have been proved to be an effective way of anastomosing the bowel. Traditional Halstedian techniques requiring inversion anastomosis have not been found to be necessary with staplers and an everted anastomosis is secure. It has not been shown that staplers save a significant amount of operative time for most anastomoses.[3, 8, 9] Laparoscopic staplers utilize techniques similar to open ones and have similar complications.[9, 10, 11, 12, 13] Intracorporeal laparoscopic anastomoses may have fewer complications and earlier return of bowel function than extracorporeal anastomosis.[14]

Circular staplers probably create a more optimal rectal anastomosis than linear staplers.[15] Before performing a stapled rectal anastomosis, it is appropriate to wash out the rectum to eliminate any stool and potential cancer cells.[16, 17] The greater the volume of irrigate, the more efficacious the washout.[18] Stricturing has been noted with an increased frequency when the circular stapler is used, though this may in part be related to the lower level of anastomosis that is typically stapled rather than hand sewn.[19] Most often, the stricture is a very thin web and can be easily dilated; it occurs in 30–40 percent of patients, but is functionally significant in only about 2 percent.

It is important to note that circular staple lines are not hemostatic, and care must be taken to confirm that there are no bleeding vessels coming through the anastomosis. If this occurs, the bleeding point must be suture ligated. In addition, the more staple lines used to make a rectal anastomosis, the greater the risk of anastomotic leakage.[20] Staplers are clearly a more costly way to anastomose the bowel, and the prudent surgeon may choose not to staple anastomoses in all situations. However, stapling techniques are clearly advantageous in specific situations and should be part of the armamentarium of all intestinal surgeons.[21, 22]

REFERENCES

1. Fraser I. An historical perspective on mechanical aids in intestinal anastomosis. *Surgery, Gynecology and Obstetrics* 1982; **155**: 566–74.
2. Ravitch MM, Ong TH, Gazzola I. A new, precise, and rapid technique of intestinal resection and anastomosis with staples. *Surgery, Gynecology and Obstetrics* 1974; **139**: 6–10.
3. Scher KS, Scott-Conner C, Jones CW, Leach M. A comparison of stapled and sutured anastomoses in colonic operations. *Surgery, Gynecology and Obstetrics* 1982; **155**: 489–93.
4. Heald RJ, Allen DR. Stapled ileo-anal anastomosis: a technique to avoid mucosal proctectomy in the ileal pouch operation. *British Journal of Surgery* 1986; **73**: 571–2.
5. Lustosa S, Matos D, Atallah A, Castro A. Stapled versus hand-sewn methods for colorectal anastomosis surgery: a systematic review of randomized controlled trials. *Sao Paulo Medical Journal* 2002; **120**: 132–6.
6. Feinberg S, Cohen F, Jamieson C et al. The double stapling technique for low anterior resection of rectal carcinoma. *Diseases of the Colon and Rectum* 1986; **29**: 885–90.
7. Grams J, Tong W, Greenstein A, Salky B. Comparison of intracorporeal versus extracorporeal anastomosis in laparoscopic-assisted hemicolectomy. *Surgical Endoscopy* 2010; **24**: 1886–91.
8. Sadahire S, Kameya T, Iwase H et al. Which technique, circular stapled anastomosis or double stapling anastomosis, provides the optimal size and shape of rectal anastomotic opening? *Journal of Surgical Research* 1999; **86**: 162–6.
9. Beart, RW, Kelly KA. Randomized prospective evaluation of the EEA stapler for colorectal anastomoses. *American Journal of Surgery* 1981; **141**: 143–7.
10. Hurst PA, Prout WG, Kelly JM et al. Local recurrence after low anterior resection using the staple gun. *British Journal of Surgery* 1981; **69**: 275–6.
11. Phillips RK, Cook HT. Effect of steel wire sutures on the incidence of chemically induced rodent colonic tumours. *British Journal of Surgery* 1986; **73**: 671–4.
12. Bannigan AE, De Buck S, Suetens P et al. Intraacorporeal rectal stapling following laparoscopic total mesorectal excision. *Surgical Endoscopy* 2006; **20**: 952–5.
13. Maeda K, Maruto M, Hanai T et al. Irrigation volume determines the efficacy of 'rectal washout'. *Diseases of the Colon and Rectum* 2004; **47**: 1706–10.
14. Akamatsu H, Omori T, Oyama T et al. Totally laparoscopic low anterior resection for lower rectal cancer: combination of a new technique for intracorporeal anastomosis with prolapsin technique. *Digestive Surgery* 2009; **26**: 446–50.
15. Heald RJ. Towards fewer colostomies – the impact of circular stapling devices on the surgery of rectal cancer in a district hospital. *British Journal of Surgery* 1980; **67**: 198–200.
16. Gertsch P, Baer H, Kraft R et al. Malignant cells are collected on circular staplers. *Diseases of the Colon and Rectum* 1992; **35**: 238–41.
17. Dziki AJ, Duncan MD, Harmom JW et al. Advantages of hand-sewn over stapled bowel anastomosis. *Diseases of the Colon and Rectum* 1991; **34**: 442–8.
18. Fukunaga M, Kidokoro A, Iba T et al. Laparoscopy-assisted low anterior resection with a prolapsing technique for low rectal cancer. *Surgery Today* 2005; **35**: 598–602.
19. Ito M, Sugito M, Kobayashi A et al. Relationship between multiple numbers of stapler firings during rectal division and anastomotic leakage after laparoscopic rectal resection. *International Journal of Colorectal Diseases* 2008; **23**: 703–7.
20. Fazio V, Jagelman D, Lavery I, McGonagle B. Evaluation of the Proximate-ILs circular stapler: a prospective study. *Annals of Surgery* 1985; **201**: 108–14.
21. Kuroyanagi H, Oya M, Yeno M et al. Standardized technique of laparoscopic intracorporeal rectal transection and anastomosis for low anterior resection. *Surgical Endoscopy* 2008; **22**: 557–651.
22. Cheung H, Leun A, Chung C et al. Endo-laparoscopic colectomy without mini-laparotomy for left-sided colonic tumors. *World Journal of Surgery* 2008; **33**: 1287–91.

Specimen handling

KIERAN SHEAHAN

INTRODUCTION

The current practice of colorectal surgery and pathology greatly benefits from the immediate triage of specimens, digital archiving of specimens, and multidisciplinary conference review. Proper handling of the specimen ensures high quality pathology reporting and greatly contributes to patient care delivered in a multidisciplinary setting.

Optimal handling of colorectal specimens is crucial for histopathological examination, cancer staging, and clinicopathological correlation. The identification of clinically significant surgical margins (e.g. the circumferential margin in total mesorectal excision (TME) specimens), depth of invasion, extent of disease, presence of precancerous lesions, as well as the number of involved lymph nodes are some of the important prognostic and therapeutic data that can be derived from the pathological examination of colorectal cancer.

Many important pathological indicators of poor prognosis in colorectal cancer are initially best assessed in the gross specimen preferably in the fresh state (e.g. tumor perforation and surgical margins), while other features are confirmed by microscopy (e.g. extent of invasion, satellite nodules). The use of neoadjuvant chemoradiotherapy in the treatment of rectal cancer heightens the responsibility for good clinicopathological correlation and review of fresh resection specimens. This is especially important because of the changes in the tumor following chemoradiotherapy. More sections need to be examined to accurately record the tumor regression grade (TRG).

Careful inspection for polyps postoperatively can help diagnose and classify polyposis syndromes. Sampling lesions with a high suspicion for malignancy contributes to better patient management. A precise diagnosis ensures optimal counseling and screening of family members.

The macroscopic examination of inflammatory bowel disease colectomy specimens in the fresh state is essential to the histopathological interpretation. Special attention should be paid to the extent and distribution of the inflammatory process, as well as to sampling areas suspicious for dysplasia or cancer.

Tissue biobanking is now an important responsibility of the pathologist working in an academic research environment. Proper organization with standard protocols is required.

COLONIC CARCINOMA

Ideally, the colonic specimen should be delivered fresh to the laboratory, within minutes of the resection. In the author's laboratory, this is assisted by a specialist colorectal medical scientist who is available to receive the specimen immediately from the operating room and trained to prepare the specimen.

Macroscopic examination

- Immediate opening and cleansing of the colorectal specimen of any fecal material. The colon is recognized by its large diameter, the presence of longitudinal muscle bands (tenia coli), sacculations, and appendices epiploicae (**Figure 1.10.1**). The colon should be opened along the anterior tenia coli and the small intestine (if present) along the mesentery. Immediate opening of the entire bowel including the area of tumor allows gross inspection and gross morphological classification of the lesion from the luminal aspect (**Figure 1.10.2**). This may be increasingly appropriate in smaller mucosal-based and early stage tumors. However, traditionally for larger tumors, the bowel is left intact at the level of the tumor. Formalin-fixed gauze wicks can be placed across the tumor to aid fixation. The appendix should always be examined.
- Immediate photography with digital archiving, to ensure optimal correlation with the microscopic examination and to facilitate discussion at a multidisciplinary meeting.

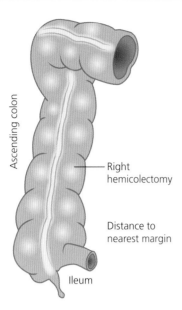

Ascending colon

Right
hemicolectomy

Distance to
nearest margin

Ileum

1.10.1 Gross examination of colonic resection specimen.

- Immediate triage of tissue for either diagnostic or research purposes.
- Fixation in formalin with an adequate tissue to formalin ratio (1:10).

The colonic cancer specimen should be fixed immediately for 24–48 hours and subsequently dissected. Instant fixation ensures optimal morphology. The mismatch repair protein antibodies used for assessing MSI status (MLHI, MSH2, PMS2, and MSH6) especially require optimal fixation. Conversely, prolonged fixation may mask antigens and diminish the quality of immunohistochemistry in certain circumstances.

The parameters listed in **Box 1.10.1** should be recorded from gross examination of a colonic specimen. Colonic cancer specimens are assessed for peritoneal involvement, tumor perforation, and margin involvement. When properly resected, proximal and distal margins of colonic

BOX 1.10.1 Parameters to be recorded from gross examination of a colonic specimen

- Type of specimen: right or left hemicolectomy/transverse/sigmoid/subtotal or total colectomy
  - size/length (cm)
- Measurements
  - length of ileum, colon, presence or absence of appendix.
- Tumor
  - size (cm)
  - site: cecal/ascending colon/transverse colon
  - shape: ulcer/infiltrating/fungating (polypoid)
  - tumor edge: infiltrative/non-infiltrative
  - peritoneal puckering: present/absent
  - distance to nearest margin (cm)
- Other lesions: metachronous/synchronous tumor, ulcerative colitis, Crohn's disease, polyps

cancer specimens are rarely involved. The mesenteric margin is infrequently involved either by discontinuous tumor spread or by in-transit metastases involving lymph nodes, vessels, nerves, or soft tissue. The colon is covered by serosa; however, the proximal ascending and sigmoid colon have a posterior non-peritonealized retroperitoneal area. As in the mesorectum, this constitutes a deep radial soft tissue resection margin, and should be assessed, inked, and sampled if at risk of involvement. The sigmoid colon ends where the tenia coli merge with the muscularis propria of the rectum.

Following fixation, the tumor is serially sliced from the luminal aspect to the peritoneum and sequential slices examined to determine the local extent of tumor (**Figure 1.10.3**). The serosal surface is meticulously examined for any evidence of peritoneal penetration (**Figure 1.10.4**). There is debate on whether inking the peritoneum is advisable or not, given that it is not a surgical margin. It is the author's practice to ink the peritoneum with yellow ink, which does not obscure cellular detail and has the advantage of highlighting the peritoneal lining microscopically and separating true positivity from artifact (**Figure 1.10.5**).

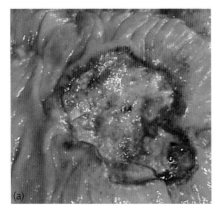
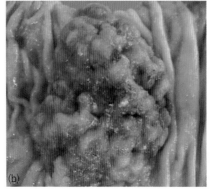
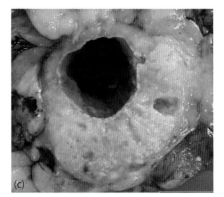

(a)   (b)   (c)

1.10.2 Three main gross morphologic patterns of colon cancer: ulcerating (a), polypoid (fungating) (b), infiltrating (annular stenosing) (c).

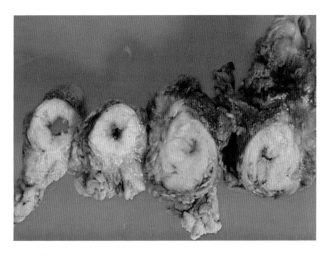

1.10.3 Serial sectioning of the tumor provides the best view of tumor invasion.

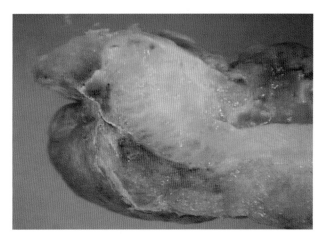

1.10.5 Yellow inking highlights the peritoneal covering.

The specimen is cut into serial transverse slices 4–5 mm thick, laid out in order, and relevant slices selected for blocking. A minimum of five blocks of tumor and bowel wall is necessary to assess the pT stage adequately and to detect extramural vascular invasion.

The presence or absence of polyps in the non-cancer-bearing area of the colon should be highlighted. Increasingly, the number and type of polyps encountered in a colectomy specimen are significant determinants of the underlying genetic conditions. For example, MYH polyposis can be suspected if more than 15 adenomas are present in a resection specimen of colon (**Figures 1.10.6** and **1.10.7**).

Hyperplastic polyposis syndrome is an underdiagnosed entity that clearly can only be diagnosed by meticulous examination of all polyps. Many of the hyperplastic polyps or sessile serrated adenomas are small, sessile lesions, which blend with normal mucosal folds, especially in the fixed specimen.

Lymph node dissection and yield

The yield of lymph nodes varies considerably. Several studies have demonstrated that there are many variables. Lymph nodes are more easily found in right colectomy specimens and more difficult to locate in anterior resection specimens, especially those treated with long-course neoadjuvant chemoradiotherapy. Optimal fixation is important. An increased nodal yield may be seen with longer periods of fixation. Thus, sectioning into mesenteric fat after receipt of the specimen may be beneficial in aiding more rapid fixation of adipose tissue (**Figure 1.10.8**).

FAT-CLEARING TECHNIQUES

Various techniques have been published which suggest that clearing the fat with chemical agents allows greater visualization and thus a greater yield of lymph

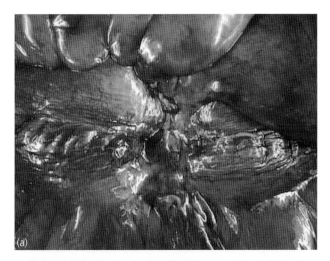

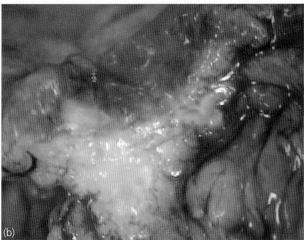

1.10.4 Peritoneal puckering (a) correlates with the invasive edge of the tumor (b) on sectioning.

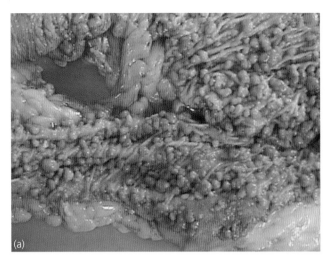

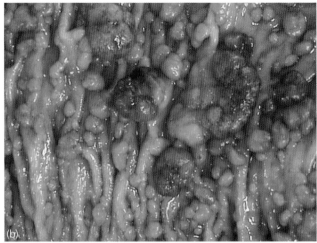

1.10.6 Familial adenomatous polyposis. Thousands of polyps can be found in the colonic specimen (a). These polyps are adenomatous microscopically, with increased risk of transformation to invasive carcinoma (b).

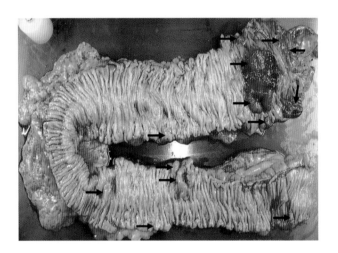

1.10.7 Diagnosis of MYH polyposis can be highly assumed if more than 15 adenomas are detected grossly (arrows point to some adenomas).

nodes. Most departments do not use these techniques, either because the chemicals are potentially toxic, the technique is cumbersome and expensive, or the fixative potentially interferes with optimal fixation and subsequent immunohistochemistry.

Complete mesocolic excision

Recent publications indicate better outcome if complete mesocolic excision (CME) combined with central vascular ligation (CVL) is performed in colon cancer surgery.[1] This approach yields more lymph nodes and may improve five-year survival rates in colon cancer patients. Assessment of the completeness of mesocolic excision will be a challenge for the pathologist in the future and will require a standardized approach.

Obstruction

Clinical presentation with obstruction is an adverse factor leading either to direct tumor perforation (pT4), proximal dilatation, ischemia and perforation (especially in the cecum), and obstructive enterocolitis. The latter can mimic inflammatory bowel disease with continuous and skip lesions of transmural inflammation either adjacent to or distant from the distal carcinoma.

Stent

Metal stenting of colonic cancers has become a common procedure to prevent bowel obstruction in a palliative setting or as a bridge to surgery. Subsequent resection specimens can pose difficulties for the pathologist. The metal stent may become embedded in the colonic wall. It may be necessary to remove the stent either intact or in a piecemeal fashion and this may be a time-consuming task (**Figures 1.10.8** and **1.10.9**).

RECTAL CARCINOMA

The parameters listed in **Box 1.10.2** should be recorded from gross examination of the rectal specimen.

The technique of total mesorectal excision has had a significant impact on the local control of rectal cancer. Neoadjuvant chemoradiotherapy can significantly reduce rectal tumors. Recent studies have shown that a complete

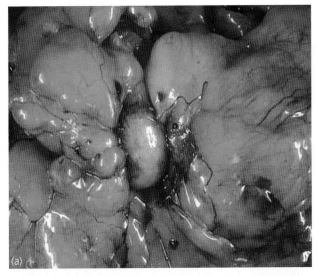

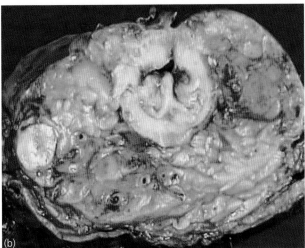

- Measurements
- Type of specimen: anterior or abdominoperineal resection (APR)
  - length of specimen
  - length of the rectum, sigmoid, and anal canal (in APR)
- Tumor
  - size (cm)
  - site: below/above peritoneal reflection
  - distance to nearest margin, to the dentate line and to anal margin (in APR)
  - shape: ulcer/polypoid or annular
  - other lesions: ulcerative colitis, polyps

pathological response in this setting predicts an overall survival benefit.[2]

Macroscopic examination

The mesorectal margin following TME and the levator ani margins following abdominoperineal resection (APR) are identified and inked (**Figures 1.10.10** and **1.10.11**). The upper anterior rectum is covered by peritoneum. The anterior mesorectum is thinner (0.75–1 cm) than the posterior mesorectum (1.5–3 cm). Where an identifiable tumor is present, the examination technique is similar to that of the colon with serial slicing of the intact specimen[3] at 5–10 mm intervals. Tumors above the peritoneal reflection should be assessed carefully for peritoneal involvement.

1.10.8 Some lymph nodes can be visible through pericolic fat (a); however sectioning into the mesenteric fat increases the yield of lymph nodes (b).

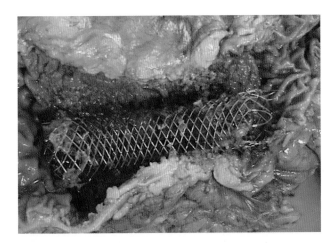

1.10.9 Metal stent *in situ* with partial embedding in the colonic wall.

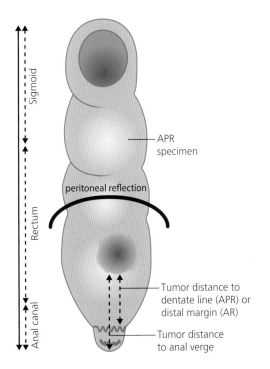

1.10.10 Gross examination of rectal resection specimen.

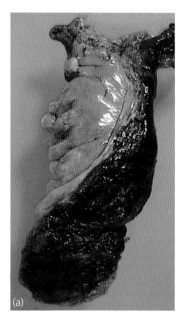

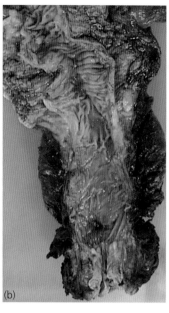

1.10.11 Inking of the non-peritonealized portion of the rectum/mesorectal plane (a), and opening of the rectum anteriorly to show the lesion in a neoadjuvant-treated case (b).

The midrectum is surrounded by the mesorectum, whereas the lower rectum is below the level of the mesorectum and is encircled by pelvic sphincteric and levator muscles. In cases where the tumor response is significant (minimal tumor, extreme fibrosis, or grossly unidentifiable tumor), the author uses a modification of the Quirke method. The bowel is opened to examine the area of regression from the luminal aspect. This area may not always be obvious and it may be necessary to liaise with the surgical team to confirm the original site of the tumor. This area is usually firm, white, and fibrotic and resembles a mucosal scar (**Figure 1.10.12**). The residual abnormal area should then be serially sliced in the normal fashion (**Figure 1.10.13**). All lesional and fibrotic tissue should be submitted for histology.

QUALITY OF TME AND APR

Assessment of the quality of surgery is an important responsibility of the pathologist and there is a standardized grading method for assessing TME specimens (**Figure 1.10.14**). Description of the three planes of sections have been published[3] and studies have confirmed the benefit of feedback to the surgical team. The mesorectal fascial plane or complete excision has a smooth surface with no defect greater than 5 mm. The intramesorectal plane or near complete excision has an irregular mesorectal surface. The muscularis propria is not visible except at the insertions of the levator ani muscles. The muscularis propria plane or incomplete excision shows little bulk to the mesorectum with deep defects extending to a visible muscularis propria. The macroscopic assessment of plane of excision is directly

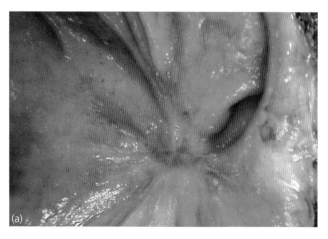

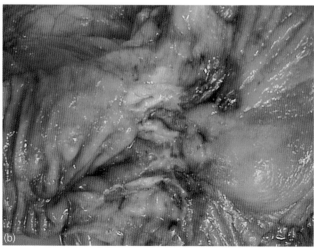

1.10.12 (a,b) Identification and sampling of regressed tumor after chemoradiotherapy can be challenging.

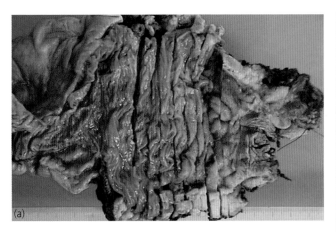

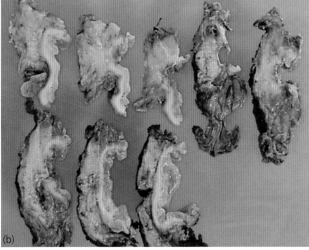

1.10.13 (a,b) Modified Quirke method in neoadjuvant cases (serial sectioning of the rectum at 5–10 mm intervals).

linked to prognosis in rectal cancers.[4] Thus, feedback to the surgeon regarding the plane of resection is vital to improve the quality of mesorectal excision.[5]

LYMPH NODE DISSECTION AND YIELD

Lymph nodes are smaller and the yield is lower in patients treated with neoadjuvant chemoradiotherapy. Fat-clearing techniques may be necessary to harvest sufficient lymph nodes for optimal staging when traditional methods fail to yield at least 12 lymph nodes. In the author's experience, alternative fixation with 100 percent alcohol may have a

significant benefit in this setting. It should be recognized that this technique hardens the mesorectal fat to a great extent and that the subsequent search for lymph nodes is more a visual than a tactile exercise.

Tumor regression grade

The author's practice uses a modified three-point grading system to assess response to chemoradiotherapy in rectal cancer. This grading system is:

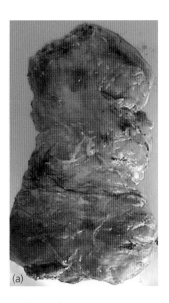

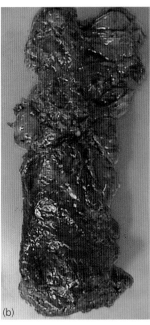

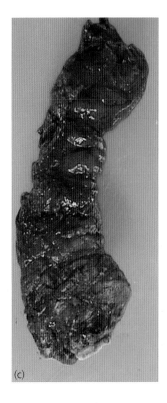

1.10.14 Examples of surgical excision planes of rectal cancer specimens (total mesorectal excision (TME)). (a) Mesorectal fascia; (b) intramesorectal; (c) muscularis propria.

- **Grade 1 (complete tumor regression).** No viable tumor cells and fibrosis extending through the bowel wall, or isolated single cell or small clusters of tumor cells scattered through fibrosis.
- **Grade 2 (partial tumor regression).** Fibrosis predominates, outgrowing residual tumor.
- **Grade 3 (no tumor regression).** Residual tumor outgrowing fibrosis and extensive residual tumor without fibrosis. Thus far, only complete tumor regression correlates with improved survival.[6]

LOCAL EXCISION SPECIMENS

Endoscopic polypectomy and endoscopic mucosal excision

Cancerous polyps will be increasingly seen as colorectal cancer screening programs are established, and proper handling and assessment is important. Lesions removed intact by both these methods require special attention in the laboratory. Polyps need to be inked at the base, bisected along the long axis of the stalk and entirely embedded. A proforma reporting system is advised.[5]

Transanal excision specimens

This surgical approach is increasingly seen as an alternative to an open procedure in patients with localized superficial rectal lesions. Ideally, these should be sent to the laboratory

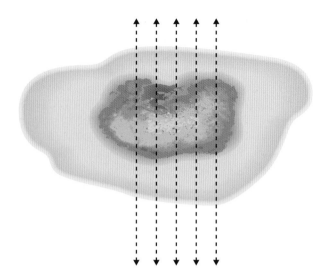

1.10.15 Illustration of transanal mucosal resection of a rectal tumor. Dashed lines show the blocking of the tumor and radial margins. Inking of the underlying surface is essential.

in the fresh state. The surgeon should mark the specimen with sutures to orient the specimen and designate the relevant margins. This will allow the mucosal resection to be stretched out and pinned on a corkboard (**Figure 1.10.15**). This is ideal for subsequent examination of surgical margins. The margins should be differentially inked and generally the entire specimen is embedded. A proforma reporting format is advised (**Table 1.10.1**).

Table 1.10.1 Transanal excision proforma.

Macroscopy	Bowel measuring	__ cm × __ cm × __ cm
	There is a tumor, __ cm situated __ cm from the nearest resection margin	
	The tumor is annular/ulcerated/plaque-like	
	The tumor invades _____	
Microscopy	Invasive well/moderately/poorly differentiated adenocarcinoma, __ cm in greatest dimension, is present in rectum	
	The tumor is 0–10/10–50/>50% mucinous	
	There is contiguous adenoma	Yes/No
	The tumor invades lamina propria/submucosa/muscularis propria/perirectal tissue	
	The tumor margin is expansile/infiltrative	
	Kikuchi level (for sessile tumors)	sm1/sm2/sm3
	Haggitt level (for polypoid tumors)	1/2/3/4
	Lymphovascular invasion	Present/absent
	Neural invasion	Present/absent
	The radial mucosal margins	Involved/uninvolved
	The deep margin	Involved/uninvolved
	Adenomas and hyperplastic polyps present	
	Tumor budding	Present/absent
pTNM stage (7th edition)		pT__ N__
Complete resection of all margins		Yes/R0; No/R1 or R2

PROFORMA REPORTING OF COLORECTAL CANCER

Standardized reporting of colorectal cancer should be performed as a matter of routine (**Tables 1.10.2** and **1.10.3**).

The RCPath dataset[5] provides detailed guidance on the reporting of pathological parameters. Controversies persist with regard to some aspects of the TNM staging system.[7] The updated seventh edition of the TNM has been published and recent changes are highlighted in **Table 1.10.4**.

New prognostic and predictive markers

New prognostic and predictive markers have emerged which have the potential to improve patient management.

TUMOR BUDDING

A strong prognostic morphological marker appears to be the presence of tumor budding. Tumor budding is defined as isolated tumor cells or clusters of <5 cells at the invasive tumor front. The author's group has found that high budding is associated with an infiltrative growth pattern and lymphovascular invasion, and five-year survival was significantly poorer in high compared with low budding groups of colorectal cancer in pT3N0 patients with colon cancer.[8]

K–RAS MUTATION STATUS

The presence of a K-Ras mutation predicts resistance to cetuximab therapy and a poorer survival.[9] Selection of tumor tissue for K-Ras analysis is the responsibility of the pathologist. In resected specimens, care must be taken to select the appropriate paraffin block, and review the H&E section to ensure that there is sufficient tumor tissue (usually >70 percent tumor). The tumor tissue may be enriched by microdissection. On occasions, the only tissue available for K-Ras evaluation is biopsy material. The clinician must biopsy an adequate amount of invasive carcinoma (avoiding adenomatous and normal mucosa, if possible). Subsequently, the pathologist must ensure that only the invasive portion of the biopsy material is microdissected for molecular analysis.

Table 1.10.2 Colon cancer proforma.

Macroscopy	Length of bowel/colon measuring __ cm including terminal ileum, __ cm, appendix, __ cm	
	There is a tumor, __ cm situated __ cm from the nearest resection margin	
	The tumor is annular/ulcerated/plaque-like	
	The tumor invades submucosa/muscularis propria/pericolic tissue/visceral peritoneum/other organs or structures	
	There is/no peritoneal puckering	
	Tumor perforation is/is not present	
	The remaining bowel shows _____	
Microscopy	Invasive well/moderately/poorly differentiated adenocarcinoma, __cm in greatest dimension, is present in the cecum/ascending/transverse/descending/sigmoid colon	
	The tumor is 0–10/10–50/>50% mucinous	
	There is a contiguous adenoma	Yes/No
	The tumor invades submucosa/muscularis propria/pericolic tissue/visceral peritoneum/other organs or structures	
	Maximum distance beyond muscularis propria	__ cm
	The tumor margin is expansile/infiltrative	
	Lymphovascular invasion	Present/absent
	Extramural vascular invasion	Present/absent
	Neural invasion	Present/absent
	Tumor perforation	Present/absent
	The peritoneum is involved/uninvolved	
	The proximal and distal margins are involved/uninvolved	
	__ of regional lymph nodes are negative/positive for metastatic carcinoma	
	Satellite pericolic tumor nodules are present/absent	
	__ adenomas and hyperplastic polyps present	
	Tumor budding	Present/absent
pTNM stage (TNM edition)		pT __ N __
Dukes stage		
Complete resection of all margins		Yes/R0; No/R1or R2

Table 1.10.3 Rectal cancer proforma.

Macroscopy	Segment of sigmoid colon and rectum __ cm, including __ cm of anus	
	There is a tumor __ cm situated __ cm proximal to the dentate line/__ cm from distal margin	
	The tumor is at/above/below the peritoneal reflection and is _____	
	The TME grade is _____	
	The tumor invades _____ and there is/no peritoneal puckering and/or tumor perforation	
	The tumor is __ mm from the radial resection margin	
	The remaining bowel shows _____	
Microscopy	Invasive well/moderately/poorly differentiated adenocarcinoma, __ cm in greatest dimension is present in the upper/middle/lower rectum	
	The tumor is 0–10/10–50/>50% mucinous	
	There is contiguous adenoma	Yes/No
	The tumor invades submucosa/muscularis propria/perirectal tissue/visceral peritoneum/other organs or structures	
	Maximum distance beyond muscularis propria	__ cm
	The tumor margin is expansile/infiltrative	
	Lymphovascular invasion	Present/absent
	Extramural vascular invasion	Present/absent
	Neural invasion	Present/absent
	Tumor perforation	Present/absent
	The peritoneum	Involved/uninvolved
	Tumor budding	Present/absent
	The proximal and distal margins are involved/uninvolved	
	The circumferential radial margin is involved/uninvolved	
	__ of regional lymph nodes is/are negative/positive for metastatic carcinoma	
	Satellite pericolic tumor nodules are present/absent	
	__ adenomas and __ hyperplastic polyps present	
	Tumor regression grade (TRG) is 1/3 (complete regression) or 2/3 (partial regression) or 3/3 (no regression)	
pTNM stage (TNM edition)		(y) pT N
Dukes stage		
Complete resection of all margins		Yes/R0 ; No/R1or R2

INFLAMMATORY BOWEL DISEASE

Ulcerative colitis

MACROSCOPIC EXAMINATION

Specimens are collected and triaged as described for colorectal cancer. The mucosal aspect of the specimen is photographed in a panoramic view and in a segmental fashion (e.g. proximal to distal) (**Figure 1.10.16**). This allows a photographic reconstruction of the entire specimen with the ability to review specimens for focal lesions that may subsequently become apparent on microscopy. In addition, areas of dysplasia or DALM (dysplasia-associated lesion or mass) can be visualized. This technique also allows documentation of unusual forms of irritable bowel disease (IBD), e.g. left-sided colitis or segmental colitis with an associated patch of cecitis.[10]

Crohn's disease

MACROSCOPIC EXAMINATION

The discontinuous inflammatory change traditionally recognized in Crohn's disease is often much more evident on macroscopic examination than apparent on microscopy (**Figure 1.10.17**). Examination in the fresh state is preferred. Prior fixation in formalin has a detrimental effect on the macroscopic appearance of colectomy specimens involved by Crohn's disease; the entire specimen contracts making the mucosal aspect of the specimen extremely difficult to examine. Small strictured areas, even malignancies, can be missed if the fresh specimen is not examined in detail.[10]

Table 1.10.4 TNM staging of colorectal cancer (7th edn).

Tis	Carcinoma *in-situ*: intraepithelial (within basement membrane) or invasion of lamina propria (intramucosal) with no extension through muscularis mucosae into submucosa	
T1	Tumor invades submucosa	
T2	Tumor invades muscularis propria	
T3	Tumor invades beyond muscularis propria into subserosa or non-peritonealized pericolic/perirectal tissues	
T4	Tumor directly invades other organs or structures and/or perforates visceral peritoneum	
	T4a	Perforates visceral peritoneum
	T4b	Directly invades other organs or structures
N0	No regional lymph node metastasis	
N1	Metastasis in 1 to 3 regional lymph nodes	
	N1a	1 node positive
	N1b	2–3 nodes positive
	N1c	Satellites (tumor deposits) in subserosa, without regional node metastasis
N2	Metastasis in 4 or more regional lymph nodes	
	N2a	4–6 nodes positive
	N2b	7 or more nodes positive
M1	Distant metastasis	
	M1a	One organ
	M1b	>One organ or peritoneum
Resection		
R0	Tumor completely excised locally	
R1	Microscopic involvement of margin by tumor (within 1 mm)	
R2	Macroscopic tumor left behind or gross involvement of margin	

Changes in TNM 7 compared to TNM 6 are highlighted in bold.

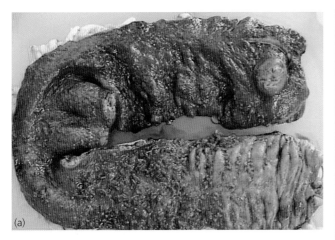
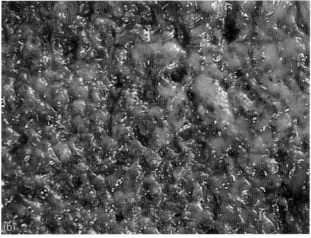

1.10.16 The colon in ulcerative colitis shows continuous (non-patchy, no skip lesions) inflammation (a), with ulcers, hyperemia, and pseudopolyps (b).

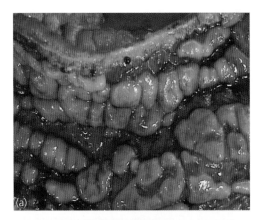

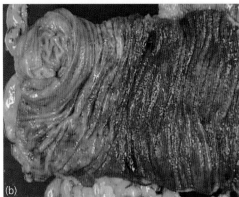

1.10.17 Crohn's disease: typical cobblestone appearance of the mucosa (a) and atypical gross features, where differentiation between ulcerative colitis and Crohn's is difficult (b).

Intestinal pouches

PROCTECTOMY FOR POUCH RECONSTRUCTION

Proctectomy specimens are common in clinical practices where ileal pouch reconstruction is performed. It is important to fix these specimens in a timely fashion and treat as outlined previously for all bowel resections. The most common finding in this setting is mucosal disease secondary either to residual IBD or diversion colitis. It is unusual to see transmural or mesorectal change and, if present, these areas need to be specifically examined.

Pouch excision

Excision of an ileal pouch which has failed is not uncommon. Examination of these specimens can be difficult. Recognition of the anatomy of these specimens is important. The afferent and efferent loops need to be identified and sampled separately. It is important not to overdiagnose these patients as having Crohn's disease. Severe pouch inflammation can be due to infection and/ or anastomotic failure and knowledge of this prior to examination is important.

Examination of vascular lesions

Vascular lesions are notoriously difficult to assess in a resected specimen due to the collapse of these lesions postoperatively. Different techniques have been used to improve their recognition (e.g. injection with barium); however, none has gained widespread acceptance (**Figure 1.10.18**).

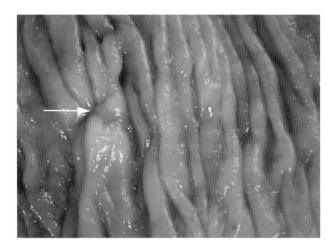

1.10.18 Collapsed vascular lesion, with submucosal haemorrhage and a mucosal scar (arrow).

ACKNOWLEDGMENT

I would like to thank Dr Osma Sharaf Eldin and Mr Robert Geraghty for their assistance with the images and figures.

REFERENCES

1. West NP, Hohenberger W, Weber K *et al*. Complete mesocolic excision with central vascular ligation produces an oncologically superior specimen compared with standard surgery for carcinoma of the colon. *Journal of Clinical Oncology* 2009; **28**: 272–8.

2. Wang LM, Sheahan K. Pathological assessment of post-treatment gastrointestinal and hepatic resection specimens. *Current Diagnostic Histopathology* 2007; **13**: 222–31.

3. Quirke P, Morris E. Reporting colorectal cancer. *Histopathology* 2007; **50**: 103–12.

4. Quirke P, Steele R, Monson J *et al*. Effect of the plane of surgery achieved on local recurrence in patients with operable rectal cancer: a prospective study using data from the MRC CR07 and NCIC-CTG C016 randomised clinical trial. *Lancet* 2009; **373**: 821–8.

5. Loughrey MB, Quirke P, Shepherd NA. *Dataset for colorectal cancer histopathology reports*, 3rd edn. London: Royal College of Pathologists, 2014. Available from: www.rcpath.org/index. asp?PageID=1153.

6. Ryan R, Gibbons D, Hyland JM *et al*. Pathological response following long-course neoadjuvant chemoradiotherapy for

locally advanced rectal cancer. *Histopathology* 2005; **47**: 141–6.

7. Puppa G, Sonzogni A, Colombari R, Pelosi G. TNM staging system of colorectal carcinoma: a critical appraisal of challenging issues. *Archives of Pathological and Laboratory Medicine* 2010; **134**: 837–52.

8. Wang LM, Kevans D, Mulcahy H *et al*. Tumor budding is a strong and reproducible prognostic marker in T3N0 colorectal

cancer. *American Journal of Surgical Pathology* 2009; **33**: 134–41.

9. Lievre A, Bachet JB, Boige V *et al*. KRAS mutations as an independent prognostic factor in patients with advanced colorectal cancer treated with cetuximab. *Journal of Clinical Oncology* 2008; **26**: 374–9.

10. Warren BF. Classic pathology of ulcerative and Crohn's colitis. *Journal of Clinical Gastroenterology* 2004; **38**: S33–S35.

2

Proctology

Office/outpatient set-up

ALEXANDER HEROLD

INTRODUCTION

The purpose of an office or outpatient facility is to facilitate diagnosis and treatment of minor diseases and the follow-up of patients with colorectal disease. A great deal of treatment can be delivered on an outpatient basis, but not all patients and not all colorectal disorders are suitable for ambulatory management. Local health care organization and the methods of reimbursement available dictate to a great extent what can be delivered. The purpose of this chapter is to demonstrate how a proctologic office may be organized. It is understood that the design must be adapted to individual and local situations depending on resources available, thus the office set-up may be designed for diagnostic evaluation alone or be equipped for both diagnosis and minor surgical procedures.

TECHNICAL PRECONDITIONS

Electronic patient administration system

A modern specialized medical facility must be designed for use of paper-free documentation in the form of an electronic patient record. Therefore, appropriate hardware tools and suitable software programs are necessary.

It is essential to have networked terminals in every room of the office. The software must, on the one hand, organize medical patient data and, on the other, facilitate organization and administration of the office: patient insurance data, waiting room lists, patient appointment lists, measuring and billing, etc. Modern practice management software also provides audit and outcome data to be readily recorded and analyzed.

Most baseline patient demographic and clinical information can be derived from well-designed patient questionnaires provided ahead of the first clinic visit. These may be completed on line ahead of the patient's visit or input by administrative staff at the time of the first visit.

Results from each patient interaction and examination are integrated online from the different examination rooms producing a complete electronic patient record.

Location and space

The size of the office should be comfortable, not too small, and easy to reach. It depends on the number of physicians whether other offices are in the same building and whether facilities or equipment is shared with others. The office should be accessible for disabled people and emergency transportation, e.g. elevator, ramp access, etc.

ENVIRONMENT

Reception desk

The reception desk is the first point of patient contact (**Figure 2.1.1**). This is the nerve center of the office

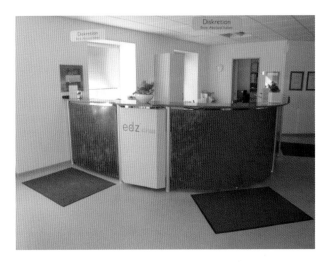

2.1.1 Reception desk.

network. From here the entire administration is managed and controlled. Primary data are collected and from here the patient is directed to the appropriate consultation or procedure room. Depending on the size of the office, other duties and functions can be delivered at this point too, e.g. call center, printing, typing.

Administration

The more patients seen and the more physicians and nurses working within the office, the more administrative support becomes mandatory. Thus the size and staffing of this part of the office is highly dependent on local requirements. If necessary, elements of the administration and organization may be outsourced.

Call center

A well-organized appointment system is essential. While the telephone may still be the most common means of making an appointment, internet and email appointment systems are rapidly becoming standard. Good communication is essential, especially for specialized colorectal centers, where patients come considerable distances. The first contacts with the office serve as a business card of the institution. Communication is important and starts here.

Consultation/examination room

In most specialties, the physician's office serves as the consulting room. For patients with colorectal symptoms a separate consultation room is optional as the majority of patients will require abdominal and/or proctological examination. It is therefore more convenient for both patient and surgeon if the office can also serve as an examination room.

LAYOUT

Examination table

For abdominal examination, an adjustable flat examination table is recommended. The table height should be adjusted for both patient mobility and physician comfort. For examination of the anorectal region, the left lateral position is recommended. The patient is positioned with the buttocks placed slightly over the side of the table, so that a rigid rectoscopy or sigmoidoscopy can be inserted. The knee–elbow position (prone) can be used, however the majority of coloproctologists use the left lateral or lithotomy position.

Examination chair

For examinations in the lithotomy position, special commercially available examination chairs are available

(**Figure 2.1.2**). This position is very convenient for both the patient and the examiner. The patient just has to lie comfortably on his back. The patient is covered except for the perineum so that it is not necessary to undress completely – letting down the trousers is quite sufficient. All instruments should be easy to reach and not directly visible to the patient.

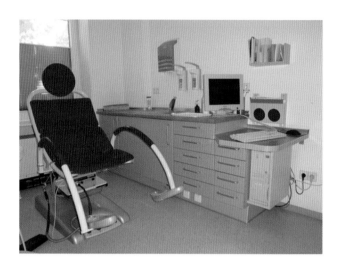

2.1.2 Examination chair.

Lighting

For efficient examination of the anorectal region, appropriate lightning is important (see above). Several types of lamps are available. If the patient is likely to be in a reproducible position, the lights can be fixed to the wall or the ceiling. If not, moveable lamps on a stand can be used. For all technical examinations (proctoscopy, rectoscopy, endoscopy) special lightning is usually connected or included into the examination tool.

Washing sink

Every single examination room needs a washing sink – in Germany this is a legal directive. Soap and disinfection dispensers are mandatory. No reusable towels and no fabric surfaces are allowed due to hygiene regulations.

INSPECTION

Inspection of the anorectal region should always precede any other examination. Appropriate lightning is important.

Inspection should include the genital, inguinal, gluteal, and presacral areas. The cheeks of the buttocks are gently spread to gain good exposure looking for scars, excoriation, dermatologic changes, external hemorrhoids, skin tags, anal and vaginal prolapse, fistulae, and fissures. The perineum is examined at rest and then during squeezing and straining. Movement is compared in relation to the ischial tuberosities. During straining, additional disorders may become visible, e.g. rectocele, cystocele, polyps, and other intra-anal diseases. Parting the buttocks may show a typical anal fissure without any instrumentation. If a rectal prolapse is suspected, the patient should be asked to strain while sitting on a toilet or commode, or a specially designed toilet chair with a mirror underneath can be used (**Figure 2.1.3**).

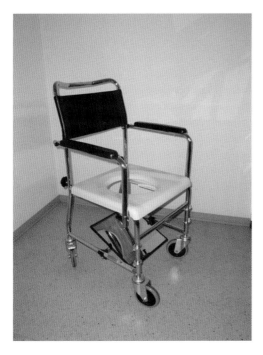

2.1.3 Toilet chair with mirror.

ANOSCOPY/PROCTOSCOPY

The examination of the anal canal is facilitated with a proctoscope. Many different instruments are available – taking all pros and cons into consideration, the physician should make an individual choice (**Figure 2.1.4**).

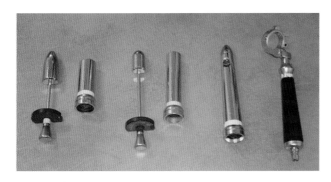

2.1.4 Different proctoscopes.

EQUIPMENT

All instruments and equipment should be kept in special designed drawers within easy reach of the surgeon (**Figure 2.1.5**).

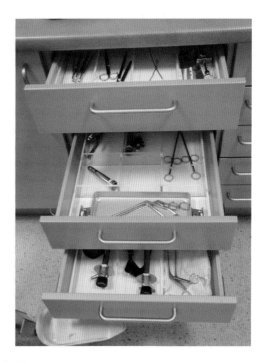

2.1.5 Combination of drawers with all instruments for a proctologic examination.

SUCTION SYSTEM

Depending on the preparation of the patient, a suction system will be necessary, more or less often. Therefore, suction should be accessible in every examination room in which proctosigmoidoscopy is undertaken.

ELECTROCAUTERY

For minor surgical procedures, a special operating room is not necessary. Any examination room is suitable for resection of polyps, skin tags, anal warts, condylomas, perianal thromboses, small abscesses, etc. The majority can be done under local anesthesia. A modern electrocautery device is mandatory when undertaking such procedures and should be available in any room in which minor procedures are undertaken. There are many good units on the market.

INSTRUMENTS

In addition to the above equipment, some special instruments are needed. A variety of probes (straight, right angulated, hook-like angulated) (**Figure 2.1.6**) is particularly useful as are sclerotherapy syringe (disposable), rubber band ligator (reusable) and a number of retractors. (See also Chapters 2.2 and 2.3.)

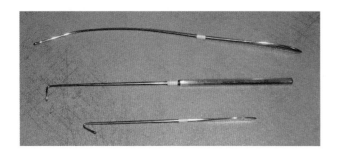

2.1.6 Different examination probes.

SPECIAL EQUIPMENT

Depending on the local requirements and the focus of the department, special instruments and examinations may be necessary, such as endoanal ultrasound, anorectal manometry, and neurophysiologic equipment. These examinations can easily be included into a general examination room. Nowadays, all radiologic examinations (transit time studies, dynamic defecography, magnetic resonance imaging, computed tomography) are performed in radiology departments, therefore no proctologic office needs to offer these.

WASHING MACHINE AND STERILIZATION SYSTEM

In a modern office, it is mandatory to use highly effective, specially designed washing machines for the cleaning of all instruments. For all instruments that penetrate skin or mucosa, a sterilization process is mandatory. In many countries this is regulated by law.

Outpatient operating room

Details are presented in Chapters 1.2 and 1.3.

Endoscopic examination room

Details of endoscopy are presented in Chapter 2.3.

Toilet

A toilet should be readily available from each examination room, especially if laxatives, suppositories, or enemas are used for the preparation of the patient. Toilets have to have enough space and at least one toilet for disabled people is necessary. In patients with suspected rectal prolapse, a toilet wheel chair with a flexible mirror underneath is very comfortable to use.

Depending on the spectrum of disease and patient profile the office arrangement described allows up to 50 patients per day to be seen. If stoma care or anorectal manometry is also available, an additional examination room may be necessary.

Proctosigmoidoscopy

SHASHANK GURJAR AND IAN LINDSEY

PRINCIPLES AND JUSTIFICATION

Proctoscopy (or anoscopy) is the inspection of the anorectal junction and the anal canal. It examines the external appearances of the anoderm, and when properly inserted, will allow visualization of the lowest part of the rectal mucosa.

Rigid sigmoidoscopy is the direct visualization of the rectum and rectosigmoid junction. The term 'sigmoidoscopy', which is used in Europe and Australasia, can be quite misleading. While the instrument may occasionally be passed beyond the rectosigmoid junction, it is usually only an adequate examination of the rectum. In the United States, 'proctoscopy' is the preferred terminology for this procedure, while 'anoscopy' is reserved for investigation of the anal canal.

A flexible sigmoidoscope exceeds the utility of a rigid sigmoidoscope. Performed by a trained endoscopist, flexible sigmoidoscopy allows definitive assessment of the rectum, sigmoid, and left colon, as well as enabling endoscopic intervention.

Indications

Proctoscopy is frequently performed in conjunction with rigid sigmoidoscopy and flexible endoscopy. Any patient presenting with symptoms suggestive of anal or perianal disease will require a proctoscopic evaluation. Common presenting symptoms include bright red per rectal bleeding, pruritis ani, perianal discharge, or a palpable lesion.

Rigid sigmoidoscopy is a very useful outpatient assessment tool and enables rapid assessment of rectal pathology. Biopsies can be taken and a simple polypectomy performed. A crucial adjunct is the determination of tumor height and quadrant in low-lying rectal cancers.

Flexible sigmoidoscopy has a role in clinically selected patients with isolated left-sided symptoms, such as bright rectal bleeding where left colonic pathology is suspected. It is also of use in inspection of a distal anastamosis.

Contraindications

Patients with severe anal pain or those who cannot tolerate digital rectal examination are unlikely to be able to undergo proctosigmoidoscopic assessment. Anal pain may be the result of a range of conditions including fissure-in-ano, abscess (e.g. perianal, intersphincteric), complex hemorrhoidal disease, or rectal prolapse. Anal stenosis is an important contraindication. Such patients are unlikely to tolerate digital rectal examination, and consequently proctoscopy is not an option. These patients may need formal examination under (general) anesthetic to establish a diagnosis and initiate treatment.

Flexible sigmoidoscopy should be avoided in patients with acute symptoms, such as acute diverticulitis with local sepsis and threatened perforation or severe inflammatory bowel disease. The procedure is a relative contraindication in patients with ascites or on peritoneal dialysis, as there can be transient release of bowel organisms into the bloodstream and peritoneal cavity during its passage. Prophylactic antibiotics may be indicated in the immunosuppressed or patients with valvular heart disease.

PREOPERATIVE

Proctoscopy

Bowel preparation is not required.

Sigmoidoscopy

The use of a pre-procedure bowel preparation is a matter of debate. Some feel that viewing the rectum without prior enemas allows visualization of the mucosa in its natural state and avoids a diagnosis of idiopathic proctitis. It allows inspection of the contents of the upper rectum, which may be of diagnostic benefit when patients present with rectal bleeding. The main disadvantage is that views may be obscured which may limit the extent of the examination.

When bowel preparation is offered, a single phosphate enema given at least 30 minutes before the procedure is preferred. This should result in adequate clearance of the left colon and rectum.

Flexible sigmoidoscopy

The patient is offered a phosphate enema 30 minutes before the procedure. It is worth noting that some patients may experience vasovagal problems after phosphate enemas: post-procedure supervision is required. The majority of patients will tolerate the procedure without sedation.

OPERATION

A digital rectal examination must always be performed to ensure there is no significant obstructive pathology immediately within the anal canal, and to aid in determining the angle of the rectal canal, for the purposes of insertion of the instruments. This avoids the risk of inadvertent trauma. The perineum must also be carefully inspected for scarring or evidence of other pathology.

General patient positioning

The patient is placed in the left lateral decubitus or Sims' position (**Figure 2.2.1**), ensuring that the buttocks just hang over the edge of the bed – this allows better access to insert the instrument effectively and improve views. The 'knees to elbows' or all fours approach, favored in the US is an alternative position (**Figure 2.2.2**). This is best achieved using a purpose-built tilting examination couch.

For flexible sigmoidoscopy, the left lateral position is preferred.

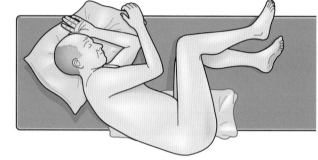

2.2.1

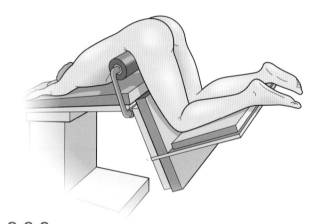

2.2.2

Proctoscopy

INSTRUMENTS

Most modern proctoscopes are disposable, with a beveled end to facilitate optimal viewing of the anal canal and allow access for treatments such as banding of hemorrhoids (**Figure 2.2.3**). Variable sizes and types are available (e.g. pediatric usage).

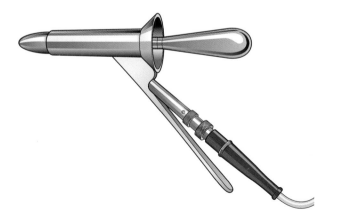

2.2.3

INSERTION AND PROCEDURE

The proctoscope is generously lubricated, with the obturator in place. The anal canal initially passes anteriorly for a few centimeters and then angles back sharply towards the hollow of the sacrum. Therefore, the proctoscope must first be passed, with firm pressure into the anal canal, in a direction towards the umbilicus. Once the instrument has traversed the sphincter mechanism, it is directed more posteriorly and passed to its fullest extent. The obturator is then withdrawn. The proctoscope is held steady with the left hand while the right hand can be used to either swab away excess mucus or suction away liquid stool.

The lower rectal mucosa and anal canal can be fully assessed by carefully rotating the instrument or by reinsertion if necessary. The anorectal mucosa is carefully inspected for lesions (rectal tumors) or inflammation (proctitis). As the instrument is gently withdrawn, hemorrhoids will prolapse into the lumen and the dentate line will become evident. Fissures, fibroepithelial polyps, and internal fistulous openings may be diagnosed. Conservative treatments for hemorrhoids (e.g. banding, infrared coagulation, injection sclerotherapy) can be performed.

With respect to assessment for pelvic floor dysfunction, a good clinical impression of internal rectal prolapse can sometimes be gained with the patient asked to bear down as the proctoscope is retracted through the anus.

Rigid sigmoidoscopy

INSTRUMENTS

The standard Lloyd-Davies sigmoidoscope, measuring 25 cm in length (internal diameter, 19 mm), is the most commonly used version (**Figure 2.2.4**), although narrower and shorter scopes are available. Older designs have a reusable built-in light source and bellows for insufflation of the rectum. More modern instruments utilize fiber-optic light sources, and can be designed to be completely disposable. This may address a possible risk of cross-contamination due to reusable parts: the cost–benefit still remains unclear. Availability of sterile long-handled biopsy and grasping forceps is mandatory, together with cotton-wool swabs and suction tubing to help clear the lumen of fluid rectal contents.

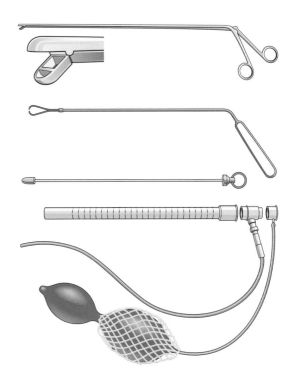

2.2.4

INSERTION AND PROCEDURE

The initial steps of insertion are similar to those of a proctoscope. As soon as the sphincter mechanism is crossed, the instrument is directed posteriorly and the obturator is removed. Dependent on design, the light source and bellows are then fitted to the end of the sigmoidoscope (**Figure 2.2.5**). Throughout the examination, the instrument is held in the left hand, while the right hand holds the inflation bellows and the bulb, which can be gently squeezed between the thumb and index finger to control the degree of inflation.

The remaining length of the scope is passed under direct vision. At this stage, a combination of careful insufflation and angling of the proximal end of the instrument to keep the intestinal lumen in view, will help to pass the sigmoidoscope into the upper rectum. The

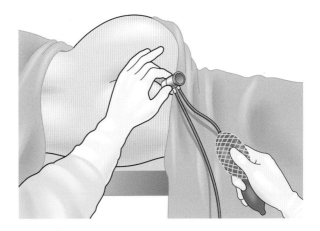

2.2.5

first few centimeters pass posteriorly towards the hollow of the sacrum. Subsequently, an anterior direction will be required to achieve full insertion. The patient may experience discomfort during these steps and should be forewarned of an urge to pass a bowel motion or wind. A long cotton bud can be useful if the lumen becomes obscured with feces. With care, the rectosigmoid junction can be successfully negotiated in the majority of cases.

Inspection of the mucosa is best achieved by rotating the instrument during its removal, taking care to ensure that lesions hidden behind rectal folds are not missed. Biopsies can be easily taken under direct vision using biopsy forceps. Excess bleeding can usually be controlled by pressure from a long cotton bud, soaked in topical adrenaline (1:1000) if necessary. Polypectomy is best reserved for a flexible sigmoidoscope, which allows superior views and can safely utilize diathermy and snaring techniques. Small benign-looking rectal polyps can be excised with a rigid sigmoidoscope and appropriate forceps.

In the acute setting, a rigid sigmoidoscope, in conjunction with a flatus tube, can be very useful in decompression of a sigmoid volvulus. Once a clinical diagnosis has been made, the instrument can be carefully inserted up to the point of torsion and gentle pressure applied to help 'untwist' the volvulus. A flatus tube can then be fed through the lumen into the sigmoid colon and taped to the buttocks to hold it in place. If ischemia is directly visualized, then sigmoidoscopic decompression should be abandoned and a laparotomy performed.

INSERTION AND PROCEDURE

Informed consent is initially obtained. Patients adopt the left lateral position and a digital rectal examination is performed to exclude low lesions and lubricate the anal canal. Local anesthetic gel may help if digitation proves painful.

All functions of the sigmoidoscope should be pre-checked before insertion. The tip is well lubricated and inserted 'sideways' with slight finger pressure for a short distance. Initially, a red blur is seen on the screen; gentle insufflation with slight instrument withdrawal will bring the lumen into view. By using a combination of maneuvers involving suction and insufflation, the instrument can be carefully advanced through the rectum. Negotiation of the rectosigmoid junction is often the trickiest part of the procedure (Figure 2.2.7), and is usually more difficult in patients with a history of previous pelvic surgery (e.g. hysterectomy). It is best attempted under direct vision, with minimal insufflation and torque applied to the shaft of the instrument. Gentle careful withdrawal, coupled with use of torque, can help straighten out a loop and speed up progress. Over-angulation using the control knobs is best avoided. If the patient begins to complain of discomfort or progress is not being made, it may be useful to briefly

Flexible sigmoidoscopy

INSTRUMENTS

The modern fiberoptic flexible sigmoidoscope is 65–70 cm in length and allows visualization of rectum, sigmoid colon, and left colon (Figure 2.2.6). A variety of manufacturers exist: all essentially provide similar capabilities that allow visualization, biopsy, brush cytology, polypectomy, and tattooing with India ink.

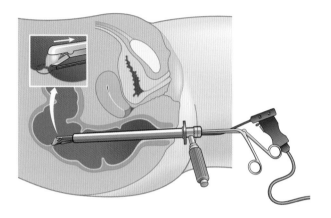

2.2.6

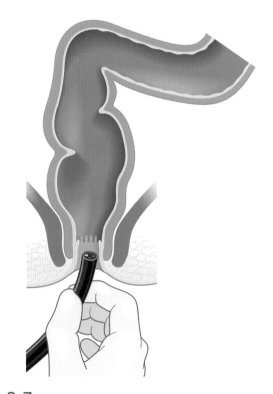

2.2.7

stop mid-procedure, consider an alteration of the patient's position or employ use of gentle pressure on the abdomen (left lower quadrant) to assist passage of the scope.

In skilled hands, a sigmoidoscope can be passed to the splenic flexure with characteristic views of the triangulated folds of the transverse colon. It should be remembered that pelvic adhesions could make the examination impossible. There is a (small) risk of perforation and in circumstances where the patient is not tolerating the procedure, and no progress is occurring, it is better to abandon the examination.

The major part of the procedure is slow withdrawal and full visualization of the entire lumen of the distal colon. Biopsies can be taken, a polypectomy performed and tattooing achieved. Retroversion in the rectum is useful to ensure that the entire capacious rectum is visualized as well as the top of the anal canal. During the withdrawal process, it is good practice to aspirate as much air as possible to increase the patient's comfort.

Proctological examination under general anesthetic

The accurate assessment of the perineum, anal canal, and rectum is an important skill in a surgeon's armamentarium.

Examination under anesthetic (EUA) may be indicated when a patient has not tolerated assessment, usually due to pain. Proctoscopy, rigid and flexible sigmoidoscopy, and relevant interventions (e.g. banding of hemorrhoids, injection of botulinum toxin for fissures) can be carried out as part of an EUA.

There are also situations when an EUA may yield more useful diagnostic information. This is especially important in the context of pelvic floor dysfunction. A patient who has undergone a full pelvic floor work up (endoscopy, radiology, anorectal physiology, and ultrasound) may still benefit from a formal EUA to confirm a finding of internal rectal prolapse.

Informed consent is obtained from the patient prior to the procedure. Once the patient is under general anesthetic, the extreme lithotomy position is adopted. A perianal block is extremely useful – within minutes of an effectively administered block, the anus appears relaxed and patulous. A circular anal dilator can be placed with ease, and if necessary, sutured into place. The obturator is removed and the lower rectum can be properly visualized. A Rampley sponge-holding forceps (loaded with a small sponge) or a Babcocks forceps, can be used to demonstrate evidence of full-thickness internal rectal prolapse into the anal canal, or occult external prolapse.

Flexible endoscopy

PIERRE H CHAPUIS AND D BRIAN JONES

INTRODUCTION

High-quality, flexible endoscopy using modern video technology is the method of choice both for the investigation and treatment of patients with a wide spectrum of large bowel disorders. It is an integral part of the comprehensive practice of surgery of the colon and rectum.

DEFINITIONS AND CONCEPTS

Colonoscopy is defined as visual inspection of the lumen of the entire colon and rectum. To achieve this, the operator must be familiar with the normal anatomy and the variation in the lengths of individual anatomical segments which contribute to natural blind spots and may also explain differences in site distribution of polyps and cancers in the adult.[1] Colonoscopy is best performed with either a 160- or 180 cm instrument.

Flexible sigmoidoscopy using the shorter 130 cm instrument permits a more limited examination of the sigmoid and descending colon when full colonoscopy is considered unnecessary. The use of a shorter 60 cm scope offers little advantage, although it is undoubtedly less cumbersome to use if combined with laser therapy or argon plasma coagulation (APC) when treating a rectal or sigmoid lesion. The splenic flexure is commonly not reached with a 60 cm scope, often because of the formation of an N-loop causing patient discomfort.

Sigmoidoscopy is performed with the patient in the knee–chest position on an electric tilt table or alternatively, in the left lateral or Sims' position with the patient's buttocks drawn to the very edge of the table and with the patient's hips and knees flexed. Preliminary inspection, including digital palpation, is performed before proceeding with the examination.

Sigmoidoscopy is invaluable as part of the patient's initial assessment and is usually conducted in an ambulatory setting without the need for formal bowel preparation or sedation. It is particularly useful for patients who are over the age of 40 years and who present with hemorrhoidal symptoms to exclude left-sided synchronous pathology.[2]

INSTRUMENTATION

The current generation of videoendoscopes has attained a high level of sophistication based on the original charge-coupled device (CCD) or silicon chip technology which electronically transmits clear, real-time, true-to-life color images of the lumen of the large bowel on to a television monitor. In all other respects, these instruments resemble the previous generation of fiberoptic endoscopes, but without the need for a viewing lens. In this way, the advantages of videoendoscopy are immediately apparent, namely that all team members may simultaneously view the screen, while the endoscopist has a clear and unobstructed view. It also allows greater comfort to the endoscopist as they may stand more comfortably when examining the patient and as there is no need to hold the instrument close to the eye, the likelihood of the examiner being contaminated by spills or splashes from the air or water channels are eliminated.

A range of colonoscopes are available, with insertion tip diameters ranging typically between 11.3 and 13.2 mm, with working channels of 3.2 mm and up to 170° angle of field of view. The quality of endoscopic visualization involves both magnification and resolution, and there has been a move towards the use of high definition colonoscopes in recent years. High resolution colonoscopy may be combined with chromoendoscopy (indigo carmine or methylene blue spraying) to enhance subtle mucosal changes. Several studies have shown magnification chromoendoscopy to have in excess of 90 percent accuracy for differentiating neoplastic from non-neoplastic colonic lesions less than 10 mm in size.

Narrow Band Imaging® (NBI; Olympus Medical Systems, Japan) and Multiband Imaging® (MBI; Fujinon,

Japan) are real-time, on-demand endoscopic imaging techniques designed to enhance visualization of the vascular network and surface texture of the mucosa without the need for dye spraying. They can be used for enhanced detection of colonic neoplasia including flat or depressed lesions (**Figure 2.3.1**). Commercially available NBI and MBI videocolonoscopes enable the user to alternate rapidly between white light and NBI or MBI viewing modes by the touch of a button on the handle of the colonoscope. A prospective randomized study has demonstrated similar accuracy of NBI and indigo carmine chromoendoscopy in differentiating neoplastic from non-neoplastic polyps, both being superior to conventional white light colonoscopy.[3]

CO_2 insufflation

The rapid absorption of CO_2 from the bowel lumen into the circulation makes it ideal for use with either colonoscopy or flexible sigmoidoscopy, so that either procedure can be effectively combined with a double-contrast barium enema to visualize the right side of the colon. CO_2 insufflation does reduce pain both during and after examination. This improves patient compliance for those enrolled in long-term endoscopic surveillance. It may also reduce the risk of an intraluminal explosion when performing polypectomy.

No respiratory depression has been reported with the use of CO_2.

Hemostatic devices

Colonoscopic hemostatic devices include contact thermal devices (heater probe, multipolar electrocautery, hemostatic graspers), non-contact thermal devices (such as APC), injection needles, and mechanical devices (clips, banders, and loops). Thermal devices generate heat directly or indirectly by passage of electrical current through tissue leading to edema, coagulation of tissue protein, and contraction of vessels.

Bipolar electrocautery (Gold Probe®, Boston Scientific, Natick, MA, USA; Bicap Superconductor®, ConMed, Utica, NY, USA) delivers thermal energy by completion of an electric current between two electrodes on the tip of a probe as current flows through non-desiccated tissue (**Figure 2.3.2**). In contrast to monopolar electrocautery, no grounding pad is needed. As the targeted tissue desiccates, there is a decrease in electrical conductivity limiting the depth of injury. A port at the tip delivers water for irrigation, and the probe may also incorporate an injector for intralesional injection of adrenaline. A foot pedal controls the delivery of energy, with a maximum power setting of no more than 50 W.

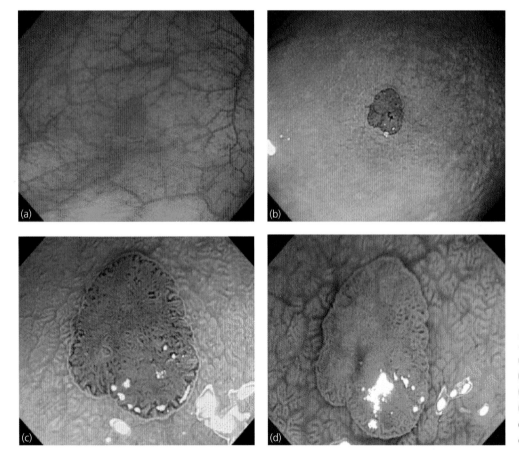

2.3.1 (a) Sessile polyp under white light endoscopy; (b) narrow band imaging (NBI); (c) NBI magnification; (d) magnification after dye spraying with indigo carmine.

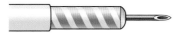

2.3.2 Gold Probe bipolar electrocautery device (reproduced with permission from Boston Scientific Inc).

Heater probes consist of a Teflon-coated, hollow, aluminium cylinder with an inner heating coil. A thermocoupling device at the tip maintains a constant temperature. The mechanism of tissue coagulation is direct heat transfer.

Hemostatic graspers are similar to conventional biopsy forceps which transmit monopolar electrocautery.

Argon plasma coagulation involves non-contact electrocoagulation using high frequency monopolar alternating current conducted to target tissue through ionized argon gas. The gas is only ignited where there is a short distance between the tip of the APC probe and the surface tissue. Coagulation depth is dependent on the generator power setting, duration of application, and distance from probe tip to tissue (2–8 mm). A typical setting for APC would be a gas flow rate of 1 to 1.5 L/min at a setting of 40–50 W.

Endoscopic clipping devices have three components, a metal double- or triple-pronged preloaded clip, a delivery catheter, and a handle to deploy the clip (**Figure 2.3.3**). The catheter is passed down the working channel, the clip is extended to open up the jaws, which are then closed around visible vessels and deployed (**Figure 2.3.4**).

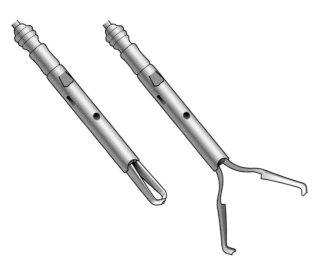

2.3.3 Endoscopic clipping device (reproduced with permission from Boston Scientific Inc).

Detachable loops are similar to snares. The loops are placed around the stalks of large polyps and deployed to strangle them and reduce their blood supply prior to snare polypectomy.

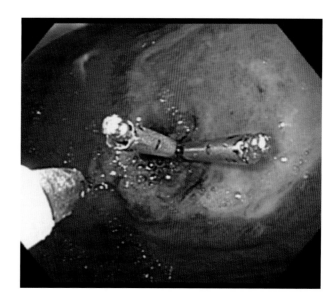

2.3.4 Deployed clips on bleeding lesion.

FACILITIES AND STAFFING

A dedicated endoscopy suite appropriately staffed by specially trained nurses, together with adequate support technicians for cleaning and maintenance of instruments should be available for all examinations. Safe and effective colonoscopy requires the availability of:

- adequately trained and certified endoscopists;
- adequately trained nursing staff;
- serviced and functioning high resolution colonoscopes;
- high level disinfection systems;
- equipment and drugs for safe sedation and anesthesia;
- spacious procedure rooms with ancillary equipment (oxygen, suction, etc.).

Most colonoscopy is performed as a day-only procedure, but may occasionally need to be performed in the operating room. In terms of desirable physical space, equipment (endoscopes, processors, television monitors, patient monitoring, anesthetic, and recovery equipment), and disinfection facilities, suitable guidelines have been formulated.[4]

Ideally, there should be at least two nursing assistants present for each procedure room, one to assist the colonoscopist and one to assist the sedationist or anesthetist. Minimum acceptable staffing requirements are covered in the guidelines.[5]

INFORMED CONSENT

Informed consent is a combination of disclosure of the substantive information necessary to make a reasoned and voluntary decision by the patient. Procedures which are scheduled, invasive, complex, requiring sedation or an anesthetic, or are associated with significant risk of harm should always require written informed consent. By these criteria, all flexible endoscopic procedures require written informed consent.

COLONIC PREPARATION

Colonoscopy and flexible sigmoidoscopy require thorough bowel cleansing for safe and effective completion of the procedure. In the case of colonoscopy, inadequate preparation is responsible for up to a third of incomplete examinations. The ideal colon preparation would:

- rapidly and reliably cleanse the colon of fecal material;
- have no effect on the macro- or microscopic appearance of the mucosa;
- require a short period for ingestion and effect;
- cause minimal discomfort, be palatable, and relatively inexpensive;
- produce no significant fluid or electrolyte shifts.

Generally, oral bowel preparations can be divided into three types.

1 Isosmotic preparations (Golytely®, Glycoprep®, Colyte®, and Nulytely®) usually contain polyethylene glycol (PEG) and are osmotically balanced, high volume, non-absorbable, and non-fermentable electrolyte solutions. They cleanse the colon by the mechanical effect of large volume lavage. The conventional dose is 3–4 L given as divided doses over a period of some hours. They may also be administered via a nasogastric tube at a rate of 20–30 mL/min. In the case of afternoon lists, it may be preferable to institute a split-dose regimen the afternoon before and early on the morning of the procedure. Low volume PEG solutions are available, combined with stimulant laxatives or ascorbic acid (Halflytely®, Moviprep®).

2 Hyperosmotic preparations draw water into the bowel lumen which stimulates peristalsis and evacuation. Although small volume, these preparations can cause significant fluid and electrolyte shifts. Sodium phosphate (Fleet Phospho-Soda®, Osmoprep®, Fleet®) and sodium sulfate (Picoprep®) preparations are available.

3 Stimulant laxatives include senna, an anthracene derivative, which stimulates colonic peristalsis. Bisacodyl is a diphenylmethane derivative which is poorly absorbed in the small intestine, but following hydrolysis by endogenous estersases its metabolites stimulate colonic motility.

The main impediment to successful bowel preparation is volume and taste. There is little difference between isosmotic and hyperosmotic solutions, but the smaller volume solutions have higher completion rates compared to the larger volume isosmolar preparations.

In patients suspected of having inflammatory bowel disease (IBD) who present with diarrhea, flexible sigmoidoscopy should be performed preferably without prior preparation. For other patients, administration of a disposable enema will usually suffice. These may be simple tap water or commercially available enemas which contain sodium phosphate (Fleet) or sodium citrate (Microlax®).

PATIENT SELECTION

An accepted list of indications for colonoscopy is shown in **Box 2.3.1**.[6]

Contraindications to colonoscopy are few and generally of a relative rather than absolute nature. Colonoscopy should not be performed where the risks of the procedure outweigh the potential benefits. Care needs to be exercised in elderly patients, those with significant cardiorespiratory comorbidities, patients with active IBD, those who may be compromised by bowel preparation, or those who have had previous pelvic surgery or have known abdominopelvic pathology which may make colonoscopy difficult or hazardous, e.g. severe stenosing diverticulosis coli, previous pelvic radiation, or extensive adhesions.

BOX 2.3.1 Indications for colonoscopy[6]

1 Abnormality on imaging study of a clinically significant lesion (filling defect or stricture)
2 Evaluation of gastrointestinal hemorrhage
   a hematochezia
   b melena with normal upper gastrointestinal endoscopy
   c positive fecal occult blood test
3 Unexplained iron deficiency anemia
4 Screening and surveillance of colorectal neoplasia
   a screening of average risk (50 years old and older) population
   b screening of patients with family history of colorectal cancer or polyps
      i familial adenomatous polyposis syndromes, hereditary non-polyposis colorectal cancer (HNPCC)
      ii sporadic colorectal cancer
   c examination for proximal synchronous cancers and polyps in patients with distal cancer
   d postcancer resection for metachronous polyps and cancers
   e postpolypectomy follow-up
   f surveillance for dysplasia in long-standing chronic inflammatory bowel disease.
5 Chronic inflammatory bowel disease to assess disease extent, activity, and diagnosis
6 Chronic diarrhea
7 Intraoperative identification of a lesion not apparent at surgery (e.g. polypectomy site)
8 Treatment of bleeding lesions, such as vascular malformations, neoplasia, polypectomy site
9 Foreign body removal
10 Excision of colonic polyp
11 Decompression of acute nontoxic megacolon or volvulus
12 Balloon dilatation of colonic strictures
13 Palliation of colorectal neoplasms (stenting, laser therapy)
14 Localization of lesions with tattoo prior to surgery

SPECIAL CONSIDERATIONS

Managing moderate to large volume lower gastrointestinal bleeding by colonoscopy

Lower gastrointestinal bleeding (LGIB) or hematochezia is defined as bleeding emanating distal to the ligament of Treitz. The causes of LGIB are summarized in **Box 2.3.2**.

> **BOX 2.3.2 Causes of lower gastrointestinal bleeding**
>
> - Diverticulosis coli
> - Ischemic colitis
> - Vascular ectasia
> - Hemorrhoids
> - Neoplasm
> - Inflammatory bowel disease
> - Infectious colitis
> - Non-steroidal anti-inflammatory drugs (NSAID)-induced colopathy
> - Radiation colopathy
> - Meckel's diverticulum
> - Rectal varices
> - Aortoenteric fistula

Patients with acute, severe LGIB must be assessed clinically and stabilized prior to proceeding to colonoscopy and should be considered early in the management algorithm. It is best performed after colonic preparation with polyethylene glycol. This facilitates visualization and improves the diagnostic yield. The diagnostic yield in emergency colonoscopy for acute, severe LGIB ranges from 50 to 90 percent. The timing of colonoscopy in this situation ranges from 12 to 48 hours after initial presentation.

The most common cause of large volume LGIB is diverticulosis coli. Sometimes, a bleeding source can be identified within a diverticulum. A combination of adrenaline injection and thermal contact devices can be used in such a situation with good results. Similarly, use of endoscopic laser therapy or APC to treat vascular ectasia is highly successful. Endoscopic clips may be used for patients presenting with a postpolypectomy bleed, if the site can be adequately demonstrated. Surgery should be considered in patients with continuing LGIB that requires more than six units of packed cells in 24 hours.

Colonoscopy in inflammatory bowel disease

The role of flexible endoscopy in the management of IBD is summarized in **Box 2.3.3**. Patients with long-standing ulcerative colitis (UC) or Crohn's colitis are at an increased risk of colorectal cancer (CRC) which may be predated by dysplasia. The risk of CRC in patients with IBD relates to

---

> **BOX 2.3.3 Role of flexible endoscopy in inflammatory bowel disease**
>
> - Initial diagnosis of inflammatory bowel disease
> - Differentiating ulcerative colitis (UC) and Crohn's disease
> - Assess disease extent (proctitis, proctosigmoiditis, left-sided colitis, pan-colitis, segmental colitis, ileitis)
> - Assess disease activity (mild, moderate, severe)
> - Monitor response to therapy
> - Surveillance for dysplasia and neoplasia
> - Provide endoscopic therapy, such as stricture dilation

---

disease duration, severity of disease, family history of CRC, young age at onset of IBD, presence of backwash ileitis, and coexistence of primary sclerosing cholangitis. Although patients with proctitis are not at increased risk of CRC, left-sided colitis does confer an increased risk and these patients should also have colonoscopic surveillance. It is recommended that patients with chronic UC and Crohn's colitis (affecting more than one-third of the colon) should undergo surveillance colonoscopy every one to two years, beginning eight to ten years after disease onset. Mucosal biopsies should be taken in four quadrants every 10 cm from the cecum to rectum, to obtain a minimum of 32 specimens. The yield of finding dysplasia-associated lesions or mass (DALM) is increased using high magnification endoscopy, NBI, and chromoendoscopy. Diagnosis of dysplasia should be confirmed by a second, independent experienced gastrointestinal pathologist.

Management of antithrombotic agents and anticoagulants

Antithrombotic agents include anticoagulants (warfarin and heparin) and antiplatelet agents (aspirin and clopidogrel). They are used to reduce the risks of thromboembolic events in susceptible individuals (e.g. atrial fibrillation with or without valvular heart disease). Before performing colonoscopy in patients on antithrombotic agents, one should consider the risks of:

- bleeding related to the antithrombotic agents;
- bleeding related to an endoscopic procedure, such as polypectomy;
- thromboembolic event arising from withholding the antithrombotic agents.

SEDATION AND ANESTHESIA

Although colonoscopy without sedation is not recommended as a routine practice, it is a viable option in selected patients including those who require sigmoidoscopy. Music during the procedure may also reduce required quantities of intravenously administered drugs.

Preprocedure assessment of the fitness of patients undergoing endoscopy with sedation is essential. Cardiovascular, respiratory, and neurological comorbidities should be assessed and knowledge of patient allergies and reactions to drugs and sedative agents, smoking history, alcohol intake, and medication use are important. Those administering sedative agents and monitoring their effects should be aware of the nature of the proposed procedure and in particular its likely duration and potential complications. Intravenous sedation for colonoscopy should only be administered where there is adequate space to permit easy movement of personnel and equipment.

Patients undergoing intravenous sedation for colonoscopy must be monitored clinically and with pulse oximetry and regular blood pressure determinations. There should be ready access to intravenous reversal agents and intravenous fluids. All patients should have an intravenous cannula in place. The full range of equipment and drugs used in advanced life support must be available.

Sedation with propofol leads to better quality sedation without compromising safety. Propofol can be administered safely by non-anesthetists in selected patients undergoing colonoscopy. Where there is significant likelihood of airway obstruction and for those patients with high American Society of Anesthesiologists grades, assistance from a specialist anesthetist is advisable, particularly if it is anticipated that the procedure will be of long duration or endoscopically exacting. Such assistance may also be advisable if there have been difficulties with intravenous sedation on a previous occasion. Due to their pharmacological profiles, midazolam, fentanyl, and propofol are among the most commonly used drugs for intravenous sedation for colonoscopy.

ACCREDITATION

When performing flexible endoscopy, good technique is essential and necessitates a period of supervised training and practice to acquire the necessary skills to perform a safe and complete examination. Today, 'self-teaching' is no longer acceptable and professional accreditation is required as a necessary prerequisite to practice. Training must include regular attendance at hospital biopsy meetings to ensure close collaboration and feedback from the pathologist and for correct identification, orientation, and interpretation of endoscopic findings. An understanding of the principles of cleaning and disinfection of endoscopes is also a necessary part of training.

PROCEDURE TIPS AND TRICKS

Essential 'one-person' technique

The examination should aim to be appropriate, complete to the cecum in at least 90 percent of attempts and performed with minimum sedation to allow for patient safety, comfort, and rapid recovery postprocedure. It must be performed gently at all times and with patience. It is important to appreciate that if any maneuver does not work then one should adapt and be prepared to alter one's technique or the patient's position to better deal with the problem.

The one-person method of performing either sigmoidoscopy or colonoscopy is preferred. This approach allows the operator to control all aspects of the examination without needing to rely on an assistant. This is especially important when applying torque to the shaft to change direction of the instrument tip and to derotate loops with safety and when performing polypectomy.

The examination is usually started with the patient in the left lateral position. The thumb, index and middle fingers of the dominant hand are needed to apply torque and the shaft of the instrument should be held with a gauze square for necessary traction. The vertical and horizontal controls of the tip are worked with the other thumb. Keeping the instrument short, using minimal insufflation, regularly pulling back and then advancing the shaft forwards in small increments and only when there is an adequate view of the lumen makes for a safe technique. Intubation is continuously adjusted by rotating the shaft between fingers and thumb and aligning the scope in the direction of the mucosal folds aimed at the center of the lumen to thread the shortened colon over the instrument. Total colonoscopy to the cecum is usually possible by advancement of the shaft for 70–80 cm from the anal verge, providing all major loops of the colon have been reduced. Gentle targeted abdominal palpation by an assistant to better control a redundant sigmoid or transverse colon is useful, as is intermittent suction to collapse the proximal colon when negotiating the hepatic flexure to enter the ascending colon.

The modern design and use of the variable stiffness setting available in current instruments have virtually eliminated the need for 'overtubes' or an image intensifier to overcome troublesome loop formation or to locate the position of the instrument tip. However, as the light intensity is less than in previous fiberoptic instruments, transillumination in the right iliac fossa (RIF) to confirm the position of the cecum is unreliable. It is far better to photograph the caput cecum with its characteristic anatomy, including the origin of the teniae coli (so-called 'crow's foot'), the appendiceal orifice, the ileocecal valve and intubation of the terminal ileum (**Figures 2.3.5, 2.3.6, and 2.3.7**). The presence of feces in the cecum obscuring the view can be largely resolved by using a foot-pedalled, 'fine-flushing' device which produces a high pressure water jet to wash away residual fecal material. Taking note of other key landmarks during examination will orientate and thus assist the endoscopist to judge progress.

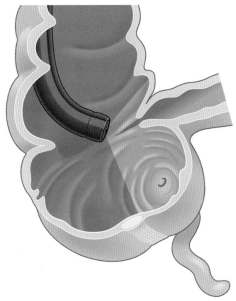

2.3.5 Caput cecum, appendiceal orifice, and ileocecal valve.

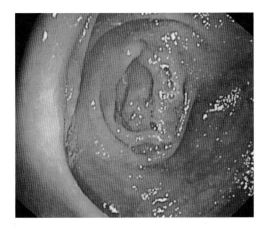

2.3.6 Endoscopic view of cecum and ileocecal valve.

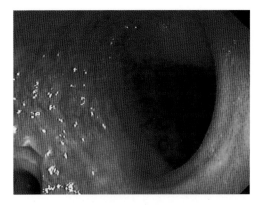

2.3.7 Endoscopic view of terminal ileum.

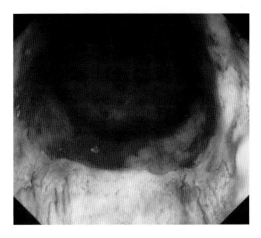

2.3.8 Endoscopic view of anal canal and dentate line.

Anal canal

The transition from the upper anal canal to the rectum is clearly identified by the presence of the dentate line, the hemorrhoidal cushions, and the gradual change in appearance from stratified squamous, non-keratinized to columnar mucus-secreting epithelium, including a variable transition zone (**Figure 2.3.8**). The anal canal is best examined with a proctoscope rather than by retroflexing the tip of the colonoscope, which is both unnecessary and potentially hazardous.

Rectum

The rectal lumen is characterized by the presence of the three semilunar valves of Houston prior to negotiating the rectosigmoid junction and distal sigmoid. A distended rectal lumen is capacious and time should be taken to carefully inspect the whole of its surface. Locating the distal edge and distance of a lesion from the anal verge is best performed, whenever possible, with the patient lying in the left lateral position using a rigid sigmoidoscope as measurements taken at flexible endoscopy are notoriously inaccurate.

Rectosigmoid

The rectosigmoid is the first difficult segment to engage and in this situation performing 'slide by', that is, blindly advancing the instrument with forceful stretching of the rectal wall causing mucosal blanching and loss of the vascular pattern should be avoided. The key is to keep to the center of the lumen, keep the instrument short, and advance with gentle torque and insufflation.

Sigmoid

The sigmoid lumen is characterized by narrowing and mucosal crowding, tortuosity, and often the presence of multiple diverticula (**Figures 2.3.9** and **2.3.10**). This is variable depending on the degree of shortening and

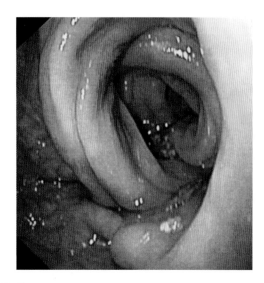

2.3.9 Endoscopic view of sigmoid colon.

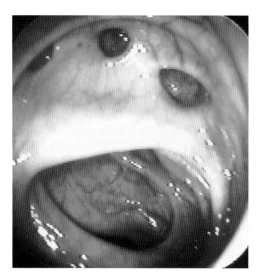

2.3.10 Endoscopic view showing diverticular disease with muscle trabeculation and multiple diverticula.

muscle hypertrophy from associated diverticular disease. Muscle trabeculation and wide-mouth diverticula can add to the disorientation of the examiner and care must be taken to ensure a clear proximal view before advancing the instrument. Any persistent angulation with loss of lumen and a sensation of rigidity or fixation must be appreciated. This is important in women who have had a hysterectomy. In this situation, if the patient is restless or uncomfortable, the procedure is best abandoned and the patient re-examined using either a barium enema or computed tomography (CT) colography.

Descending colon – splenic flexure

The lumen of the descending colon is usually relatively straight and easily traversed (**Figure 2.3.11**). The

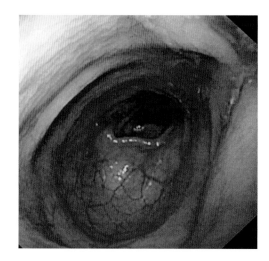

2.3.11 Endoscopic view of descending colon.

splenic flexure is thin walled and often identified by the transilluminated shadow of the inferior pole of the spleen. Its angulation depends on the degree of laxity of attachment of the phrenocolic ligament and in some patients difficulty in negotiating the flexure usually implies poor control of the sigmoid colon due to looping. This is overcome by shortening the instrument to straighten the lower left colon assisted by gentle abdominal palpation to splint the sigmoid or else rotate the patient to the supine position.

Transverse colon – hepatic flexure

The transverse colon is clearly demarcated by its triangular outline due to the orientation of the three teniae coli and the extent of circular muscle hypertrophy (**Figure 2.3.12**). Passage under the liver is recognized by noting the distinct

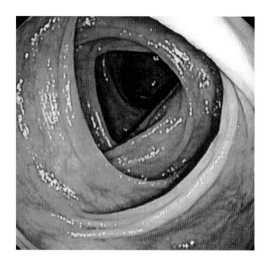

2.3.12 Endoscopic view of transverse colon.

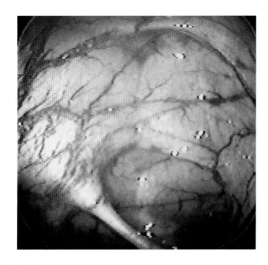

2.3.13 Endoscopic view of hepatic shadow.

transilluminated shadow through the thin colonic wall (**Figure 2.3.13**).

Negotiating the hepatic flexure to enter the ascending colon is assisted by palpating the upper mid-abdomen and occasionally rotating the patient into the supine or the right semi-prone position, while applying suction to deflate the colon and draw it on to the scope.

Polypectomy and other considerations

It is important to confirm the diagnosis of an adenomatous polyp. In the case of small polyps, even experienced clinicians are not always able to correctly distinguish between a hyperplastic polyp and an adenoma based solely on the endoscopic appearance.[7] Ideally, all polyps should be removed for histology using either a 'hot' biopsy forceps or diathermy snare. High resolution and high magnification colonoscopy, together with chromoendoscopy, will significantly improve the detection of flat or depressed lesions. This technique is also increasingly preferred as the method of choice for long-term endoscopic surveillance for dysplasia in patients with chronic ulcerative colitis.[8]

Multiple polyps

Small flat polyps are best removed when they are first encountered as they may easily be missed on extubation. Larger lesions may be more easily removed during scope withdrawal after completion of the examination. The colon is then straighter, allowing better tip control to maneuver the snare. If multiple polyps are observed, especially if confined to one anatomical segment, consideration should be given to bowel resection to achieve a 'clean' colon rather than repeating numerous examinations and polypectomies.

Diminutive sessile polyps

For diminutive (≤ 5 mm), sessile polyps found incidentally at diagnostic colonoscopy in an elderly patient, the presence of comorbidities will influence the decision to perform a polypectomy. Care must be taken to avoid a full thickness burn with delayed perforation or secondary hemorrhage when using hot biopsy forceps to remove small lesions. The polyp is best grasped at its tip and pulled away from the mucosal surface before applying a brief burst of current to achieve coagulation (**Figure 2.3.14**). A blanching effect will be apparent indicating coagulative necrosis and most of the polyp will then slough leaving a shallow, healing ulcer.

Taking a deep bite by pushing the cups of the forceps firmly against the bowel wall will include deeper tissue and increase the risk of perforation. This is more likely to occur depending on the intensity and the duration of current application. Following a hot biopsy, one must ensure that the colon is adequately deflated to avoid unnecessary distension, particularly if the biopsy has been taken from the thin-walled right colon. Alternatively, these polyps can be safely removed with a mini-snare.

Larger sessile polyps

Sessile polyps between 1 and 2 cm in size are usually removed by snaring, making sure to 'tent' the polyp into the lumen and avoid inadvertent contact with surrounding tissue.

Polyps which are greater than 2 cm in diameter may be removed piecemeal beginning with the distal portion of the polyp (**Figure 2.3.15**). A submucosal injection of saline, combined with adrenaline to produce a bloodless 'bleb' or fluid cushion which lifts the mucosal lesion off the underlying circular muscle will provide a safe plane on

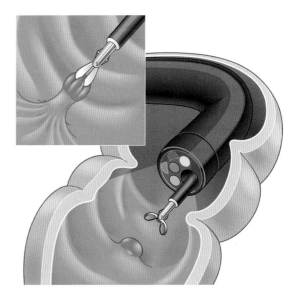

2.3.14 Application of hot biopsy forceps.

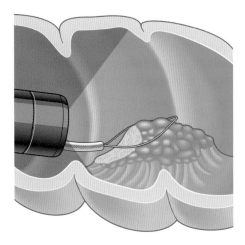

2.3.15 Piecemeal removal of polyp.

which to perform the polypectomy reducing the risk of a full thickness burn (**Figure 2.3.16**). With very flat polyps, care should be taken to avoid injecting directly into the underlying muscularis propria so as not to obscure the submucosal plane making it difficult to apply a snare.

Endoscopic mucosal resection (EMR) with saline lift is an effective technique for dealing with large, flat lesions extending beyond one-third of the circumference of the

bowel wall with a minimal spreading margin. Polyps involving more than two haustral folds or extending on to the ileocecal valve or when there is visual suspicion of invasive malignancy may be better managed by bowel resection.

EMR is time-consuming and there is an appreciable risk of bleeding, perforation, and long-term stricture formation, as well as the risk of persistent polyp. Furthermore, multiple examinations may be necessary to achieve complete clearance and this can be a concern for patients with right-sided lesions and significant distal diverticular disease, making subsequent colonoscopy technically demanding. The chance of any complication occurring when resecting a right-sided polyp is of the order of 12 percent. During prolonged EMR, intravenous antibiotic cover to safeguard against the risk of bacteremia is recommended.

Careful patient selection is most important if deciding to use this technique and, if in doubt, the patient should be referred to an experienced endoscopist or a laparoscopic resection should be considered. Tattooing to indicate the site of the polyp is particularly helpful in this situation.

The pedunculated polyp

Stalked polyps are best removed with a diathermy snare. The snare must be precisely positioned over the head of

2.3.16 (a) Sessile polyp; (b) post-injection with indigocarmine, saline, and adrenaline; (c) snare polypectomy; (d) residual post-resection defect. (Courtesy of Dr Michael Bourke, Westmead Hospital, Sydney, Australia.)

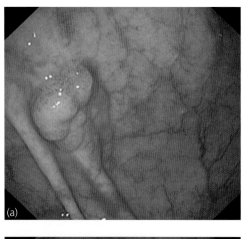

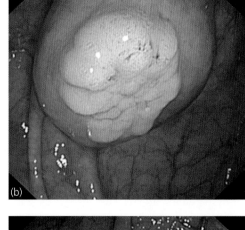

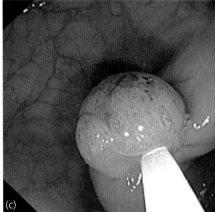

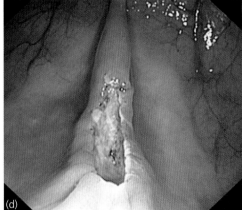

the polyp and adjusted to fit just below the junction of the head and stalk and away from the bowel wall (**Figure 2.3.17**). To accurately place the snare, the patient's position may need to be changed. Small bursts of current at the lowest setting (15–20 W) in coagulation mode should be applied to the stalk to produce mucosal blanching. Moving the lassooed polyp around when transecting the stalk should avoid inadvertent contralateral mucosal burns. If necessary, once the stalk has been cut it can be resnared and further coagulation performed to achieve hemostasis. Preinjecting a thick stalk with 1:10 000 dilute adrenaline and applying the snare above the blanched area will also lessen the risk of reactionary bleeding at the time of polypectomy (**Figure 2.3.18**).

Retrieving and handling the specimen

All specimens should be recovered for histopathology.

Small specimens are easily suctioned through the scope and collected into a dedicated polyp trap. Larger polyps may be retrieved by suction on to the tip of the scope and withdrawing the specimen and scope together. Otherwise, a large polyp may need to be resnared or entrapped using three-pronged grasping forceps, a Dormia basket, or a nylon net. If the polyp is temporarily lost, then irrigating the lumen with water and aspirating will identify the specimen. Alternatively, the patient will need to use a bedpan as a last resort.

Malignant polyps

Close communication between endoscopist and pathologist is most important in the management of patients who have had a 'malignant' polyp treated by endoscopic polypectomy. Here, the pathologist must have adequate clinical information on which to base the final report.

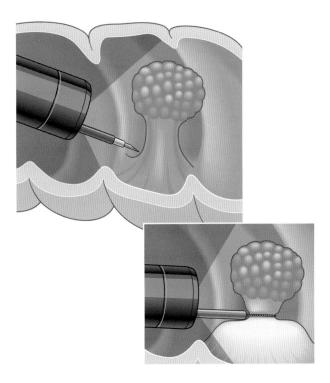

2.3.18 Basal injection of 1:10 000 adrenaline solution.

Whenever possible, histological slides should be reviewed conjointly and a consensus reached so that the report is issued using clear, unambiguous terminology. To ensure this, the request form should include an estimate of size, as well as location, together with information on the shape, mobility, and presence or absence of surface ulceration. When multiple polyps are removed, each should be placed in its own clearly labelled specimen jar. For pedunculated polyps, the stalk should be identified and preferably the specimen should be pinned out on to backing using a fine hypodermic needle before immersing the specimen into 10 percent formalin. This will greatly assist the pathologist to orientate the specimen correctly.

The pathologist should describe the villous content, the degree of dysplasia, extent of clearance of diathermy margins, and the presence of pseudoinvasion which may occasionally cause confusion in interpreting the true level of invasion in a 'malignant' polyp. Also, clear distinction between a small polypoid carcinoma and malignant invasion in an adenoma is particularly important, as the former invariably will require a colectomy, while the latter may be managed conservatively in the absence of other adverse features. For patients with multiple polyps, the index adenoma is usually defined as that with the most severe dysplasia or the largest of two or more equally dysplastic adenomas. The characteristics of the index polyp will usually determine management, the need, and the frequency of subsequent endoscopic surveillance.

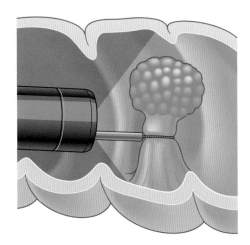

2.3.17 Correct application of diathermy snare.

Associated procedures

COLONIC TATTOOING PRIOR TO LAPAROSCOPY

Laparoscopic colectomy is a useful alternative to EMR for the management of patients with large flat polyps. Undoubtedly, these can be effectively removed by a competent endoscopist and the decision to proceed in either direction should be made in a multidisciplinary setting with review of the relevant histology. If a laparoscopic approach is used, accurate preoperative identification of the site by tattooing the segment of bowel is essential. This is best and reliably performed by using Indian ink (SPOT®, GI Supply, Camp Hill, PA, USA) during the initial diagnostic procedure.

ENDOSCOPIC LASER THERAPY

Endoscopic laser therapy (ELT) is a useful adjunct to colonoscopy and depending on the wavelength and power setting it may be used in a controlled, precise manner to produce coagulation, carbonization, or vaporization of tissue. It is commonly used to produce hemostasis and to debulk tumors. It can be combined with radiotherapy to palliate advanced cancers or combined with colonoscopic balloon dilatation to open short segment fibrous strictures. Generally, the neodymium yttrium aluminum garnet (NdYAG) laser with a 1064-nm wavelength using a non-contact probe passed through the biopsy channel of the colonoscope is the most useful method of delivering ELT to treat large bowel pathology.

For hemostasis, a low power setting of 10–30 W for 0.5 s at a working distance of 1.0 cm is sufficient to treat angiodysplasia by blanching the mucosal surface. Treatment should begin at the periphery of the lesion if greater than 5 mm in diameter and then be directed to its center. The colon must then be deflated to avoid delayed perforation. Hemostasis in the right colon may also be achieved by APC using a non-contact technique to produce a superficial burn not exceeding 2–3 mm in depth.

Combined endoscopic NdYAG laser treatment with external beam radiotherapy or with brachytherapy using iridium-192 necessitates close cooperation with a radiation oncologist. The aim of this treatment is to debulk tumors and create an adequate lumen, achieve hemostasis, and dry up mucus discharge using both coagulation and vaporization. This technique has the advantage of reducing the symptomatic relapse rate compared to patients treated by laser alone,[9] and provides effective palliation of patients with advanced, inoperable rectal cancer with minimal morbidity and can be performed as an outpatient procedure. The laser is delivered preferably via a 60 cm sigmoidoscope aimed at 0.5–1.0 cm from the target with the machine enabled at 40–80 W of power, set at a pulse-mode of 0.5–1.0 s.

ELT is also used to perform a stricturotomy combined with balloon dilatation to open tight fibrous strictures, using a non-contact probe with the machine enabled at 40 W and a 1-s pulse mode. One, two, or more transverse cuts are made in the circumference of the stricture and the lumen is then dilated under direct vision with an endoscopic balloon.

Balloon dilatation

The current generation of 'through the scope balloon catheters' (CRE™ Wireguided, Boston Scientific) are available in a range of diameters (12–20 mm) produced by controlled radial expansion and varying lengths of 180–240 cm. These catheters are designed to pass through the working channel of the scope specified on the package label and positioned across the stricture. It is useful to prelubricate the instrument channel with a silicon spray before introducing the catheter. The balloon is inflated under direct vision using an Alliance™ II single-use syringe/gauge system. The gauge is graduated in both atmospheres (12 ATM) and kilopascals (1200 Pa) maximum (Boston Scientific). The balloon must be completely deflated using this device prior to its withdrawal.

Stenting

Colonoscopic placement of self-expandable metal stents (SEMS) under fluoroscopic control is generally well tolerated and an effective palliation for patients with incurable, metastatic cancer presenting with obstruction (**Figure 2.3.19**). However, stent-related perforation (reported in up to 20 percent of patients) remains an important concern. Where preliminary dilatation is considered necessary for stent placement, a decision not to proceed necessitates careful consideration given the risk of stent migration, occlusion, and perforation, especially in those patients who are likely to survive for more than a few weeks.

Self-expandable metal stents combined with palliative

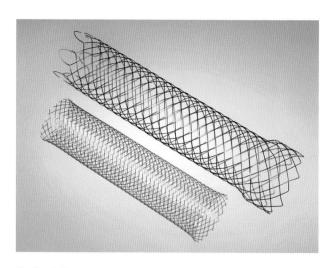

2.3.19 Deployed enteric Wallstents (reproduced with permission from Boston Scientific Inc.).

chemotherapy to avoid laparotomy in patients with advanced disease remains controversial.[10]

PATIENT RECOVERY AND MANAGEMENT OF COMPLICATIONS

Most complications can be foreseen and largely prevented. They may be general and related to the sedation used or they may be specific to colonoscopy per se. Elderly frail patients are best examined with the assistance of an anesthetist. After examination, the responsibility remains with the endoscopist to review the patient prior to discharge to ensure that they are recovered adequately to be allowed home safely with a responsible carer. The procedure should be briefly discussed with the patient in the predischarge area and arrangements made for a more formal consultation later when the final pathology can be discussed and a decision made about further management or surveillance, where appropriate.

It is useful to give a simple discharge instruction sheet to the patient which includes contact telephone numbers and specific directions of what is normal postprocedure, and what to be aware of and how to reach the endoscopist over the ensuing 24 hours should a problem arise.

Indications for a possible overnight admission to hospital include poor recovery from sedation, a technically difficult polypectomy, or multiple polypectomies in a patient who complains of pain or bleeding or who is generally frail or who may be socially isolated or without an escort. After colonoscopy, careful observation is necessary, taking particular note of vital signs and any complaints of abdominal pain or bleeding. The two most likely complications that may occur are perforation or hemorrhage.

Perforation

Bowel perforation can be classified as mechanical, pneumatic, or thermal when associated with polypectomy. Mechanical perforation implies a disruption to the bowel wall due to direct trauma from forceful advancement of the instrument often without a clear view of the lumen. Not infrequently, there is associated pathology which puts the patient at risk because of a fixed angulation or tortuosity secondary to IBD, phlegmonous diverticular disease, ischemic colitis, or previous irradiation. This may be further complicated by poor vision resulting from inadequate bowel preparation.

The onset of pain, a change in the patient's vital signs, difficulty in maintaining luminal distension or the recognition of a peritoneal structure (mesenteric fat) during the examination will confirm that a full thickness tear has occurred. However, presentation in association with an incomplete tear or a subserosal antimesenteric hematoma especially in the rectosigmoid and sigmoid with signs of peritonitis may not be apparent until hours or even days later.

Pneumatic perforation is due to overforceful distension with a high intraluminal pressure sufficient to rupture the thin-walled colon, most commonly in the cecum (in accordance with the Law of LaPlace). Thermal perforation is due to full thickness coagulative necrosis occurring during polypectomy using either a snare or hot biopsy forceps. On occasions, this can also complicate endoscopic laser or APC procedures.

Post-polypectomy syndrome refers to an incomplete injury or a local leak with signs of localized abdominal pain or tenderness, but without evidence of spreading peritonitis or free gas on a plain abdominal x-ray.

REFERENCES

1. Chapuis PH, Faithfull GR, Dent OF. Large bowel segment lengths and the distribution of colorectal cancer. *Australia and New Zealand Journal of Surgery* 1982; **52**: 385–90.
2. Vening W, Willigendael EM, Tjeertes EKM *et al.* Timing and necessity of a flexible sigmoidoscopy in patients with symptoms suggestive of haemorrhoids. *Colorectal Disease* 2010; **12**: 109–13.
3. Song LM, Adler DG, Conway JD *et al.* Narrow band imaging and multiband imaging. *Gastrointestinal Endoscopy* 2008; **67**: 581–9.
4. Anon. *Standards for endoscopic facilities and services*, 3rd edn. Gastroenterological Society of Australia, 2006. Available from: www.gesa.org.au.
5. Anon. *Guidelines on sedation and/or analgesia for diagnostic and interventional medical or surgical procedures.* Australian and New Zealand College of Anaesthetists, 2008. Available from: www.anzca.edu.au.
6. Rex DK, Petrini JL, Baron TH *et al.* Quality indicators for colonoscopy. *American Journal of Gastroenterology* 2006; **101**: 873–85.
7. Chapuis PH, Dent OF, Goulston KJ. Clinical accuracy in the diagnosis of small polyps using the flexible fiberoptic sigmoidoscope. *Diseases of the Colon and Rectum* 1982; **25**: 669–72.
8. Efthymiou M. Endoscopic surveillance in colitis in 2010: time for a change? *Australia and New Zealand Journal of Surgery* 2010; **80**: 125–6.
9. Chapuis PH, Yuile P, Dent OF *et al.* Combined endoscopic laser and radiotherapy palliation of advanced rectal cancer. *Australia and New Zealand Journal of Surgery* 2002; **72**: 95–9.
10. van Hooft JE, Fockens P, Marinelli AW *et al.* Early closure of a multicenter randomized clinical trial of endoscopic stenting versus surgery for stage IV left-sided colorectal cancer. *Endoscopy* 2008; **40**: 184–91.

Treatment of uncomplicated hemorrhoids

CAROLINE WRIGHT

HISTORY

Topical treatment of hemorrhoids dates back to 1700BC and the first surgical treatment was described in 460BC[1] in the Hippocratic Treatises. The principles of treatment of hemorrhoids have changed little over the centuries, even if the techniques have evolved. John Morgan first used sclerotherapy in 1869 in Dublin to obliterate hemorrhoids by using iron persulfate.[2] Although ligation of the hemorrhoidal mass has been the basis of many treatments over the centuries, band ligation was first described by Blaisdell in 1954;[3] the technique was later modified by Barron in 1963.[4] Neiger described the use of infrared coagulation to treat hemorrhoids in 1979.[5] Newer coagulative techniques continue to evolve. A more recent technique, Doppler-guided transanal hemorrhoidal dearterialization (HAL) may bridge the gap between nonsurgical techniques and excisional hemorrhoidectomy (open, closed, or stapled). HAL was first described by the Japanese surgeon, Kazumasa Morinaga in 1995.[6]

PRINCIPLES AND JUSTIFICATION

Hemorrhoids are fibrovascular 'cushions'[7] found in the subepithelial space. The cushions contain blood vessels supported by a framework of connective tissue, elastic tissue, and smooth muscle. The blood vessels comprise arteriovenous communications between the terminal branches of the superior and middle rectal arteries and the superior, middle, and inferior rectal venous systems. Hemorrhoids are divided into internal and external components dependent on whether they originate above or below the dentate line. There are three main cushions in the left lateral, right anterior, and right posterior positions; this is the recommended terminology because it is not dependent on the position of the patient. Varying degrees of secondary hemorrhoids, between the main complexes, may also be found.

Internal hemorrhoids are covered with columnar epithelium, which is viscerally innervated, therefore insensate to pain, touch, or temperature. External hemorrhoids have normal sensation as they are covered by modified squamous epithelium (anoderm).

The Goligher system is the most widely used classification system of hemorrhoids. There are four grades:

1 First-degree hemorrhoids bleed, but do not prolapse.
2 Second-degree hemorrhoids bleed and prolapse, but reduce spontaneously post-defecation.
3 Third-degree hemorrhoids prolapse and need to be manually reduced.
4 Fourth-degree hemorrhoids are irreducible.

First-degree, second-degree, and small third-degree hemorrhoids can be readily treated in the outpatient/office setting using non-excisional techniques because internal haemorrhoids are insensate. All methods, except HAL, predominantly work by producing submucosal fibrosis and thereby fix/re-anchor the apex of the hemorrhoid in place to reduce symptoms. Rubber band ligation, in addition, results in fixation with tissue excision. Each technique has advantages in specific circumstances, and may be performed as an individual procedure or in combination with other procedures.

Surgical hemorrhoidectomy techniques are reserved for fourth-degree hemorrhoids and symptomatic third-degree hemorrhoids that have not responded to outpatient treatment. These techniques are described elsewhere.

Indications

Contrary to popular belief, hemorrhoids are a normal part of human anatomy. The hemorrhoidal plexus has a role in the maintenance of continence; it is estimated to contribute up to 15–20 percent of the resting anal pressure and is important in providing a watertight seal.[7] Treatment should only be undertaken for symptom control. The type of treatment depends on the degree of prolapse and severity of symptoms, with the aim of minimizing adverse effects.

Common symptoms include bleeding per rectum and prolapse/protrusion from the anal verge. Bleeding, often associated with defecation, is not always associated with prolapse and can be a result of localized mucosal trauma and damage to the underlying vasculature. Prolapse occurs as the connective tissue support of the hemorrhoidal complex deteriorates with age and is compounded by straining, and the anal cushion is displaced caudally.

Secondary symptoms due to prolapse include mucus discharge, pruritus, difficulty with anal toilet, and fecal soiling. Loss of the watertight seal formed by the blood-filled cushions can lead to seepage of fecal material and/or flatus and disordered sensation. Anal pain is not a feature and when present suggests either a complication of hemorrhoids, such as thrombosis, or other pathology, such as an anal fissure or perianal sepsis.

Operations

Non-surgical treatments include:

- **Rubber band ligation**: this is the gold standard for the treatment of internal uncomplicated hemorrhoids. It is particularly useful for second- and third-degree hemorrhoids.
- **Injection sclerotherapy** is effective for controlling bleeding, particularly if the hemorrhoid is not bulky (first- and small second-degree hemorrhoids). It may also be used to supplement banding, or for recurrent bleeding post-hemorrhoidectomy. It can be used in patients who are on anticoagulants.

Both rubber band ligation and sclerotherapy are simple, inexpensive procedures and quick to perform. The instruments required are simple and universally available in their various forms.

- **Coagulative therapies** include infrared photocoagulation, electrocoagulation, radiofrequency ablation, and cryotherapy. These techniques are most suited to bleeding first- and small second-degree hemorrhoids. They all rely on the coagulation, occlusion, or sclerosis of the hemorrhoidal vascular pedicle. Following tissue destruction, the area sloughs leaving an ulcer that forms fibrotic tissue at the treatment site. Their main limitation is the need for specialized more expensive equipment which tends to be available only in more major centers or those which have developed an interest in the technique. Of the coagulative therapies, infrared coagulation is the most widely used. It can be used in hepatitis B or C, or HIV-positive patients as it does not cause bleeding, and is particularly useful in patients who are receiving anticoagulants, who are immunocompromised or are pregnant.

- **Doppler-guided transanal hemorrhoidal artery ligation**, also called the hemorrhoidal artery ligation operation (HALO), or transanal hemorrhoidal dearterialization (THD), is relatively new minimally invasive therapeutic technique, which can be performed in the outpatient setting, and appears to be a potential treatment option for second- and third-degree hemorrhoids.

Contraindications

Treatment should be deferred in the presence of thrombosis or sepsis, active inflammatory bowel disease, or in bleeding associated with immunodeficiency disorders, such as acute leukemia. Injection is best avoided during pregnancy. Injection may be repeated, but it is not advisable to do so within 3 weeks because of the risk of causing injection ulcers, which can bleed profusely. Banding should not be used for external hemorrhoids.

Conservative management

Conservative management should be discussed with all patients, whether or not further surgical intervention is undertaken. The aim is to optimize defecatory function and anal hygiene to help prevent recurrence. Adequate fiber (25–30 g/day) and fluid intake should normalize the stool to give a soft but formed stool. Psyllium, sterculia, guar gum, and methylcellulose are commonly used fiber supplements. Patients should be educated in good defecation dynamics and to avoid straining and spending prolonged periods sitting on the toilet. Stool softeners may also be used to minimize straining. Over-the-counter topical agents include simple analgesic ointments, astringents, steroid-containing agents, and antiseptics. These tend to have a soothing effect, but do not actually cure the underlying condition. Long-term use of these agents should be discouraged, particularly steroid-containing preparations, because of the risk of local reactions and sensitization of the skin. In Europe, venotonics, such as flavoids, are available and popular, and may work by improving venous tone, reducing hyperpermeability, and have anti-inflammatory properties;[8] however, studies of effectiveness are inconsistent.

PREOPERATIVE ASSESSMENT

A thorough history and examination including inspection of the perineum, rectal examination, and proctosigmoidoscopy should be undertaken prior to any treatment to exclude other anorectal pathology, including fissures, fistulae, anal skin tags, hypertrophied anal papillae, anal warts, and rectal prolapse. In particular, inflammatory bowel disease, rectal polyps, or carcinoma should be excluded. If proximal colonic pathology is suggested by the history and examination findings, or the patient is over 50 years of age, a colonoscopy or alternative method of visualizing the colon, is indicated. Hemorrhoid disease in association with the symptoms of soiling and fecal incontinence may require anorectal physiology studies and an endoanal ultrasound prior to any intervention.

PREPARATION

No special preparation is required, although an enema or suppositories may be used to facilitate the view if the rectum is loaded with soft feces. Dependent on the relative risk–benefit profile, it is advisable to cease anticoagulation therapy, including warfarin and antiplatelet agents, and non-steroidal anti-inflammatory agents prior to treatment, because of the increased risk of post-treatment bleeding. These can usually be reinstated after 10 days, once the main risk of secondary hemorrhage has passed. It is recommended, however, that the above is discussed with the patient's cardiologist or primary care physician. Sclerotherapy, or one of the other coagulative therapies, may be preferred to rubber band ligation if a patient is unable to stop taking anticoagulant therapy.

Antibiotic prophylaxis is indicated for patients with valvular heart disease or immune deficiency, because of the risk of transient bacteremia after banding and injection sclerotherapy.

ANESTHESIA

These treatments can be performed in the office or out-patient setting and, except for HAL, do not require anesthesia. They are often, however, performed as an adjunct to another procedure, such as a flexible sigmoidoscopy or colonoscopy, in which conscious sedation is used. Although the focus area of treatment is the insensate mucosa overlying internal hemorrhoids, patients often experience some discomfort or sphincter spasm afterwards – particularly those with high anal tone and good sphincter function. Prospective randomized trials assessing the use of local anesthetic injection into or around the ligation site, however, have failed to demonstrate any benefit in terms of reducing post-banding discomfort.[8] It is the author's practice, however, to use a local anesthetic gel (such as 2 percent lidocaine gel) as the lubricant for the proctoscope, or to insert this into the anal canal at the end of the treatment.

Doppler-guided HAL can be performed under intravenous sedation (midazolam or propofol) and local anesthesia, using 2 percent lidocaine, which is locally injected at the 3 and 9 o'clock positions.

POSITION OF THE PATIENT

HAL is performed best in the lithotomy position. All the other procedures, however, are usually performed with the patient in the left lateral Sims position. Alternatively, the patient may be placed in the semi-inverted (jack-knife) position on a proctological table.

PROCEDURES

Rubber band ligation

INSTRUMENTS (Figure 2.4.1)

There are many versions of hemorrhoidal ligators, but they tend to all have the same basic design, including a barrel or suction cap to trap/pull down the hemorrhoidal tissue and a triggering mechanism to deploy/fire the rubber bands. Banding removes excess hemorrhoidal tissue by strangulation. The remaining ulcer scars, and the internal hemorrhoid remnant is anchored back in place.

The hemorrhoids may be grasped using angulated forceps, for example the McGivney ligator, or suctioned using one of the suction band ligators. The non-suction techniques require an assistant to hold the proctoscope, as the primary operator has to hold both the ligator and the grasping forceps. The suction band ligators have the advantage of not requiring an assistant. Suction ligators include the non-disposable McGown ligator, or one of the many brands of disposable suction ligators; these are increasingly used because of the risk of transmissible diseases. Proprietary brands include the KilRoid™ suction ligator, which is attached to wall suction, or the O'Regan™ ligator, which is combined with a syringe to produce suction.

TECHNIQUE

One or two rubber bands are loaded on to the band applicator. A well-lubricated lighted proctoscope/anoscope is passed through the anal canal into the rectum, and then withdrawn slowly until the hemorrhoidal tissue prolapses into view. An anoscope with a beveled end allows the hemorrhoid to more readily prolapse into the lumen of the scope. The suction device or grasping forceps (such as Allis forceps) are applied to the base of the hemorrhoid about 2 cm above the dentate line. If the patient feels significant pain, the hemorrhoid has been grasped too caudally where there is sensate mucosa, and should be regrasped more proximally (**Figure 2.4.2**).

The rubber band(s) is then deployed (**Figure 2.4.3**). Up to a maximum of three sites can be banded in one sitting and is the author's practice. Some surgeons, however, prefer to band only two sites per sitting because there is a higher rate of pain and vasovagal symptoms with triple ligation in one setting.

For large volume hemorrhoidal prolapse, serial bands (one above the other) can be placed to reduce the degree of prolapse, in which case it is definitely advisable to band only one or two complexes in one sitting.

The tissue usually necroses in 7–10 days, when the band and hemorrhoid slough. Rebanding can be easily performed for recurrent symptoms with minimal morbidity. When banding small hemorrhoids, a small volume of sclerosant or local anesthetic can be injected into the ligated mass to make it tenser and encourage sloughing. Band ligation can also be performed endoscopically using a flexible scope. Hemorrhoidal banding using this method is performed

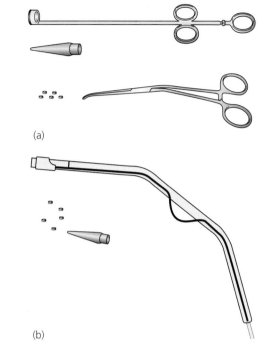

(a)

(b)

2.4.1

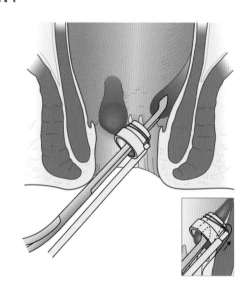

2.4.2

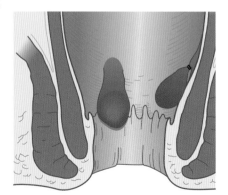

2.4.3

the same way as banding esophageal varices. The bands are deployed with the scope retroflexed, giving a clearer view.

COMPLICATIONS

Complications (<1%–3% of patients) include the following:

- Bleeding: secondary hemorrhage can be significant after the rubber band has sloughed. Patients should be warned that a small amount of bleeding per rectum is common post-procedure; this tends to occur 7–10 days post-banding as the band sloughs. However, patients should be advised to seek medical attention if they experience more significant bleeding, in which case bleeding may be controlled with an adrenaline-soaked or alginate anal pack. If the bleeding point is not controlled with pressure, the bleeding point can be suture ligated under a general anesthetic.
- Discomfort: this is caused by anal sphincter spasm, and is associated with an urge to defecate. It can last a varying length of time, but is generally worse in the first 24 hours, and may be relieved by warm sitz baths. Pain developing slowly 1–2 days post-banding may be from ischemia. Severe pain is caused by an application too close to the dentate line and the band should be removed.
- Vasovagal syncope.
- Urinary retention.
- Thrombosis of the external component.
- Chronic ulcer.
- Necrotizing pelvic sepsis is a rare, but serious complication. It should be suspected if there is the clinical triad of severe increasing pain, pyrexia, and urinary retention. In this situation, an examination under anesthesia is recommended, with drainage of any abscess and antibiotic treatment.
- Band slippage.

Injection sclerotherapy

INSTRUMENTS (Figure 2.4.4)

The most popular sclerosant is 5 percent phenol in almond or arachis oil; other sclerosants used include 5 percent quinine and urea, hypertonic saline, and sodium tetradecyl sulfate. Following injection, the vessels thrombose, there is sclerosis of the connective tissue, and shrinkage and fixation of the overlying mucosa. Because of the increased prevalence of transmissible diseases, a 10 mL disposable plastic syringe is preferred to the traditional Gabriel glass syringe. A wide bore drawing up straw is required to draw up the thick oily sclerosant into the syringe.

TECHNIQUE

Using a well-lubricated lighted proctoscope 2–3 mL sclerosant is injected into the submucosal plane at the apices of the hemorrhoidal complexes, avoiding the lumen of the vessel (Figure 2.4.5).

The injection should produce a swelling with a pearly appearance/wheal. By moving the injection slightly during injection, intravascular injection should be avoided. All three primary hemorrhoids can be injected at the same time. Injection should be painless. If pain is experienced, then the needle has been placed too low or, if resistance is felt, the needle is in the wrong plane. If a wheal is not

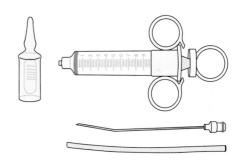

2.4.4

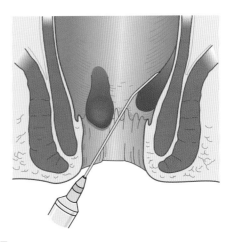

2.4.5

observed the injection is too deep, and if there is blanching of the mucosa the injection is too superficial (**Figure 2.4.6**).

After injecting, delay removing the needle for a few seconds to help lessen the escape of solution. If bleeding occurs, pressure can be applied; if this does not control the bleeding, a rubber band can be used to ligate the bleeding point.

COMPLICATIONS

They include mucosal necrosis and ulceration, local infection and abscess formation, prostatitis, epididymo-orchitis, erectile dysfunction (if parasympathetic nerves are damaged), and urinary retention (from misplaced injections that are too anterior), and portal pyemia. It can cause chest and upper abdominal pain if injected directly into the hemorrhoidal vein.[8] Stricture formation and scarring can occur with repeated procedures.

Both banding and sclerotherapy are relatively cheap procedures, that are easy to perform and teach.

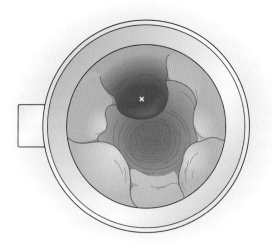

2.4.6

Coagulative therapies

The following techniques are more expensive because they require specialized equipment and therefore are not so commonly performed, except in units with special expertise and interest in the technique.

Infrared coagulation

INSTRUMENTS (Figure 2.4.7)

Infrared coagulation (IRC) coagulates the vessels and fixes the hemorrhoidal tissue by converting light to heat, resulting in tissue destruction. The infrared coagulator has a 15 V tungsten-halogen light as the infrared energy source, which is applied on to the hemorrhoid tissue via a polymer probe tip.[9] The temperature at the tip reaches 100°C. Varying the optical wavelength of the coagulator or the time of exposure varies the depth of penetration and coagulation. The automatic timer range is 0.5–3.0 s, giving a coagulation depth range of 0.5–2.5 mm. The working setting is between 1 and 1.5 s to give a depth of 1 mm of coagulated protein.

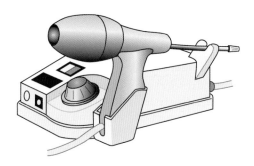

2.4.7

TECHNIQUE (Figure 2.4.8)

Through a well-lubricated lighted proctoscope, the base of the hemorrhoid is identified. The tip of the coagulator is placed in firm contact with the base of the hemorrhoid using light pressure. The instrument is then fired to the end of each automatically timed setting. Three to five exposures are recommended in a triangular or semicircle shape around the base of the hemorrhoid, allowing a gap of a few millimeters between each. The area treated should appear as a white spot after the procedure. At the end of the procedure, the tip of the coagulator should be wiped clean.

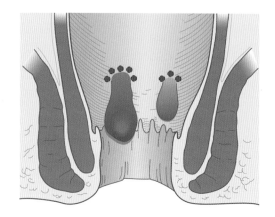

2.4.8

This is one of the most expensive forms of treatment in the outpatient setting because of the cost of the IRC probe.

COMPLICATIONS

IRC is a painless procedure and complications are rare[8] because the effects on the tissues of the anal canal are controlled and reproducible.

Electrocoagulation

Electrocoagulation may be used for first- and second-degree hemorrhoids.

- Bipolar-electrocautery is applied in 1-second pulses of 20 W until the underlying tissue coagulates, which often takes <30 seconds.
- Direct current electrocoagulation requires the prolonged application (up to 10 minutes) of 110 V direct current up to 15 mA and is therefore not popular.

Complications include pain, bleeding, fissure, or spasm. Multiple applications to the same site are often required. It does not eliminate prolapsing tissue.

Electrocoagulation has relatively low complication rates.

Radiofrequency ablation

INSTRUMENTS

This is a technique that converts radiofrequency waves to heat. The radiofrequency unit comprises a transformer that converts the main voltage to a high voltage, very high frequency radiowave of 4 MHz. This is delivered at low temperature through radiofrequency microfiber electrodes. The tissue rather than the electrode serves as the resistance, therefore, there is no heating of the radiofrequency electrodes. Tissue fluids are vaporized without generating heat, resulting in cellular volatilization, which in turn produces coagulation and shrinkage of the tissues. There is no danger of shock or burn injury to the patient, and there is controlled and minimal lateral tissue damage.

TECHNIQUE

Using a lighted lubricated anoscope, the hemorrhoid complex is coagulated from its base by gradually rotating a ball electrode attached to a handle held by the operating surgeon. Shrinkage and gradual change of the hemorrhoid to a dusky white color (blanching) indicates satisfactory coagulation necrosis. The coagulation should be kept above the dentate line to avoid pain during the application of the electrode. Coagulation generally takes between 5 and 10 seconds.

COMPLICATIONS

Complication rates including postoperative pain, swelling, and risk of infection are reported to be lower than other procedures because of the low level of tissue destruction and controlled direction of the radiowave current.

Cryotherapy

Cold coagulation uses nitrous oxide or liquid nitrogen to cause cellular destruction through rapid freezing (−60 to −80°C), followed by rapid thawing. Mentioned for completeness, this technique is no longer recommended for the treatment of hemorrhoids because of its associated morbidity and the availability of alternative treatments associated with fewer complications. Cryotherapy is associated with profuse watery discharge and a foul smell, and can cause pain due to necrosis; in addition, it can cause necrosis of the internal sphincter resulting in anal stenosis and incontinence.

Doppler-guided transanal hemorrhoidal artery ligation

INSTRUMENTS

This technique utilizes a specially designed lighted proctoscope which incorporates a Doppler transducer to identify the terminal branches of the superior rectal artery, of which there is an average of five (range, 1–8). At the distal end of the Doppler transducer, there is also a lateral ligation window, which allows the surgeon to selectively ligate the arteries. The primary aim of the treatment is to reduce the arterial inflow to the hemorrhoidal plexus, leading to shrinkage of the hemorrhoidal cushion and subsequent symptomatic improvement. The potential advantage of this technique is that dearterialization is guided by a Doppler probe, rather than being undertaken blindly.

TECHNIQUE (Figure 2.4.9)

The perineal skin region is cleaned and covered with a sterile drape. Intravenous sedation is given and local anesthetic is infiltrated. Following gel lubrication, the special proctoscope is inserted through the anal canal into the lower rectum and rotated to identify the main arterial trunks. These are then suture ligated in a figure-of-eight fashion. A 2-0 synthetic braided absorbable suture, such as polyglycolic acid, with a 5/8-inch needle is used. When the suture is pulled on, the Doppler signal should be abolished or significantly reduced confirming successful ligation of the artery. Once all the arteries are ligated, an anal sponge covered with lidocaine gel is inserted into the anal canal.

COMPLICATIONS

Complications include anal discomfort, bleeding, thrombosis caused by closure of the venous system, fissures, and submucosal fistula formation. There is also the possibility of revascularization and therefore recurrence of symptomatic hemorrhoids.

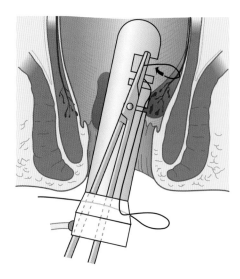

2.4.9

GENERAL POSTOPERATIVE CARE

No special care is required. Patients, however, should be advised what to expect after the procedure, and a patient information sheet is recommended. In particular, patients should be warned of the potential for minor bleeding, and discomfort which may be relieved by warm (40°C) sitz baths and simple analgesics, such as paracetamol. The sitz baths will help reduce tissue edema and sphincter spasm. In addition, patients should be advised to take a fiber supplement to optimize defecatory function, if required.

Outcome

A meta-analysis of 18 distinct randomized controlled studies that compared rubber band ligation, infrared coagulation, sclerotherapy, cryotherapy, hemorrhoidectomy, internal sphincterotomy, and manual dilation of the anus for patients with first-, second-, or third-degree hemorrhoids concluded that rubber band ligation was the initial procedure of choice in this group of patients. Rubber band ligation is associated with a lower recurrence rate, but with more immediate discomfort than sclerotherapy or infrared coagulation.[10] The literature reports a success rate of 75–90 percent for rubber band ligation. About 20 percent of patients develop recurrent symptoms requiring repeat banding and about 2 percent fail to respond to banding.[8] The technique of endoscopic band ligation is at least as effective as conventional rubber band ligation using a rigid proctoscope.[8]

Dietary fiber supplementation increases the long-term cure rate after banding.[8] Infrared coagulation may be as effective as rubber band ligation and sclerotherapy in the treatment of first- and second-degree hemorrhoids.[11] Infrared coagulation is significantly less painful than rubber band ligation, but requires more sessions to relieve symptoms, has a higher recurrence rate, and is more expensive.[10] Electrocoagulation has similar success rates to those of infrared coagulation.[8] There is currently insufficient evidence to judge the effectiveness of radiofrequency ablation compared with other methods.[11, 12]

Transanal hemorrhoidal dearterialization appears to be a potential treatment option for second- and third-degree hemorrhoids, but its role needs to be clarified with clinical trials of longer follow-up to assess its effectiveness in comparison with other established treatments.[11] The majority of studies are low level evidence observational studies, but report a reduction in bleeding in about 90 percent of patients.

REFERENCES

1. Hardy A, Chan CL, Cohen CR. The surgical management of haemorrhoids – a review. *Digestive Surgery* 2005; **22**: 26–33.
2. Morgan J. Varicose state of saphenous haemorrhoids treated successfully by the injection of tincture of persulphate of iron. *Medical Press and Circular* 1869: **29**.
3. Blaisdell PC. Office ligation of internal hemorrhoids. *American Journal of Surgery* 1958; **96**: 401–4.
4. Barron J. Office ligation treatment of hemorrhoids. *Diseases of the Colon and Rectum* 1963; **6**: 109–13.
5. Neiger A. Haemorrhoids in everyday practice. *Proctology* 1979; **2**: 22–8.
6. Morinaga K, Hasuda K, Ikeda T. A novel therapy for internal hemorrhoids: ligation of the hemorrhoidal artery with a newly devised instrument (Moricorn) in conjunction with a Doppler flowmeter. *American Journal of Gastroenterology* 1995; **90**: 610–13.
7. Thomson WH. The nature of haemorrhoids. *British Journal of Surgery* 1975; **62**: 542–52.
8. Chong PS, Bartolo DC. Hemorrhoids and fissure in ano. *Gastroenterology Clinics of North America* 2008; **37**: 627–44, ix.
9. Sneider EB, Maykel JA. Diagnosis and management of symptomatic hemorrhoids. *Surgical Clinics of North America* 2010; **90**: 17–32.
10. MacRae HM, McLeod RS. Comparison of hemorrhoidal treatment modalities. A meta-analysis. *Diseases of the Colon and Rectum* 1995; **38**: 687–94.
11. Reese GE, von Roon AC, Tekkis PP. Hemorrhoids. *Clinical Evidence (Online)* 2009.
12. Rivadeneira DE, Steele SR, Ternent C, Chalasani S, Buie WD, Rafferty JL. Practice Parameters for the Management of Hemorrhoids (Revised 2010). *Dis Colon Rectum* 2011; **54**(9)1059–64.

Excision of perianal thrombosis

BARD C COSMAN

TERMINOLOGY

The terms 'perianal haematoma' (British) and 'thrombosed external hemorrhoid' (American) are synonymous, but neither is sufficiently accurate. 'Perianal hematoma' suggests an extravascular bleed and subsequent collection rather than a discrete venous clot, and 'thrombosed external hemorrhoid' associates this condition with internal hemorrhoids when in fact they are only tangentially related. Both these terms have such wide recognition that a Commonwealth practitioner might puzzle over the American shorthand 'TEH', while a reader of American texts might wonder why one would ever excise a perianal hematoma. The compromise term 'perianal thrombosis', both concise and accurate, is used here.

PRINCIPLES AND JUSTIFICATION

A perianal thrombosis usually develops suddenly when a hemorrhoidal vein at the anal verge thromboses, with consequent inflammation. The inciting event of this thrombosis is usually unknown, but it may accompany straining, some change in bowel habit, or instrumentation such as ligation of internal hemorrhoids. The most prominent feature is swelling, both from the space-occupying blood clot and from inflammation. Physical examination reveals a bluish lump in one quadrant of the anal verge, covered with hairless skin (anoderm), and typically appearing to obliterate the anal opening. Spreading the buttocks moves the lump to one side, revealing an intact distal anal canal. There is occasional necrosis of the overlying anoderm, exposing and sometimes even extruding the clot. Perianal thromboses are usually solitary, but occasionally multiple. The natural history of perianal thrombosis is of an acutely painful anal verge lump which persists for several days to a few weeks, slowly subsiding as the clot is organized and inflammation runs its course. During this period, the clot has acted as a skin expander, so when it resorbs, the patient is left with a skin tag. Many of the skin tags that accumulate with aging are the result of resolved perianal thromboses.

INDICATIONS

The usual course is spontaneous resolution over 2–4 weeks, so there is no absolute indication for surgical intervention. The later in the typical course the patient presents, the stronger the case to do nothing. Surgical intervention eliminates the painful perianal hematoma, replacing it with a painful incision and its attendant inflammation. Therefore, operative treatment is most logical when the patient is seen early and still has pain and edema overlying the clot, usually within 2 days of onset. When the anoderm over the clot is soft and supple, the patient should be warned that excision will cause another cycle of inflammation like the one that he or she has just suffered.

Even after the inflammation has resolved, patients may be disturbed by the subcutaneous clot and want it removed. This is often reasonable, because distressing clots can be removed at minimal risk (though not without significant pain) and because the overlying skin tag may cause hygiene problems.

CONTRAINDICATIONS

Because doing nothing surgically is often a reasonable choice, hardware at risk for infection (e.g. prosthetic heart valve) is a relative contraindication to excising a perianal thrombosis. Because of the uncontrolled nature of the subsequent open wound, anticoagulation (e.g. warfarin) is a relative contraindication. If perianal thrombosis appears incidental to a malignancy, such as leukemia, the underlying problem takes priority.

PREOPERATIVE

No preparation at all is required. A stool-filled rectum does not pose a significant risk of infection. This is an office procedure and requires only local anesthesia, so no preprocedure work up is needed, other than to check for the rare local anesthetic allergy.

ANESTHESIA

The excision is performed under local anesthesia, e.g. lidocaine 1 percent with adrenaline/adrenaline 1:200 000. The anxious patient may benefit from moderate sedation, although the same anxiety may well produce a flurry of postoperative concerns and calls. If a patient requires general anesthesia, the practitioner may consider not doing the procedure at all and managing the patient conservatively.

OPERATION

Position of patient

The left lateral position is ideal for the right-handed practitioner, as is the right lateral for the left-handed surgeon. The upper buttock may be held back by an assistant or by the patient.

Injection of local anesthetic

The skin is cleaned with an antiseptic solution. A thin (e.g. 30-gauge) needle is used for the local anesthetic injection, with infiltration deep to the clot and including the surrounding skin. Infiltration into the clot itself is not helpful. (**Figure 2.5.1**)

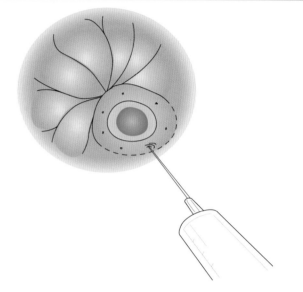

2.5.1

Excision of thrombus and overlying anoderm

A short incision, 1–2 cm long, is made on the anoderm overlying the clot. The thrombus can then be squeezed out or removed with a forceps. The venous lining and redundant anoderm forming the 'sac' around the clot are excised with fine scissors (**Figure 2.5.2**). Alternatively, the clot and overlying anoderm can be excised together using fine, curved scissors, with the convex surface of the blades pushing back against the underlying tissue. This maneuver is analogous to the use of Buie scissors in a conventional hemorrhoidectomy.

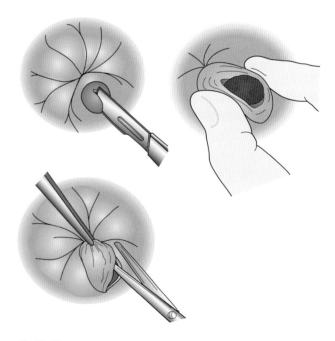

2.5.2

There is no need for irrigation or curettage, once the offending large clot has been removed. The wound is left open and the resulting scar further inhibits skin tag formation (**Figure 2.5.3**).

Postoperative care

The wound is dressed by tucking small gauze pad between the buttocks to catch the few drops of drainage, protecting the patient's clothing. The patient is instructed to place a gauze pad or toilet paper between the buttocks to absorb the drainage for as long as it occurs. Warm sitzbaths are optional, but the patient is advised to bathe or shower once a day, letting water run over and into the wound. Excessive bathing and washing, in a counterproductive attempt to prevent infection (see below), may lead to skin maceration and pruritus ani. Oral analgesics are prescribed for a week, although patients often take them for 2–3 days only. Stool softeners may be prescribed to counteract the hardening effect of oral analgesics.

COMPLICATIONS

Infection, abscess formation, and fistula

If a wide open wound is left as depicted, there should be no question of wound infection. This type of wound can be pointed out to patients (and to students) as an example of an open wound that essentially never becomes infected, regardless of a daily dousing with stool. If an abscess should form in defiance of this principle, then it of course is incised and drained, preferably in the operating room under general or spinal anesthesia. Another possible consequence of an insufficiently open wound is a superficial wound fistula, distinct from an anal fistula in that it does not pass behind any muscle, and analogous to the fissure–fistula that occasionally follows the healing of an anal fissure. This is laid open, again under general or spinal anesthesia.

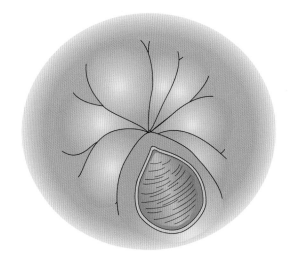

2.5.3

Repeat thrombosis

Since the cause of perianal thrombosis is unknown, its recurrence in a different location cannot be prevented. The vein that thrombosed initially has been partially excised and becomes obliterated: when one excises the clot and sac, the minimal bleeding is presumably due to clinically silent upstream thrombosis. However, elsewhere under the anal verge are other veins which may suffer the same fate, sooner or later. It is fairly common for a patient to have more than one perianal thrombosis in his or her lifetime, and it is even more common to find evidence of several old thromboses (in the form of tiny clot residua) on routine anal examination of the asymptomatic patient.

FURTHER READING

Keighley MRB, Williams NS (eds). Haemorrhoidal disease. In: *Surgery of the anus, rectum and colon*, 2nd edn. London: WB Saunders, 1999, 351–427.

Open hemorrhoidectomy

P RONAN O'CONNELL

PRINCIPLES AND JUSTIFICATION

Background

Hemorrhoids are vascular cushions found in the anal canal. Whether these contribute to the effective sealing of the canal and indirectly to continence is unclear. The great majority of hemorrhoids are asymptomatic. The incidence increases with age and men are more commonly symptomatic than women.

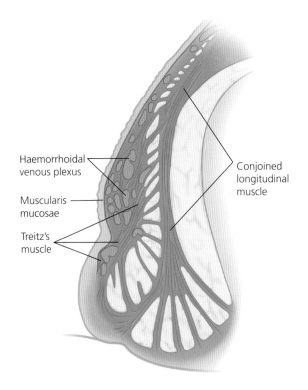

2.6.1 Reproduced with permission from Thomson WH. The nature of haemorrhoids. *British Journal of Surgery* 1975; **62**: 542–52.

The pathophysiology of hemorrhoids is poorly understood, but probably relates to venous engorgement during straining coupled with stretching or disruption of Treitz's muscle (fibromuscular bands that arise partly from the internal anal sphincter and partly from the conjoined longitudinal muscle and which tether the anal mucosa at the dentate line). For a more comprehensive discussion, the reader is directed to the excellent articles by Parks[1] and Thomson[2] on the subject

Open hemorrhoidectomy as an operation evolved from an operative description by Sir Ernest Miles in 1919 that involved scissors dissection of the hemorrhoidal tissue beginning at the perianal skin and extending to, but not beyond, the mucocutaneous junction. The pedicle so created was suture ligated but not excised, leaving the hemorrhoidal tissue to slough.[3] In 1937, Milligan *et al.*[4] described a low ligation technique with excision of the dissected hemorrhoid, but which was otherwise very similar to that described by Miles. They surmised that the ligated pedicle was tethered to the lower part of the anal canal by Treitz's muscle fibers and therefore did not retract leaving a large raw surface that could later stricture. The technique with slight modifications became the standard operation in the UK and elsewhere and is described below.

Indications

Hemorrhoidectomy is an operation with a bad reputation for postoperative pain and discomfort. Yet it offers the best chance of permanent cure of prolapsing internal hemorrhoids, particularly when accompanied by external hemorrhoids or skin tags, so called 'mixed hemorrhoids'. In addition, formal hemorrhoidectomy is of value when other non-operative treatments, such as phenol injection or band ligation, have failed. Occasionally, one large hemorrhoid is dominant and single quadrant hemorrhoidectomy is a reasonable option that is associated with less postoperative discomfort. However, it is important to be sure that

Labels on figure: Haemorrhoidal venous plexus; Muscularis mucosae; Treitz's muscle; Conjoined longitudinal muscle

the symptoms causing the complaint can reasonably be attributed to hemorrhoidal disease, as the majority of patients presenting with proctological symptoms will attribute the symptoms to 'piles'. Therefore, the surgeon must exercise careful judgment before recommending a formal hemorrhoidectomy.

Anemia is an unusual consequence of hemorrhoidal bleeding, but can occur particularly in men in the third and fourth decade. If other causes of gastrointestinal hemorrhage have been excluded, formal hemorrhoidectomy is appropriate.

Symptomatic hemorrhoids are relatively common in pregnancy, particularly in the third trimester. Symptomatic and expectant management is usually sufficient, however, prolapse with thrombosis can occur, especially late in pregnancy and urgent hemorrhoidectomy may on rare occasions be necessary.

Contraindications

Hemorrhoidectomy is best avoided in patients with Crohn's disease or patients who are immunosuppressed. It is important that coexisting proctological conditions be treated in the first instance (fungal infections, pruritis ani). Difficulties can arise when large internal hemorrhoids coexist with a symptomatic anal fissure or anal fistula. It is the author's practice to treat the more symptomatic condition first and to avoid combining hemorrhoidectomy with lateral internal sphincterotomy or fistulotomy. On occasion, synchronous operation is unavoidable, in which case a single quadrant excision of the largest (usually most symptomatic) hemorrhoid or excision of the hemorrhoidal tissue that might interfere with the planned primary surgery should be sufficient.

DIAGNOSIS

All patients with a presumed diagnosis should have a digital rectal examination and rigid proctosigmoidoscopy performed to confirm the diagnosis and exclude other anorectal and distal colonic pathology. If flexible sigmoidoscopy or left colonoscopy is performed, hemorrhoidal disease is best assessed using a rigid proctoscope which should be inserted at the end of the endoscopy. If the source of bleeding is unclear, if it is associated with a change in bowel habit or if there is a family history of colorectal cancer then a full colonoscopy, computed tomography (CT) colonography or other imaging must be performed to exclude significant colonic pathology. It is also unwise to accept a diagnosis of hemorrhoidal bleeding in older patients without screening the colon as there may be coincident but asymptomatic neoplasia.

Preoperative assessment

No specific preoperative assessment is required other than the standard institutional protocol for day case or overnight admission. The latter is determined by the patient's overall medical condition, age, social circumstances and distance travelled to the hospital. There is some evidence to support preoperative administration of a mild laxative, such as lactulose for 2 days prior to operation.[5] It is the author's practice to request that a phosphate enema be administered at least 1 hour preoperatively. Prophylaxis against thromboembolism is not normally required and the use of broad-spectrum antibiotics is not routine. There are conflicting data regarding the potential benefits of perioperative administration of metronidazole.[5, 6]

Postoperative urinary retention is not uncommon, particularly in men over the age of 50. Where prostatic hypertrophy has been detected preoperatively, particularly if the patient has symptoms of bladder outlet obstruction, pre-emptive consultation with a urologist may be advisable. Patients should be advised to pass urine before leaving the ward for the operating room prior to operation.

Anesthesia

Hemorrhoidectomy is generally performed under general anesthesia but it is quite possible to comfortably perform the operation using spinal, epidural, or caudal anesthesia. The latter is particularly useful if the operation is performed in the prone jack-knife position. Local anesthetic is possible, however, it is the author's preference to use local anesthesia as an adjunct to general anesthesia. A recent systematic review confirmed that local anesthetic infiltration, either as a sole technique or as an adjunct to general or regional anesthetic are recommended.[7]

OPERATION

Position of patient

The operation is usually performed in the full lithotomy position with the buttocks lifted over the edge of the table. The illustrations that follow assume that the patient is in the lithotomy position, however, the operation may equally well be performed in the prone jack-knife position.

Once the patient is positioned, perianal hair can be shaved and the buttocks strapped apart. Prior to skin preparation, a 'time out' safety check is undertaken. The skin is then prepared using a povidone iodine or chlorhexidine solution. If electrocautery is to be used, alcohol-based solutions should be avoided.

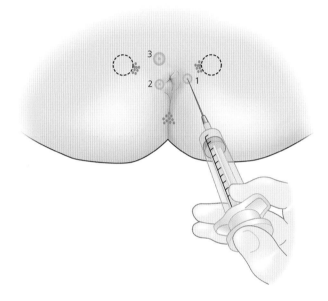

2.6.2

Injection of local anesthesia

A local anesthetic solution containing adrenaline may be usefully injected prior to starting the dissection. The author routinely uses 20 mL 1 percent lidocaine with 1:100 000 adrenaline. If the hemorrhoids are edematous or recently thrombosed, the addition of 1500 IU hyaluronidase facilitates diffusion of the anesthetic and significantly reduces tissue edema.

Local anesthetic solution is injected subcutaneously and submucosally into each hemorrhoidal mass. Usually 2–3 mL at each of the three primary hemorrhoidal sites is sufficient. The remaining local anesthetic can be injected into each ischiorectal fossa just medial to the ischial tuberosity to obtain a block of the inferior rectal branches of the pudendal nerves as they pass to the top of the anal canal in the 3 and 9 o'clock positions. It is advisable to wait several minutes after local anesthetic infiltration to allow the full hemostatic and anesthetic effects to develop.

Display of the operative field

Spencer Wells or Dunhill artery forceps are placed on the perianal skin just outside the mucocutaneous junction opposite each primary hemorrhoidal cushion (left lateral, right anterior, and right posterior; 3, 7, and 11 o'clock). Skin tags should be included in the area of perianal skin to be removed. Gentle traction on the forceps then brings each hemorrhoidal mass into view.

At this stage, a careful note is made of the areas of skin and mucosa (skin bridges) which should remain between each area from which the hemorrhoidal cushions are to be dissected. It is usual to leave a skin bridge between each excised hemorrhoidal cushion and these should be greater than 1 cm wide to avoid a significant risk of postoperative anal stenosis.

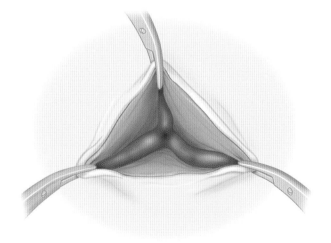

2.6.3

Triangle of exposure

As the internal hemorrhoids are pulled down, a second pair of forceps is placed on the main bulk of each hemorrhoidal mass; further traction exposes the pedicles of the hemorrhoids and produces the so-called 'triangle of exposure' which is caused by the stretching of pink columnar cell mucosa between the apices of each taut pedicle. When the second pair of forceps is clipped to each hemorrhoid, care must be taken not to include the internal sphincter muscle by taking too deep a bite. Intervening small hemorrhoids may be taken with separate forceps and approximated to the nearest primary forceps so that they are included with the main hemorrhoid in the subsequent section.

Once the triangle of exposure has been achieved, the hemorrhoids are ready to be dissected and removed. It is a mistake to carry the pedicle dissection higher than this exposure allows because there is a risk of narrowing the upper anal canal if too much mucosa is gathered at the anorectal junction, and the excision of large amounts of anal epithelium will result in reduced anal sensation.

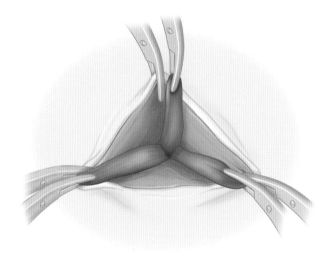

2.6.4

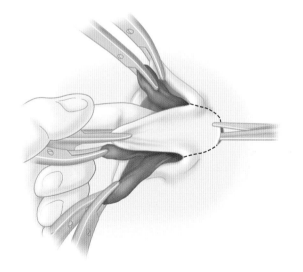

2.6.5

Start of dissection

The hemorrhoids are dissected in turn. For a right-handed surgeon, it is convenient to start with the left lateral hemorrhoid, the others being temporarily held out of the way with slight traction by the assistant. The two forceps are held in linear fashion in the palm of the left hand, with the left forefinger in the anal canal on the pedicle of the hemorrhoid pressing lightly outwards to stretch the pedicle gently over the pulp of the finger. Dissection is usually performed with electrocautery, however it can also be performed using a pair of blunt-nosed scissors. Dissection begins at each edge of the base, as seen from the cutaneous aspect and the tissues divided towards the median plane until the incisions meet. The subcutaneous space superficial to the lowest (white) fibers of the internal sphincter and deep to the external (red) sphincter muscle is then exposed and can be opened up.

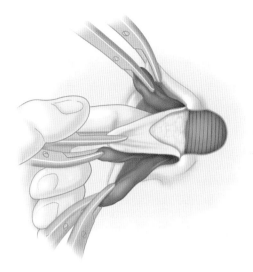

2.6.6

Further dissection

Dissection is continued in a coronal plane superficially at first, but almost at once this is changed to medial to the internal sphincter muscle and is directed towards the pedicle of the hemorrhoids in the submucosal plane. The borders of the dissection taper towards the base of the hemorrhoids and upward mobilization is not continued more than is necessary to allow easy control of the pedicle as previously defined by the triangle of exposure.

Ligation of pedicle

As the pedicle is exposed by dissection, traction on the hemorrhoid should be eased. Once the hemorrhoid has been defined, the pedicle is suture ligated with a slow dissolving suture material (e.g. 2-0 Vicryl) with the knots tied on the luminal aspect. It is not necessary to use very strong material for the pedicle ligation; a large knot of non-absorbable material can excite a foreign body reaction and even cause a fistula.

Once the pedicle has been secured and traction on the pedicle released to check that vessels have been safely controlled by the ligature, the pedicle is cut through, leaving a good cuff. The ends of the ligatures are left long so that the pedicle can easily be identified and recovered to control persistent oozing. The pedicle is then allowed to retract to its normal position in the upper anal canal.

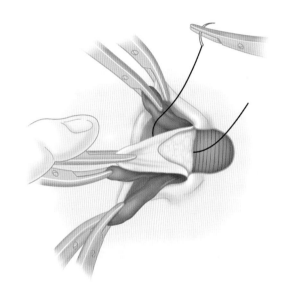

2.6.7

Procedure for remaining hemorrhoids

The other hemorrhoids are removed in a similar fashion. The right anterior hemorrhoid is usually the smallest and easiest to deal with, and is frequently left until last because, when the patient is in the lithotomy position, bleeding from the front of the anal canal may obscure subsequent dissection posteriorly. If the patient is prone, the sequence should be reversed. Intact bridges between perianal skin and anal mucosa must be preserved between each dissection site, and should be not less than 1 cm wide.

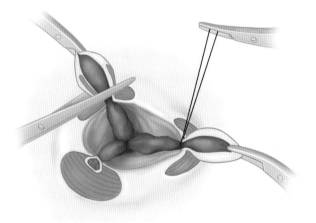

2.6.8

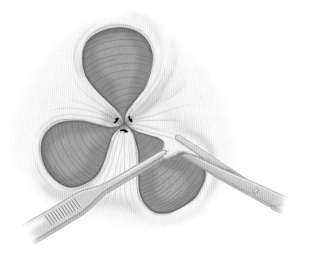

2.6.9

Trimming of wounds

After all the pedicles have retracted into the upper anal canal, the mucosal defects are critically inspected for persistent bleeding and for redundant flaps of mucosa or perianal skin. Any redundant tags of skin are removed, and puckering of the skin bridges can be reduced by anchoring sutures of slowly dissolving 3-0 suture material. Hemostasis of any small bleeding points, either from the mucosal edges or from the raw area of the mucosal wounds, is controlled by light application of diathermy or by ligation with 3-0 Vicryl sutures. Occasionally, in the presence of diffuse bleeding, the application of a swab soaked in adrenaline solution (1:1000) is preferred to excessive diathermy.

Final appearance and dressing

The final appearance of the operated area should resemble a clover leaf and the wounds should be completely dry before a dressing is applied. Dressings are a matter of personal choice, except that greasy or oily materials should be avoided as they prevent proper drainage of serosanguineous exudate from the raw anal mucosal defects. Dressings, such as cellulose mesh, which dissolve spontaneously can be lightly tucked in over each raw area. Bulky anal packs should be avoided because they are uncomfortable. The wound should be dry at the end of the procedure and there should be no need for anal tamponade. In occasional cases, where packing is thought to be justified because of difficulty with hemostasis, the use of gelatin sponge is beneficial because it provides some initial tamponade and hemostasis, but decomposes quite quickly. This avoids the risk of hurting the patient which occurs when a non-absorbable pack is removed from the anal canal.

A thick pad of cotton wool is then laid over the perineum and held in place by either a T bandage or Tenafix pants.

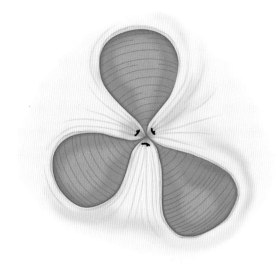

2.6.10

POSTOPERATIVE CARE

In the modern era, hemorrhoidectomy is performed in the majority as a day-case procedure. By the time the patient is due for hospital discharge, the effects of local anesthetic injected at the time of operation will have begun to wear off. Therefore, pre-emptive analgesia should be administered prior to discharge and written instructions given regarding regular pain management over succeeding days. A combination of non-steroidal anti-inflammatory drugs, paracetamol and oral opiates is recommended.[7] A gentle laxative, such as lactulose syrup, and a stool softening agent containing ispaghula husk (Fybrogel®, Isogel®, Regulan®, Metamucil®) or sterculia gum (Normacol®) should be taken daily until bowel movements are comfortable.

It is the author's preference to use a gelatin sponge dressing rather than any formal packing of the anal canal. The patient should be aware that the dressing will disintegrate and pass spontaneously. An on-lay pad dressing will be needed for 7–10 days.

Patients at risk of urinary retention should remain in hospital on the night following the operation. It is the author's practice to advise discontinuation of perioperative intravenous fluids and mild restriction of oral fluid intake until urine is passed.

A warm bath once or twice a day will assist hygiene and ease anal sphincter spasm. Written contact details should be provided in case of difficulty and an outpatient clinic review scheduled for 3–4 weeks after the procedure. A digital rectal examination should be performed to assess healing and rule out stenosis.

Postoperative complications

The most common postoperative difficulties relate to pain management, urinary retention, and fecal impaction. If the postoperative care regime described is adhered to, it is rare for a patient to require readmission for pain relief or impaction of feces, itself often due to inadequate pain management. If retention of urine is suspected, bladder distension is checked by ultrasound and if more than 200 mL residual urine is found, a catheter should be passed. This usually can be successfully removed within 24 hours.

Bleeding is a relatively rare complication of open hemorrhoidectomy. When it occurs within the first 24 hours, it is due to bleeding from small vessels that were not noted at the time of operation, usually due to vasospasm occasioned by the subcutaneous injection of adrenaline, or to slippage from a ligature. Bleeding may also occur at the time of first bowel movement if the stool is forced and the ligated pedicle is traumatized. It is important to be aware that the volume of blood passed is an unreliable guide to the actual volume of bleeding, as blood may pass proximally into the rectum and distal colon. Tachycardia should not be attributed to pain and syncope as the patient tried to get to the bathroom is indicative of serious hemorrhage. In this circumstance, rapid resuscitation and early return to the operating room for resuturing is required.

Postoperative septic complications are rare, but can be life threatening. Severe pain, coupled with signs of systemic sepsis must be acted upon and broad-spectrum antibiotics administered. A CT scan of the pelvis is advisable and drainage or debridement of the infected area undertaken.

Anal stenosis is a potential long-term complication that reflects excessive removal of perianal skin at the time of operation. This usually responds to a program of anal dilatation, however on occasion it may require formal anoplasty (see Chapter 2.13).

OUTCOMES

The operation described has been in widespread use for decades and despite the disadvantages of postoperative discomfort and an average time off work of 2 weeks, it continues in widespread use. Recurrence rates are low; however, one long-term study did identify long-term functional disturbances, such as soiling, as being an important and underestimated outcome.[8] It is likely that difficulties in continence after hemorrhoidectomy relate to damage to the internal anal sphincter muscle during operation, either through excessive stretching or direct injury, and not to excision of the hemorrhoidal tissue per se.

In North America particularly, a modified technique in which the hemorrhoidectomy wound is closed as described by Ferguson is more widely used (see Chapter 2.7). Despite several randomized trials, there appears to be little difference in outcome.[7] Stapled hemorrhoidopexy (see Chapter 2.8) is associated with less postoperative discomfort and an earlier return to work than open hemorrhoidectomy.[9] However, a Cochrane review has concluded that if hemorrhoid recurrence and prolapse are the most important clinical outcomes, then conventional hemorrhoidectomy (open or closed) remains the 'gold standard' in the surgical treatment of internal hemorrhoids.[10]

REFERENCES

1. Parks AG. The surgical treatment of haemorrhoids. *British Journal of Surgery* 1956; **43**: 337–51.
2. Thomson WH. The nature of haemorrhoids. *British Journal of Surgery* 1975; **62**: 542–52.
3. Miles W. Observations upon internal piles. *Surgery, Gynecology and Obstetrics* 1919; **29**: 496.
4. Milligan ETC, Morgan CN, Lionel EJ, Officer R. Surgical anatomy of the anal canal, and the operative treatment of haemorrhoids. *Lancet* 1937; **230**: 1119–24.
5. Carapeti EA, Kamm MA, McDonald PJ, Phillips RK. Double-

blind randomised controlled trial of effect of metronidazole on pain after day-case haemorrhoidectomy. *Lancet* 1998; **351**: 169–72.

6. Balfour L, Stojkovic SG, Botterill ID *et al.* A randomized, double-blind trial of the effect of metronidazole on pain after closed hemorrhoidectomy. *Diseases of the Colon and Rectum* 2002; **45**: 1186–90.

7. Joshi GP, Neugebauer EA. Evidence-based management of pain after haemorrhoidectomy surgery. *British Journal of Surgery* 2010; **97**: 1155–68.

8. Johannsson HO, Graf W, Pahlman L. Long-term results of haemorrhoidectomy. *European Journal of Surgery* 2002; **168**: 485–9.

9. Tjandra JJ, Chan MK. Systematic review on the procedure for prolapse and hemorrhoids (stapled hemorrhoidopexy). *Diseases of the Colon and Rectum* 2007; **50**: 878–92.

10. Jayaraman S, Colquhoun PH, Malthaner RA. Stapled versus conventional surgery for hemorrhoids. *Cochrane Database of Systematic Reviews* 2006; (**4**): CD005393.

Closed hemorrhoidectomy

STANLEY M GOLDBERG

HISTORY

Over 200 years ago, the French anatomist, Petit,[1] first attempted to eradicate hemorrhoids without denuding the lower anal canal of its mucosa. The technique, modified by many surgeons and popularized in the United States by Ferguson[2] and Fansler[3] involves saving the anoderm, removing hemorrhoidal tissue, and replacing the anoderm into its normal position. The advantages over open hemorrhoidectomy are that the anal canal is covered with its own anoderm, postoperative dilatations are not required and primary healing is secured, resulting in much less discomfort for the patient. Frykman (unpublished) modified the partially closed technique of Fansler to a completely closed technique. Fansler advocated closing the wound only to the dentate line; however, Frykman extended closure to include the undercut and mobilized perianal skin. The same technique, used by the author's group of surgeons for 40 years, is described in this chapter.

PRINCIPLES AND JUSTIFICATION

Indications

Since the advent of the rubber band ligature technique for bleeding internal hemorrhoids, indications in this unit for closed hemorrhoidectomy have been limited to prolapse, pain, bleeding not controlled by rubber band ligature or injection, and association with other surgical conditions of the anal canal, e.g. fissure and fistula.

The most frequent indication for hemorrhoidectomy in our practice today is rectal mucosal prolapse associated with prolapsing mixed hemorrhoids. Pain associated with hemorrhoids is always associated with thrombosis. When thrombosis is extensive, hemorrhoidectomy is indicated although the majority of painful thrombosed hemorrhoids can be handled with simple excision of

the entire hemorrhoidal complex under local anesthesia. When surgery is required for fissures or fistula associated with hemorrhoids, hemorrhoidectomy may be added at that time.

PREOPERATIVE

All patients undergoing hemorrhoidectomy undergo preoperative sigmoidoscopy at the time of their first examination; if they are older than 40 years and their symptoms suggest additional pathology, colonoscopy is indicated. Special care is always taken with any patient who has a history of soft stools or diarrhea to rule out the possibility of undiagnosed inflammatory bowel disease, which is a specific contraindication for hemorrhoidectomy.

Almost all hemorrhoidectomies are now performed on a day surgery basis. The patient should refrain from any heavy lifting for a period of 2 weeks after surgery. He is advised that complete healing will not occur for a period of approximately 3–4 weeks, and that his chance of returning to the operating room for a complication related to surgery is usually about 1 percent.

Oral preoperative preparation is not indicated for this technique. One disposable packaged enema is given the evening before surgery and another approximately 1 hour before surgery. Neither laxatives nor antibiotics are used before operation or during the procedure.

Position of patient

Anorectal procedures have traditionally been performed in the lithotomy position or the left lateral position as favored in certain parts of North America. However, the semiprone or jack-knife position is preferred, with soft rolls under the hips and ankles of the patient ensuring that the patient is comfortable on the table (**Figure 2.7.1**). The advantages of this position are that any bleeding that

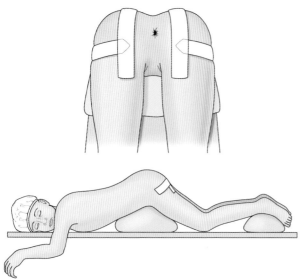

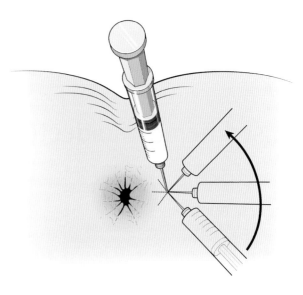

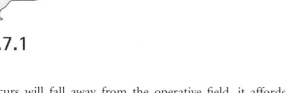

2.7.1

2.7.2

occurs will fall away from the operative field, it affords comfort for the operating surgeon and superior access to the operative field.

Skin preparation

No attempt is made to sterilize the skin other than using povidone-iodine (Betadine). The operative area is not shaved and adhesive tapes are applied to the buttocks to provide lateral traction.

Anesthesia

The prone position lends itself well to a combination of general and local anesthesia (**Figure 2.7.2**). Infiltration of local anesthesia (see below) commences after the establishment of monitored intravenous sedation with propofol and midazolam. Regional anesthesia, either spinal or caudal, can be used in this position; however, local anesthesia is preferred. With certain patients, it is necessary to use an endotracheal tube in the prone position; however, in all cases, local infiltration with bupivacaine and adrenaline is employed.

It is very important that the infiltration of local

anesthetic be carried out correctly, especially when it is administered without intravenous sedation. A dose of 20–30 mL of a 0.5 percent lidocaine and 1:200 000 adrenaline solution is injected through a No. 30 needle into the skin, picking up the cutaneous nerves. After this, a direct injection of 0.25 percent bupivacaine with 1:200 000 adrenaline into the muscle, as illustrated, is performed to pick up the branches of the inferior rectal nerve, resulting in immediate relaxation of the sphincter muscle; neither manual dilatations nor stretching of the sphincter muscle are carried out. No specific attempt is made to inject the anoderm directly in the area of the hemorrhoids or to 'balloon up' the mucosa. The anesthetic usually lasts for 60–180 minutes, more than sufficient for the operative procedure, and it also provides considerable relief in the immediate postoperative period. Elderly patients with hypertension or cardiovascular problems present no difficulty with the low concentration of adrenaline.

Another important point regarding anesthesia is the use of minimal volumes (less than 50 mL) of intravenous solutions during surgery, a principle which has helped to keep the catheterization incidence in this unit under 3 percent. The author's group believes that by keeping patients dehydrated in the postoperative period their bladders are not distended, resulting in spontaneous voiding within the first 20 hours.

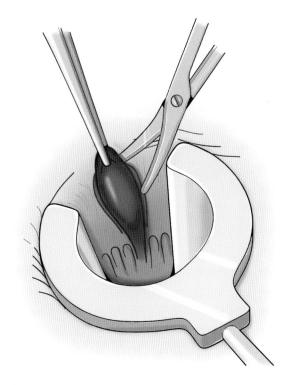

2.7.3

OPERATION

After the introduction of local anesthesia to relax the sphincter, the anal canal is examined digitally and then by a Pratt bivalve speculum introduced into the anal canal, examining carefully the specific hemorrhoidal areas; the operation is planned in greater detail at this point. Dilatations are not carried out with the bivalve speculum. The largest hemorrhoidal complex is removed first; the quadrants usually involved are the left lateral, right posterior, and right anterior. No suction is necessary during the procedure. Small 7.5 cm² gauze sponges which fit through the operative anoscope are used as an alternative to suction. Having examined the area with the Pratt bivalve speculum, the Fansler operating anoscope is then used.

Dissection is started on the perianal skin. No attempt is made to remove all the tissue in one motion. An elliptical incision is made with fine dissecting scissors (**Figure 2.7.3**), removing skin and hemorrhoidal tissue down to the underlying internal sphincter (**Figure 2.7.4**).

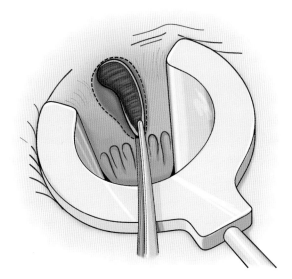

2.7.4

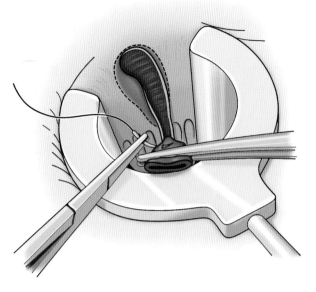

2.7.5

Redundant rectal mucosa is excised high up to and sometimes even beyond the first valve of Houston to correct rectal mucosal prolapse. No crown suture is placed on the pedicle. Most of the bleeding occurs from the edges of the mucosa; individual bleeding vessels in the mucosa are coagulated using diathermy (**Figure 2.7.5**).

At this point, the mucosa is elevated, hemorrhoidal tissue is dissected from beneath the mucosal flaps, other bleeding points are electrocoagulated, and the anodermal flaps are undercut adequately so that they can be closed without tension (**Figure 2.7.6**).

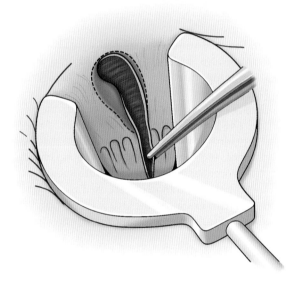

2.7.6

After dissecting the secondary hemorrhoidal vessels from beneath the anodermal skin flaps and controlling the bleeding, the wound is closed, starting at the apex using a running suture of 3-0 chromic catgut. The mucous membrane is sutured down to the underlying sphincter mechanism in an attempt to create a longitudinal scar which will prevent further prolapse. Trimming of excess skin is performed, but it is essential that the wounds be closed without tension. A loose knot is tied at the completion of the procedure. Rarely is any clamping of vessels necessary, and no pile clamps are used (**Figure 2.7.7**).

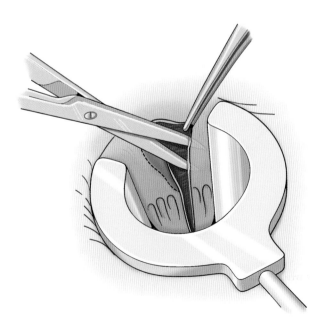

2.7.7

The procedure is carried out in three major areas and in as many additional areas as necessary. In certain cases of prolapsed thrombosed hemorrhoids, as many as six areas may be excised and primarily closed (**Figure 2.7.8**).

At the completion of the procedure, all quadrants are examined carefully and blood clots are removed. No packing or dressing is placed in the anal canal or perianal area. The average operating time is 35 minutes (**Figure 2.7.9**).

POSTOPERATIVE CARE

After the operation, patients are encouraged to take only sips of water until such time as they void spontaneously. Since the institution of this program of dehydration, the catheterization rate on all patients has been under 3 percent. Once postoperative voiding has taken place, patients are allowed fluids and food as desired.

Early activity is encouraged. Warm packs are applied to the perineum during the immediate postoperative period. After 24 hours, patients are encouraged to take as many sitz baths as required for cleanliness and comfort. A small cotton dressing is put in the perianal area to collect whatever discharge or drainage may be present. No other local treatment is carried out. Patients are discharged home with oral analgesics and a fiber supplement. Because patients receive only a small (100 mL) packaged enema the evening before surgery and the morning of surgery, they usually have their first bowel action on the second or third postoperative day. If they do not, a tap water enema is given on the third postoperative day using a soft rubber catheter.

Complications

Skin tags may result from any operative procedure on the perianal area; however, no greater incidence of skin tag formation occurs with the closed technique. A large skin tag can be removed under local anesthesia in the clinic; however, the author likes to have a 'pleat' so that the patient does not split the perianal skin when the anal canal opens at the time of defecation.

Anal stenosis and stricture have been reported after the closed technique, and usually result from the removal of too much normal skin in the perianal area. With attention to detail, however, these complications have not been a problem.

OUTCOME

Patients return to the clinic 10–14 days after surgery, but digital and anascopic examinations are deferred until healing is complete. It is apparent at this time that a percentage of the wounds have failed to remain closed; however, the majority have healed primarily. Secondary hemorrhage occurs in 0.3 percent of cases. Less than 1

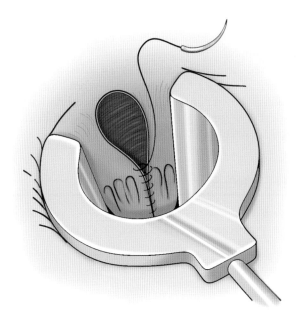

2.7.8

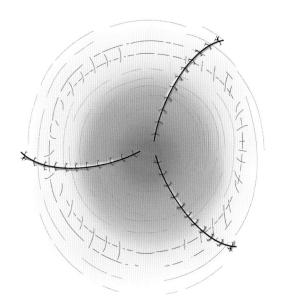

2.7.9

percent of patients return to the operating room for a second operative procedure resulting from an unhealed wound or a persistent sinus tract. Postoperative infection is uncommon.

Closed hemorrhoidectomy is an effective and safe alternative to open hemorrhoidectomy, resulting in rapid healing and minimal postoperative discomfort for the patient. The use of the prone position and infiltration of local anesthetic facilitate the procedure.

REFERENCES

1. Petit JL. *Traité des maladies chirurgicales et des opérations qui leur conviennent*, vol. 2. Paris: Didot, 1974: 137.

2. Ferguson JA, Mazier WP, Ganchrow MI, Friend WG. The closed technique of hemorrhoidectomy. *Surgery* 1971; **70**: 480–4.

3. Fansler WA. Surgical treatment of hemorrhoids. *Minnesota Medicine* 1934; **17**: 254–5.

FURTHER READING

Bleday R, Pena J, Rothenberger DA *et al.* Symptomatic hemorrhoids: current incidence and complications of operative therapy. *Diseases of the Colon and Rectum* 1992; **35**: 477–81.

Parks AG. Haemorrhoidectomy. *Advances in Surgery* 1971; **5**: 1–50.

Stapled hemorrhoidopexy

PER-OLOF NYSTRÖM

HISTORY

Stapled hemorrhoidopexy was conceived by Dr Antonio Longo of Palermo in Italy in the early 1990s. Other surgeons had attempted using a circular stapling device for hemorrhoidectomy, however Longo's operation was different in that he performed a 'prolapsectomy' with the distinct intention of preserving the hemorrhoids (anal cushions), but excising the concomitant prolapse of loosened rectal mucosa immediately cranial to the hemorrhoids. Initially, Longo also thought that the excision of a column of mucosa would also divide the arterial supply to the hemorrhoids which would result in shrinkage. The mature operation is an antiprolapse operation intended to reposition the hemorrhoidal cushions in their normal anatomical position at the top of the anal canal. The scar of the mucosal anastomosis binds the hemorrhoids to their normal anatomical position. The operation is correctly termed 'hemorrhoidopexy' or 'anopexy' to distinguish it from operations where the hemorrhoids are excised.

PRINCIPLES AND JUSTIFICATION

As a surgical disease, 'hemorrhoids' are one part of a mucoanal prolapse involving the distal rectal mucosa, hemorrhoid pedicles, and anoderm. The traditional grading mode assigns a grade III to the prolapse that requires manual repositioning by the patient after passing a motion. If manual reduction is not required, a grade II prolapse is assigned. The symptoms are similar for both grades of prolapse, including bleeding and pain caused by entrapment of the prolapse in the anal canal, while soiling and pruritus reflect disturbance of the anal closing mechanism. By reversing the prolapse, these symptoms will be much less frequent. There is only minor difference in outcome compared with conventional hemorrhoidectomy.

The ideal patient has grade II or III prolapse with no or only minor anodermal skin tags that are soft. Soft skin tags will often be smoothed as the prolapse is lifted and fixed. Any remaining tag of appreciable size can be excised in its extension outside the anal verge (lower margin of the internal sphincter). Patients with a large anodermal component of fixed polyps are less suitable. Patients with a large protrusion of prolapse or eversion of the entire anal canal, which will require a more extensive procedure such as the stapled transanal rectal resection (STARR), are not suitable.

Stapled hemorrhoidopexy is well tolerated with less pain, as well as faster resolution of pain compared with conventional hemorrhoidectomy. The gain is about 1 week. About half the patients will be able to return to work, or will rate themselves as 'normal', within a week.

PREOPERATIVE ASSESSMENT AND PREPARATION

As with all anal surgery, bowel habits should be medically regulated as far as possible before the operation. In young patients with typical symptoms of hemorrhoids, a rigid rectoscopy or flexible sigmoidoscopy is sufficient. A full colonoscopy is advisable in any patient with additional bowel symptoms.

A small enema should evacuate the rectum in the morning of surgery. There is no evidence that antibiotic prophylaxis is needed.

Position of the patient

Lithotomy (Lloyd-Davies) position or prone positions can both be used. In lithotomy position, the hemorrhoids are filled and the prolapse protrudes more clearly which some surgeons prefer. In the prone position, with a pillow under the hips and the table broken at the level of the hips, the hemorrhoids are empty and the mucosal prolapse will need to be demonstrated with forceps or a swab. It is also possible to perform the operation with the patient in the left lateral position (for the right-handed surgeon) making sure that the buttocks reach beyond the side of the table and hips and the knees are flexed.

The anesthetist providing a general anesthetic will usually prefer the lithotomy position. Surgeons using perianal local block will find this easier to apply with the patient in the prone position.

Anesthesia

The operation will take about 25 minutes which allows several modes of anesthesia, such as general, spinal, epidural, or perianal local block with conscious sedation. The operating room time will be about 1 hour. No premedication is necessary. Closing and firing of the stapler can be quite painful which currently requires rather deep anesthesia. A trick that abolishes this painful moment is to inject small amounts of a local anesthetic agent in the submucosal space under the purse-string suture (e.g. 8–10 mL of ropivacaine 2 mg/mL) before applying the stapler. A further advantage of this practice is that the immediate postoperative pain is relieved.

OPERATION

The operation is demonstrated with the patient in the prone position (**Figure 2.8.1**). The patient who is intended for a perianal local block is fully awake and can find a comfortable position that can be endured for up to an hour. The legs are held together with a pillow under the hips to elevate the buttocks. The table is broken at the level of the hips to further elevate the buttocks, which can also be taped apart to expose the anus.

The draping can be made simply by covering the patient with a non-woven single-use sheet in which a hole is cut to expose the anus. The surgical team can use clean fabric, but non-sterile gowns.

The additional instruments should include an anal speculum (e.g. Eisenhammer), diathermy, and suction device. It is preferable to use rather long anatomical forceps and needle holder (e.g. 24 cm) so that the surgeon's hands do not hinder exposure of the work.

The right-handed surgeon stands on the patient's left side and the assistant, or nurse, on the opposite side.

There are now several manufacturers of staplers and kits for the stapled hemorrhoidopexy.

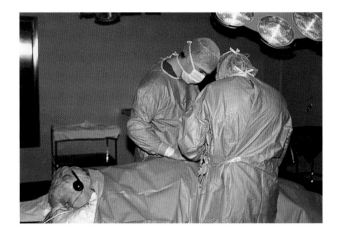

2.8.1

The perianal block is applied with a 20-mL syringe fitted with a 60 mm intramuscular needle (**Figure 2.8.2**). A suitable local anesthetic agent is Naropin® (ropivacaine) 5 mg/mL using 40–50 mL in total for the block. The intention is to administer the agent immediately peripheral to the external sphincter and reaching to the levator ani under which the terminal branches of the nerves to the sphincters and anus emerge. The mid-distance between the tip of the coccyx and the anus is pierced by the needle and advanced full length. A column of 5 mL of the anesthetic agent is applied while retracting the needle. The needle is then advanced 45° anterolaterally, immediately peripheral to the external sphincter for a new 5-mL column, and then on the opposite side.

Anteriorly, the mid-perineum is pierced for the same injections, but the fibrous condensation of the transverse perineal muscles is painful to inject. Therefore, a slow advancement of the needle while injecting minute amounts of the agent is advisable until the resistance dissolves when the needle tip is above this fibrous condensation. Further injections are made 45° anterolaterally on each side. The final injections of 5-mL columns are made on each side of the anus. Altogether, eight columns have been applied. The take time is about 5 minutes. The perianal skin will be anesthetized about 3 cm peripheral to the anal verge. The anus will be relaxed and accept dilatation without pain.

The pathology is reassessed with the patient under anesthesia using the Eisenhammer speculum to inspect the anal canal and the lower rectum (**Figure 2.8.3**). The presence of anodermal prolapse (skin tags), the position of the dentate line and the detachment of the hemorrhoid pedicles is observed by gentle testing with forceps. A swab can be inserted into the rectum and pulled out to mimic the passage of a fecal bolus. It will display the degree of mucosal and hemorrhoidal prolapse. Alternatively, a large swab on a stick can be used to pick up the rectal mucosa and retract it towards the anus. The diameter of the anus is also assessed to make sure it will accept the instruments. Occasionally, the anus will be too narrow in which case the procedure is converted to a conventional hemorrhoidectomy.

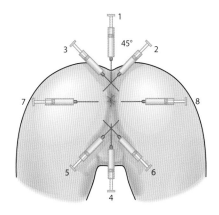

2.8.2

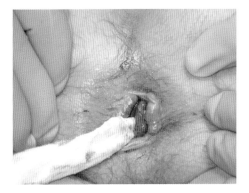

2.8.3

The obturator is introduced into the anal canal to assess that the anus is sufficiently wide and the prolapse can be reduced with it (**Figure 2.8.4**a). The circular anal dilatator CAD is then mounted on the obturator (**Figure 2.8.4**b) and introduced (**Figure 2.8.4**c) and sutured to the perianal skin (**Figure 2.8.4**d). Care is taken to introduce the CAD

sufficiently far to cover the dentate line, preferably 0.5–1 cm beyond it (**Figure 2.8.4**e). If insufficiently introduced, the hemorrhoids will protrude and obliterate the view, which makes the correct insertion of the purse-string suture considerably more difficult.

The purse-string suture is applied using 2-0 prolene

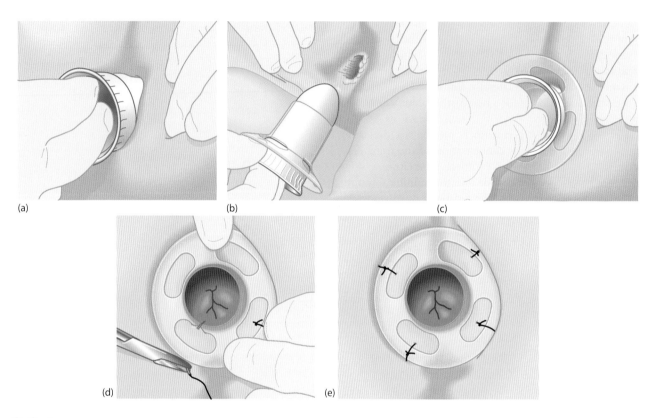

(a)

(b)

(c)

(d)

(e)

2.8.4

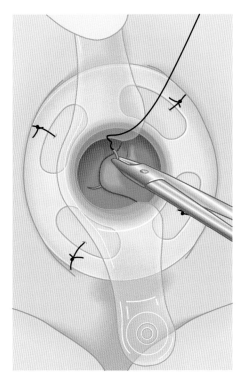

2.8.5

with a 25 mm needle (**Figure 2.8.5**). The suture should commence at the site of the most pronounced prolapse as identified from the examination of the anatomy. The reason for this is that the traction on the purse-string will produce the largest excision at this site. The purse string anoscope is introduced to flatten the hemorrhoidal pedicle and mucosal surface proximal to the dentate line. The needle is introduced between 3 and 4 cm above the dentate line. The lower suture placement is selected for larger hemorrhoids that must be securely lifted and fixed, while the higher position is better if there is richness of mucosa in need of excision.

The suture is applied in the submucosal plane beginning each new bite at the site of exit of the previous bite. It is advisable to attempt as long bites as possible and observe that the needle is advanced strictly parallel to the dentate line. About eight bites with the needle will suffice to produce a submucosal suture completing the circumference without skips. The final bite can exit 0.5 cm proximal or distal to the starting point to further enlarge the excision at the starting point.

Once the purse-string suture has been applied, it is best to confirm correct insertion as follows. First, an index finger is inserted through the suture and the surgeon pulls slightly on the free ends to bring it down on to the finger (**Figure 2.8.6**a). It will be possible to ascertain that the suture has not skipped part of the circumference and a sensation of the depth of the suture in the submucosal plane is obtained. The suture may be too superficial, in which case the excised doughnut will be inadequate at this site. The suture may also be inappropriately deep into the bowel wall and result in a full thickness excision.

The second test is to retract the index finger and pull on the free ends of the suture so it closes completely (**Figure 2.8.6**b). The index finger then probes the depth of the mucosal 'pockets' peripheral to the suture. If the pockets are deeper than 1 cm, it indicates that the suture has been placed too high (**Figure 2.8.6**c).

There is a learning process in recording these observations and comparing them with the specimen and the distance above the dentate line of the final staple line, as well as the extent of prolapse control with a swab test repeated after stapling.

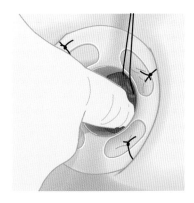

(a)

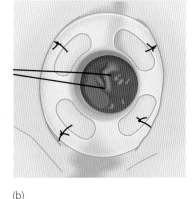

(b)

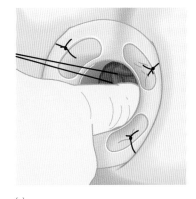

(c)

2.8.6

If one part of the circumference has a too superficial or too high purse-string suture, it may be appropriate to insert a second suture immediately distal to the previous suture. The second suture covers only the faulty segment, but not the entire circumference. After the stapler has been applied, the first suture is tied first followed by the second suture, both being tied around the stapler rod to secure the excision of more mucosa. The two pairs of free ends are then brought out each through one of the channels of the stapler head and all clamped together externally to allow equal traction on the mucosa.

The stapler is opened fully (**Figure 2.8.7**a). A little gel on the stapler may assist the insertion through the suture line. The free ends of the suture are held in one hand without traction while the stapler is pushed forward through the purse string. This should involve no undue force. If passage is not easy, the stapler should be removed and the purse string is again examined to ensure that it is correctly positioned. Once the stapler anvil has passed, the surgeon pulls on the free ends of the suture to close the purse string and brings the mucosa snugly down on the stapler rod (**Figure 2.8.7**b). While maintaining traction on the suture, the stapler is retracted to show that the mucosa has been circumferentially closed around the stapler rod. An index finger may be introduced to feel that the suture is securely applied around the central rod (**Figure 2.8.7**c). The suture is then tied with one throw, which is sufficient to avoid tearing the mucosa when applying traction on the suture (**Figure 2.8.7**d). Each of the free ends is brought through one of the channels of the stapler head using the purse string threader and clamped together externally (**Figure 2.8.7**e).

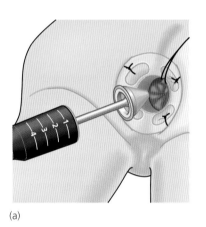

(a)

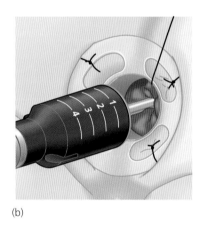

(b)

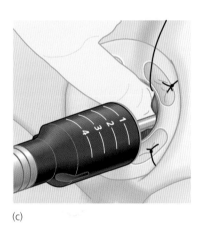

(c)

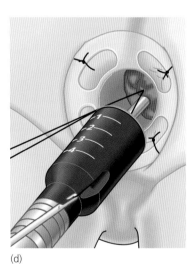

(d)

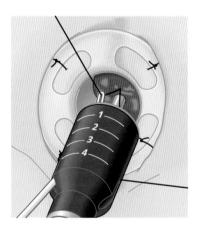

(e)

2.8.7

The stapler is held in the left hand with the thumb on the safety plate and the index finger hooking the free end of the purse-string suture (**Figure 2.8.8**a). The stapler is aligned with the midline (the patient's spine) and the direction of the anal canal (pointing towards the umbilicus in the prone patient). No force should be necessary for this alignment. Once the surgeon is convinced that the correct position of the anvil above the suture line is confirmed, the stapler is fully closed with moderate traction on the suture with the index finger (**Figure 2.8.8**b). The stapler head has a scale that is gradually advanced through the CAD and anal canal. When fully closed, the number 4 should be level with the anal verge meaning that the staple line will be approximately 2 cm above the dentate line.

In a female patient, the posterior vaginal wall is palpated while slightly rotating the closed stapler from side to side. The vaginal wall must be free. Only when the operator is convinced that the posterior vaginal wall is free should the stapler be fired. It has been recommended that the stapler is kept closed for up to a minute before firing with the expectation that staple line bleeds will be fewer. There is no formal evidence to support the practice, however as with all intestinal stapling, the stapler should be closed for 15 seconds before being fired to accomplish tissue compression and displacement of tissue water. This is the time needed to check the vaginal wall and ensure that all aspects are correct before firing the stapler (**Figure 2.8.8**c).

Once fired, the stapler is opened one half turn and removed. It is important not to open the stapler further because it will hook onto the CAD and be difficult to remove.

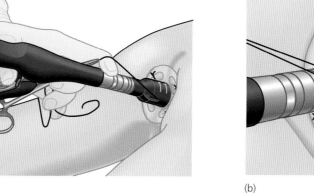

(a)

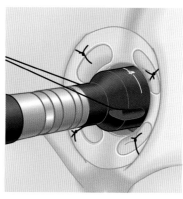

(b)

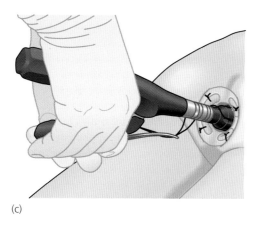

(c)

2.8.8

After removal of the stapler, the purse-string anoscope is introduced to inspect the staple line circumferentially (**Figure 2.8.9**a). The distance of the staple line above the dentate line is recorded (to the nearest half centimeter) in each quadrant. Any bleeding point along the staple line is secured with a resorbable suture (e.g. 4-0) and tied for hemostasis. About 40 percent of the operations will require one or more sutures. The ideal staple line is situated 2 cm above the dentate line immediately on top of the hemorrhoids that should be securely fixed when tested with forceps. Any additional redundancy of mucosa above the staple line is recorded because it can potentially prolapse through the staple line.

The doughnut is removed from the stapler (**Figure 2.8.9**b) and inspected for width and amount of muscular wall that is attached (**Figure 2.8.9**c). All the information about the various steps of the operation is integrated in a learning process that aims at increasing the precision and reproducibility of the procedure. These steps are important because the final stages of the operation are performed blindly once the stapler begins to close.

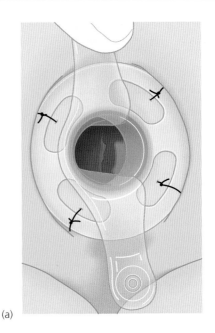

(a)

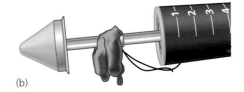

(b)

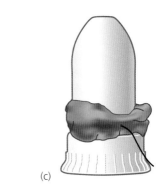

(c)

2.8.9

Technical errors

In the early days, this procedure was afflicted by some serious technical errors by insufficiently trained surgeons. It is a relatively easy procedure to perform, but it is also a very precise procedure with narrow margins for success. It is recommended that training is obtained from a surgeon who has acquired experience with the technique before embarking on performing it. The learning process consists of around 20 procedures, not for managing the technique but for applying the technique to the variety of pathology seen in patients with hemorrhoids.

The following serious complications have been described:

1 **Tearing of the rectal wall**. This is usually the result of undue force being applied during insertion of the stapler. However, the underlying problem may also have been due to misinterpretation of the anatomy. If the purse-string suture is placed too high, there is the potential for inserting the purse string in the anterior rectal wall only. This can result in obstruction to insertion of the stapler, leading to use of excess force.

2 **Obliteration of the rectal lumen**. The mechanism for this is less obvious but again it likely involves misinterpretation of the anatomy with a faulty placement of the purse-string suture that was attempted too high.

3 **Rectovaginal fistula**. This outcome results from too deep insertion of the purse-string suture in the anterior aspect in a female patient combined with failure to check that the vaginal wall is free once the stapler is closed, but before it is fired. In the normal procedure, this complication is very rare but has been described as a late complication several months after an apparently correctly executed hemorrhoidopexy.

4 **Resection of the internal anal sphincter**. This involves applying the purse string too low and too deep with two possible outcomes. The hemorrhoids, the dentate line, and the upper part of the internal sphincter can be excised. Second, if the CAD devise is not used (e.g. in cases where there is difficulty with insertion), there is the possibility that the stapler head is not fully inserted into the anal canal and that the lower part of the internal anal sphincter is hooked on the margin of the stapler head. If this is not recognized and the stapler is fired, part of the internal anal sphincter will be excised.

5 **Fragmentation of the internal anal sphincter**. There are few patients (about 2 percent) whose anal canal is too narrow to accommodate the CAD. The procedure should then be aborted and converted to a conventional excision hemorrhoidectomy. Performing a stapled hemorrhoidopexy without using the CAD requires long experience with the procedure and increases the risk of the above-mentioned serious technical errors. It is advisable to have obtained the patient's prior consent for conversion.

POSTOPERATIVE CARE

Day surgery is appropriate in more than 90 percent of patients. A telephone call the next day will assure that the course is normal and that pain control is adequate. Patients will frequently report disturbed defecation (urgency) and minor voiding difficulty in the first days after surgery. Minor bleeding with stool is also common. Patients are generally well and need no specific care other than provision of a contact telephone number to call if problems arise.

The degree of pain in the recovery room and later is quite variable for reasons that are not well understood. Younger males tend to have more pain and elderly female patients less pain, perhaps reflecting variable density of their tissues. With initial experience, it was believed that postoperative pain was related to inclusion of the rectal wall in the staple line as opposed to rectal mucosa alone. However, nearly all excised specimens have evidence of inclusion of rectal muscularis propria. Pain is undoubtedly greater in patients with a low staple line and less with a higher staple line. The ideal staple line is about 2 cm above the dentate line. A lower staple line will inadvertently excise part of the hemorrhoids and a higher line will not lift the prolapse and fix the hemorrhoids in their normal position. In both situations, there is increased risk of a failed operation with remaining mucosal prolapse above the low staple line or remaining hemorrhoidal prolapse below the high staple line.

In patients with a perianal local block, the patient is usually free of pain for several hours. Some patients will remain pain-free for as long as 10–12 hours, but the more common period is 2–4 hours. This allows the patient to return home without pain.

For patients who remain in hospital, morphine-based agents injected subcutaneously may be preferred. It is particularly useful to alleviate returning pain after a local block. After discharge, a combination of diclofenac 50 mg three times a day and paracetamol 1 g four times a day will suffice in the majority.

The risk of important postoperative bleed is 1–2 percent, but depends on careful control of bleeding points along the staple line. About 5 percent of patients will experience voiding problems but a single urinary catherization is usually sufficient to resolve it.

Defecatory urgency is common in the first weeks and hence patients do not need postoperative laxatives.

OUTCOME

The final result should be evaluated at a visit no earlier than three to six months after surgery. The need to manually reduce prolapse will have been cured in approximately 90 percent of patients and the overall preoperative symptoms will be much reduced in the great majority. There should be no anal pain. Bowel habits should have returned to a normal pattern without urgency. However, as with formal hemorrhoidectomy, as many as 40 percent of patients will report that they experience occasional episodes of one or more of the cardinal symptoms. This also includes occasional symptoms of disturbed continence, such as involuntary gas passage and soiling. Using a questionnaire to capture remaining symptoms after one year or longer showed that 11 percent had remaining or recurrent prolapse and 17 percent had daily or weekly symptoms attributable to hemorrhoids.

The reintervention rate is about 10 percent including a redo stapled hemorrhoidopexy, conventional hemorrhoidectomy, excision of symptomatic skin tags, or rubber band ligation.

Procedure-related complications

The incidence of postoperative bleeding from the staple line reflects the degree of attention to control all bleeding spots at the operation. About 1–2 percent will need reoperation for bleeding.

Thrombosis of retained hemorrhoids below the staple line is a procedure-specific complication that will be seen in about 2 percent of patients. If troublesome, the thrombosis can be excised or otherwise left to resolve spontaneously.

Stenosis of the staple line is rare, but may need dilatation. Separation of part of the staple line is also rare and needs no more than observation.

The staples are expected to discharge from the mucosal anastomosis, but sometimes they will be retained and can lead to inflammatory polyps of the staple line. Such granulomas can cause protracted defecatory bleeding and pain. It is suggested that the granulomas are excised and retained staples are removed if the problem remains several months after the operation.

Rarely, a small pocket can form in the staple line, within what has been termed a 'mucosal exclusion pocket'. It is probably the result of a double folding of the mucosa when closing the stapler. A fecal pellet can be retained in the pocket, which is the reason for its postoperative diagnosis. The pocket can be excised if it is believed to cause any problem.

The operation leads to defecatory urgency in much higher frequency than experienced in conventional hemorrhoidectomy. The reason is not well understood. It has been speculated that the staple line engages a trigger zone of the low rectum. About 30–40 percent will report some degree of this problem, but it will resolve spontaneously within the first weeks. After one year, less than 5 percent report this problem. At its peak, some patients will report urgency incontinence which resolves as the urgency settles.

Rare or serious complications

There will be the rare patient with excessive pain that can result in troublesome spasm of the anal sphincters and pelvic floor. Such patients experience a deep, intense, and highly unpleasant cramp, which sometimes needs relief with a combination of morphine and a benzodiazepine over several days. A continuous low epidural has been needed in some. It is advisable to ascertain that that there is no underlying healing problem, necrosis, or infection involved. These patients typically present 3–5 days after the operation.

There have been rare reports of necrosis of the staple line and development of Fournier's gangrene engaging the anus and distal rectum. There are also rare reports of pelvic emphysema that may extend in the retroperitoneal plane to the diaphragm. Although very rare, such events emphasize that any patient with unexpectedly severe postoperative pain or voiding difficulty needs to be carefully reviewed to exclude a serious complication.

ACKNOWLEDGMENTS

Figure 2.8.3 is reproduced with permission from Nyström PO, Derwinger K, Gerjy R. Local perianal block for anal surgery. *Techniques in Coloproctology* 2004; **8**: 23–6.

FURTHER READING

Burch J, Epstein D, Baba-Akbari A *et al*. Stapled haemorrhoidectomy (haemorrhoidopexy) for the treatment of haemorrhoids: a systematic review and economic evaluation. *Health Technology Assessment* 2008; **12**: 1–193.

Fueglistaler P, Guenin MO, Montali I *et al*. Long-term results after stapled hemorrhoidopexy: high patient satisfaction despite frequent postoperative symptoms. *Diseases of the Colon and Rectum* 2007; **50**: 204–12.

Gerjy R, Lindhoff-Larson A, Sjödahl R, Nyström PO. Randomised trial of stapled haemorrhoidopexy under local perianal block or general anaesthesia. *British Journal of Surgery* 2008; **95**: 1344–51.

Longo A. Stapled anopexy and stapled hemorrhoidectomy: two opposite concepts and procedures. *Diseases of the Colon and Rectum* 2002; **45**: 571–2.

Nyström PO, Qvist N, Raahave D *et al*. on behalf of the STOPP trial study group. Randomised trial of symptom control 1-year after circular stapler anopexy or diathermy excision for prolapsed haemorrhoids. *British Journal of Surgery* 2010; **97**: 167–76.

Shao WJ, Li GC, Zhang ZH *et al*. Systematic review and meta-analysis of randomized controlled trials comparing stapled haemorrhoidopexy with conventional haemorrhoidectomy. *British Journal of Surgery* 2008; **95**: 147–60.

Perianal sepsis

JEAN-CLAUDE R GIVEL AND MICHAEL H COTTON

PRINCIPLES AND JUSTIFICATION

Perianal sepsis corresponds to a spectrum of conditions very commonly encountered in surgical practice. Its presentation may be acute, in the form of an abscess, or chronic as a fistula. Even if most perianal sepsis is simple and easy to manage, a thorough understanding of the etiology and anatomy is required to avoid persistence or recurrence of the disease or impairment of fecal continence. Inadequate attention to detail may lead to serious consequences, in particular necrotizing fasciitis.

Etiology

Most perianal sepsis has a cryptoglandular origin and begins as an intermuscular abscess secondary to infection of an anal gland. Extension of this downwards, between the internal and external anal sphincters or through the lowermost fibers of the external anal sphincter produces a perianal abscess. Extension medially into the submucosal plane produces a high intermuscular or submucosal abscess. Extension laterally into the ischiorectal fossa produces an abscess in this large fatty space. Extension upwards may give rise to a supralevator abscess (**Figure 2.9.1**).

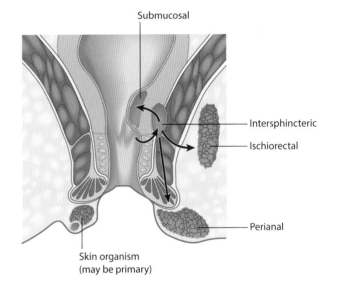

Submucosal

Intersphincteric

Ischiorectal

Perianal

Skin organism
(may be primary)

2.9.1

Diagnosis

The diagnosis of perianal abscess is usually obvious. The patient complains of a lump and the severity of pain is such that the history is short. Examination shows perianal swelling, usually with skin erythema and local tenderness to palpation. Less frequently, the diagnosis is delayed when the patient complains of pain but there is neither obvious swelling nor erythema. Rectal examination is then very uncomfortable. In such a situation, it is possible to miss the true diagnosis of high submucosal sepsis. Any patient who complains of perianal pain of short duration, with or without fever, in whom no fissure is visible should undergo imaging or examination under anesthesia to identify the cause of their symptoms, which will frequently be a high submucosal abscess. A bilateral ischiorectal abscess may, by contrast, present with urinary retention. In the differential diagnosis of perianal sepsis, consideration should be given to abscesses arising nearby, e.g. perineal or periurethral, each of which usually requires a different approach. Pilonidal abscesses and hidradenitis suppurativa (Verneuil's disease) likewise merit specific consideration and therefore should be distinguished from classical perianal sepsis.

The only effective treatment of perianal abscess is surgical. It should be governed by etiology and relieve the immediate symptoms, prevent recurrent sepsis, and minimize healing time. Information for consent should include the possibility of recurrent disease, fistula formation, and rarely, incontinence.

PREOPERATIVE ASSESSMENT AND PREPARATION

In most cases, no specific preoperative assessment or imaging is required, except in patients where deep-seated collections are suspected, or when unusual etiology is present. For example, a rectal examination is advised to exclude the presence of a tumor or an impacted foreign body. Preparation does not include bowel cleansing but, in special situations, antibiotics and thromboembolic prophylaxis may be indicated. Careful positioning of the patient on the operating table in either the lithotomy or the jack-knife position is mandatory. In certain instances, the lateral position may be used.

Usually, surgery for significant perianal sepsis is performed under general anesthesia. Some surgeons use local anesthetic, mostly for small lesions.

OPERATION

Taking note of the anatomy and microbiology is of paramount importance. Nevertheless, at the time of presentation no bacteriological data are usually available.

Examination

Visual examination and then careful palpation define the extent of induration and determine whether an external abscess is perianal, or ischiorectal; a large area of erythema does not necessarily indicate ischiorectal sepsis. The anal canal is then inspected using a speculum, to look for pus draining into it through an internal opening at the dentate line. Gentle pressure on the abscess from outside may help to identify the internal opening by the appearance of pus.

Incision and drainage

Incision and drainage is necessary to evacuate pus. Adequate linear incision over the point of maximal tenderness or induration releases the pus which is sent for microbiological examination. The incision may be radial or circumanal (**Figure 2.9.2**). If radial, it should be superficial to prevent damaging the underlying anal sphincter muscles. The line of incision should reflect the direction of any potential fistula track. A perianal abscess will probably be associated with a low fistula track running directly towards the anal canal, for which a radial incision is indicated. An ischiorectal abscess may be associated with a 'high' fistula running posteriorly, or sometimes anteriorly, and a circumanal incision is then preferred.

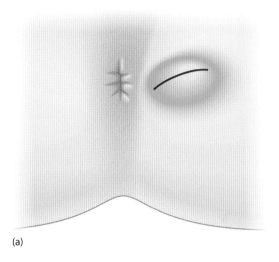

(a)

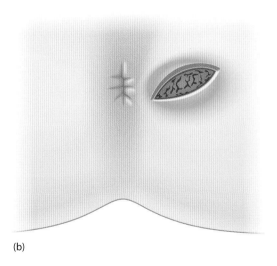

(b)

2.9.2

Curettage

The cavity is curetted, and a small drain may be left *in situ*, or the wound may be lightly packed with an antiseptic dressing.[1] This technique will relieve the immediate symptoms and minimize healing time but will do nothing to prevent recurrent sepsis if a fistula is present. Excision of the overlying skin may be necessary to allow good persistent drainage.

Perianal sepsis may present with bilateral abscesses where the cavities connect in the midline and are usually associated with a posterior fistula. Drainage of such a 'horseshoe' abscess will require at least one incision on either side, depending on the extent of the sepsis. (**Figure 2.9.3**). Such incisions should not cross the midline.[2]

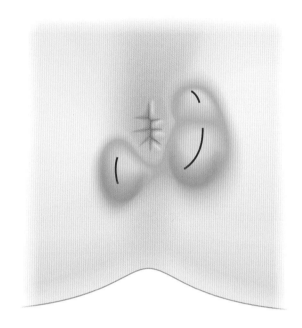

2.9.3

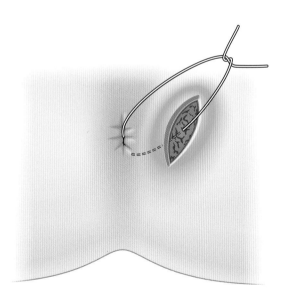

2.9.4

Debate still exists concerning the management of a fistula, if present.[3] If it is superficial and easy to delineate with a probe, it may be excised or deroofed concurrently (**Figure 2.9.4**). Otherwise, a fine loose rubber seton is passed through the fistula for drainage.

More complicated or multiple fistulae are best left alone at this stage. Vigorous probing of a fistula track may cause a false passage and exacerbate the sepsis. In children, it is especially worth looking for and treating a fistula (see Chapter 2.10).[4]

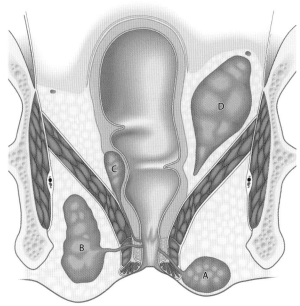

A: Superficial perianal abscess
B: Ischeorectal abscess
C: High intersphincteric abscess
D: Supralevator abscess

2.9.5

High perirectal abscesses

A high submucous or intersphincteric abscess requires a different approach. The diagnosis is made either at anorectal palpation, imaging, or instrumentation, which may itself cause the abscess to rupture. Localization of the abscess cavity by needling may be necessary at speculum examination. The entire extent of the abscess, which usually extends longitudinally, is deroofed intrarectally and its edges marsupialized to ensure proper drainage. Such drainage should never be attempted exteriorly as a high fistula will result (**Figure 2.9.5**).

The higher, more complex, supralevator abscess is likewise drained through the rectum, provided it does not arise from a pelvic septic process (such as appendicitis, gynecological sepsis, or diverticulitis) or from extension of an ischiorectal abscess. These two latter rare types of supralevator abscess are best drained through the perineum, vagina, or abdominal wall, or via the ischiorectal fossa itself (**Figure 2.9.6**).

In contrast, the deep postanal space abscess, which is palpable between the coccyx and the anal margin, should not be approached through the anorectum, but directly through the skin.

Purulent drainage found in the anal canal may not arise from a submucous abscess, but be caused by gonorrhea, inflammatory bowel disease, fungal infection especially related to HIV infection, tuberculosis, schistosomiasis, or amebiasis. Occasionally, sepsis arises secondary to coexisting tumors, condylomata, or unsuspected trauma.

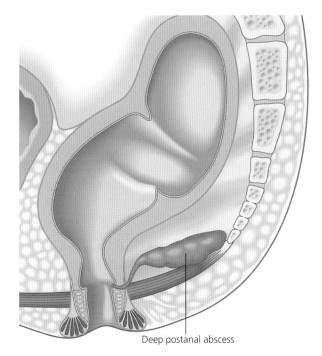

Deep postanal abscess

2.9.6

POSTOPERATIVE CARE

Non-constipating analgesia will be required, but patients with an abscess or abscess and fistula rarely experience as much pain as those who have undergone hemorrhoidectomy.

Following examination and drainage, if no fistula is found, the abscess cavity should be packed as necessary for hemostasis with antiseptic solution, such as povidone iodine or chlorhexidine in the dressing. This will be removed the following day and then renewed with an alternative comfortable dressing. In the presence of residual infection, an alginate dressing with silver can be used. The patient should be discharged home either with instructions on wound management or followed up in an ambulatory care unit.

The patient should shower at least twice a day and after each bowel motion. The wound will be daily irrigated with antiseptic solution and normal saline. Then a suitable dressing is applied into the cavity. It should not be tightly packed and ribbon gauze should only exceptionally be used. The anal dressing should be held in place with close-fitting elastic underwear which holds the dressing comfortably in place. Altogether the dressing should be kept simple, to allow the patient independence as soon as possible.

With adequate surgical drainage of the abscess there is no place for antibiotics in postoperative management, except in those few cases with fulminating gangrene, tuberculosis, or immunosuppression.

Normal bowel action should be encouraged from the first postoperative day. A high-fiber diet combined with mild laxatives will ensure that the patient will have normal and easy bowel movements.

OUTCOME

The outcome after surgery for acute perianal sepsis is usually straightforward. Three main complications may however occur: (1) recurrent sepsis due to incomplete drainage or persistent fistula; (2) fecal incontinence; and (3) spreading sepsis leading to necrosis. For recurrent or spreading sepsis, the causes are usually either insufficient initial surgery or the presence of associated special conditions. Among the latter, three have to be considered: Crohn's disease, immunosuppression, above all HIV infection, and tuberculosis.[5]

Recurrent sepsis

The management of perianal sepsis in these situations must include treatment of the underlying disease. Certain principles should be kept in mind: (1) perianal sepsis is always associated with a fistula which should be managed by conservative means, e.g. a seton; (2) a course of appropriate antibiotics is advised in addition to surgical treatment; (3) radical surgery should be avoided as large anal wounds do not heal quickly.

Incontinence

Incontinence after such intervention may include simple soiling, flatus, and urge incontinence or gross fecal spillage. The former may be managed by dietetary control and sphincter exercises. Complete fecal incontinence usually requires a temporary defunctioning colostomy and careful examination to elucidate its cause. Treatment is often complex, and may include sphincter reconstruction.

Necrotizing fasciitis

Necrotizing fasciitis is a rapidly spreading infection caused by a combination of obligate anaerobes.[6] Infection is then often associated with gas production, bad odor, and rapid proliferation to adjacent planes, especially subcutaneous tissues or subfascial planes. Thus infection may spread to the perineum, scrotum, abdominal wall, thigh, and buttocks. This is a surgical emergency which requires resuscitation for septic shock, immediate treatment with large-spectrum intravenous antibiotics, extensive debridement to include surrounding unaffected tissues (regardless of the extent), and often a defunctioning colostomy once the initial catastrophic circumstances have resolved. Frequent repeated desloughing procedures are often required.

Hidradenitis suppurativa (Verneuil's disease) syn. acne inversa

Hidradenitis suppurativa is a chronic low-grade sepsis of the skin and subcutaneous tissues, whose pathogenesis remains unclear. The anatomical distribution of the disease is mainly in the axillary and anogenital areas, and appears to be the result of occlusion of hair follicles, leading in turn to inflammation of apocrine glands.[7]

It occurs after puberty, more commonly in smokers and the obese, and sometimes as a result of lithium or oral combined estrogen–progesterone contraceptive therapy.

The patient presents with typical multiple discharging lesions with interconnecting sinus tracts in the skin, associated with attempts at healing resulting in pitted scars, fibrous bands, and indurated plaques. There is variable secondary infection which may result in considerable inflammation, offensive odor, and decreased mobility.

The diagnosis should be differentiated from donovanosis (granuloma inguinale), which produces ulceration rather than fistulae, and Crohn's disease, where the fistulae are deeper and often associated with diarrheal symptoms.

Treatment of the condition is often prolonged (up to 20 years), frustrating, and with poor results. A conservative approach is recommended for early and mild disease: cessation of smoking, avoidance of perspiration and friction from clothing, and promotion of weight loss. The use of clindamycin or rifampicin, possibly with the addition of anti-androgens, may induce a remission, but the disease is very likely to relapse in time.

Surgical intervention is necessary for chronic, relapsing, and severe disease: this entails excision of the affected area of skin and subcutaneous tissues, including fistula tracks, as far as soft normal tissue, leaving adjacent and deep margins of 2 cm well beyond active disease. As a principle, the wound should be left open to heal by secondary intention, but skin grafting and transposition flaps may be useful in exceptional situations.

REFERENCES

1. Tonkin DM, Murphy E, Brooke-Smith M *et al.* Perianal abscess: a pilot study comparing packing with nonpacking of the abscess cavity. *Diseases of the Colon and Rectum* 2004; **47**: 1510–4.

2. Whiteford MH, Kilkenny J 3rd, Hyman N *et al.* Standards Practice Task Force; American Society of Colon and Rectal Surgeons. Practice parameters for the treatment of perianal abscess and fistula-in-ano (revised). *Diseases of the Colon and Rectum* 2005; **48**: 1337–42.

3. Juviler A, Hyman N. Perianal abscess and fistula. *Surgical Technology International* 2008; **17**: 139–49.

4. Murthi GV, Okoye BO, Spicer RD *et al.* Perianal abscess in childhood. *Pediatric Surgery International* 2002; **18**: 689–91.

5. Mardini HE, Schwarz DA. Treatment of perianal fistula and abscess: Crohn's and non-Crohn's. *Current Treatment Options in Gastroenterology* 2007; **10**: 211–22.

6. Ledingham IMcA, Tehrani MA. Diagnosis, clinical course and treatment of acute dermal gangrene. *British Journal of Surgery* 1975; **62**: 364–72.

7. Buimer MG, Wobbes T, Klinkenbijl JHG. Hidradenitis suppurativa. *British Journal of Surgery* 2009; **96**: 350–60.

Anal fistula

TOBY M HAMMOND AND PETER J LUNNISS

HISTORICAL

Anal fistulae are chronic pathological connections between the anal canal and the skin of the perineum or buttocks, which do not heal spontaneously. They usually pass through a variable proportion of the anal sphincter complex. They are subject to either persistent discharge or recurrent episodes of painful abscess formation, eased by either spontaneous drainage or repeated hospital admissions for surgical drainage. Failure of adequate and sustained drainage may lead to a more complicated situation, as secondary tracks and abscesses develop. The majority of anal fistulae can be managed, without significant compromise to anal sphincter function, by a conventional approach, but a substantial minority can present a major challenge to both patient and surgeon. Indeed, in the concluding remarks of his address to the Royal Society of Medicine in 1929, Mr JP Lockhart

Mummery stated, 'Probably more reputations have been damaged by the unsuccessful treatment of cases of fistula than by excision of the rectum or gastroenterostomy.' The difficulty resides in the balance between eradication of the pathology and preservation of function (continence). Over the last 30 years, efforts have been increasingly directed towards sphincter preservation, but almost certainly at the expense of long-term surgical cure. The contribution of Sir Alan Parks to the etiology, classification, and principles of management of anal fistulae remains highly pertinent today.

The relevant anatomy of the anal region is shown in **Figure 2.10.1**. It is important to appreciate that the pelvic floor and sphincter complex are funnel shaped, and thus the apex of the ischiorectal fossa lies above the anorectal junction, and that the sling-shaped puborectalis muscle is absent anteriorly.

PRINCIPLES AND JUSTIFICATION

The multiplicity of reported techniques designed to achieve the dual aims of fistula eradication and preservation of continence is testament to the fact that no single method is universally effective at achieving both. The following principles dictate approach:

- Define the etiology of the fistula.
- Classify the anatomy of the fistula in relation to the primary track and, if present, any secondary tracks and collections. This must involve an appreciation of the fistula's vertical, horizontal, and circumferential dimensions.
- Determine the structural and functional integrity of the sphincter complex through which the fistula passes.
- Determine the patient's bowel habit (stool frequency and form).
- Assess the individual patient's expectation of treatment based on the degree to which they are prepared to accept sphincter damage and its functional outcome. This is

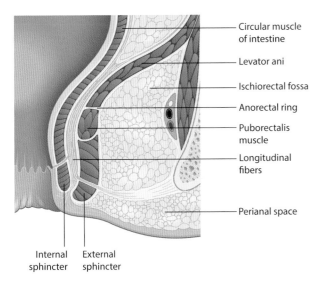

Circular muscle of intestine

Levator ani

Ischiorectal fossa

Anorectal ring

Puborectalis muscle

Longitudinal fibers

Perianal space

Internal sphincter   External sphincter

2.10.1

often determined by the severity of symptoms and the number of previous attempts at cure. Most patients are prepared to accept minor degrees of soiling (mucous or feculant) as a reasonable alternative to chronic pain and sepsis (itself associated with soiling in the form of discharging pus, inflammatory exudate, and occasionally feces).

- Before surgical intervention, clarify what the surgical strategy should be, including whether the ultimate aim is palliation or cure.

Etiology

CRYPTOGLANDULAR HYPOTHESIS

Anal fistulae may be found in association with a variety of conditions, but the majority (>90 percent) seen in the United Kingdom are classified as nonspecific, cryptoglandular, or idiopathic, in which the diseased anal gland in the intersphincteric space is deemed central. Intersphincteric anal gland ducts traverse the internal sphincter to open into the anal canal lumen, at the lower end of the anal crypts of Morgagni. The function of anal glands is uncertain, although they do secrete mucin. Parks hypothesized, with histological evidence, that intersphincteric gland dilatation (congenital or acquired) is a precursor to mucin accumulation, which renders the gland prone to infection from ascending enteric bacteria via the openings of the anal ducts. The infected intersphincteric gland is unable to drain spontaneously back into the anal canal, because of inflammatory obstruction of its connecting duct across the internal sphincter, and thus infection spreads along the plane of least resistance, the fibers of the conjoined longitudinal muscle (**Figure 2.10.2**).

Sepsis can spread inferiorly via the intersphincteric space to emerge at the skin as a perianal abscess, laterally through the external sphincter to form an ischiorectal abscess, superiorly to form a supralevator abscess, as well as circumferentially to form a horseshoe extension (**Figure 2.10.3**).

Parks further proposed that following subsidence of the initial abscess within the intersphincteric anal gland, the diseased gland becomes the seat of chronic infection and subsequently a persistent fistula. The fistula is therefore a track, lined by granulation tissue, that is maintained by the infecting source, the chronically infected anal gland deep to the internal anal sphincter. Whether fistula persistence is secondary to chronic infection of a diseased anal gland or to epithelialization of the fistula tract (as in fistulae found at other sites in the body) is debated, but nonetheless the importance of the intersphincteric component in relation to the management of the fistula must not be ignored.

SPECIFIC ETIOLOGY

The remainder of anal fistulae may be seen in association with inflammatory bowel disease (commonly, but not exclusively, Crohn's disease), tuberculosis, pilonidal disease, hidradenitis suppurativa, malignancy (anal canal cancers, rectal cancer, and cancer arising in an anal gland), trauma, foreign bodies, and sexually transmitted diseases. These specific fistulae primarily require treatment (systemic or local) of their underlying pathology, and will not be addressed further.

Classification

The most practical and widely used classification is that proposed by Sir Alan Parks, based upon the centrality of intersphincteric space infection, and the relation of the primary track to the external anal sphincter (EAS). The classification divides fistulae into four main groups: (1) intersphincteric and (2) trans-sphincteric (which together constitute about 95 percent of fistulae), (3)

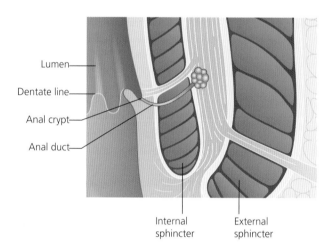

Lumen
Dentate line
Anal crypt
Anal duct
Internal sphincter
External sphincter

2.10.2

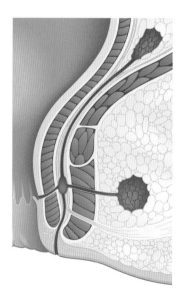

2.10.3

suprasphincteric, and (4) extrasphincteric. These groups can be further subdivided according to the presence and course of any extensions or secondary tracks.

Intersphincteric fistulae are usually solitary primary tracks which pass caudally through the intersphincteric space to the perianal skin (**Figure 2.10.4**a). As the most inferomedial fibers of the subcutaneous EAS often lie beyond the distal border of the internal anal sphincter, intersphincteric fistulae may actually cross some voluntary muscle (a detail that has little implication in the management). However, some intersphincteric fistulae may have a high blind intersphincteric secondary extension, and very rarely a secondary high opening into the rectum (**Figure 2.10.4**b). Equally rarely, there may be a track extending cephalad to end in a supralevator abscess, and there may not be an external opening (**Figure 2.10.4**c).

Trans-sphincteric fistulae cross the external sphincter to pass through the ischiorectal fossa to reach the gluteal skin (**Figure 2.10.5**a). They may be subdivided into 'high', 'mid', or 'low' dependent on the point at which the track crosses the EAS in relation to the dentate line (above, level with, or below, respectively). This is not always at the same level that the track crosses the internal anal sphincter (IAS). Fistulae may consist of the primary track, or have a blind high secondary track terminating below or (rarely) above the pelvic floor (**Figure 2.10.5**b).

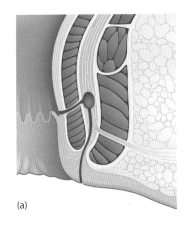

(a)

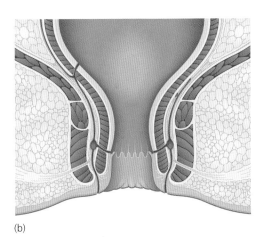

(b)

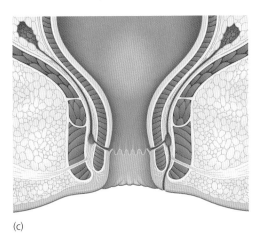

(c)

2.10.4

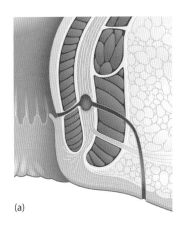

(a)

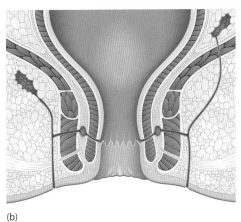

(b)

2.10.5

Suprasphincteric fistulae run cephalad in the intersphincteric space to a level above the puborectalis muscle leading to a supralevator abscess (**Figure 2.10.6**). The fistula gains access to the ischiorectal fossa and buttock skin through the levator ani muscle. The advent of magnetic resonance imaging (MRI) has led to a decrease in the prevalence of fistulae so classified (as opposed to high trans-sphincteric), and many believe them to be iatrogenic rather than a natural result of cryptoglandular pathology.

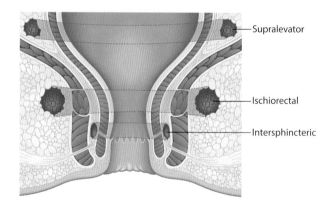

2.10.6

Extrasphincteric fistulae run without specific relation to the anal sphincters, are not cryptoglandular, and are classified according to their pathogenesis (such as pelvic sepsis (diverticular, appendicular, gynecological), Crohn's disease, tuberculosis (TB), malignancy, and iatrogenic) (**Figure 2.10.7**).

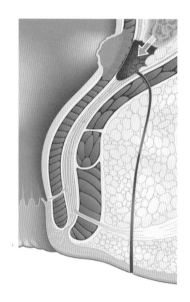

2.10.7

In addition to horizontal and vertical spread, sepsis may spread circumferentially, in a (hemi- or full) horseshoe pattern, within any of the three spaces: intersphincteric, ischiorectal, or supralevator (**Figure 2.10.8**).

PREOPERATIVE ASSESSMENT

CLINICAL

A full history and examination including proctosigmoid-oscopy are essential in all cases. The history should detail:

- Perineal/anal events leading up to the current presentation (abscesses and treatment thereof) and symptomatology: is this typical for idiopathic fistula or suggestive of specific etiology? Has the patient suffered abscesses at other skin sites (groins or axillae) suggestive of hidradenitis suppurativa, or other dermatological pathology? Is the discharge purulent or feculent (indicative of rectal or large anal internal opening)? How much do the symptoms interfere with quality of life?
- Bowel habit (frequency and stool form).

Supralevator

Ischiorectal

Intersphincteric

2.10.8

- Assessment of continence (anal soiling may be difficult to assess in the presence of fistula discharge), obstetric history in women, and any previous fistula, or other anal or gastrointestinal surgery.
- Personal or family history of bowel disease.
- When indicated, HIV and BCG status.

Following a general examination, local clinical assessment is directed at the fistula and the sphincters. Fistula assessment involves five essential points: (1) location of the external opening(s), (2) location of the internal opening, (3) the course of the primary track, (4) the presence of any secondary extensions, and (5) the presence of other diseases complicating the fistula.

Goodsall's rule generally applies (**Figure 2.10.9**). Exceptions include anterior openings greater than 3 cm from the anal verge, which may be anterior extensions of posterior horseshoe fistulae, or fistulae associated with other diseases, such as Crohn's disease and malignancy.

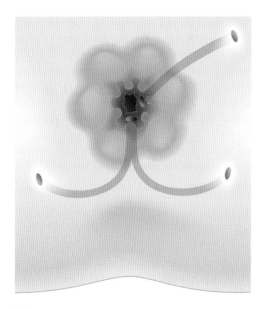

2.10.9

The entire perianal region is initially inspected for the presence of an external opening(s). A well-lubricated gloved index finger should feel around the anus for the presence and direction of an indurated cord extending from the external opening to the anal verge (**Figure 2.10.10**). If a track can be palpated, it suggests a relatively low fistula, and the direction (radial or circumferential) will often indicate the location of the internal opening. If induration cannot be felt in proximity to the anus, it is probable that the track crosses the sphincter at a higher level. To identify the internal opening by palpation, the examining index finger is placed within the anal lumen while the thumb applies counterpressure on the perianal skin. Indentation or induration tends to mark its position, which usually lies at the dentate line.

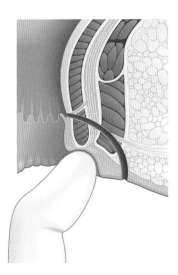

2.10.10

The index finger is then advanced into the distal rectum to assess for supralevator induration (it feels like bone, and if unilateral is palpably different from the contralateral side) (**Figure 2.10.11**). Induration at this level usually arises from the upward extension of a trans-sphincteric track (either terminating at the roof of the ischiorectal fossa or passing through the levators), a high primary transsphincteric track, or rarely a suprasphincteric extension of an intersphincteric track. Digital examination cannot distinguish between these scenarios.

Global pelvic floor strength can be judged by the surrogate of perineal position at rest and degree of descent at strain. The length and bulk of the anal sphincter complex, the resting tone of the internal sphincter, and the strength and duration of voluntary muscle squeeze can

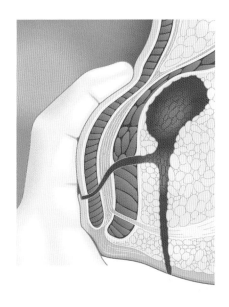

2.10.11

be, at least subjectively, assessed digitally. Depending on the clinical assessment of the fistula, it may be possible to judge how much functioning muscle would remain if the fistula were to be laid open. The suppleness (as opposed to woodiness) of the sphincters, and the presence of other anal pathology (e.g. fissures, large haemorrhoids, warts, etc.) should be assessed, as these factors may influence management.

Finally the surgeon should perform proctosigmoidoscopy to assess the anorectal mucosa and hopefully to see the internal opening.

Imaging

Although careful examination will be sufficient for the majority of newly presenting fistulae, there are situations in which imaging, to define fistula topography, is helpful in planning management. These include patients in whom previous surgery has led to scarring, fibrosis, and deformity; the primary track is not palpable; high induration is evident; and those with external openings either side of the midline. In these circumstances, MRI of the perineum using appropriate protocols (including STIR (short T1 inversion recovery) sequencing, and nowadays with gadolinium enhancement) is the most useful to counsel patients as to potential problems in management and to plan surgical strategy. In those patients with suspected extrasphincteric fistulae, pelvic imaging combined with fistulography may be useful in determining the underlying etiology.

Physiological

Complete division of the sphincter complex including the puborectalis sling and upper external sphincter (the anorectal ring) in extrasphincteric and suprasphincteric fistulae results in total incontinence to all rectal contents. Below this level, the term 'incontinence' becomes relative, dependent more on subjective values of the patient (and its impact on individual quality of life) than on objective measurements obtained in a physiology laboratory. However, it is reasonable to assume that the higher the level at which the primary track crosses the sphincter complex (i.e. the more sphincter tissue enclosed by the fistula), the greater the possibility and severity of impaired function after surgical division; and the weaker the sphincters before surgical intervention, the greater the likelihood of such morbidity. Preoperative anorectal physiology assessment can be used to identify patients at risk of incontinence, and thus guide surgical treatment, but it does not necessarily predict postoperative functional outcomes. It is important to acknowledge that, in a condition in which adequate drainage of the intersphincteric space has been deemed central to success, internal sphincter division to the dentate line may have a functional price (about a 1 in 4 chance of occasional soiling and passive flatus leakage).

PATIENT PREPARATION

- **Consent**. The details of informed consent obviously depend on the nature of the agreed procedure, whether it is part of a staged surgical strategy, and whether sphincter division is planned. If the latter, consent necessarily must involve a discussion of the risks to sphincter function. The patient should also be informed of the likely postoperative course. Pain is normally well controlled by a combination of paracetamol and sodium diclofenac (if not contraindicated). Postoperative bleeding is rare, but may necessitate return to hospital and further procedure under anesthetic to control it. Wound care will depend upon the procedure performed. Postoperative stool softeners and bulking agents are employed to overcome the fear of pain associated with defecation in the early postoperative course.
- **Bowel preparation and antibiotics**. These are usually only indicated if an advancement flap is to be created.
- **Venous thromboembolic prophylaxis**. Compression stockings, intraoperative pneumatic calf pumps, and prophylactic doses of low molecular weight heparin are used according to the patient's level of risk, renal function, and hospital policy.
- **Anesthesia**. The preference is general anesthesia, although rarely, regional anesthesia may be used. It is essential, however, that the patient does not move from the position they are placed in before surgery begins, as retraction of the perineum away from the surgeon will make the procedure much more difficult.
- **Patient position**. The lithotomy position is preferred, with the buttocks clear of the end of the table, the lumbosacral spine well supported, and the legs in Lloyd Davies stirrups (rather than standard lithotomy poles) to allow hip abduction and easy surgical access. A slight head-down position improves the operator's visual and manual comfort. The prone jack-knife position is perhaps more popular in the United States, and possibly provides better access to anterior fistulae.
- **Shaving**. Shaving of the perineum with a large scalpel blade and lubricant (Savlon) makes examination under anesthesia more informative, surgery more esthetic, and wound care easier.

OPERATIVE PRINCIPLES

Equipment. The instruments that are required include a set of Lockhart-Mummery fistula probes and lachrymal probes. Lachrymal probes may provide the only means with which to negotiate narrow, fibrosed tracks. Hand-activated monopolar diathermy, tenotomy scissors, mosquito forceps, a small self-retaining retractor and an Eisenhammer proctoscope should also be available. We use 2 mm silastic setons (the knot reinforced with 2/0 Ethibond™) for short-term drainage and as cutting setons, due to the comfortable nature of the material and its elasticity, respectively. 1/0 Ethibond™ is employed for long-term palliative drainage, as it is durable and comfortable.

The preoperative assessment of the fistula is confirmed at examination under anesthesia (EUA). This involves a repeat examination as performed in the clinic (including proctosigmoidoscopy), confirmation of the presence of the fistula and site of internal opening, and course of the primary track with the gentle use of probes. An Eisenhammer anal retractor is inserted into the anal canal, the blades gently separated and the internal opening sought. Downward or lateral traction of the dentate line may expose concealed openings, or reveal dimpling of the mucosa which suggests a tethered opening. Massage of any induration may release a bead of pus at the internal opening. Instillation of dilute hydrogen peroxide through the external opening (which should be performed before any operative intervention, and with the blades of the Eisenhammer proctoscope opened minimally to avoid track compression) will confirm the site of the internal opening. Submucosal bulging indicates the site of an epithelialized internal opening.

One of a variety of straight or angled probes (depending upon ease of passage) is passed through the external and/or internal opening to determine the course of the fistula track (**Figure 2.10.12**). If the internal and external openings can be detected but the probe fails to traverse the fistula track, there may be a high extension, or an acute angulation. This can occur in the intersphincteric space if the fistula crosses the external sphincter at a different level to that at which it traverses the internal sphincter, or in the roof of the ischiorectal fossa, where the fistula having crossed the external sphincter takes a sharp downward turn towards the skin of the buttock. Such fistulae can sometimes be negotiated by passing probes through both openings, and feeling for their metallic clash ('fencing'). Care should always be taken and probes never unduly forced lest an iatrogenic track be created. If the fistula cannot be successfully probed, the track has to be followed as it is cored out, until the angulation is overcome and probing possible.

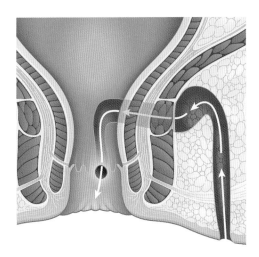

2.10.12

Following EUA, the surgeon must decide whether it is reasonable to perform a one-stage sphincter dividing procedure (fistulotomy or cutting seton) on the basis of the level at which the primary track crosses the IAS ± EAS. If the primary track is relatively short, or the external opening remote but the extrasphincteric component of the track superficial, then a one-stage procedure is indicated. If the primary track is long and deeper, or if there are secondary extensions deep in the ischiorectal fossa, the situation should be simplified such that the extrasphincteric parts of the track are eradicated, and that part of the track crossing the sphincters drained by a loose seton.

To ensure wound healing following this procedure, with no recurrence of the previously sited external opening, then rather than simply laying open the extrasphincteric components of the fistula, they are cored out (along with their fibrous surround) using diathermy (**Figure 2.10.13**). Although resulting in a larger wound and longer healing time, such a strategy allows a more accurate determination of the level at which the primary track crosses the EAS (evident as the core out reaches the sphincter's lateral border). Once the wound has fully healed, the seton-enclosed sphincteric component of the fistula track can be dealt with at a second stage.

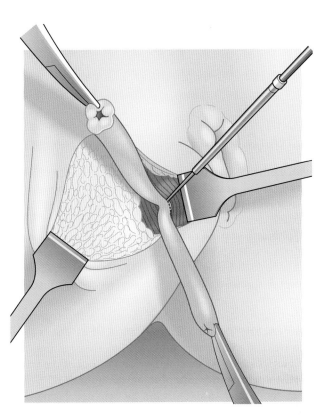

2.10.13

Intersphincteric horseshoe extension/high intersphincteric blind extension (Figure 2.10.14). In the chronic situation, these rarely resolve simply by placement of a draining seton, and require internal sphincterotomy from the internal opening to the anal margin and simple curettage of the intersphincteric extension. The functional consequences of a long internal sphincterotomy are such that this strategy is best avoided unless there is persistence following curettage.

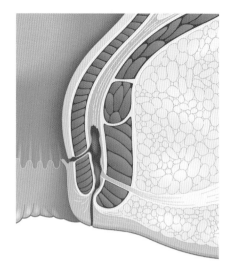

2.10.14

If there is a secondary rectal internal opening, then the circular muscle will need to be divided to that point (**Figure 2.10.15**).

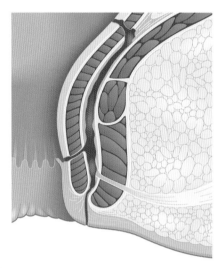

2.10.15

Posterior horseshoe fistula running high under the roof of the ischiorectal fossa (Figure 2.10.16). In this situation, it is often not initially possible to negotiate probes along the length of the fistula because of an acute bend in its course at the roof of the ischiorectal fossa. A probe should be passed through the external opening(s) to the presumed apex of the angulation, the edge of the external opening is then grasped with a pair of mosquito forceps, traction applied and a circumferential incision made around the opening. The track is cored out until the apex of the bend is reached. The incision may need to be enlarged and a small self-retaining retractor applied to facilitate the dissection. A probe can then be used to follow the track as it passes medially, to reach the track passing up from the similarly mobilized contralateral hemi-horseshoe. The extrasphincteric component of track in the posterior midline is then laid open with diathermy. This may require dislocation of the posterior sphincter from the anococcygeal ligament, and entry into the retrosphincteric space. This will allow the sphincteric component of the fistula to be negotiated with a probe.

High blind secondary extension from a transsphincteric fistula which penetrates the levators to reach the pelvis. Such extensions cannot be cored out. With the non-dominant index finger transanally abutting the rectal wall, the limit of the extension is assessed with the end of a curette (safer than a probe), the passage through the levators enlarged laterally (this usually requires division

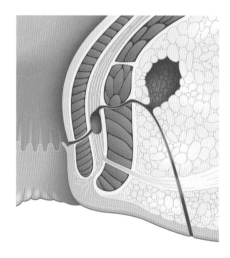

2.10.16

with diathermy), and the extension carefully but completely curetted of all granulation tissue. Widening the hole in the levators enables access, and also allows wound dressings to reach the wound apex and thus satisfactory healing.

Sphincter-sparing surgery. Central to the success of all techniques which avoid sphincter division (advancement flaps and use of biomaterials) are the elimination of acute sepsis and the eradication of any secondary fistulous extensions by the techniques described above, such that there is a loose draining seton through a short primary track. At the second (curative) stage, it is essential to remove all granulation or epithelial tissue lining the primary track, either by curettage or core out of the track.

Histological and microbiological appraisal. Tissue from the fistula should always be sent for histological appraisal, and if there is suspicion, also for microbiological culture, including that for *Mycobacterium tuberculosis*.

Although the overall pick up is low for specific etiologies, failure to look for them can lead to protracted misery for the patient.

A record of the operative findings should be documented diagrammatically. The authors' preference is the St Mark's Hospital fistula operation sheet (**Figure 2.10.17**).

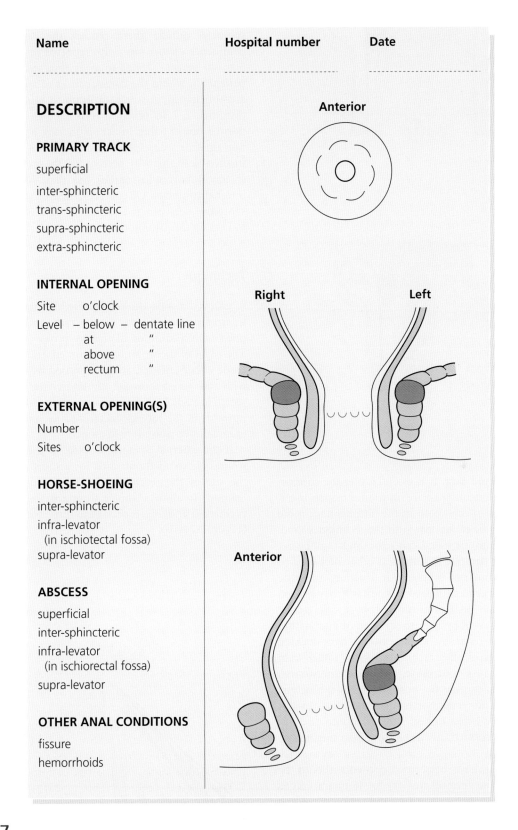

Name

Hospital number

Date

DESCRIPTION

PRIMARY TRACK

superficial

inter-sphincteric

trans-sphincteric

supra-sphincteric

extra-sphincteric

INTERNAL OPENING

Site   o'clock

Level – below – dentate line
        at   "
        above   "
        rectum   "

EXTERNAL OPENING(S)

Number

Sites   o'clock

HORSE-SHOEING

inter-sphincteric

infra-levator
  (in ischiotectal fossa)
supra-levator

ABSCESS

superficial

inter-sphincteric

infra-levator
  (in ischiorectal fossa)
supra-levator

OTHER ANAL CONDITIONS

fissure

hemorrhoids

Anterior

Right   Left

Anterior

2.10.17

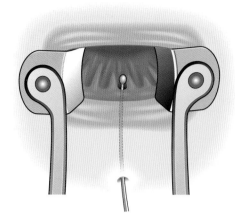

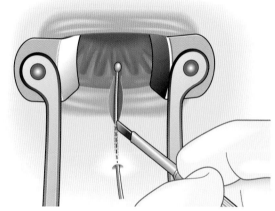

2.10.18

Details of wound care. It is essential that the surgeon is explicit in documenting advice on wound management, as those involved in care, both in the hospital and in the community, may be unfamiliar with the techniques used. For example, it must be stated that setons must not be cut and removed, in contrast to sutures at other sites used to close wounds primarily. Similarly, instructions must be given in the management of deep wounds, which may need irrigation and daily digitations (possibly by a willing carer or partner) to prevent premature bridging of granulation tissue (and thus recurrent sepsis), before light tucking of the wound (especially reaching its apex) rather than traditional packing. On occasion, the size of the wound, particularly after surgery for posterior trans-sphincteric fistulae with ischiorectal horseshoe extensions, means it may take many weeks to heal, but the resulting scar is surprisingly less cosmetically displeasing than might have been anticipated.

If biomaterials have been used, patients should be advised to keep the perineal area dry for 48 hours, and to avoid any activity which may disrupt this region, including swimming, cycling, horse-riding, and sexual activity, for at least 2 weeks following surgery.

FISTULOTOMY

This technique involves surgically dividing the tissue enclosed by the fistula and allowing the wound to heal by secondary intention. It remains the most effective way of eradicating fistulae, but through division of the enclosed sphincter muscle fibers, renders the patient at risk of continence disturbance, with reported rates ranging from 5 to 40 percent. Fistulotomy is thus indicated in those patients in whom the consequences of sphincter division are anticipated, at worst, to result in minimal functional disturbance – in practical terms, in an individual with normal bowel habit, intact sphincters, and a fistula (but not anterior trans-sphincteric fistulae in women) which involves less than 30 percent of the external sphincter (below puborectalis) and/or less than 30 percent of the internal sphincter. Of course, failure of other techniques, symptom persistence, and patient agreement extends the indication for fistulotomy.

Technique

A grooved fistula probe is passed from the external to internal opening of the fistula track, and the fistula laid open with a knife or diathermy probe (**Figure 2.10.18**). The edges of the wound are trimmed, and the granulation tissue either curetted away or excised by sharp dissection with care taken to avoid any underlying muscle. Careful search is made for any extensions of the fistula, particularly upwards in the intersphincteric plane, and if present, the granulation tissue curetted away.

If the external opening is close to the anal verge, the wound is extended outwards for a short distance beyond the site of the (excised) external opening (back-cut of Salmon) to allow adequate wound drainage and prevent premature bridging, especially in those with large buttocks (**Figure 2.10.19**).

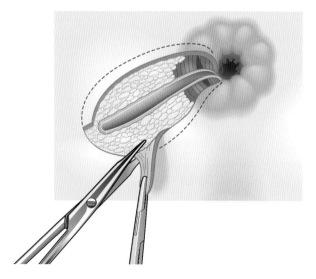

2.10.19

Marsupialization involves suturing the divided wound edges to the edges of the opened curetted fistula track with absorbable sutures (**Figure 2.10.20**). Although marsupialization may lead to a smaller defect and more rapid healing, worse cosmesis can result.

THE LOOSE SETON

The term 'seton' is derived from the latin word '*seta*', meaning a bristle. Setons are used in fistula surgery in various ways. They are classified as loose or cutting (tight, snug, or chemical) according to their different properties and modes of action. The loose seton can be used for different reasons in the management of anal fistulae. A loosely tied thread can be used to drain sepsis and to allow subsidence of acute inflammation, as a drain for the primary track following eradication of secondary extensions before subsequent definitive surgery, or as a long-term palliative measure aimed at symptom control (by preventing the fistula track from occluding, and allowing sepsis to drain, thereby avoiding recurrent abscess formation and covert spread of sepsis). It can also be used as a marker to help determine the amount of muscle enclosed by the fistula, perhaps because scarring from previous surgery or relaxation under anesthesia makes assessment during surgery difficult. In such circumstances, the proportion of enclosed sphincter above and below the fistula may be more accurately determined when the patient is awake and the track marked by the seton.

Technique

Various materials are suitable, including a braided or monofilament non-absorbable suture or silastic. The extrasphincteric component of the track is cored out or laid open, and a probe is negotiated through the sphincteric component of the track. Lockhart-Mummery probes are designed with a groove, along which a suture can be negotiated. If used, a length of 0-0 nylon (employed as it has sufficient rigidity) is passed along the groove, and a more appropriate material (either silastic or Ethibond™) is then tied securely to one end of the nylon, and the other end pulled through such that the seton then traverses the track. If a probe with an eyelet is utilized then the seton can simply be passed through the aperture, secured, and then the probe pulled out leaving the seton positioned through the sphincteric component of the fistula (**Figure 2.10.21**).

THE CUTTING SETON

The first recorded description of this technique is credited to Hippocrates, who recorded the use of a horse hair thread, tightened intermittently 'until the enclosed flesh was eaten through'. The rationale is similar to that of the

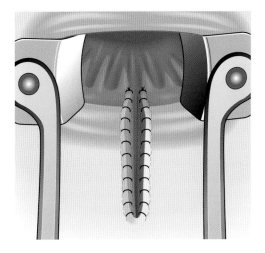

2.10.20

now infrequently employed staged fistulotomy (in which the sphincter below the fistula is divided surgically in stages, with a loose seton applied and further division performed upon adequate healing of the previously created wound), in that the sphincter complex is gradually severed, by repeated tightening or replacement of the seton, with the advantage of less retraction of the divided muscle. The technique certainly works, but when applied (more historically) to 'high' fistulae it is associated with high rates of both major and minor incontinence. Additionally, the technique may be associated with considerable patient discomfort and there is the need for repeated replacement/ tightening of the seton, of which a number of different types have been described. These include Penrose drains, stainless steel rubber bands or their elastic equivalent, braided synthetic suture, silk, prolene and nylon sutures, and plastic cable ties.

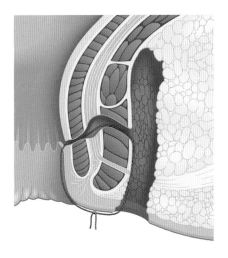

2.10.21

The literature indicates that rates and severity of incontinence seem to be proportional to the speed, as well as amount, of sphincter division, and it is intuitive that the slower the division, the lower the risk to continence. Modifications to the cutting seton technique can thus be employed to take advantage of its excellent fistula eradication rates, while reducing continence disturbance (a 25 percent incidence of occasional leakage of flatus and soiling in our experience), the requirement for repeat tightenings, and patient discomfort. A 'snug' rather than tight seton can effect a slower more gradual severance of tissue; and a silastic seton may not only be more comfortable, but also reduces the requirement for replacement or retightening, as its elastic recoil allows a slow caudal migration. The authors recommend the 'snug' seton in those patients with idiopathic fistulae, and good preoperative function, with intersphincteric or trans-sphincteric tracks involving up to two-thirds of the sphincters below puborectalis (excluding anterior trans-sphincteric fistulae in women in whom more than one-third of the external sphincter is involved).

Technique

Any acute sepsis or secondary tracks should have already been adequately dealt with (as previously described), leaving a single primary track. Any remaining component of the extrasphincteric primary track should be excised by core fistulectomy, or laid open, using diathermy. The primary track traversing the sphincter should be thoroughly curetted. Sharp division of the skin and anoderm is then performed to denude the sphincter below the track, but with no internal sphincter division. A 2 mm silastic seton (silicone nerve vessel retractor, Medasil®) can then be drawn into position by either using one end of an existing loose seton (cut and with clips applied to each end to prevent it falling out of the fistula), or by passing a 0-0 nylon suture along a grooved fistula probe, and tying the silastic seton to one of the loose ends. The silastic seton is 'snugly' tied around the sphincter muscle, so that it abuts the enclosed tissue, with minimal tension. In over half of cases, the seton will eventually cut out spontaneously; in the remainder, the minimal amount of tissue (usually skin and a few muscle fibers) enclosed can be simply laid open.

SPHINCTER-PRESERVING STRATEGIES

Sphincter-preservation techniques, such as advancement flaps and the use of biomaterials, are generally associated with lower success than those strategies which divide the sphincters, especially in the longer term. Therefore, they only tend to be indicated in those patients in whom the potential consequences of sphincter division are either unacceptable, irrespective of perceived severity, or in whom sphincter division cannot be recommended on the basis of poor preoperative continence, and level of the fistula (suprasphincteric or trans-sphincteric fistulae involving more than two-thirds of the sphincter complex).

It is likely that the initial key to the success of sphincter-preservation techniques is in providing the correct environment for healing to occur. Previous eradication of secondary extensions and acute sepsis are a prerequisite for success. Attention to the primary track is also necessary to optimize the chances of fistula eradication. Failure to adequately remove all granulation or epithelial tissue lining the fistula tract, possibly in conjunction with incomplete removal of the presumed source (the diseased intersphincteric anal gland), will inhibit healing and lead to fistula recurrence. Interestingly, combining advancement flaps with the application of biomaterials tends to worsen rather than improve outcomes.

Advancement flaps

Advancement flaps have been used to treat anal fistulae for a century. The key principles include separation of the track from the communication with the anal canal, adequate closure of that communication (by anastomosis of a healthy tension free flap to a site well distal to the previous internal opening), and eradication of all diseased tissue in the anorectal wall. There is little consensus as to whether the flap should be mucosal or include part if not all of the underlying internal sphincter. Mucosal advancement flaps seem to be associated with higher rates of fistula recurrence, whereas full or partial thickness advancement flaps can have an unpredictable effect on resting pressures, and potentially severe functional consequences in the event of breakdown. Overall mean success rates are between 50 and 60 percent. Advancement flaps are contraindicated in the presence of large internal openings (>2.5 cm), due to the risk of anastomotic breakdown, and a heavily scarred, indurated, woody perineum which precludes adequate exposure and flap mobilization. Conversely, as the authors have been taught by Professor Robin Phillips, those patients with an internal rectal prolapse lend themselves to such a technique, as the intussuscepting tissue can be relatively easily mobilized and anastomosed without tension.

TECHNIQUE

Acute sepsis, secondary extensions, and the primary track should have been treated as previously described. The extrasphincteric portion of the track is cored out to the intersphincteric space, or laid open to the lateral border of the EAS, and the granulation tissue within the residual track curetted away. An Eisenhammer retractor is then placed in the anal canal, and a rectal flap marked out with diathermy. It should have a broad proximal base (twice the width of the apex), the distal end needs to incorporate the internal opening, and the flap should be of sufficient length (at least 3 cm) to ensure adequate closure without tension. The submucosal or intersphincteric plane can be infiltrated with 1:300 000 adrenaline to saline solution. This facilitates flap elevation, dependent on whether a mucosal or full-thickness flap is planned. The flap is then carefully dissected free from the underlying tissue, from the free distal end to its proximal base (**Figure 2.10.22**).

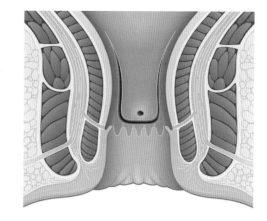

2.10.22

The internal opening is excised at the distal end of the flap and the granulation tissue curetted out (or epithelium excised by sharp dissection with tenotomy or Miltex scissors) where the track pierces the internal sphincter (**Figure 2.10.23**).

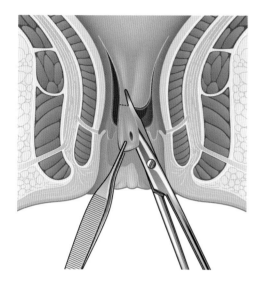

2.10.23

The defect in the internal sphincter is sutured with interrupted 3-0 Vicryl sutures, double breasting the IAS if there is rectal redundancy. Careful hemostasis is crucial to prevent a flap hematoma and subsequent dehiscence. The flap is then advanced and secured around its margins with interrupted 3-0 Vicryl sutures (**Figure 2.10.24**).

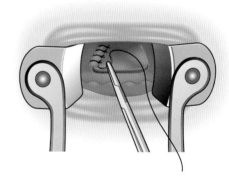

2.10.24

The extrasphincteric wound is left open to drain, and an intra-anal absorbable sponge dressing (e.g. Spongostan™) inserted to reduce the risk of hematoma (**Figure 2.10.25**). If the internal opening is at the level of the dentate line (i.e. not high in the anus), it may be easier to construct a distally based cutaneous flap, which is advanced proximally (as in an advancement flap anoplasty for anal fissure).

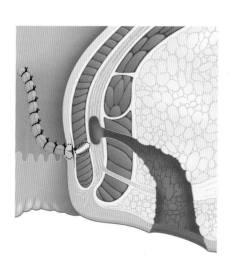

2.10.25

Biological materials

For a procedure to be truly sphincter-preserving, there should be no division or excision of any part of the sphincter complex. Adequate track preparation and simple closure of the internal opening (by stitch or mucosal advancement) is however often insufficient. Theoretically, an infill material is therefore required, which not only bridges the defect left by excision of the track, but also allows full host tissue incorporation and neovascularization, while withstanding premature degradation and bacterial colonization. To date, two novel materials have been used for the treatment of anal fistulae, fibrin glue and lyophilized porcine-derived small intestinal submucosa (Surgisis®, AFP™ (anal fistula plug)). Both have been reported to have widely variable success rates, with an overall clinical success rate of 50–60 percent, and with no reported incidences of functional disturbance. Proposed reasons for failure include those that are also associated with recurrence after conventional therapy, early extrusion of the biomaterial, and those specific to their biology. Nonetheless, these treatments may be useful therapies as they are simple to perform, may provide full or partial symptomatic relief, are repeatable, and do not seem to compromise future alternative attempts at cure.

TECHNIQUE

Fibrin glue

As with all advanced techniques, acute sepsis, secondary extensions and the primary track should have been previously treated. At the time of glue instillation, the track must be rid of granulation tissue and epithelium. The glue is then made up and instilled through the external opening.

To make the glue (the authors' preference is the 1.0-mL Tisseel Kit®: two component fibrin sealant, Baxter Healthcare, Newbury, UK), there are individual active components that are mixed and warmed, then drawn up into two syringes (syringe 1: fibrinogen, factor XIII, aprotinin, and fibronectin; syringe 2: thrombin and calcium chloride solution), which are subsequently placed in a two-syringe clip, which shares a common plunger. A plastic double-lumen, Y-connector joins the two syringes. This apparatus is then attached to a 21-gauge cannula (passed along a grooved fistula probe), the tip of which should be visualized at the internal opening. On injection, the components combine at the cannula tip to form the fibrin glue. Slow withdrawal of the cannula during instillation, and visualization of the mixture extruding from both internal and external openings ensures tract filling. The clot should be allowed to set for up to 5 minutes, as it takes this long for the fibrin glue to adhere firmly to the surrounding tissue; at 10 minutes, it reaches 70 percent of its maximum strength and full strength occurs after 2 hours. Excess clot from each opening can then be removed with scissors, and the internal opening closed with 3-0 Vicryl. The external opening is only partially closed, using 3-0 Vicryl, so as to allow drainage of any inflammatory exudate. Gauze and mesh pants are used to protect the wound.

Anal fistula plug

A recently published consensus statement on the correct technique for employing the anal fistula plug (AFP) suggested that debridement, curettage or brushing of the fistula track are not advised, and eradication of secondary tracks not advocated (both seemingly counter-intuitive), as such strategies may lead to a larger track and risk expulsion of the plug. A 2-0 Vicryl suture is placed at the narrow end of the plug, which is then pulled from the internal to the external opening until the plug is snug. Excess plug should be trimmed from the internal opening, and an absorbable suture placed, incorporating the internal sphincter, to close the opening and anchor the plug. The excess external end of the plug is then excised flush with the skin, and the external opening left open to allow drainage of any exudate.

Rectovaginal fistula repair

TRACY L HULL

PRINCIPLES AND JUSTIFICATION

Women with symptoms of ano- or rectovaginal fistula (RVF) usually present with air or stool from the vagina or perineum. The initial step is always to ensure that any associated abscesses are adequately drained. If needed, an examination under anesthesia and seton placement are the first steps. Full evaluation is required to plan surgical management. The fistula location and etiology must be delineated. While most fistulae are cryptoglandular or obstetrical in origin, fistulae from diverticulitis, radiation, cancer, and Crohn's disease require specific considerations which will be discussed later. For fistulae in the colon or upper rectum an abdominal approach is chosen and will not be discussed further. Similarly, fistulae from a low pelvic anastomosis will not be discussed. For low rectal or anal vaginal (or perineal) fistulae the approach can be transanal, transperineal, or transvaginal. The tissue must be soft before considering any repair. Therefore, a traumatic fistula such as from an obstetrical injury may require three to six months post-injury for the tissue to become appropriate for repair.

Patients must be apprised of the risk of recurrence and infection. For transanal repairs there could be deterioration in fecal control due to muscle stretch or internal sphincter damage during mobilization. All repairs could result in postoperative dyspareunia, but the risk is more likely with transperineal or transvaginal repair.

Distal RVF from radiation therapy or cancer should be approached with caution and recurrent cancer must be excluded. The tissue usually has some woody changes, particularly following radiation therapy. It may never reach the mandatory soft and supple state. Evaluation of the rectum and anal canal is done looking for inflammation and scarring resulting from the radiation.

Crohn's-related RVF can be considered for surgical treatment if the rectum has minimal inflammation and the anal canal is relatively soft and supple. Surgical repair of fistulae associated with ulcerations of the anal canal and large Crohn's skin tags should be approached with caution. The surgeon should have a low threshold to place a seton to drain any infected collections. Seton placement also permits delineation of the fistula track during an awake examination in the office.

PREOPERATIVE ASSESSMENT AND PREPARATION

Before planning surgical intervention, the fistula tract is delineated. If either the external or internal openings are not seen, an examination under anesthesia is needed. This also allows assessment of induration in the rectovaginal septum, the course of the tract, and its relation to the sphincter complex. The surgeon should have a low threshold to place a seton both to drain infected collections and to examine the course through the muscle when the woman is awake. Sometimes when the patient is anesthetized, the course through the muscle and rectovaginal septum is difficult to assess and may be delineated by gentle traction on the seton, during an awake examination in the office. There are some reports that seton placement for 3–4 weeks before definitive repair increases the chances of success.

Screening colonoscopy is considered for women 50 years of age or older. For patients with known or suspected Crohn's disease full evaluation of the small and large bowel may guide treatment. Particular attention is paid to the rectum to evaluate inflammation and scarring. Medical optimization in consultation with gastroenterologists is invaluable. If there is ulceration or inflammation of the anus and/or rectum, aggressive treatment may decrease the disease and allow for surgical intervention. Fistulae due to radiation or cancer require biopsies to ensure no cancer is currently involved.

Any cause of fistula can also lead to significant sphincter damage and loss. Most sphincter defects usually require repair in conjunction with the fistula repair for optimal results. If there is any question regarding the status of the muscle, anal endosonography should be performed.

SURGICAL PROCEDURES

The approach for surgery usually depends on the training of the surgeon, but also is influenced by the specific fistula anatomy and etiology. Anesthesia is typically general, but regional can be used in select instances.

Bowel preparation is controversial. While some surgeons use no preparation or enemas, the author prefers a full mechanical colon prep. Intravenous antibiotics are given just before the incision. While there are no definitive guidelines for postoperative antibiotics, the author's routine is 24 hours of intravenous antibiotics and 5–6 days of oral antibiotics after the procedure.

During the procedure, the author typically irrigates the open wound with tetracycline irrigation (1000 mg diluted in a liter of hot saline; the saline must be hot for the tetracycline to dissolve). However, the author would not use this type of antibiotic irrigation with a biologic implant due to concern of damage to the biologic material.

Transanal approach

RECTAL ADVANCEMENT FLAP

Rectal advancement flap is the most popular repair typically described. For consideration of this approach the sphincter muscle should be intact. The prone position is preferred since it optimally exposes the anterior anorectum. However, some surgeons do prefer the lithotomy approach.

To expose the anal area, anal everting sutures or the Lone Star™ retractor is placed. The author's preference is for four anal everting sutures.

The tract is delineated. The author does not typically inject any adrenaline into the area. Just distal to the opening, an approximately 180° circular flap is marked out (**Figure 2.11.1**). The author does not use a 'U' or trapezoid flap, but prefers a curved incision that follows the dentate line. This flap dissection begins just distal to the internal opening. The mucosa is removed from the anal canal, being careful to avoid internal sphincter injury. Dissection is continued cephalad to involve the full thickness of rectal wall, being very careful not to create a 'button hole' injury. Once the dissection is cephalad to the sphincters and into the rectovaginal septum, the dissection becomes easier. Cephalad dissection continues until the flap easily advances to cover the fistula opening and reach the distal incision without tension. Meticulous hemostasis is necessary to limit oozing beneath the flap after the procedure is completed.

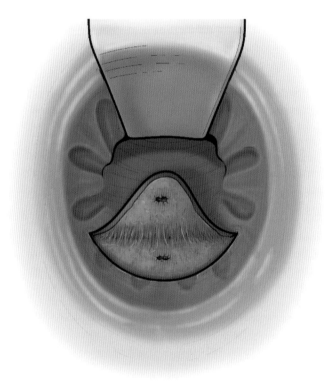

2.11.1

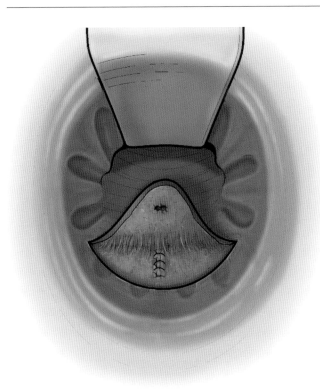

The fistula tract is cored out keeping the size of the opening as small as possible. The electrocautery usually works well to remove the superficial lumen of the tract. The fistula defect is closed in layers with 2-0 polyglactin sutures on a 5/8 circle curved needle. The curve of this needle allows precise placement of sutures in the confined space of the anal canal. Whether to close the opening horizontally or vertically depends on the opening's relation to the sphincter.

Note: **Figure 2.11.2** shows a vertical closure. Undermining the distal lip of the incision line facilitates closure and separates the sutures of the tract closure from those of the flap closure. The defect on the vaginal side is left open for drainage.

2.11.2

3-0 polyglactin sutures are placed from the undersurface of the flap to the raw surface of the rectovaginal septum to close the dead space and relieve tension on the flap (**Figure 2.11.3**).

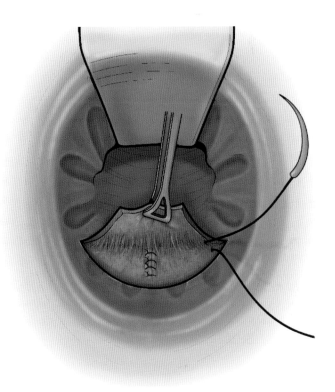

2.11.3

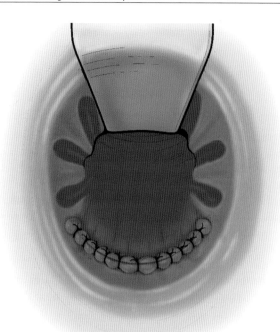

2.11.4

The flap is then advanced down and the tip is trimmed to excise the fistula opening. The flap is sewn to the distal incision with interrupted 2-0 or 3-0 polyglactin sutures. When failure occurs it is most typically at the tip of the flap, and meticulous alignment is essential (**Figure 2.11.4**).

SLEEVE ADVANCEMENT FLAP

One option for a failed flap repair with an intact sphincter muscle or RVF from Crohn's disease with scarred anal canal tissue is a sleeve advancement flap. The advantage of using a sleeve of the rectal wall for the flap is that there seems to be less tension and better elimination of dead space. A stoma is almost always placed when performing a sleeve advancement. A circular 360° mucosal incision is made just distal to the fistula (**Figure 2.11.5**).

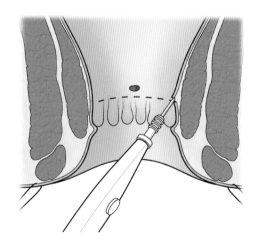

2.11.5

The anal canal mucosa or scar is dissected from the internal anal sphincter taking care not to injure the internal sphincter muscle (**Figure 2.11.6**). The rectal wall is transected and dissection continued in the intersphincteric plane until above the puborectalis. Circumferentially, the dissection continues cranially along the external aspect of the rectal wall.

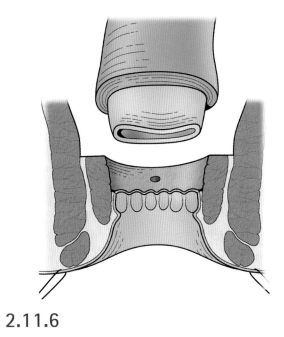

2.11.6

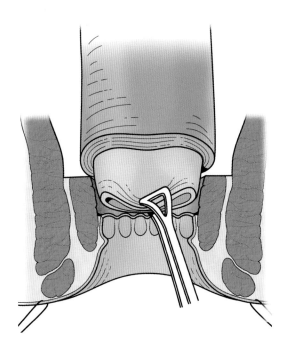

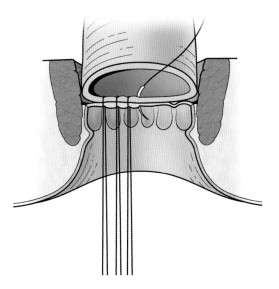

Dissection is carried cephalad until the rectal wall will advance down to the cut distal edge without tension. The fistula defect is closed as described above. The fistula is excised from the advancement flap and the rectal wall is then sewn to the cut edge with interrupted 2-0 or 3-0 polyglactin sutures (**Figure 2.11.7**).

Occasionally, the sleeve cannot be adequately mobilized from the anal approach and abdominal mobilization is required. Therefore, the surgeon must always be prepared for this possibility and discuss it preoperatively with the patient. After the anal dissection is completed, the rectum is mobilized in its anatomic plane and is divided at the pelvic floor. After closing the fistula from the anal side, there are two choices for anastomosis: immediate and delayed.

2.11.7

Immediate anastomosis

The rectum is advanced through the anal canal and a coloanal anastomosis is performed using 2-0 or 3-0 polyglactin sutures on a 5/8 circle needle, reinforced with short segments of running polyglactin suture (**Figure 2.11.8**).

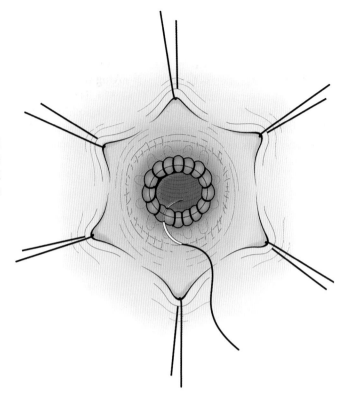

2.11.8

Delayed anastomosis

If the closed internal opening is in close proximity to the sutured anastomosis, a delayed anastomosis is performed. This allows the raw surface of the anal canal to fuse to the outer wall of the rectum. After full rectal mobilization, eight 2-0 or 3-0 polyglactin sutures are placed through the anoderm and internal sphincter muscle at the cut edge, equidistant around the anal area (**Figure 2.11.9**).

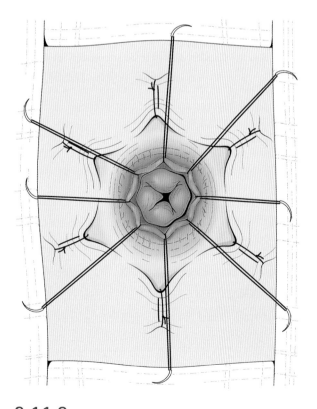

2.11.9

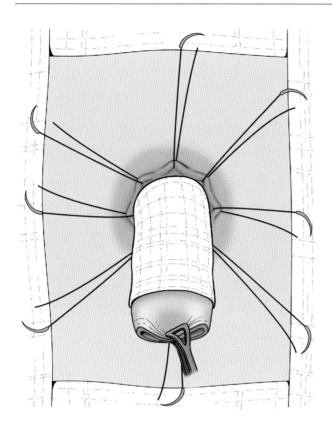

2.11.10

The rectum is advanced out of the anal canal and extruded 5–6 cm. Gauze is wrapped around the extruded rectum, including in the wrap the sutures that were placed through the anal muscles and skin, with the needles still attached (**Figure 2.11.10**).

Approximately 5–7 days later, the patient is returned to the operating room. The gauze is carefully unwrapped and the sutures are untangled and splayed out (**Figure 2.11.11**).

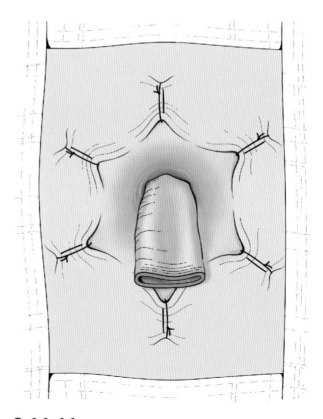

2.11.11

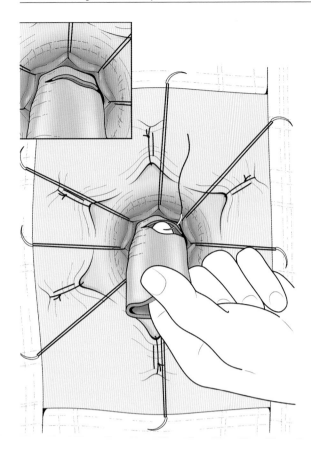

The rectum is amputated just at the anal verge, being cautious not to resect too far into the anal canal to avoid disruption of the adherent rectum from the internal fistula opening. (**Figure 2.11.12**).

2.11.12

There should be enough rectal wall left for easy suturing to the distal cut edge. The previously placed anal sutures are placed full thickness through the new cut edge of the rectal wall and tied down (**Figure 2.11.13**).

Further short segments of running polyglactin sutures are used to reinforce this anastomosis.

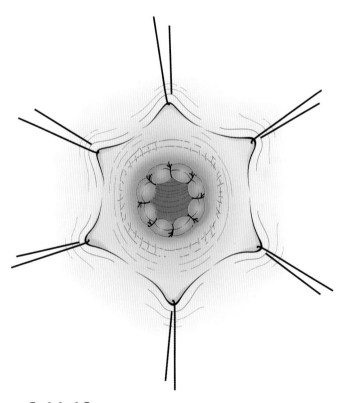

2.11.13

2.11.14

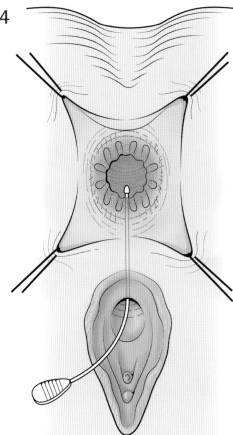

EPISIOPROCTOTOMY

If the sphincter is not intact (especially after an obstetrical injury), an episioproctotomy is a preferred approach. The author prefers the prone position. The buttocks are taped apart. A probe is placed in the fistula and the track is laid open, creating a fourth degree perineal laceration (**Figure 2.11.14**).

A lighted Hill-Ferguson retractor can be used to optimize exposure.

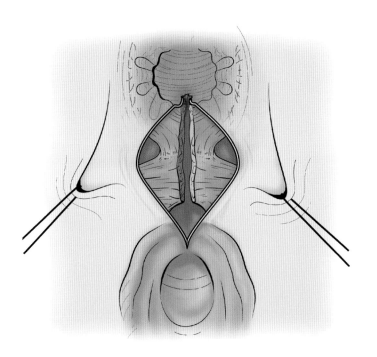

Next, each limb of the sphincter is dissected laterally into the ischiorectal fossae until there is enough mobility to perform a sphincter muscle overlap. The rectovaginal septum is also dissected 1–2 cm cephalad to the fistula tract to allow enough mobility to overlap the muscle (**Figure 2.11.15**).

2.11.15

The rectal mucosa must be reapproximated with mattress sutures of 2-0 or 3-0 polyglactin suture prior to the muscle overlap (**Figure 2.11.16**). (If the muscle is overlapped first, it is impossible to view the apex of the rectal mucosa due to the constraints of the overlap.)

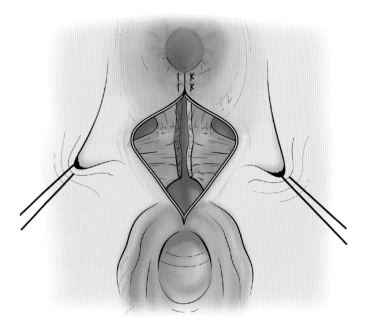

2.11.16

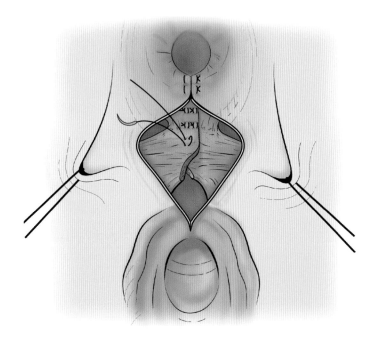

The rectal mucosa is closed to accurately approximate the dentate line. Sometimes it is easiest to begin the overlap after the initial mucosal sutures are placed, keeping in mind the goal is to close the muscle but eliminate dead space as the rectal mucosa is closed (**Figure 2.11.17**).

2.11.17

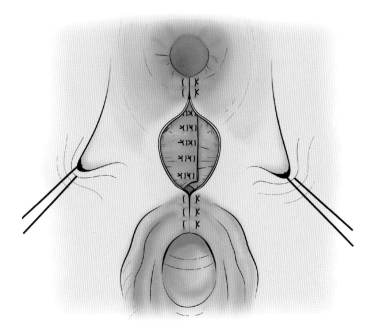

2.11.18

Once the muscle and mucosa are sutured, the vaginal closure is done. Starting at the apex of the proximal vagina, mattress sutures are placed (**Figure 2.11.18**). It is important to attempt to accurately restore the hymnal ring.

Full closure of the perineal body is not necessary. Leaving the mid-portion open allows for drainage of any fluid that accumulates. Drains are not routinely used, but a 0.25-inch Penrose drain is occasionally placed laterally to avoid fluid accumulation. This drain is removed on the first postoperative day.

Transperineal repairs

Rectovaginal fistula repair can be accomplished with a transperineal approach. Proponents feel it limits sphincter stretch (and thus damage) while allowing limited repair of the muscle. For patients with a thick perineal body, this may be an approach to consider. An incision is placed transversely across the perineal body. A probe is placed through the fistula to allow easier identification of the tract (**Figure 2.11.19**).

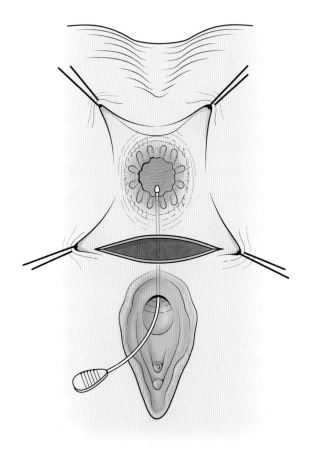

2.11.19

Proximal dissection can be performed either in the intersphincteric groove or between the external anal sphincter and the posterior vaginal wall. However, dissection in the intersphincteric plane can be extremely difficult and should only be considered if the fistula is small and minimal muscle defect exists. The probe is encountered in the fistula, the tract divided and the probe removed. The dissection is carried at least 1 cm proximal to this location. The fistula margins are debrided and the anal and vaginal openings are closed with simple or figure-of-eight 2-0 or 3-0 polyglactin suture (**Figure 2.11.20**).

There are several options for closure of the rectovaginal septum.

PRIMARY CLOSURE

The lateral tissue can be approximated, usually imbricating the anal canal opening. Care is taken to avoid changing the vaginal contour as this could lead to dyspareunia. A drain may be placed to decrease fluid accumulation and some surgeons reapproximate the vaginal and anorectal tissue. The skin is loosely closed with simple absorbable sutures to allow drainage.

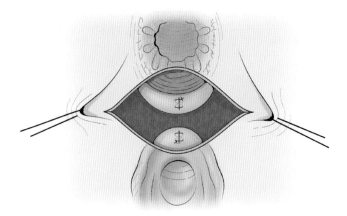

2.11.20

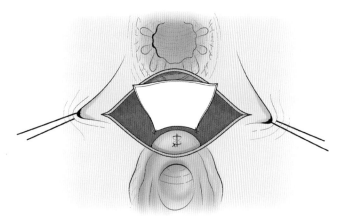

2.11.21

BIOLOGIC MESH INSERTION

The use of biologic mesh to aid repair and reinforcement of tissue in the perineum has been gaining acceptance. Some advocate its use to close the septum. After the anal and vaginal openings have been closed, measurement is taken of the rectovaginal space. A piece of biologic material is cut to conform to this space, making sure there is an overlap of at least 1 cm in each direction from the closed anal opening (**Figure 2.11.21**). Absorbable suture is placed in the two cephalad corners. The suture is then placed through the corners of the biologic mesh and tied down.

Several additional sutures are placed to anchor the biologic material (**Figure 2.11.22**). The distal portion of the biologic is trimmed so it just reaches the cut edge of the skin. The perineal skin is approximated by taking a bite of each edge of skin including some of the biologic mesh.

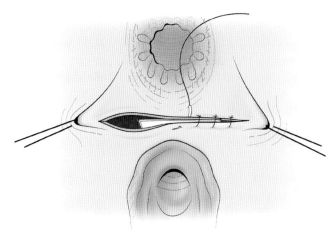

2.11.22

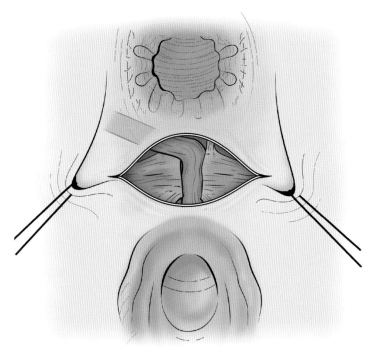

Gaps are left between the sutures for drainage which can last up to 3 weeks. If the skin edges are closed tightly the fluid accumulates over the mesh which can lead to seroma, infection, and failure.

INSERTION OF MUSCLE OR FAT

To separate the two fistula openings, various tissues from the patient have been used. Transposition of the fat of the labia is termed a Martius flap and is discussed in Chapter 7.3. The gracilis muscle is another option. The muscle is mobilized via one or more medial thigh incisions and its tendon divided at its insertion at the knee. The neurovascular bundle is left intact at the origin. The muscle is then delivered through a subcutaneous tunnel into the rectovaginal septal space (**Figure 2.11.23**). The muscle is fixed in place with absorbable sutures with the goal of complete coverage of the rectal side of the fistula.

The skin is closed, over a suction drain if there is a large amount of dead space. A drain is nearly always placed in the donor site of the medial thigh. Gracilis interpositions are virtually always done under the cover of a diverting stoma.

2.11.23

Transvaginal approach

Fistula closure via the vaginal approach is usually done with the patient in the lithotomy position. The fistula tract is excised and the vaginal mucosa is elevated (**Figure 2.11.24**). This is typically done transversely to avoid shortening the vagina.

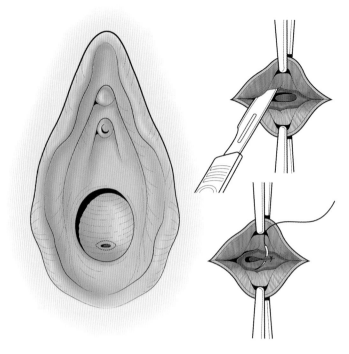

2.11.24

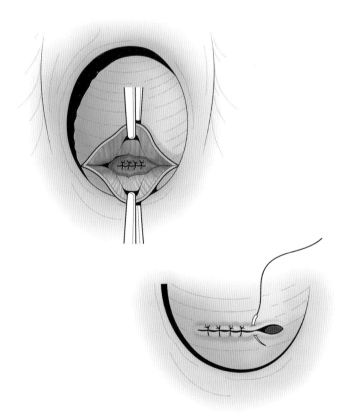

The anorectal opening is closed with interrupted 3-0 polyglactin sutures. Care is taken to exclude the mucosa from the depths of the wound. The vaginal wall is then closed with interrupted 3-0 polyglactin sutures, again being careful to avoid imbricating mucosa (**Figure 2.11.25**).

2.11.25

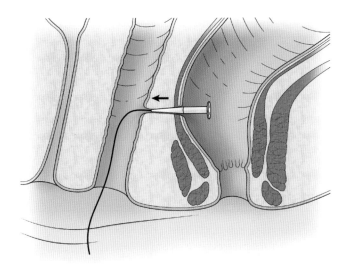

2.11.26

Biologic plug

Plug devices of rolled biological material have been manufactured for anal fistula closure. Due to the short nature of many rectovaginal fistula tracts, plugs have been specifically designed for rectovaginal fistula repair with a button to allow fixation on the anal side. Biologic plugs are not ideal for short rectovaginal fistulae or thin rectovaginal septa. Minimal manipulation is done of the tract and cleaning is usually performed by instilling hydrogen peroxide. If the tract is completely epithelialized, the lining should be excised. The tract diameter is measured to choose the correct size and preparation of the plug is carried out as per the manufacturer's recommendation (some require hydration for a specific amount of time). The tapered end of the plug is threaded through the fistula starting at the anal side and pulled toward the vaginal side (**Figure 2.11.26**).

The button is sewn in place with 2-0 polyglactin suture. The suture should pass through the button hole, the anorectal wall and also through the flange of the plug (**Figure 2.11.27**). The button must be flat against the anorectal wall after the sutures are placed.

The excess plug is trimmed from the vaginal side. There should be sufficient room around the plug at the vaginal opening to allow for drainage.

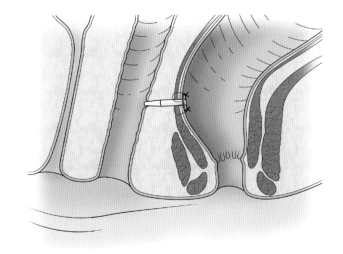

2.11.27

POSTOPERATIVE CARE

There is no established protocol for the postoperative care of women after rectovaginal fistula repairs. Patients that require a stoma, transabdominal mobilization, or gracilis mobilization will require admission. Some surgeons keep patients confined in bed for several days after a gracilis mobilization. Less complex surgery can be performed and the patient discharged on the same day, according to surgeon preference. The author's preference is to admit patients for 24–48 hours for observation and intravenous antibiotics. For episioproctotomy, the author irrigates the wound with saline using a 22-gauge plastic catheter. If patients are admitted after an anal advancement flap or episioproctotomy (without a stoma), they typically are not fed until just prior to discharge (to reduce the chance of mucous washing over the anal wound).

For patients who are not diverted avoidance of constipation is critically important. When a diet is instituted, patients are instructed to take adequate fiber and are given mineral oil (1 oz orally) each morning for the first several weeks. If a patient does not defecate for 2 days, they are instructed to take 1 oz of milk of magnesia daily until they have a bowel action. Patients are placed on oral antibiotics for 5–6 days after discharge and the wound is assessed on a weekly basis.

OUTCOMES

Successful rectovaginal fistula closure depends on the etiology, condition of the anal sphincter and surrounding tissue, degree of scarring, and number of previous repairs. Before a repair, women are warned that closure may not be accomplished after the first repair, and some rectovaginal fistula are never successfully closed. For transanal repairs, the reported success rate ranges from 50 to 100 percent.

At our institution the healing rate for obstetrical or cryptoglandular rectovaginal fistula is 78 percent for episioproctotomy and 62 percent for advancement flaps.[1] These figures are similar to our previous published results.[2,3]

The reported success rates of biologic interposition and plug closure vary by series but average around 60 percent.[4,5] The other tissue interposition repairs also have varied success rates of up to 75 percent.[6,7]

REFERENCES

1. El-Gazzaz G, Hull TL, Mignanelli E et al. Obstetric and cryptoglandular rectovaginal fistulas: long-term surgical outcome; quality of life; and sexual function. *Journal of Gastrointestinal Surgery* 2010; **14**: 1758–63.
2. Hull TL, Bartus C, Bast J et al. Success of episioproctotomy for cloaca and rectovaginal fistula. *Diseases of the Colon and Rectum* 2007; **50**: 97–101.
3. Sonoda T, Hull T, Piedmonte MR. Outcomes of primary repair of anorectal and rectovaginal fistulas using endorectal advancement flap. *Diseases of the Colon and Rectum* 2002; **45**: 1622–8.
4. Schwandner O, Fuerst A, Kunstreich K, Scherer R. Innovative technique for closure of rectovaginal fistula using Surgisis mesh. *Techniques in Coloproctology* 2009; **13**: 135–40.
5. Ellis CN. Outcomes after repair of rectovaginal fistulas using bioprosthetics. *Diseases of the Colon and Rectum* 2008; **51**: 1084–8.
6. Lefevre JH, Bretagnol F, Maggiori L et al. Operative results and quality of life after gracilis muscle transposition for recurrent rectovaginal fistula. *Diseases of the Colon and Rectum* 2009; **52**: 1290–5.
7. McNevin MS, Lee PY, Bax TW. Martius flap: an adjunct for repair of complex, low rectovaginal fistula. *American Journal of Surgery* 2007; **193**: 597–9.

Anal fissure

JOHN H SCHOLEFIELD

INTRODUCTION

Anal fissure is a linear tear or ulcer in the lining of the distal anal canal below the dentate line. It is a common condition that may affect all age groups, but it is particularly seen in young and otherwise healthy adults, with equal incidence across the sexes.[1] Many consider anal fissures to be ischemic in origin, but other causes of anal ulceration must be considered, especially in the presence of a low or normal anal sphincter tone.

DIAGNOSIS

The classical symptoms are of anal pain during or after defecation accompanied by the passage of bright red blood per anus. The pain is often severe and may last for a few minutes during, or persist for several hours after, defecation; bleeding is separate from the stool and usually modest. In addition, pruritus ani may accompany up to 50 percent of anal fissures.[2, 3] Symptoms from fissures cause considerable morbidity and reduction in quality of life.[4]

On examination, the fissure may be apparent as the buttocks are parted, but marked spasm of the anal sphincter often obscures the view. An early fissure, if seen, has sharply demarcated, fresh mucosal edges and there may be granulation tissue in its base. With increasing chronicity, the margins of the fissure become indurated and there is a distinct lack of granulation tissue. Horizontal fibers of the internal sphincter muscle may be evident in the base of a chronic fissure and secondary changes, such as a sentinel skin tag, hypertrophied anal papilla, or a degree of anal stenosis are often present (**Figure 2.12.1**).

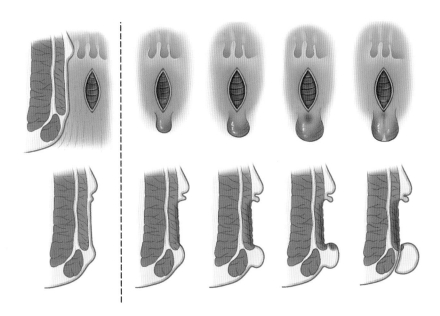

2.12.1

Occasionally, an anal fissure may be the presenting feature of Crohn's disease or an anal carcinoma. Therefore, careful clinical evaluation to exclude other pathologies is essential. This may mandate an examination under an anesthetic if there are atypical features – such as atypical site, the absence of anal spasm, or induration around the edge of the fissure.

TREATMENT

The majority of anal fissures are acute and symptoms relatively short-lived, resolving either spontaneously or with simple dietary modification to increase fiber, and stool-softening laxatives where appropriate. The distinction between acute and chronic fissures is somewhat arbitrary and cannot be made reliably solely on appearance. However, the accepted definition is that fissures failing to heal within 6 weeks despite straightforward dietary measures are designated as 'chronic'.

Although a proportion (approximately 10 percent) of chronic fissures will eventually resolve with conservative measures, most require further intervention in order to heal.[5, 6] Fissures are usually single and in the posterior midline, but 10 percent of women and 1 percent of men have anterior fissures.[7] Women with symptoms postpartum account for 3–11 percent of all chronic fissures and tend to have anterior fissures.[8, 9, 10] Multiple fissures or those in a lateral position on the anal margin may indicate underlying inflammatory bowel disease, syphilis, or immunosuppression. However, it should be recognized that most fissures occurring in the presence of inflammatory bowel disease are in the posterior midline and at least one-half are also painful. Fissures that are resistant to treatment should prompt further investigation, including examination under anesthesia and appropriate biopsy.

Chronic anal fissures are generally associated with raised resting anal canal pressure secondary to hypertonicity of the internal anal sphincter, and treatment is directed at reducing this. Traditional surgical treatments, namely manual anal dilatation or sphincterotomy, effectively heal most fissures within a few weeks, but may result in permanently impaired anal continence. This has led to the search for alternative non-surgical treatment, and various pharmacological agents have been shown to lower resting anal pressure and heal fissures without threatening anal continence.

Acute fissures will usually heal spontaneously or with conservative treatments – bathing and stool softeners. In recent years, the use of glyceryl trinitrate (GTN) ointment has become a first-line therapy providing a 'chemical sphincterotomy' in the treatment of anal fissures and is very effective in acute fissures and in some chronic fissures. The major side effect of GTN is headache, which if it occurs generally precludes use. An alternative is diltiazem, a calcium channel antagonist, that results in smooth muscle relaxation, and can also be used in topical form. The accepted definition of chronicity (6 weeks) is too short. About 80 percent of patients whose fissures have caused symptoms for 6–12 weeks will heal with chemical sphincterotomy, but in the author's experience those fissures which have been present for many months are unlikely to heal with these agents – particularly those which have been present for more than four months respond less well to chemical sphincterotomy with either GTN or diltiazem.

Botulinum toxin is preferred by some surgeons in the primary treatment of anal fissures, while others use it to treat fissures that have not responded to topical GTN or diltiazem. However, the success rates are variable and randomized trials have failed to show a significant benefit for one non-surgical treatment over another. It is the author's view that there is an overall failure rate of 20–40 percent with non-surgical treatment and that, in these cases, a well-performed lateral internal sphincterotomy will resolve the patient's symptoms in the vast majority of cases without long-term side effects.

SURGICAL TREATMENT OF ANAL FISSURE

Anal sphincterotomy is not advised in patients with a risk of incontinence, particularly women with a history of obstetric trauma. Similarly, sphincterotomy is not recommended for anal fissures in patients known to have Crohn's disease. Although surgical sphincterotomy has gained something of a bad reputation for causing incontinence, this is largely based on historical data when surgeons undertook a sphincterotomy over the full length of the anal sphincter. All patients undergoing sphincterotomy should be warned of the risk of flatal or fecal incontinence. These symptoms are usually transient. The risk of long-term fecal incontinence is low (probably around 5 percent[9]), but the incidence of leakage of flatus is higher (20 percent). While some surgeons have moved away from surgical treatment for anal fissures, in the author's experience symptoms of transient impairment of continence following a 'tailored' sphincterotomy are rare and permanent impairment of continence is even more uncommon, such that a tailored internal sphincterotomy is the procedure of choice for most chronic fissures which have failed chemical sphincterotomy. The exception to this rule is the low pressure chronic fissure which sometimes occurs – an advancement flap is probably advisable in such cases.

Tailored internal sphincterotomy

The tailored sphincterotomy should extend from the anal margin for the length of the fissure and then 2–3 mm proximally.

The author prefers not to use bowel preparation, but broad-spectrum prophylactic antibiotics should be given at induction of anesthesia. The procedure is usually performed under general anesthesia, although spinal anesthesia or local anesthesia are preferred by some surgeons. The patient is placed on the operating table in the lithotomy position with the buttocks hanging over the free edge of the table to allow good access to the anal canal. A Parks' anal retractor is preferred to a bivalve speculum as the Parks' retractor is self-retaining, gives good exposure, and provides tension on the internal sphincter that facilitates identification of the intersphincteric groove at the anal margin (**Figure 2.12.2**). The author prefers a closed to an open technique as the latter increases the risk of a gutter deformity.

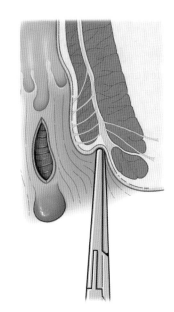

2.12.2

After making a stab incision at the anal margin in the intersphincteric groove (**Figure 2.12.3**), blunt dissection with a small hemostat or McIndoe scissors isolates the internal sphincter from the mucosa medially and the external sphincter laterally (**Figure 2.12.4**). The author then applies the hemostat over the length of the fissure to crush the muscle fibers of the internal anal sphincter

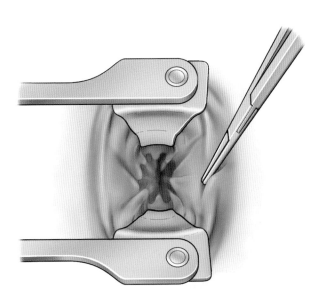

2.12.3

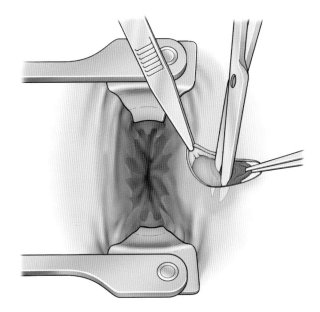

2.12.4

for about 1 minute (**Figure 2.12.5**). Crushing the muscle makes it ischemic and reduces the bleeding when the muscle fibers are divided with McIndoe scissors (**Figure 2.12.6**). Alternatively, a scalpel blade can be used, either a No. 11 blade or a Beaver iridectomy scalpel (**Figure 2.12.7**). The blade may be introduced deep to the mucosa, parallel to the sphincter, and then rotated 90° to incise the internal sphincter. Some surgeons prefer to insert the blade in the

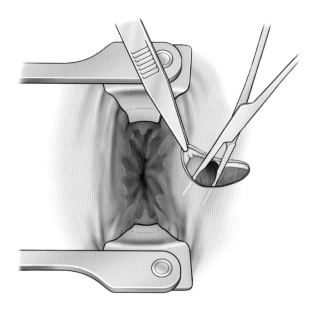

2.12.5

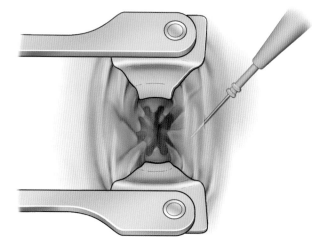

2.12.7

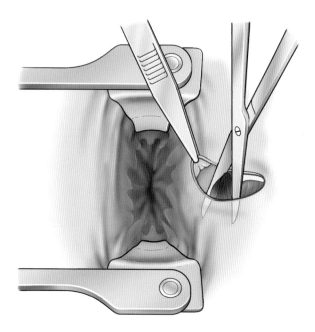

2.12.6

intersphincteric plane and divide the internal sphincter from the deep aspect. This has the advantage of reducing the risk of injury to the external anal sphincter, but carries some risk of incising the mucosa. If this occurs, it may be sutured with an absorbable suture. Hemostasis is achieved relatively easily by direct pressure over the sphincterotomy site with a swab or by rotating the Parks' retractor through 90° for a few minutes. The wound is left open (**Figure 2.12.8**).

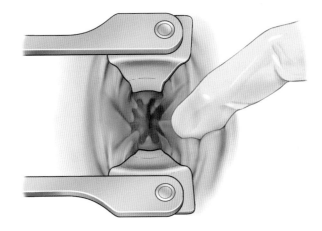

2.12.8

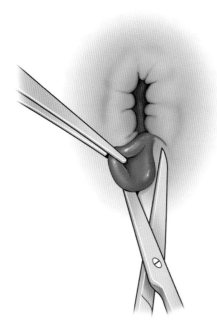

2.12.9

Excision of any sentinel tag is recommended, but not essential. The tag should be excised without damaging any adjacent sphincter tissue, but removing the minimum of healthy perianal skin (**Figure 2.12.9**). Many patients find that the site of the tag excision is more troublesome in the postoperative period than the sphincterotomy site itself. If left alone, the sentinel tag will usually shrink within a matter of a few weeks.

Any associated hypertrophied anal papilla at the dentate line should be excised at the end of the procedure.

Postoperative care

Once hemostasis is achieved, no dressing is required. Very little postoperative analgesia is required, but stool softeners for a week or two are recommended. Patients should be warned of a slight discharge from the wound for approximately 1 week. Bathing the area in clean water two or three times a day is said to aid healing.

Alternative sphincterotomy techniques

OPEN SPHINCTEROTOMY

Open sphincterotomy is briefly described here, but is not recommended by the author as it causes more postoperative pain than closed sphincterotomy and carries an increased risk of gutter deformity (leading to fecal incontinence), particularly if carried out through the fissure itself. Open sphincterotomy may be performed under local, regional, or general anesthesia in either the Lloyd Davies or prone jack-knife position. The sphincterotomy may be performed either laterally or through the fissure itself (not recommended). With the anal sphincter under slight tension, the anoderm is incised at the level of the anal margin for around 2 cm in length. The anoderm is freed from the underlying internal sphincter (avoid creating a buttonhole injury to the anoderm). The internal anal sphincter muscle fibers are then divided under direct vision for the length of the fissure plus a few millimeters. After achieving hemostasis, the skin wound can then be closed with an absorbable suture or left open.

FISSURECTOMY

Some surgeons advocate excising the chronically inflamed skin either side of the fissure, curettage of the base of the fissure which may then be left to heal or covered with a skin flap.[8] While this avoids dividing any sphincter muscle and some authors claim success, there are no published randomized trials.

DIFFICULT ANAL FISSURES

Women with chronic anal fissures present an interesting therapeutic challenge because their sphincters are shorter than those of men. In addition, up to 20 percent of women who have had children may have an occult sphincter injury. For these reasons, many surgeons believe that a sphincterotomy should not be performed in a woman of childbearing age without checking the sphincter's integrity preoperatively by endoanal ultrasound and manometry. Manometry is useful to confirm that this is a high pressure sphincter and therefore that a sphincterotomy is likely to be therapeutic.

Women (and less commonly men) with an anal fissure, but normal anal tone, should not be subjected to sphincterotomy. Other causes for perianal skin ulceration should be considered, such as Crohn's disease, anal herpes, and drugs which cause anal ulceration, such as nicorandil. Treating the underlying cause will lead to healing in most of these cases. If the fissure fails to heal by these measures, then rather than a sphincterotomy an anal skin advancement flap should be considered. Advancement flaps can easily be created in the perianal skin and advanced into the anal canal; they are often referred to as V–Y flaps. The skin of this flap relies on its blood supply in the underlying subcutaneous fat so a good pedicle of skin and fat needs to be moved to cover the defect (**Figure 2.12.10**).

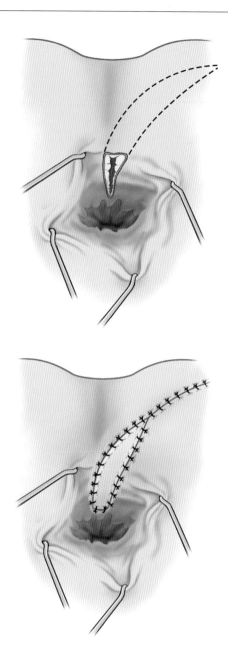

2.12.10 The V–Y island advancement flap for anal fissure.

ANAL STENOSIS

In patients with a long-standing fissure, there is sometimes a degree of fibrosis in the internal sphincter; this is often referred to as an 'anal stenosis'. Such patients are unlikely to have a good result from chemical sphincterotomy, but the problem resolves with a tailored sphincterotomy.

This type of anal stenosis should be distinguished from the type of anal stenosis which might follow a badly performed hemorrhoidectomy or radiotherapy for an anal cancer, where the anal skin is abnormally scarred. In this latter type of anal stenosis, the patient requires a house or similar flap to bring healthy skin into the anal canal.

In these patients, a sphincterotomy will not help and may make any subsequent incontinence worse.

FISTULA ASSOCIATED WITH ANAL FISSURE

Occasionally, a superficial fistula can occur in the sentinel tag associated with a fissure. These are usually very superficial fistulae with little muscle involvement. They can be laid open or excised with the tag, taking care not to damage underlying sphincter tissue. The sphincterotomy should be performed in the lateral position to reduce the risk of a keyhole deformity.

REFERENCES

1. Bennett RC, Goligher JC. Results of internal sphincterotomy for anal fissure. *British Medical Journal* 1962; **2**: 1500–3.

2. Sailer M, Bussen D, Debus ES *et al.* Quality of life in patients with benign anorectal disorders. *British Journal of Surgery* 1998; **85**: 1716–19.

3. Lund JN, Scholefield JH. A randomised, prospective, double-blind, placebo-controlled trial of glyceryl trinitrate ointment in the treatment of anal fissure. *Lancet* 1997; **349**: 11–14.

4. Maria G, Cassetta E, Gui D *et al.* A comparison of botulinum toxin and saline for the treatment of chronic anal fissure. *New England Journal of Medicine* 1998; **338**: 217–20.

5. Keighley M, Williams N. *Surgery of the anus, rectum and colon*, vol. 1, 3 edn. London: WB Saunders, 2007: 364–86.

6. Sweeney JL, Ritchie JK, Nicholls RJ. Anal fissure in Crohn's disease. *British Journal of Surgery* 1988; **75**: 56–7.

7. Jost WH. One hundred cases of anal fissure treated with botulin toxin: early and long-term results. *Diseases of the Colon and Rectum* 1997; **40**: 1029–32.

8. Nyam DCNK, Wilson RG, Stewart KJ *et al.* Island advancement flaps in the management of anal fissures. *British Journal of Surgery* 1995; **82**: 326–8.

9 Lewis TH, Corman ML, Prager ED. Long term results of open and closed sphincterotomy for anal fissure. *Diseases of the Colon and Rectum* 1988; **31**: 368–71.

10. Nelson RL. Meta-analysis of operative techniques for fissure-in-ano. *Diseases of the Colon and Rectum* 1999; **42**: 1424–8; discussion 1428–31.

Anoplasty

KAREN P NUGENT

PRINCIPLES AND JUSTIFICATION

Anoplasty is defined as a reconstructive procedure on the anus. Generally, it is a local procedure used to replace defective, poor or damaged tissues with nearby perianal skin and underlying fatty tissue. Indications for anoplasty include anal stenosis, chronic anal fissure, fistulae which are resistant or difficult to treat by more conventional methods, and occasionally to replace skin excised for anal neoplasia, either anal intraepithelial neoplasia (AIN) or after local excision of a small anal cancer.

Anal stenosis is a rare but disabling condition which is most commonly seen after previous anorectal surgical procedures. It may occur following any condition which can cause scarring of the anoderm, however, the most common cause is hemorrhoidectomy which is responsible for approximately 90 per cent of cases.[1] Stenosis can also be associated with Crohn's disease, sepsis, sexually transmitted disease, and generalized skin disorders, such as scleroderma. Patients with anal stenosis present with pain and inability to evacuate, as well as bleeding. Mild cases can be treated with laxatives or bulking agents along with anal dilatation; however, strictures that have resulted from considerable anal skin loss or concentric contraction will require some form of anoplasty.

Anoplasty for anal fistula is usually reserved for trans-sphincteric and high complex fistulae. Surgery should only be contemplated after resolution of anal sepsis and in patients in whom 'laying open' would render the patient incontinent. Usually, other less invasive procedures, for example, anal fistula plugs, have failed (see Chapter 2.10). Anoplasty for fissure in ano is reserved for patients who have completed an algorithm of medical treatment, from stool softeners to topical glyceryl trinitrate (GTN) and/or diltiazem cream, botulinum toxin injection, or sometimes a sphincterotomy (see Chapter 2.11). Anoplasty is usually reserved for those with low anal canal pressure in whom a sphincterotomy would be likely to cause incontinence or for patients who have a persistent and symptomatic fissure after other therapeutic options have failed.

There are a number of techniques used to perform an anoplasty. These range from the house advancement flap, a rhomboid flap, a Y–V anoplasty, as well as rotational flaps and simple island flaps.[2] All techniques that use a flap are designed to bring pliable anoderm into the anal canal to replace the scarred lining at that level. In cases of severe anal stenosis, more than one flap is often necessary. With all flaps used in this area, it is important to ensure that there is adequate subcutaneous tissue included in the flap in order to provide good vascularization to the skin pedicle. There should be no tension on the flap as this will lead to wound healing failure at the distal portion of the flap. It is important to remember that all these procedures are often technically challenging and problems of surgical technical failure include tension or ischemia causing necrosis at the tips of the skin flaps, as well as infection.

PREOPERATIVE

For all procedures, preoperative enemas should be given in the form of a phosphate enema, one the evening before and one on the morning of the surgical procedure. When more than one flap is to be performed, some people advocate full mechanical bowel preparation. Antibiotics normally used as bowel prophylaxis should be given at induction and as per protocol for anorectal procedures within the individual hospital.

ANESTHESIA

The procedure may be performed under a general spinal or local anesthesia depending on the patient and hospital preference. In the case of local anesthesia, bupivacaine 0.25 percent with 1:200 000 adrenaline should be used.

OPERATIONS

Position of the patient

The patient may be placed in the prone jack-knife position, which gives good access to the anus and the perianal skin and allows for easy positioning of any assistant (**Figure 2.13.1**). A Hill-Ferguson retractor allows access and easy visualization of one side of the anal canal (**Figure 2.13.2**). Alternatively, in some cases, a Lone Star™ retractor will allow circumferential visualization on the anus when resection of pathology followed by a flap advancement is required. Procedures can also be performed in the lithotomy position. If the patient is placed in the prone jack-knife position with the buttocks taped, it is essential that the tapes should be released after the flap has been designed and raised, and before the flap is sutured into position. This allows the surgeon to assess the true position of the flaps and ensures that there is minimal tension on the flap.

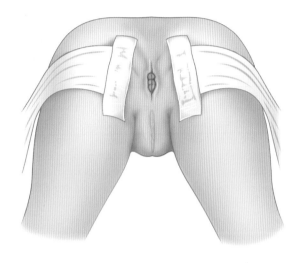

2.13.1

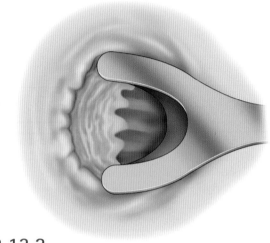

2.13.2

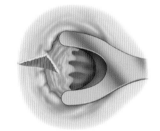

(a)

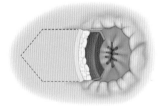

(b)

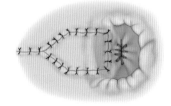

(c)

2.13.3

House flap procedure

With the use of a Hill-Ferguson retractor, an incision is made from the dentate line towards the perianal skin through the area of stenosis (**Figure 2.13.3a**). Sometimes a partial internal sphincterotomy may be needed, usually when there is coincident pathology that must be excised. The length of the incision corresponds to the length of the flap that must be advanced into the anal canal. The flap consists of skin and subcutaneous tissue that can be easily mobilized without damaging the underlying perforating blood vessels. The flap is designed in the shape of a house and the base is orientated proximally with the width of the base of the house designed to match the transverse incision within the anal canal or the mucosal defect that has resulted from an excision biopsy (**Figure 2.13.3b**). The advantages of this technique are that a wide flap is advanced into the anal canal and the donor site can be closed as a 'chimney at the top of the house' (**Figure 2.13.3c**).

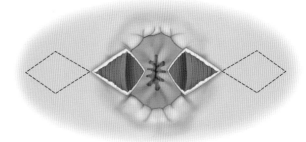

2.13.4

Island flaps

Island flaps are usually rhomboid in shape, although an ellipsoid shape can also be used (**Figure 2.13.4**). It is essential when dissecting into the fat not to undermine the edges of the flap, as this may create ischemia of the skin edges and undermine the blood supply to the flap. The flap is full thickness skin and the subcutaneous fat is incised deeply around the entire circumference of the flap, so that there is no tension when the tip is sutured into the top of the incised area within the anal canal (**Figure 2.13.5**). The flap should be approximately twice as long as it is wide. The flap should be sutured in place with absorbable sutures (Vicryl or PDS™ may be used). The area where the skin has been harvested should be closed (**Figure 2.13.6**) using interrupted sutures so that individual suture may be removed in case of infection. In the case of severe stenosis, a second flap can be brought in from the other side.

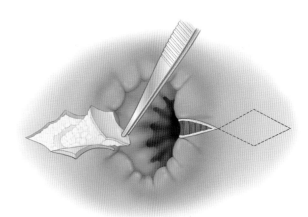

2.13.5

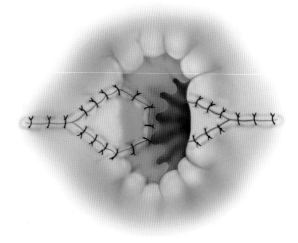

2.13.6

V–Y advancement flap

Using a Hill-Ferguson retractor, the stricture is incised or the anal pathology is excised. The incision in the anal canal constitutes the vertical stem of the Y, while the top V component of the Y is incised on the perianal skin. The limbs of the V incision should be 5–8 cm long, at a 45° degree angle from each other (**Figure 2.13.7**). The V advancement flap is created by incising through the skin and subcutaneous fat of each of the V limbs maintaining a good blood supply (**Figure 2.13.8**). The flap can then be sutured, without tension, down to the bottom on the vertical Y incision in the anal canal. Suturing should be with interrupted long-term absorbable sutures (**Figure 2.13.9**).

When this procedure is used for anal stenosis, it may be performed bilaterally; however, if used for an anal fissure it will be performed in either the posterior or anterior midline depending on the site of the fissure.

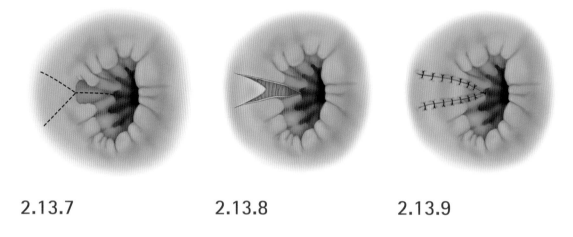

2.13.7   2.13.8   2.13.9

Rotational S flap

An S-plasty may be used in patients with severe anal stenosis or in patients with Bowen's disease or Paget's disease of the anus in whom a significant amount of anal and perianal skin needs to be excised. Although this is a more complicated procedure, with a higher morbidity and longer hospital stay, it does allow replacement of a larger amount of skin. A full mechanical bowel preparation may be required in order to prevent an early postoperative bowel movement. With the patient prone, a full thickness S-shaped flap can be made in the perianal skin with the size of the base as great as its length starting from the dentate line and extending for 8–10 cm (**Figure 2.13.10**). This flap can then be rotated and sutured to the normal skin (**Figure 2.13.11**). This can be repeated on the opposite side of the anus (**Figure 2.13.12**).

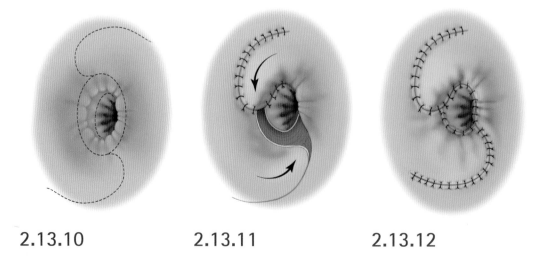

2.13.10   2.13.11   2.13.12

POSTOPERATIVE CARE

Because of the contaminated nature of perianal wounds, it is reasonable to maintain antibiotic cover perioperatively for at least three doses. Wound care can be difficult and the use of a sitz bath, as well as local hygiene, in the postoperative period is often useful. For simple procedures, patients should be started on a high fiber diet postoperatively with or without some form of bulk laxative. Patients with more complex flaps or in whom there has been extensive dissection or reconstruction may be better managed within the hospital setting for 3–5 days with bowel confinement.

COMPLICATIONS

A variety of complications have been reported in the literature after anoplasty, the most common of which is flap necrosis resulting from poor vascular supply and/or infection. Whichever flap is used, it is important to preserve as much subcutaneous fat as possible with wide mobilization. When dissecting the flap from the skin, the plane of dissection should be angled out from the skin edges in order to avoid undermining the skin flaps. Tension should be avoided at all costs as this leads to suture dehiscence. The flap tissue should be treated with respect and handling should be kept to a minimum. Absorbable sutures should be used and a minimal amount of tissue should be resected.

The choice of surgical technique for anoplasty is dependent upon the underlying pathology. There are few controlled studies comparing different techniques and the studies often use the procedures for a variety of pathologies. A recent study of 60 consecutive patients treated for anal stenosis randomized to receive a house flap, a rhomboid flap, or a Y–V anoplasty, found that the house advancement flap took significantly longer to perform than either the rhomboid flap or the Y–V anoplasty (62 minutes versus 44 or 35 minutes). However, the house advancement flap was associated with a better clinical result after one month and resulted in a larger anal canal diameter after one year than either of the other techniques. It seems, therefore, that when technically feasible, a house advancement flap has both better short- and long-term results in the treatment of anal stenosis.

REFERENCES

1. Brisinda G, Vanella S, Cadeddu F. Surgical treatment of anal stenosis. *World Journal of Gastroenterology* 2009; **28**: 1921–8.
2. Farid M, Youssef M, El Nakeeb A *et al.* Comparative study of the house advancement flap, rhomboid flap, Y–V anoplasty in treatment of anal stenosis: A prospective study. *Diseases of the Colon and Rectum* 2010; **53**: 790–7.

Perianal condylomata and anal intraepithelial neoplasia

TIM W EGLINTON AND FRANK A FRIZELLE

PRINCIPLES AND JUSTIFICATION

Pathogenesis and natural history

Anal condylomata are caused by the human papillomavirus (HPV), most commonly subtypes 6 and 11. They are usually acquired through sexual contact with an infected person, although HPV infection may be acquired in the absence of anal intercourse. Typically, condylomata will increase in size and number, although spontaneous regression does occur. These lesions are associated with the development of anal intraepithelial neoplasia (AIN) in up to 35 percent and, occasionally, a squamous cell cancer will be found among the condylomata.

The development of AIN is associated with HPV infection with high-risk subtypes (subtypes 16 and 18). AIN is classified as low (AINI), intermediate (AINII) or high grade (AINIII). The natural history of AIN remains poorly defined. AINIII probably carries a risk of progression to invasive squamous cell carcinoma of around 10 percent, whereas AINI and II will more often remain stable or regress. Both the risk of development of AIN and its subsequent progression to squamous cell carcinoma (SCC) are increased with HIV infection and immunosuppression and patients in these subgroups require closer surveillance.

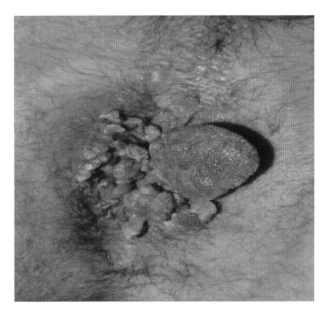

2.14.1 Anal condylomata.

Clinical features

Condylomata may be asymptomatic, but can cause perianal itch, moistness, swelling, and occasionally bleeding. Examination reveals elevated, cauliflower-like pink lesions, which may form larger plaques (**Figure 2.14.1**). It is important to accurately determine the extent of the disease because warts may be present within the anal canal and on the external genitalia. The Buschke–Lowenstein tumor is a giant condyloma acuminatum which is a locally aggressive lesion requiring surgical excision.

AIN is often asymptomatic and may be an incidental finding in histological specimens from minor anal procedures, such as hemorrhoidectomy. In contrast, the patient may present with irritation or pruritis. While there may be no specific examination features, gross lesions do occur which are raised, scaly plaques that can be white, red, or pigmented. Ulceration generally suggests invasion.

Assessment

Assessment of the patient should include a detailed sexual history and testing for other sexually transmitted diseases may be indicated. Testing and education of partners should also be undertaken where possible.

Principles of treatment

It should be noted that local treatments for condylomata do not eradicate the HPV infection and recurrence is common. Medical treatments include podophyllin which is a topical agent that can be applied to the warts in the perianal region, but not in the anal canal. In contrast, bichlorocetic acid and trichlorocetic acid are effective topical agents suitable for anal canal use. Imiquimod is an immunomodulator available as a topical cream. A number of HPV-based immunotherapies are currently under investigation.

Surgical treatment of condylomata is required for lesions that do not respond to topical therapy or for extensive involvement of the perianal skin and anal canal. Warts may be excised with diathermy or scissors. Diathermy is effective in removing the warts, however, damage to surrounding normal skin can lead to scarring and possibly anal stenosis. For this reason, many surgeons prefer scissor excision. Excised lesions should be subjected to histological examination for the presence of AIN, the exclusion of cancer and also, where indicated, viral subtyping of HPV to identify infection with subtypes associated with the development of AIN.

The treatment of AIN is controversial due to the lack of certainty regarding its natural history, the high likelihood of recurrence and the potential morbidity after significant excisions. Topical therapy with imiquimod has been shown to produce regression. AINI and -II in immunocompetent HIV-negative individuals can be managed with annual or biannual examination with biopsy of suspicious lesions. However, in patients with AINIII, immunosuppression, or HIV, many surgeons now advocate high resolution anoscopy with acetic acid application then biopsy and eradication of suspicious lesions at three to six monthly intervals.

PREOPERATIVE

A phosphate enema 1 hour preoperatively gives adequate preparation.

Anesthesia

Excision using local anesthetic infiltration for a small number of minor lesions is possible, although many patients find this difficult to endure. A caudal block will provide sufficient anesthesia and relaxation of the anal canal. However, in those who will tolerate it, and those requiring large excisions, general anesthesia is the preferred option.

OPERATION

The operator should use universal precautions against viral transmission including gloves, protective eyewear, mask, and gown. In addition, a smoke evacuation device should be used with diathermy. Marcaine 0.25 percent with adrenaline 1:100 000 is infiltrated subcutaneously into the perianal area. This is best done in quadrants so that the solution is injected in a particular area immediately before the excision is begun; if all the solution is injected initially, absorption occurs and the benefit of the 'ballooning' effect is lost.

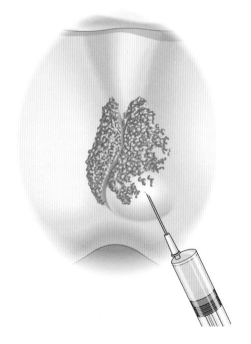

2.14.2

Warts are individually removed, preserving as much normal skin as possible using a pair of fine-toothed forceps and scissors. There is usually little hemorrhage, but a persistent bleeding point may be controlled with diathermy.

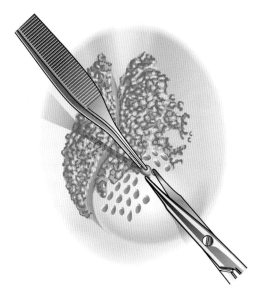

2.14.3

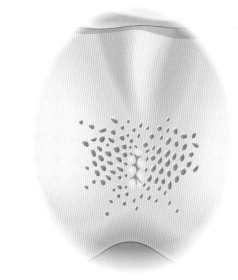

2.14.4

Removal of warts from within the anal canal

With the aid of an anal retractor, such as the Parks' or Zerney retractor, the local anesthetic solution is injected submucosally. The warts are again removed individually, preserving the mucosa between them. A large mucosal defect may be sutured with 3-0 PDS to approximate the mucosa of the lower rectum to the dentate line.

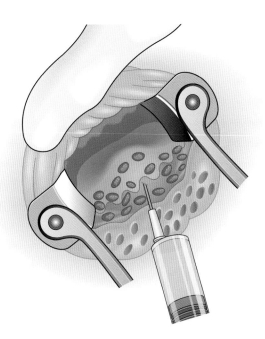

2.14.5

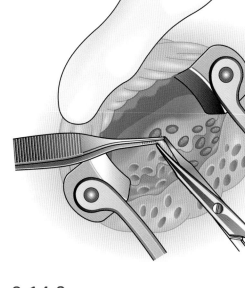

2.14.6

Circumferential lesions

Circumferential lesions may be removed in the same way. The defect, which is seldom more than 2 cm in length, is closed by approximating the distal rectal mucosa to the line of anal valves with 3-0 PDS. However, if the lesions are circumferential, excision in a staged approach may be better, so avoiding the risk of anal stenosis. A giant Buschke–Lowenstein lesion may require flap reconstruction to close the defect after excision (not shown).

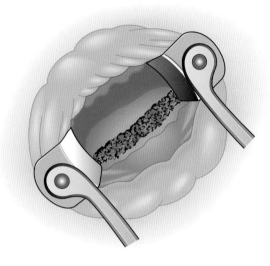

(a)

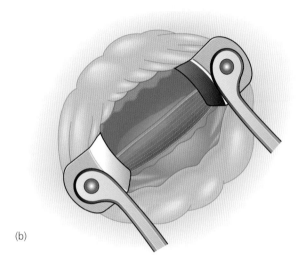

(b)

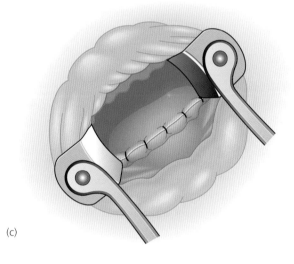

(c)

2.14.7

High-resolution anoscopy, biopsy, and eradication of AINIII

The anal canal is examined with the aid of a Parks' retractor and any gross lesions noted. A gauze soaked in 3 percent acetic acid is placed in the anal canal and a second gauze over the perianal area for 1 minute.

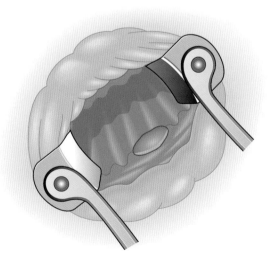

2.14.8

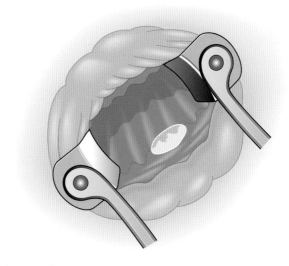

The anal canal is then reinspected for suspicious areas that will now appear white.

Using some form of magnification, such as the operative microscope, colposcope, or loops, areas of acetowhitening are identified and inspected for vascular abnormalities, including punctuate vessels or honeycomb patterns which suggest high-grade AIN. It should be noted that acetowhitening in the absence of vessel changes does not require intervention. The locations of any suspicious areas are documented and incision biopsy performed.

The suspicious areas are then fulgurated using the tip of the needle point diathermy. Ensuring the needle point is moved rapidly over the involved anoderm minimizes the damage to the underlying tissue, but still destroys the lesion which is limited to the epithelium. Normal anal mucosa and skin must be maintained between treated areas to prevent anal stenosis. A paraffin gauze dressing is applied at the conclusion of the procedure.

2.14.9

POSTOPERATIVE CARE

After excision of warts or high-resolution anoscopy (HRA) for AIN, simple oral analgesia will suffice and patients are given a fiber supplement. Daily sitz baths may provide relief. Condylomata should be submitted for histological examination. Up to a third of condyloma specimens will contain a focus of AIN and if this is the case the patient requires closer follow-up. Recurrence of perianal condyloma is common and further topical treatment and excision is often necessary.

Patients with AINIII, immunocompromise, or HIV require repeat HRA at 6–12-month intervals. Immunocompetent patients with low-grade AIN can be examined in the outpatient clinic annually.

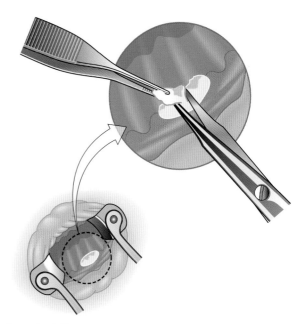

2.14.10

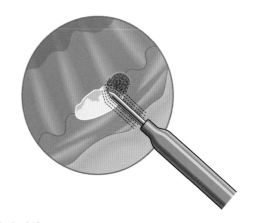

2.14.11

Perianal skin and anal cancer

JOHN MA NORTHOVER

INTRODUCTION

Anal cancer is relatively rare compared with colon and rectal cancer, but it is becoming more common, both absolutely and in relative terms: a generation ago, there were 100 cases of colorectal cancer for each anal cancer – that number has fallen to 27, while at the same time colorectal cancer has become more common. Anal cancer remains relatively much less common in Western countries than in several other locations, including parts of Brazil and India. Most tumors are epidermoid (including squamous cell, basaloid, and mucoepidermoid types); malignant melanoma is even more rare, and responds poorly to surgery and other modalities.

The rising incidence of anal cancer has occurred against a background of increasingly prevalent human papillomavirus (HPV) and human immunodeficiency virus (HIV) infection. HPV infection predisposes to premalignant anal intraepithelial neoplasia (AIN), while in turn HIV predisposes to HPV infection.

Two other important lesions that may require surgical attention are the Buschke–Lowenstein tumor (giant condyloma) and Paget's disease.

EPIDERMOID ANAL CANCER

Until the latter part of the twentieth century, anal cancer was predominantly treated surgically. Surgical series in the 1980s and 1990s described the outcomes of treatment over the previous several decades, with five-year survivals around 50–60 percent. Since then, radical chemoradiotherapy has taken over as the primary treatment in most patient groups, with similar or better survival prospects. Moreover, the avoidance of anorectal excision obviates the otherwise inevitable colostomy in the majority of cases.

Principles and justification

Despite the move away from surgery, the surgeon has a continuing role, as follows:

- initial diagnosis, including biopsy, and postoperative follow-up;
- primary treatment by local excision for small anal margin tumors;
- radical surgery following either incomplete remission after radical chemoradiotherapy or relapse after initially complete remission;
- primary radical surgery in those with major sphincter disruption or rectovaginal fistula at initial presentation;
- some cases of inguinal nodal metastasis.

INITIAL DIAGNOSIS AND POST-THERAPY ASSESSMENT

The surgeon is no longer the predominant therapeutic practitioner in most cases; nevertheless, the initial referral pathway is still usually to the surgeon. This may be because the initial referrer may not have considered this uncommon diagnosis, and passed the patient to the surgeon as the clinical presentation has suggested a 'surgical' problem.

The diagnosis, particularly obtaining biopsy proof, requires an examination under anesthesia (EUA). Ideally, the oncologist is present at this procedure.

The decision regarding completeness of remission after radical chemoradiotherapy usually still falls to the surgeon, who has particular expertise in the examination of the anal canal; complete remission is suggested if the canal epithelium feels and appears flat and soft, with no palpable extraluminal induration. If there is uncertainty, a further EUA is performed. As there is a risk of radionecrosis following biopsy, this should be avoided at EUA unless the result of digital and visual examination does not allow confident diagnosis.

PRIMARY MANAGEMENT OF SMALL MARGIN TUMORS

Small margin lesions (TNM stage T_1, <2 cm diameter) may be treated effectively by local excision alone, thus avoiding protracted chemoradiotherapy, with the accompanying risk of treatment morbidity. The treatment plan should be changed if under anesthesia there is any evidence that the lesion is more advanced than appeared at initial clinical examination.

RADICAL SURGERY AFTER FAILED PRIMARY CHEMORADIOTHERAPY

Three situations may trigger this:

1 Residual tumor
2 Complications of therapy
3 Later tumor recurrence.

Residual tumor

A minority of patients fall into this category. While the reassuring findings suggesting complete remission are reliable, histological proof of residual disease is mandatory before concluding that there is residual disease – and certainly before resorting to 'salvage surgery' – as clinical findings can be misleading: a residual lump may be found to comprise only inflammatory tissue on generous biopsy.

Complications of therapy

Severe anal pain caused by radionecrosis may necessitate surgery – a colostomy (in the often vain hope that healing may occur), or radical anorectal excision. Sometimes following successful tumor shrinkage, the sphincter has been so disrupted by the tumor prior to treatment and/ or by the effects of therapy that disabling incontinence supervenes; similarly, the rectovaginal septum may break down, producing a fistula that is unlikely to be amenable to surgical repair. Under these circumstances, radical surgery is indicated.

Tumor recurrence

Documented change in clinical findings during follow-up is likely to indicate recurrence, but again, histological proof is mandatory before proceeding to radical surgery. Further local excision may be considered in limited local relapse after primary surgery for a small margin lesion.

If this is not deemed sensible, radical chemoradiotherapy is generally preferable to immediate recourse to radical surgery.

PRIMARY RADICAL SURGERY FOR MAJOR SPHINCTER DISRUPTION OR RECTOVAGINAL FISTULA

If these features are present at initial presentation – given that they will not improve even after oncologically successful radical chemoradiotherapy, and are very unlikely to be curable by post-therapy surgical repair – primary surgery may be the best option in this group.

INGUINAL NODAL METASTASIS

Inguinal lymphadenopathy is present in 10–25 percent of cases,[1] although this is only inflammatory in half; later development of inguinal lymphadenopathy is almost always due to metastasis. In either scenario, histological evidence must be obtained by fine needle aspiration (FNA), needle biopsy, or excision biopsy before surgery is considered. Although the inguinal region is included in the standard radiotherapy fields by most oncologists, some argue that surgery is preferable, either primarily or at subsequent relapse.

Preoperative work up

An appropriate history should be taken to check for the risk of HIV infection, and after suitable counseling, HIV serology should be sought, not least as a precaution for the operating team.

As part of the evaluation of all patients – not just those requiring surgery – the following diagnostic and staging procedures will have been performed:

- EUA and biopsy.
- Computed tomography (CT) scan to check for distant spread.
- Magnetic resonance imaging (MRI) to define the anatomy of the primary lesion and to look for mesorectal and inguinal lymphadenopathy. In some units and particularly in the United States, ultrasound scan (USS) may be the more popular modality for examining the primary lesion.

OPERATIVE PROCEDURES

Local procedures

These may be performed in either the lithotomy or prone positions: the author prefers the latter.

BIOPSY

Besides initial diagnosis at presentation, this is required in all patients in whom surgery is contemplated for possible residual or recurrent disease after primary chemoradiotherapy.

Superficial biopsy in those who have undergone chemoradiotherapy should be conservative, using a size-15 scalpel blade, to minimize the risk of symptomatic radionecrosis. Deeper biopsy may be necessary in the ischiorectal fossae; for this, a Trucut needle should be used.

LOCAL EXCISION

Local excision involves complete removal of a lesion close to, or at, the anal verge and perhaps extending very slightly into the distal anal canal. Complete excision should include a 1 cm margin of normal skin beyond the circumferential edge of the lesion, and a margin of subcutaneous fat sufficient to allow at least 5 mm of deep clearance. Local excision of small canal tumors is not satisfactory treatment, as a decent deep margin would require inclusion of part of the underlying sphincter.

Subdermal 1:200 000 adrenaline injection may be used to minimize bleeding during the dissection. Although this approach should be confined to tumors at the anal margin or on the perianal skin, placement of Parks', Gelpy, or Lone Star™ retractors may facilitate excision, particularly if the medial border of the surgical specimen straddles the verge (**Figure 2.15.1**a). The incision should be vertical to the skin surface, and the deep margin must be within the subcutaneous fat (**Figure 2.15.1**b). The specimen should be pinned onto a flat piece of cork to ensure accurate orientation for the pathologist (**Figure 2.15.1**c).

In some cases, the wound can be left open to heal by second intention. Alternatively, the wound can be 'marsupialized' to speed healing, or a simple advancement flap may be fashioned to close the wound completely.

Radical surgery

Abdominoperineal excision of the rectum (APER) and anal canal is broadly the same for anal cancer as for rectal cancer (see Chapter 6.1). As more attention has been given to the disturbing excess of local recurrence after APER for rectal cancer, there has been a move towards prevention of exposure of the lateral margins of the tumor by halting pelvic dissection at the level of the origin of the levator plate, prone dissection in the perineal phase of the operation, excision of the coccyx to improve transperineal access to the low pelvis, and relative preservation of

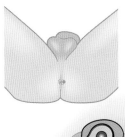

(a)

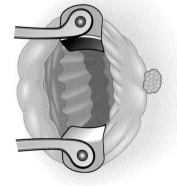

(b)

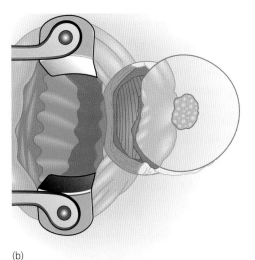

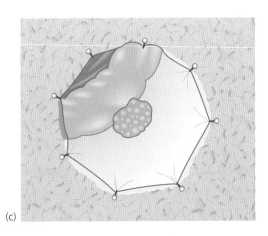

(c)

2.15.1

perianal skin and ischiorectal fat (unless the levator plate is transgressed by the tumor). For anal epidermoid tumors, however, there are certain points of difference in surgical technique that deserve special emphasis:

- Perineal skin excision should be wide enough to be clear of the tumor and, importantly, to facilitate clearance of all the ischiorectal fat. The latter is ensured by taking the dissection laterally to the ischial tuberosity, and hugging the medial surface of the ischium and obturator internus up to the bony origin of the levator muscle (**Figure 2.15.2**).
- As the operative field has been subjected to radical chemoradiotherapy, and as the defect produced by the more radical perineal phase, flap advancement to bring in healthy tissue to fill the defect should be considered the norm.
- The conventional advancement procedure is the vertical rectus abdominis myocutaneous (VRAM) flap, mobilized at the end of the abdominal phase and delivered into the pelvis prior to abdominal closure, ready for deployment at the end of the perineal phase (see Chapter 7.1). The author prefers the inferior gluteal artery perforator (IGAP) advancement flap. The two main advantages of this procedure are the avoidance of weakening of the abdominal wall musculature and the larger bulk of tissue to fill the defect. This is essentially a uni- or bilateral V–Y advancement in which a block of buttock skin, subcutaneous fat, and gluteal fascia (not muscle) is mobilized extensively on one or more IGAP branches, identified before dissection using a Doppler probe (**Figure 2.15.3a**). Once these large flaps have been mobilized, the medial several centimeters of skin is cleared of its epidermis, thus exposing the dermis; this permits the thinned skin to be buried as part of the bulky filling tissue (**Figure 2.15.3b**). If the posterior wall of the vagina has been excised, the most medial 2–3 cm of each flap can be left unstripped to allow reconstruction (**Figure 2.15.3c**). Once the flaps have been transferred medially, the standard Y-shaped lateral closure is fashioned (**Figure 2.15.3d**) (see also Chapter 7.3).

Postoperative care

Little specific care is needed after local excision. The patient should be reassured that they can continue with normal activities at an early stage, and should be reassured that the chance of wound infection is relatively low. A laxative to ensure a soft stool may help to ease any apprehension about evacuation; a shower after each bowel movement is recommended. A small dressing to cover the wound is more to protect clothing than the operation site.

Postoperative care following abdominoperineal excision is described in Chapter 6.1.

POSTOPERATIVE COMPLICATIONS

Early complications are uncommon after local excision; most infections require no more than careful cleaning

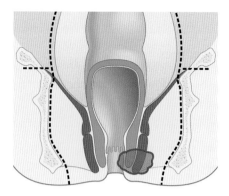

2.15.2

and dressing. The only important later complication is anal stenosis, which sometimes develops if a significant proportion of the anal margin has been excised, and the wound has been left open to heal by second intent. If recognized early, stenosis will usually respond to dilatation under anesthesia, followed by regular self-dilatation for two months.

Complications following abdominoperineal excision are described in Chapter 6.1.

Outcome

Series that describe the efficacy of surgery alone all date to the time before radical chemoradiotherapy became the treatment of choice for most anal epidermoid cancers.

ANAL MARGIN CANCER

The largest and most informative series of cases treated by local excision alone were published in the latter part of the twentieth century, describing patients treated for this rare lesion over several decades. The largest series was reported from St Mark's Hospital and included cases treated during the period 1948–84.[2] Two-thirds of 83 patients were treated by local excision alone, of whom 65 percent survived for at least five years. Of 11 treated by anorectal excision with curative intent, only four (36 percent) survived for five years. Overall five-year survival was 65 percent for T_{1-2} tumors, but only 33 percent for those at stages T_{3-4}.

A series from Copenhagen comprised 76 patients, 58 of whom were treated with curative intent.[3] This series highlighted the tendency to later recurrence than in rectal cancer, the longest interval being nine years. Twenty-four (41 percent) developed recurrent disease, all but one of which were locoregional; of 32 treated by local excision only, 20 (62 percent) developed local recurrence.

In contrast, a New York series showed a corrected five-year survival for local excision of 88 percent.[4]

ANAL CANAL CANCER

The largest series was reported by the Mayo Clinic in 1984.[5] Of 188 patients presenting in the period 1950–76, only 118 were operated radically with curative intent: of these, 81

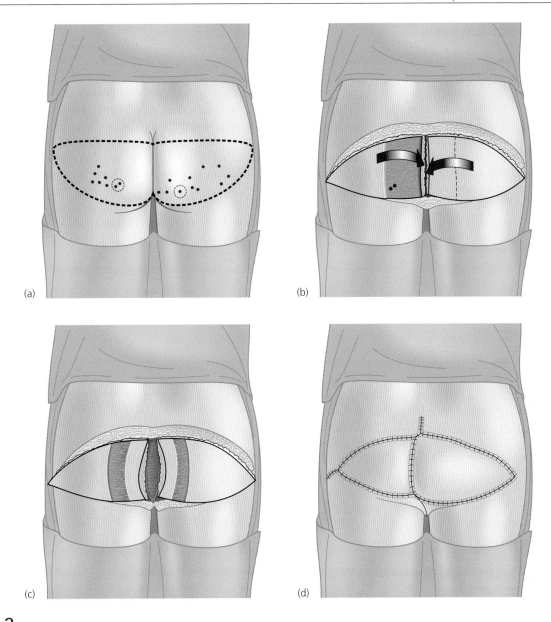

(a)

(b)

(c)

(d)

2.15.3

(69 percent) survived to five years. Thirteen (7 percent) with superficial lesions of ≤2 cm were treated by local excision, with excellent results.

Other series from the same era had less favorable results, with five-year survivals of 20–50 percent.

Non-surgical primary therapy

By the late 1990s, the evidence base for chemoradiotherapy as primary treatment in most cases was sufficiently positive to lead to the abandonment of routine primary surgery, reserving it for the case groups mentioned above. A very large randomized trial in 585 UK patients indicated significant superiority for chemoradiotherapy over radiotherapy alone, both in terms of local recurrence and

cancer-free survival.[6] In a comprehensive review of trials performed to seek improvements on the 1996 protocol, no significant advances have been demonstrated.[7]

OTHER PERIANAL AND ANAL TUMORS

Malignant melanoma

This tumor is excessively rare, accounting for less than 1 percent of anal canal tumors; no more than 20 percent of patients survive for five years. The tumor is resistant to chemo- and radiotherapy, and the outcome of radical surgery is so poor that most advocate such surgery only if disabling symptoms require it for palliation of what almost inevitably becomes generalized disease at an early stage.

Buschke–Lowenstein tumor

Buschke–Lowenstein tumor (giant condyloma, BLT) is also an unusual lesion, with only around 50 published cases. The etiology is related to HPV, as with ordinary condylomata. The lesion usually surrounds the anus completely, although when examined under anesthesia, it may become apparent that the base of the lesion is to one side of the anal orifice. It is important to remember that up to 50 percent of these tumors harbor malignancy, so careful and comprehensive biopsy to exclude malignancy is recommended before local excision is chosen.

Paget's disease

Also rare, this is a bizarre lesion: the nature, pathogenesis, and natural history remain unclear. First described as a disease of the nipple, the anus is the most common site for so-called 'extra-mammary Paget's disease'. The typical appearance is a slightly raised area of variegated red/gray discoloration of the skin around the anus. It is four times more common in women. The diagnosis is confirmed by the typical Paget's cells, with their abundant foamy cytoplasm, infiltrating the epidermis of the perianal skin. In at least 25 percent of cases, an occult adenocarcinoma will be found, usually in the rectum, but sometimes more proximally. Occasionally, Paget's disease itself can metastasize to the inguinal lymph nodes. In the absence of an associated primary adenocarcinoma, surgical treatment is usually by wide local excision and appropriate skin advancement or grafting.

Surgical management of apparently benign BLT and Paget's disease

These lesions are removed using the same principles employed in the excision of areas of anal intraepithelial neoplasia (AIN). If the tumor has a base involving a third or less of the anal verge, there is the option to leave the wound to heal by second intent. For anything larger, particularly if circumferential skin excision is necessary, either an advancement flap or a split skin graft is required; adequate access demands that the patient be placed prone. The margins for excision are as for small epidermoid cancers, as described above. It is particularly important to ensure that any extension towards the dentate line is excised, including if necessary a strip of mucosa. The mucosal margin proximal to the excision must be secured by stay sutures, while the graft or flap is being prepared.

SPLIT SKIN GRAFT

This technique should be within the skill range of a colorectal surgeon. Skin is easily harvested from the back of the thigh. The author uses intact skin rather than the widely fenestrated skin that can be taken to cover larger areas elsewhere. The skin is mounted on paraffin gauze in the standard way, and cut into four 'truncated pyramids' to allow ease of application (**Figure 2.15.4**). The pieces are shaped to fit the defect precisely; the narrow ends of the pyramids are secured with care to the four quadrants of the dentate line using absorbable sutures. The outer corners are sutured to the skin edge, and the four corner sutures on each segment are tied over proflavine-soaked cotton wool to apply gentle, molding pressure to ensure close apposition to the curved grafted bed. Some surgeons routinely use a defunctioning colostomy, but antidiarrheals and a liquid diet to discourage evacuation is an effective alternative. The patient should be nursed prone initially. Sutures are cut, releasing the dressings, at 7 days. There must be careful follow-up looking for early signs of stenosis at the dentate line, with early use of anal self-dilatation as necessary.

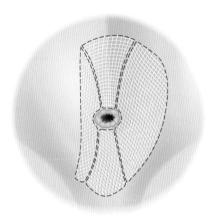

2.15.4

ADVANCEMENT FLAPS

Small advancements are straightforward, but the author prefers to work with a plastic surgeon for more ambitious tissue transfer.

These procedures are best performed with the patient in the prone position. The most frequently used methods involve V–Y advancement, in which an island of skin and subcutaneous fat is mobilized from the underlying gluteus maximus, retaining a pedicle to ensure a blood supply to the flap. The flap can then be moved medially to allow the carefully crafted medial border to be advanced to the dentate line if necessary. Again, care is required to ensure that the dentate line is re-epithelialized circumferentially to avoid stenosis. As with split skin grafting, it is usual to nurse the patient prone for several days and to discourage early bowel movements by the preferred method (see also Chapter 7.3).

REFERENCES

1. Mistrangelo M, Bello M, Mobiglia A *et al*. Feasibility of the sentinel node biopsy in anal cancer. *Quarterly Journal of Nuclear Medicine and Molecular Imaging* 2009; **53**: 3–8.

2. Pinna Pintor M, Northover J, Nicholls R. Squamous cell carcinoma of the anus at one hospital from 1948 to 1984. *British Journal of Surgery* 1989; **76**: 806–10.

3. Jensen S, Hagen K, Harling H *et al.* Long term prognosis after radical treatment for squamous-cell carcinoma of the anal canal and anal margin. *Diseases of Colon and Rectum* 1988; **31**: 273–8.

4. Greenall M, Quan S, Stearns M. Epidermoid cancer of the anal margin. *American Journal of Surgery* 1985; **149**: 95–101.

5. Boman B, Moertel C, O'Connell M. Carcinoma of the anal canal. A clinical and pathologic study of 188 cases. *Cancer* 1984; **51**: 1830–7.

6. UKCCCR Anal Cancer Trial Working Party. Epidermoid anal cancer: results from the UKCCCR randomised trial of radiotherapy alone versus radiotherapy, 5-fluorouracil, and mitomycin. *Lancet* 1996; **348**: 1049–54.

7. Fraunholz I, Rabeneck D, Weis C, Rodel C. Combined modality treatment for anal cancer: current strategies and future directions. *Strahlentherapie und Onkologie* 2010; **186**: 361–6.

Pilonidal disease

MATT RICKARD

HISTORY

Sacrococcygeal pilonidal disease is a chronic inflammatory condition of the natal cleft. It was first described by Herbert Mayo in 1833 and was named a *pilo* (hair) *nidal* (nest) sinus in 1880 by Hodge. The disease is active from the late teens and usually resolves by the age of 40–50 years irrespective of the method of treatment.

There is continued debate over the pathogenesis of pilonidal sinus disease (PSD) and subsequently different treatment methods have been developed based on the presumed etiology. The author feels that the condition is acquired when hair invades the skin because of forces in the midline natal cleft and that these hairs incite an inflammatory reaction. The pits through which the hairs enter the subcutaneous tissue may be congenital. Others believe the PSD is a condition of the epidermis that begins with forces that stretch the normal hair follicle.[1] Congenital theories include medullary canal remnants, dermal inclusions, or vestigial sex glands.

Pilonidal sinus can be confused with and can coexist with hidradenitis suppurativa. Therefore, the groins and axillae should be examined for sinuses. A posterior anal fistula is another differential diagnosis. There are at least 17 published surgical methods of managing PSD, which clearly means that there is no perfect option. In pooled data analysis[2] and a recent Cochrane review[3] lateralizing the wound is associated with better wound healing and lower recurrence rates. It is important to note that asymptomatic midline pits should not be managed surgically.

PREOPERATIVE ASSESSMENT AND PREPARATION

These are usually young healthy patients and minimal preoperative preparation is necessary. It is important to fully inform the patient of the risk of recurrence, the cosmetic appearance of a flattened natal cleft with a lateral wound and the numbness associated with flap surgery.

OPERATIONS

Acute pilonidal abscess

INDICATIONS AND CONTRAINDICATIONS

An acute pilonidal abscess presents as a red, fluctuant tender mass in or just lateral to the natal cleft. The diagnosis is usually quite clear on clinical examination. When the abscess is situated caudally in the natal cleft (which is rare), it can be confused with a perianal abscess of cryptoglandular origin.

ANESTHESIA

The abscess can be drained under local or general anesthetic. Often, a more adequate drainage can be performed with general anesthesia. Intravenous antibiotics should be given with induction and oral antibiotics continued for another 1–2 weeks postoperatively, as this is usually an acute-on-chronic situation. Another option is needle aspiration and oral antibiotics.

INCISION

The incision site is dictated by the surgeon's approach to definitive treatment of chronic PSD. Usually, the abscess has formed lateral to the natal cleft and it can be incised over the fluctuant point. This incision would then be included in the excised tissue in any subsequent Karydakis flap procedure. A small ellipse of skin can be excised to prevent premature resealing. Packing is not necessary and is quite painful. All that is necessary is an absorbent pad to protect the clothing.

OUTCOME

In some patients, although they may be left with a residual pilonidal sinus, if it remains asymptomatic, no further treatment will be necessary. However, in the majority, definitive surgical treatment will be required because of a symptomatic pilonidal sinus. The options are outlined below.

Karydakis flap

This is the author's preferred method and the technique described is an adaptation of Karydakis' original description.[4]

INDICATIONS AND CONTRAINDICATIONS

A chronic abscess/sinus, manifesting as pain or persistent drainage, is the most common form of pilonidal disease and is the usual indication for definitive surgery. The wounds are usually chronically infected despite numerous courses of antibiotics. Often, patients will have had previous surgical procedures for the pilonidal sinus, but this is not a contraindication to the Karydakis flap.

Rotation or V–Y flaps should be considered for very large, complicated PNS, or sinuses involving a track that runs very close to the anal sphincter complex.

ANESTHESIA

General anesthesia and endotracheal intubation with muscle relaxation is preferred by the author, however the procedure can be performed with a laryngeal mask and no muscle relaxation. Broad-spectrum intravenous prophylactic antibiotics are given with induction (gentamycin and metronidazole).

The prone position is preferred by the author, however the procedure can be performed in the left lateral position. This allows excellent surgical access, but does increase the potential for anesthetic complications. Paramount importance must be placed on maintaining a secure and safe airway. This relies on using a suitable intubating device and securing it appropriately. Potential complications (from the prone position), other than airway problems, include corneal abrasion, ocular pressure injury, conjunctival oedema, carotid and vertebral vessel injuries (from excessive head rotation), stretch injuries to the roots of the brachial plexus and axillary neurovascular bundles. It is important to avoid abdominal compression by placing pillows under the (bony and hence fixed) chest and pelvis.

OPERATION

The natal cleft is shaved and the incision is marked. The buttocks are separated using adhesive tape attached to the side of the operating table (this needs to be freed prior to wound closure and therefore must be accessible under the drapes). The markings are drawn such that a symmetrical vertical ellipse with the long axis centered off the midline incorporates all of the diseased tissue (Figure 2.16.1). The long axis of the elliptical incision is placed on the side of

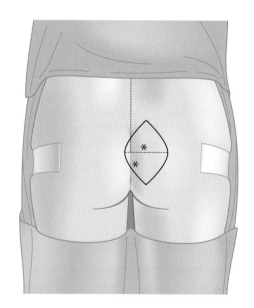

2.16.1

the dominant disease which results in a longitudinal skin wound 1.5–2 cm off the midline (**Figure 2.16.2**). If the disease is bilateral, a decision must be made as to which side encompasses more tissue and the ellipse is based on this side. It is important to make the ellipse symmetrical and this will often entail removing a large portion of normal tissue on the lateral side of the ellipse (shaded area

in **Figure 2.16.3**). If the ellipse is asymmetrical and less skin is taken laterally the mid-part of the final wound will curve towards and may even reach the midline.

The ellipse of skin, underlying fat, and pilonidal sinus is excised down to the sacrococcygeal fascia. The aim is not to see any granulation tissue associated with any tracks associated with the PNS and thus to ensure complete

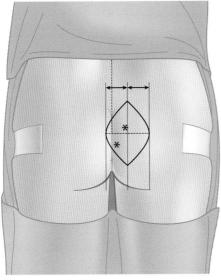

2.16.2

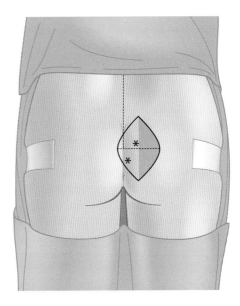

2.16.3

excision of the sinus and minimal contamination of the wound. As the incision is extended through the fat, dissection is angled slightly towards the midline on the lateral portion of the ellipse and parallel with this medially (**Figure 2.16.4**). The skin and soft tissue defects can appear quite large following removal of the specimen. On

the contralateral side, skin and subcutaneous tissue along the length of the incision are mobilized until the flap can comfortably reach across to the fixed side. This dissection is performed at the level of the sacral fascia and the fascia over the gluteal muscles (**Figure 2.16.5**). It is necessary to make this dissection quite extensive (shaded area in

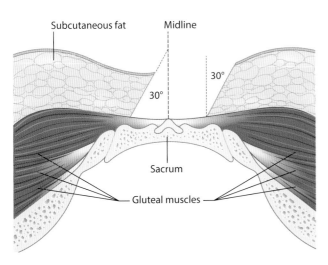

2.16.4

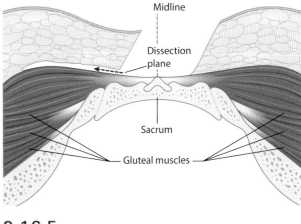

2.16.5

Figure 2.16.6). Care must be taken at the caudal end of the wound to identify and preserve the external anal sphincter which may be encountered.

At this point, the tape used to separate the buttocks should be removed and an assessment made as to whether the flap is under any tension. Further dissection can be performed if tension is present. A suction drain is placed under the flap and exteriorized cranially and away from the midline on the side of flap dissection. However, some surgeons do not drain the wound and there is no evidence for or against a drain. The wound is closed in three layers. A series of interrupted 1-Vicryl sutures are placed without tying. These sutures begin in the bulk of the flap, include a small bite of the fascia (slightly lateral to the mid-portion of the wound) and the deep subcutaneous fat of the lateral portion of the wound. The deepness of these sutures should be such that another fat layer can be performed above this layer and the skin edges will be even with no asymmetry. These sutures are then tied with the drain carefully positioned under the bulk of the flap. The subcutaneous layer is then closed with a series of interrupted 2-0 Vicryl, such that the skin edges are perfectly aligned without tension. It should almost feel like no skin sutures are necessary. Subcuticular 3-0 monocryl is used and it is the author's preference for interrupted sutures. Steristrips are carefully placed along the wound and an occlusive dressing applied (**Figure 2.16.7**).

POSTOPERATIVE CARE

The author believes that it is worthwhile to keep the patient in hospital for 3–4 days. Many surgeons perform this operation as a day-stay procedure. While in hospital, bed rest (with toilet privileges) is encouraged. Minimal hip flexion is allowed in the first week and sitting and bending is discouraged. Oral antibiotics (metronidazole 400 mg three times a day and cephalexin 500 mg four times a day) are given for 2 weeks. The drain is left in place while in hospital (3–4 days). Patients are advised to take leave from work for 2 weeks and during this time undertake minimal physical activity. It is recommended that they squat above the toilet rather than sit directly on it. Patients are advised to clean following defecation with a forward motion away from the wound.

OUTCOME AND COMPLICATIONS

In a series of 70 patients treated with this approach, our data show that 38 percent will get superficial wound breakdown, 10 percent will get complete wound breakdown. The recurrence rate was 4.2 percent at a median three-year follow-up.[4] In Karydakis' original series, the recurrence rate was less than 1 percent.[5]

Lateral drainage and pit excision (Bascom's procedure)

This can be performed as an office or outpatient procedure with local anesthetic or under general anesthesia.

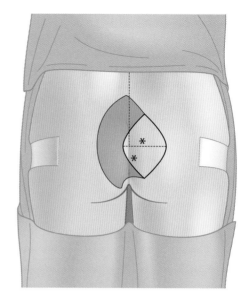

2.16.6

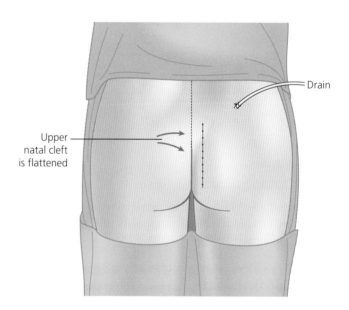

2.16.7 Final result showing wound off the midline and drain.

OPERATION

The patient is in the prone or left lateral position. An incision is made 2.5 cm to one or both sides of the midline. The incision is made long enough to be able to see inside the entire cavity quite clearly. Incision length adds nothing to disability and does not delay healing. The cavity is scrubbed with gauze to remove granulation tissue, hair, and other debris. This will often reveal a fibrous wall. Branch cavities must be sought, identified, opened, and scrubbed. It may be necessary to excise a small segment of fibrous abscess wall if it is infiltrated with hair (**Figure 2.16.8**).

The point of a hemostat is then pushed into the cavity, directing it against the underside of the midline skin and rubbed firmly. This identifies the originating follicle

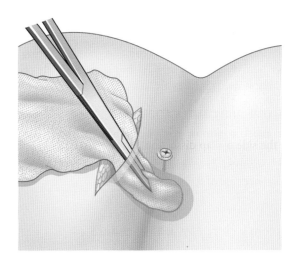

2.16.8

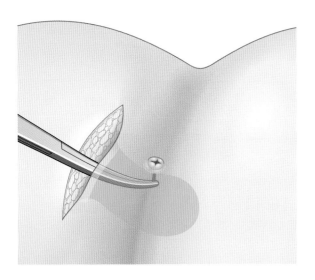

2.16.9

and other enlarged follicles that require removal (**Figure 2.16.9**).

All midline pits are identified and excised with a small diamond-shaped incision around the pit. The tip of an 11 blade is used to excise the pit by excising a piece of tissue

the size of a grain of rice (**Figure 2.16.10**). Multiple pits are excised individually as far as is feasible. It is important to inspect the deep end of the removed specimen to ensure that the whole track has been excised down to the cavity that has been entered via the lateral incision. Skin punches have also been described to excise the pits. The resulting small defects may be sutured with a subcuticular removable monofilament or allowed to heal secondarily.

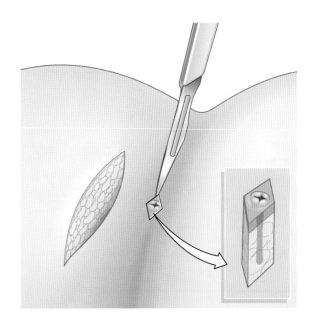

2.16.10

POSTOPERATIVE CARE

Oral antibiotics should be given postoperatively. Patients can shower normally and commence normal sitting and other activity immediately. A simple dressing to protect clothing is used. Sutures are removed on the 7th day.

OUTCOME AND COMPLICATIONS

The most common complication is a slowly healing midline wound. Bascom describes a 5 percent recurrence rate.[1] Senapati described a 7.7 percent abscess rate and a recurrence rate of 9.6 percent.[6]

Bascom's cleft closure procedure

The cleft closure was first described by John Bascom in 1982. He describes it as 'our modification of the successful method of Karydakis and Kitchen'. It obliterates the deep cleft, closes the unhealed midline wound, keeps the suture line away from the midline and reduces the tension between skin and coccyx. In this technique, it is very important that it is appreciated that skin and skin only is removed. It accomplishes a skin transfer by lifting a flap of extra skin from the donor buttock and drawing it across the midline on to the recipient buttock (**Figure 2.16.11**).[7]

OPERATION

The patient is in the prone or left lateral position. The buttocks are pushed together and the outer line of their contact is marked with a felt pen (**Figures 2.16.12** and **2.16.13**). The buttocks are then taped apart. The extent of mobilization for the donor flap (the least damaged side of

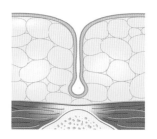
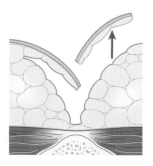
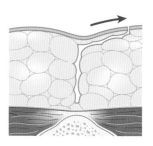

2.16.11

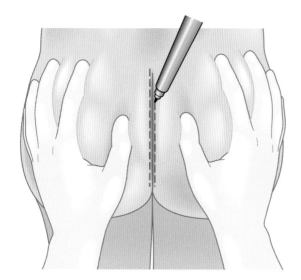

2.16.12

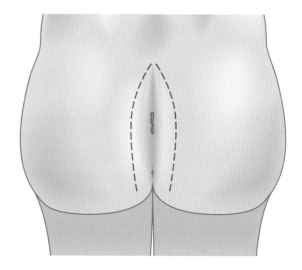

2.16.13

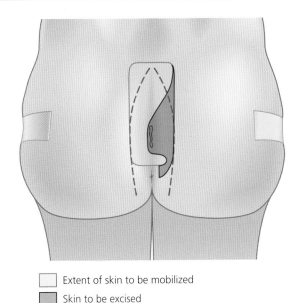

☐ Extent of skin to be mobilized

■ Skin to be excised

2.16.14

the natal cleft) should be marked. In **Figure 2.16.14**, the skin on the right of the diagram is to be removed, on the left it is undermined and shifted for the repair.[1, 8]

The incision is commenced on the recipient side, off the midline and above the top of the natal cleft. The incision should then slant down and across the midline at an acute angle just above the unhealed wound. The incision then turns sharply to cross the midline at right angles cephalad of the anus, and then it should turn again so that the

lower end of the incision points towards the anus (**Figure 2.16.15**). Mobilization of the skin medial to the wound then commences. Cephalad to the anus, the perianal skin is weak, therefore the surgeon should leave some extra subcutaneous tissue attached. It may be necessary with low-lying wounds to extend undermining of the anal flap into the subcutaneous sphincter fibers. Rotation of this anal flap will relieve tension at the anal end of the closure and prevent skin necrosis. At the upper end of the incision, undermining continues above the top of the natal cleft, because leaving the upper cleft attached to the sacrum can contribute to recurrence.

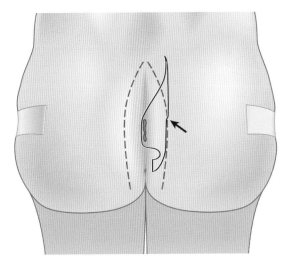

2.16.15

The recipient side is measured to mark the lateral extent of excision. (The flap has been raised, but nothing has been excised yet.) The donor flap itself is used as a template to ensure that enough skin has been mobilized. The tapes are released and the buttocks are pushed together. The donor flap is gently pulled across the midline (**Figure 2.16.16**). Any skin overlapped by the donor flap is marked for removal. A loose donor flap, which would fold down between the fat layers, should be avoided. Below the level of the end of the sacrum, the skin is marked for removal to the natural line of contact but not beyond (arrow on **Figure 2.16.15**). The removal of more skin risks postoperative discomfort from skin tension while the patient is in the sitting position.

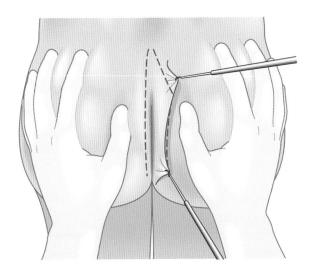

2.16.16

The skin (which will include the pilonidal sinus) is then excised (**Figure 2.16.17**). Note that the excision plane is subcutaneous. This prepares a bed to receive the flap and unroofs the unhealed wound. From the bed of the unhealed wound, granulation tissue and debris are scrubbed away with gauze. The 2–3 mm sheet of scar that forms the base of the wound is excised. Fat or muscle should not be mobilized. As much fat as possible is saved to provide padding. Hemostasis should be achieved to avoid hematoma underneath the skin flap. At this stage, the wound appears quite large, however most of the raw surface disappears as fat from the right meets fat from the left (**Figure 2.16.11**). The donor flap covers the remainder.

A suction drain is placed under the flap. Subcutaneous fat at the skin edges is closed with a 3-0 absorbable suture to position the skin for closure. Closure is started by tacking the rotated anal flap roughly into position. The skin edges should now lie together without tension. The skin is closed with subcuticular sutures. Steri-strips are placed across the wound and an occlusive dressing applied.

POSTOPERATIVE CARE

The patient can be discharged the same day. Oral antibiotics should be continued for 5–7 days afterwards. The drain is removed around day 4. Patients can resume normal activities after a week or so depending on the degree of discomfort.

COMPLICATIONS

Complications of cleft closure are uncommon. Infection responds quickly to opening the inferior 2 cm of the wound and continuing (or recommencing) antibiotics. Small patches of skin necrosis heal and do not affect the result. Hematomata respond best to evacuation under anesthesia and reclosure over a drain. Small recurrences respond to local revision and flattening.

OUTCOME

Bascom and Bascom[8] performed this procedure on a series of patients with persistent open wounds despite at least two prior pilonidal surgeries elsewhere. Sixty-nine patients had undergone 223 surgeries (average of three), with an average follow-up of 30 months. Only 52 patients were able to be contacted. Of these 52 patients, five required two 'cleft lifts' and one patient required three 'cleft lifts'. All 52 patients were healed at the time of follow-up.

Midline excision/incision

A midline incision is acceptable if it lays open the cavity through all openings, but it is not recommended as the initial treatment. If a midline incision is used, marsupialization (suturing down the edges of the wound) has been shown to speed healing. The disadvantages of midline vertical incision are the need for packing and the occasional resistant wound which does not heal. Non-

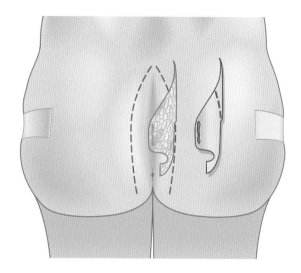

2.16.17

healing wounds can, however, be treated with a Karydakis flap or the Bascom's cleft closure technique.

Midline excision with primary closure should probably be avoided as the wounds often break down. There is no place for tension sutures or pressure packs.

Other flaps

Z PLASTY

This is an off-midline surgical technique where the whole diseased area is removed. This is followed by the skin flaps being cut in a Z-shape and moved to fill the excised diseased area.

MODIFIED RHOMBOID (LIMBERG) FLAP

This technique is similar to the classical rhomboid technique; however, the end part of the suture line is moved to the side of the midline.

VY ADVANCEMENT FLAP

The diseased area is cut away, creating a defect that is closed with a 'V'-shaped full thickness flap. The technique of raising the flap is similar to that of a rhomboid flap, only the shape is different. When the space left by the flap is closed, the sutures form a Y shape.

GLUTEUS MAXIMUS MYOCUTANEOUS FLAP

This flap is based on the superior gluteal vessels and nerve. The skin, subcutaneous tissues, and gluteus maximus muscle are mobilized and rotated medially to close the defect.

REFERENCES

1. Bascom JU. Procedures for pilonidal disease. In: Fielding LP, Goldberg SM (eds). *Operative surgery of the colon, rectum and anus*, 5th edn. Oxford: Butterworth-Heinemann, 1993: 893–906.

2. Petersen S, Koch R, Stelzner S *et al.* Primary closure techniques in chronic pilonidal sinus. A survey of different surgical approaches. *Diseases of the Colon and Rectum* 2002; **45**: 1458–67.

3. AL-Khamis A, McCallum I, King PM, Bruce J. Healing by primary versus secondary intention after surgical treatment for pilonidal sinus. *Cochrane Database of Systematic Reviews* 2010; (1): CD006213.

4. Keshava A, Young CJ, Rickard MJFX, Sinclair G. Karydakis flap repair for sacrococcygeal pilonidal sinus disease: how important is technique? *Australia and New Zealand Journal of Surgery* 2007; **77**: 181–3.

5. Karydakis G. Easy and successful treatment of pilonidal sinus after explanation of its causative factors. *Australia and New Zealand Journal of Surgery* 1992; **62**: 385–9.

6. Senapati A, Cripps NP, Thompson MR. Bascom's operation in the day-surgical management of symptomatic pilonidal sinus. *British Journal of Surgery* 2000; **87**: 1067–70.

7. Bascom J, Bascom T. Failed pilonidal surgery. New paradigm and new operation leading to cures. *Archives of Surgery* 2002; **137**: 1146–50.

8. Bascom J, Bascom T. Utility of the cleft lift procedure in refractory pilonidal disease. *American Journal of Surgery* 2007; **193**: 606–9.

3

Stomas

Ileostomy

JONATHAN M WILSON AND ROBIN KS PHILLIPS

PRINCIPLES AND JUSTIFICATION

Types of operation and indications

An ileostomy diverts small bowel contents onto the anterior abdominal wall and may be either temporary or permanent. The three main types of ileostomy are end, loop, and end-loop ileostomy, and there are differing indications for each.

END ILEOSTOMY

- Patients with inflammatory bowel disease (IBD) undergoing emergency subtotal colectomy or non-restorative proctocolectomy.
- Patients with familial adenomatous polyposis (FAP) when ileorectal anastomosis is contraindicated (significant rectal polyposis or rectal high-grade dysplasia/invasive carcinoma) and in whom a restorative ileal pouch-anal anastomosis (IPAA) is considered ill-advised or undesirable by the patient.
- Synchronous large bowel cancers that necessitate proctocolectomy where restorative IPAA is not possible.
- A 'temporary' end ileostomy may be necessary after ileal resection when a primary anastomosis is ill-advised. Subsequent restoration of intestinal continuity can be achieved at a later date. Examples include:
  - ileal/ileocecal resection for perforating Crohn's disease;
  - trauma/obstruction requiring resection of the ileocecum/right colon;
  - after complex enterocutaneous fistula surgery;
  - damage control surgery in an unstable patient.

LOOP ILEOSTOMY

A loop ileostomy may be required to provide proximal diversion in several settings:

- A distal anastomosis where there is concern over potential anastomotic leakage. For example, low colorectal/coloanal anastomosis, post-radiotherapy, and complex reconstruction, such as IPAA.

- Distal pathology where resection is inappropriate, e.g. severe perianal Crohn's disease, unresectable colorectal malignancy.

END-LOOP ILEOSTOMY

An end-loop ileostomy may be employed when there is insufficient length for the divided end of the small bowel to reach the skin and achieve a spout (e.g. obesity, bulky/short mesentery, emergency surgery with peritonitis).

Occasionally, a loop ileostomy may be converted to an end-loop stoma by transection of the efferent limb of small bowel just inside the peritoneal cavity, usually with a linear stapler (e.g. following excision of an ileal pouch where there is a satisfactory pre-existing loop ileostomy).

PREOPERATIVE ASSESSMENT AND PREPARATION

Routine preoperative assessment and optimization of comorbidities is essential. A multidisciplinary team approach involving surgeon, specialist stoma therapist, patient, and carers will adjust individual expectations and expedite postoperative recovery. Both patient and carers will benefit from reading relevant stoma-related literature preoperatively.

Siting and marking the stoma

The stoma is best marked with a permanent marker with the patient sitting (when skin creases/folds are most prominent), standing, and in the supine position. The site should be well away from skin creases, previous scars, bony prominences, and the main wound to allow for watertight appliance application. The site should be at the apex of the infraumbilical fat mound and should overlie the midpoint of the rectus abdominis muscle, although stomas lateral to this do not seem to be associated with an increased

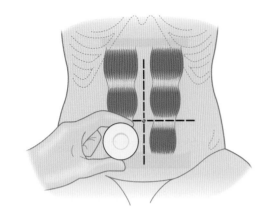

3.1.1

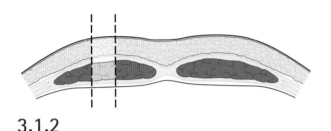

3.1.2

rate of parastomal herniation.[1] The site should be readily accessible to the patient, and in obese patients this may require placement much higher than normal to avoid the stoma disappearing 'over the horizon'. It is sensible to cover the mark with a transparent adhesive dressing, which can be removed before preparing the abdomen in the operating room, to minimize fading during the preoperative wait. The center of the marked site can then be marked using a variety of techniques, as even indelible marker pen can be rubbed off during the course of surgery. Examples of such techniques include the placement of a suture or a small cruciate score using a hypodermic needle.

ANESTHESIA

Routine general anesthesia with muscle relaxation and endotracheal intubation is employed. Broad-spectrum antibiotics with anaerobic cover should be administered on induction of anesthesia. A nasogastric tube and urinary catheter are usually required intraoperatively.

OPERATIONS

End ileostomy

PATIENT POSITIONING
The lithotomy/Trendelenburg or Lloyd-Davies position permits anorectal access, as well as giving access for a second assistant.

INCISION
Where a midline laparotomy has been used, the linea alba and dermis are retracted towards the midline at the level of the marked stoma site with tissue-grasping forceps (Littlewood or Lane). This helps to reduce any angulations of the abdominal wall aperture as it is created (**Figure 3.1.3**).

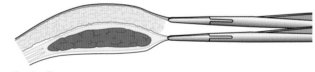

3.1.3

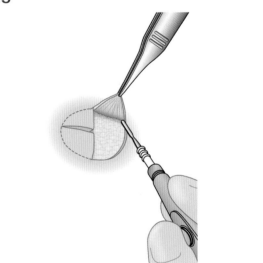

A disk of skin approximately 2 cm in diameter is excised over the marked ileostomy site, however, this will require intraoperative judgment depending on patient body habitus and the bulk of the bowel and its mesentery. This can best be done most accurately using a cruciate incision and excising the four pieces of skin to complete the circle (**Figure 3.1.4**). The transverse limb of the incision should be slightly shorter in diameter than the vertical, as the skin will naturally stretch along Langer's lines. During

3.1.4

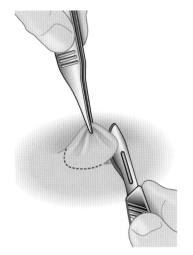

3.1.5

laparoscopic surgery, tissue retraction after release of the pneumoperitoneum should be taken into account. The alternative of picking up a piece of skin and slicing it off with a knife may result in a wound which is oval rather than round, and which has edges that in places are only a partial thickness depth (**Figure 3.1.5**).

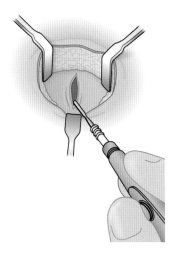

3.1.6

Only the skin is excised and the subcutaneous fat is preserved to reduce dead space and provide subcutaneous stomal support. The fat is incised and separated, taking care to obtain good hemostasis, thereby exposing the anterior rectus sheath (**Figure 3.1.6**). The dissection through the abdominal wall is aided by three equidistant Langenbeck's or phrenic retractors. A cruciate incision is made in the anterior rectus sheath and the rectus muscle is then split (**Figure 3.1.7**). If a laparotomy is being undertaken, an artery clip is then passed through the abdominal wall, and the abdominal wall everted. A cruciate incision can then be made in the peritoneum, and the finger guided through the track by placing the finger on the tip of the artery forceps as it is withdrawn. The size of the fascial aperture is a matter of intraoperative judgment with adjustment taking into account the bowel diameter, mesenteric bulk, abdominal wall tissues and pathologies encountered. An end ileostomy in individuals of normal build may need a tunnel through the abdominal wall the width of a male thumb, although in obese individuals a much larger opening may be necessary. Parastomal herniation is seen much more frequently than stenosis suggesting that laxity, rather than tightness, is a greater problem. It follows that it is prudent to start small and extend the incision as is necessary.

The inferior epigastric vessels may be inadvertently damaged during this step, therefore tension on the abdominal wall should be released slightly, and the abdominal wall defect carefully inspected for bleeding.

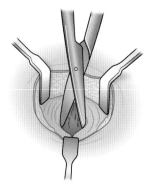

3.1.7

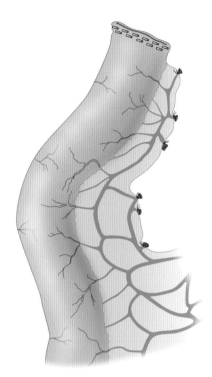

3.1.8

A Babcock forceps is passed through the stomal aperture to grasp the closed end of the prepared ileum and the bowel is gently delivered through the abdominal wall without undue traction, as this may damage the bowel or its mesentery. The ileal mesentery should lie in a cephalad direction and a 6 cm length of exteriorized ileum prior to excision of the staple/suture line is optimal (**Figure 3.1.9**).

Some authors advocate closure of the lateral mesenteric defect ('lateral space') by suturing the free edge of the mesentery to the lateral abdominal wall or falciform

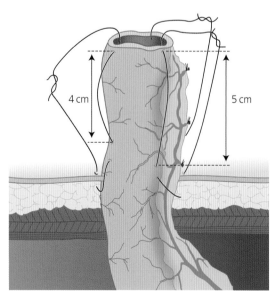

3.1.10

FASHIONING THE STOMA

The terminal ileum is prepared for drawing through the aperture by dividing the mesentery 0.5–1.0 cm from the bowel wall preserving the marginal vessels close to the bowel wall. This reduces the bulk of the mesentery. Sufficient length of bowel should be prepared to pass though the abdominal wall and protrude by 6 cm beyond the level of the skin (**Figure 3.1.8**).

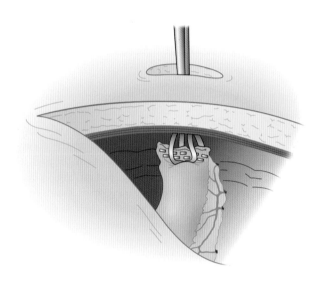

3.1.9

ligament, or by fashioning a tunneled extraperitoneal ileostomy. This can be done in an attempt to reduce the incidence of small bowel volvulus around the stomal limb, stomal prolapse, and parastomal herniation. However, there is little evidence in the literature to support this practice.[1]

MATURATION OF AN EVERTED 'BROOKE' ILEOSTOMY

The main incision is first closed and protected from contamination. The closed end of the ileum is held vertically by two Babcock clamps and the staple line is excised using cutting electrocautery. In order to direct the spout slightly caudally into an appliance, we recommend a '554' technique.[2] Sutures are inserted through the full thickness of the bowel edge, then through a proximal seromuscular bite at the future skin level before passing through the subcuticular dermis in such as way as to bury the knots (**Figure 3.1.10**). We recommend using a 2-0 Vicryl suture.

The diagram is orientated so that the 'head end' is to the right of the picture. At 10 and 2 o'clock on either side of the mesentery, sutures are placed with 5 cm distances between the bowel edge and the proximal seromuscular bite, but at the 6 o'clock position this distance is only 4 cm. On tying these sutures, the stoma will evert with a spout which is 2.5 cm superiorly, but only 2 cm inferiorly. To facilitate eversion of the ileum, sutures can be snugged down over the atraumatic end of an upturned Langenbeck retractor. Interrupted sutures in the gaps are then placed between the bowel (full thickness) and subcuticular dermis with buried knots.

Loop ileostomy

The stoma is sited and the trephine created as described for the end ileostomy. The piece of small bowel selected should be a sufficient length proximal to either an intact ileocecal valve or to the small bowel pathology/anastomosis being defunctioned, so as to avoid undue tension on the stoma. At laparotomy, a nylon tape is passed through a small window in the mesentery close to the bowel wall of the selected loop to act as a retractor (**Figure 3.1.11**), or a Babcock forceps can be used to deliver the loop in the desired orientation (usually afferent limb cranially) through the abdominal wall aperture (**Figure 3.1.12**). There is the potential to twist the loop (180–360°) during subsequent closure of the abdominal wall which needs to be guarded against.

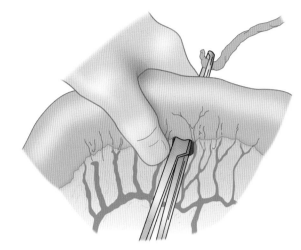

3.1.11

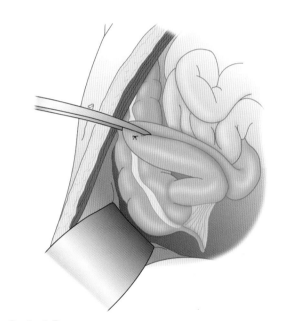

3.1.12

With regards to a 'bridge' or 'rod', it really depends on whether there is any tension on the loop ileostomy. Such tension may arise in the morbidly obese and is frequent when defunctioning an ileoanal pouch. The reason for the tension in a pouch is that the small bowel mesentery is pulled back along the posterior abdominal wall to permit the pouch to reach the anus, effectively drawing in the loop ileostomy. When defunctioning a low colorectal anastomosis, there is no tension on the small bowel mesentery, permitting a bridge to be omitted. Any bridge will delay independence with stoma care and can be removed 3–5 days after surgery, determined by the initial tension on the stoma (**Figure 3.1.13**).

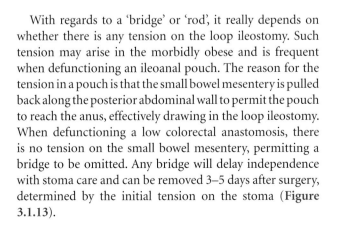
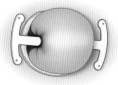

3.1.13

During laparoscopic surgery, it is sensible to mark the afferent and efferent limbs of the loop in such a way that the orientation is obvious once the trephine has been made and the loop delivered. There are several techniques to choose from. One example is laparoscopically to place one ligaclip proximally and two clips distally on the peritoneal surface of the adjacent mesentery. In addition, before making the trephine, the medial side of the mesenteric apex of the marked loop is grasped with an atraumatic instrument (e.g. Yohan grasper) via a left-sided abdominal port and the ratchet applied, thereby maintaining the correct orientation during the subsequent formation of the trephine.

The abdominal wounds are closed and protected before stomal maturation. A generous transverse enterotomy is made (to facilitate spout eversion) parallel to the skin on the caudal aspect of the loop using cutting electrocautery (**Figure 3.1.14**). This incision should stop a few millimeters short of the mesentery on both sides to minimize bleeding and mucocutaneous tension at these points. Bleeding is welcomed and judicious diathermy should be reserved for arterial bleeding points so as to minimize thermal injury to the bowel.

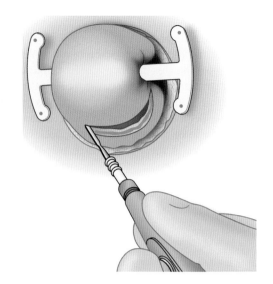

3.1.14

Sutures are placed in the 9, 12, and 3 o'clock positions on the afferent limb incorporating the full thickness of bowel edge, a seromuscular bite 5 cm proximally, and the dermis (as described for the end ileostomy). The bowel is everted as these sutures are tied, creating the afferent limb spout, and additional interrupted sutures are placed in the gaps. The edge of the defunctioned efferent limb is sutured flush with the skin with interrupted sutures with the knots buried (**Figure 3.1.15**).

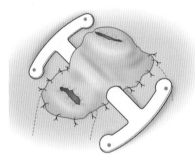

3.1.15

END-LOOP ILEOSTOMY

When it proves difficult to achieve an end stoma in an obese patient or in the presence of marked peritonitis, an end-loop ileostomy should be raised. The distal end is closed with a linear stapler and, a few centimeters proximally, a loop stoma is matured over a rod in a similar fashion to a loop ileostomy described above.

POSTOPERATIVE CARE

General management

The general care of the patient will be governed by the indications for performing the ileostomy, whether or not surgery was performed on an elective or emergency basis, and should take into account patient factors, such as comorbidity. In the elective setting, much of the traditional dogma concerning perioperative surgical management following resectional surgery with anastomosis is gradually being refined in the light of the growing body of evidence underpinning 'enhanced recovery after surgery (ERAS)/ fast track surgery' protocols. These protocols encompass many individual evidence-based strategies to improve patients' experience and postoperative outcomes, the details of which are beyond the remit of this chapter. However, salient examples include early reintroduction of postoperative fluids and diet, abandonment of routine use of nasogastric tubes and intra-abdominal drains, early removal of urinary catheters, and early mobilization.[3]

Care of the ileostomy

An appliance is fitted in the operating room after stoma construction. Transparent pouches are desirable in the immediate postoperative period to facilitate easy inspection of stoma viability. In elective surgery where the need for a stoma has been anticipated, stoma therapist-led educational programs and appliance training should be commenced preoperatively, thereby expediting recovery and patient confidence in the postoperative period.

Early complications

ISCHEMIA

Edema of the stoma or venous congestion are common early findings relating to surgical trauma and abdominal wall compression of the mesenteric venous return. These are usually self-limiting and rarely require intervention. Vascular compromise or excessive tension on the stoma may result in frank ischemia. This may be limited to the mucosa, which can be managed expectantly, however, mucosal sloughing and healing by secondary intention may result in late stomal stenosis or retraction. If the ischemia is full thickness or extending deep to the fascia (as demonstrated endoscopically) immediate revision of the stoma will usually be required.

HIGH OUTPUT

As postoperative paralytic ileus resolves and ileostomy function begins (usually third or fourth postoperative day), the daily output volume will initially be greater than after small bowel adaptation has occurred. During this high output phase, there is potential for dehydration and electrolyte imbalance and careful monitoring and appropriate replacement is essential. Occasionally, it may be necessary to slow the small bowel transit pharmacologically with antimotility drugs, such as codeine or loperamide. High output may be more problematic after significant ileal resection and may require long-term replacement.

SKIN IRRITATION

Skin irritation is a common complication with an ileostomy due to the liquid alkaline and enzymatically active effluent. Precise surgical technique, individualized preoperative siting, and thorough appliance training by experienced stoma therapists will minimize the risk of significant skin problems. Superimposed fungal infection, allergic reaction to appliance materials, and exacerbation of pre-existing skin conditions should be managed appropriately.

SMALL BOWEL OBSTRUCTION

In the early postoperative period, there may be hesitant function due to either paralytic ileus or to the early postoperative adhesions that usually clear over the ensuing 6–12 weeks. Both will usually resolve without surgery. Clearly, a tight fascial aperture or inadvertent 180–360° twist will need surgical correction after either clinical or radiological diagnosis. Otherwise, normal ileostomy function will resume in the majority of patients with non-operative management, and patience should be exercised along with any necessary nutritional supplementation in order to avoid the occasional disastrous complications that can follow too early relaparotomy.

Late obstruction may be due to adhesions, volvulus, parastomal herniation, or food bolus impaction.

ILEOSTOMY PROLAPSE AND PARASTOMAL HERNIATION

Given the limited size of the abdominal wall fascial aperture, ileostomy prolapse in the early postoperative period is unusual and can be managed non-operatively. Persistent prolapse or parastomal herniation may require late stomal revision.

ILEOSTOMY RETRACTION

Retraction of the stoma may be due to poor surgical technique or follow complications, such as ischemia and infection. The condition can often be managed non-operatively by an experienced stoma therapist, although stoma revision may be required if this approach is unsuccessful and skin complications ensue.

REFERENCES

1. Leong AP, Londono-Schimmer EE, Phillips RK. Life-table analysis of stomal complications following ileostomy. *British Journal of Surgery* 1994; **81**: 727–9.
2. Hall C, Myers C, Phillips RK. The 554 ileostomy. *British Journal of Surgery* 1995; **82**: 1385.
3. Gouvas N, Tan E, Windsor A *et al.* Fast-track vs standard care in colorectal surgery: a meta-analysis update. *International Journal of Colorectal Disease* 2009; **24**: 1119–31.

Colostomy

KATHERINE GRANT AND ROBIN KS PHILLIPS

PRINCIPLES AND JUSTIFICATION

Types of operation and indications

A colostomy diverts fecal flow on to the anterior abdominal wall and may be either temporary or permanent. A temporary stoma is often used to protect a distal anastomosis, or with certain anal operations. A permanent colostomy is created in association with operations to excise the rectum or when managing some patients with idiopathic fecal incontinence.

The main types of colostomy are:

- loop colostomy;
- terminal colostomy;
- end-loop colostomy.

These stomas may be created at laparotomy, or via a minimal access approach (trephine or laparoscopic colostomy). The double-barreled and divided (Devine) colostomy are principally of historical interest and will not be covered here.

LOOP COLOSTOMY

This is the most usually formed temporary colostomy. Its site depends on the reason for its construction and may be either in the transverse or in the sigmoid colon. In principle, a loop of colon is brought out to the surface, secured by a mucocutaneous suture, and often held in place by a rod until it becomes adherent (usually 3–5 days) when the rod can be removed.

Loop stomas are now less commonly constructed in cases of obstruction or complicated diverticular disease than in the past, as the majority of surgeons now embark on immediate intestinal resection. Furthermore, in cases of malignant obstruction, colonic stenting may alternatively be employed as a bridge to surgery. The majority of loop stomas are used to defunction a distal anastomosis or to provide symptomatic relief/prevent obstruction in patients undergoing long-course neoadjuvant treatment for locally advanced rectal cancer. They may also be used with certain anal operations (rectovaginal fistulae or some anal sphincter repairs, particularly in cases of Crohn's disease).

The advantages of a transverse loop colostomy include its ease of construction and ease of closure. The disadvantages are its site in the right upper quadrant (however, the surgeon may mobilize the hepatic flexure so the stoma can be sited in the more convenient right iliac fossa); a tendency to prolapse; the vulnerability of the marginal artery during closure (and hence of the distal colonic blood supply if the inferior mesenteric artery has previously been ligated at its origin). Because of these disadvantages, many surgeons prefer to construct a loop ileostomy to defunction a distal anastomosis after total mesorectal excision (TME) surgery.

For cases of malignancy where laparotomy is not required, a laparoscopic approach carries the advantage over trephine colostomy of being able to assess and biopsy intraperitoneal disease. Trephine colostomy, however, may be performed under regional anesthesia, and is therefore of use in the unfit patient.

TERMINAL COLOSTOMY

This end stoma is usually constructed in association with operations to excise the rectum or when performing a Hartmann's operation. It may be necessary, however, in cases of irremediable fecal incontinence, where a trephine incision or laparoscopic approach may be employed. Great care must be taken not to inadvertently close the proximal colon and mature the distal limb. The colostomy is formed from the sigmoid colon, which is brought out through an incision in the left abdominal wall.

END-LOOP COLOSTOMY

An end-loop colostomy may be employed principally in the emergency situation (but also in some morbidly obese individuals), where tissue edema in the mesentery does not allow adequate length to bring out an end stoma. The bowel end is stapled closed, following which a more easily delivered loop of colon a few centimeters upstream is brought out as a loop stoma.

Preoperative

STOMA SITING

The optimal position for the stoma should be marked preoperatively by a stoma therapist, and then checked by the surgeon. The stoma site should be placed over the rectus muscle at least 4 cm from any midline incision. Bony landmarks and skin creases should be taken into consideration to avoid placing the stoma either in a 'dip' where it may leak, directly on the belt line, or where the patient cannot see the stoma. Siting is facilitated by examining the patient sitting, lying, and standing.

BOWEL PREPARATION

When circumstances allow, the authors prefer a full bowel preparation. This will avoid a column of stool in the defunctioned segment, and an empty colon may be easier to deliver through the abdominal wall. Some of the conditions, however, for which a loop stoma is constructed are 'urgent' or 'emergency' in nature, which may preclude bowel preparation. Perioperative antibiotics are given against aerobic and anaerobic organisms.

ANESTHESIA

General anesthesia is preferred because traction on the mesentery causes pain and nausea. It is possible, however, to perform a trephine colostomy under local or general anesthesia.

PATIENT POSITIONING

The lithotomy/Trendelenburg or Lloyd-Davies position permits anorectal access, as well as giving room for a second assistant.

OPERATIONS

Loop colostomy

INCISION

The sites of incision for a transverse colostomy and a left iliac fossa sigmoid colostomy are shown in **Figure 3.2.1**. The ideal site for a transverse colostomy is in the right iliac fossa, but the hepatic flexure must be mobilized in order to achieve this. If a transverse colostomy is to be performed using a trephine approach, then the incision must be in the right upper abdomen, midway between the umbilicus and the costal margin, and placed just over the rectus abdominus muscle but extending just lateral to its lateral margin.

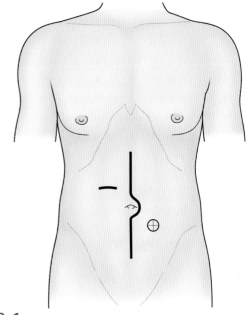

3.2.1

The incision is deepened through the anterior rectus sheath. The rectus abdominis may either be divided or split in the line of its fibers, and then the abdomen is opened (**Figure 3.2.2**).

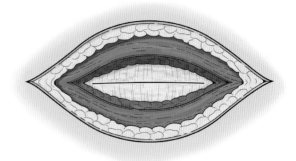

3.2.2

PREPARATION OF THE COLON

A transverse colostomy may be prepared either by making a window in the omentum, or by lifting the free edge of the omentum upwards, and dissecting the intact omentum from its largely avascular attachment to the colon. A nylon tape is passed through the mesentery in order to draw the colon up to the surface where the tape is substituted with a plastic rod (**Figure 3.2.3**).

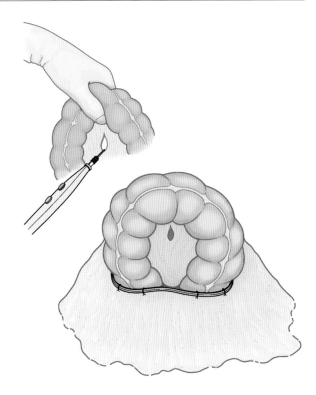

3.2.3

OPENING THE COLOSTOMY

The colon may be opened longitudinally or transversely. A transverse incision is preferred, as it damages fewer of the encircling vessels in the colonic wall, it is easier to secure, and it may be easier to close (**Figure 3.2.4**).

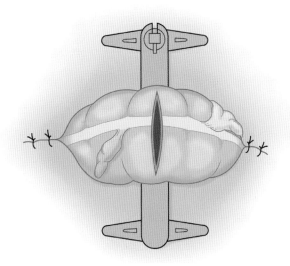

3.2.4

MUCOCUTANEOUS SUTURE

Once open, the colostomy is sutured to the skin with interrupted sutures of 2-0 or 3-0 absorbable material mounted on a taper-cut needle. The stitch should penetrate the entire thickness of the intestinal wall, but only pass through the subcuticular layer of the skin. The wound is cleaned and a stoma appliance is fitted immediately (**Figure 3.2.5**).

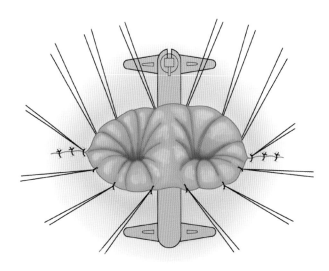

3.2.5

Terminal colostomy

INCISION

A disk of skin approximately 2 cm in diameter is excised over the marked colostomy site. This can best be done most accurately using a cruciate incision and excising the four pieces of skin to complete the circle. The transverse limb of the incision should be slightly shorter (**Figure 3.2.6a**) in diameter than the vertical, as the skin will naturally stretch along Langer's lines. The alternative of picking up a piece of skin and slicing it off with a knife should be avoided as it results in a wound which is oval rather than round, and which has edges that in places are only a partial thickness depth (**Figure 3.2.6b**).

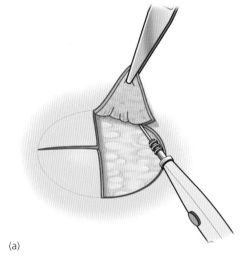

(a)

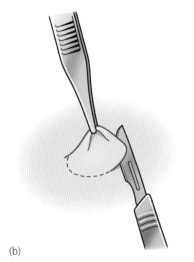

(b)

3.2.6

The fat is incised and separated, taking care to obtain good hemostasis, therefore exposing the anterior rectus sheath. The dissection through the abdominal wall is aided by three equidistant Langenbeck's or phrenic retractors. A cruciate incision is made in the anterior rectus sheath and the rectus muscle is then split. If a laparotomy is being undertaken, an artery clip is then passed through the abdominal wall, and the abdominal wall is everted. A cruciate incision can then be made in the peritoneum, and the finger guided through the track by placing the finger on the tip of the artery forceps as it is withdrawn. An end colostomy in individuals of normal build may need a tunnel through the abdominal wall two fingers wide, although in obese individuals a much larger opening may be necessary. The inferior epigastric vessels may be inadvertently damaged during this step, therefore tension on the abdominal wall should be released slightly, and the abdominal wall defect carefully inspected for bleeding (**Figure 3.2.7**a–d).

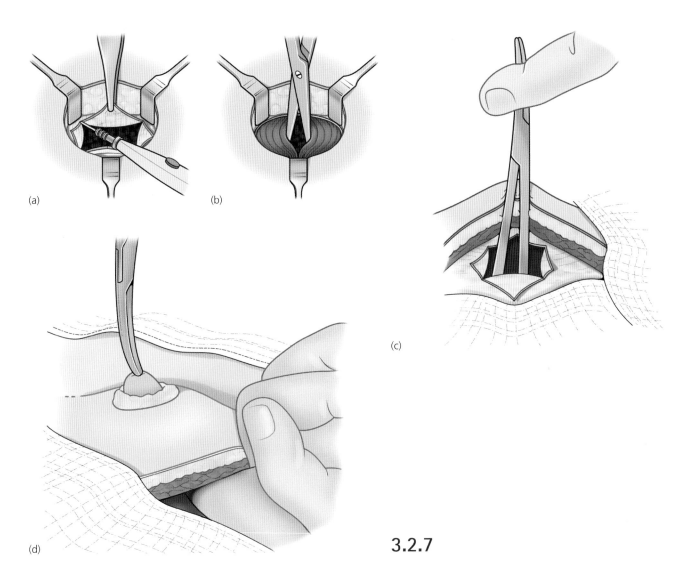

(a)

(b)

(c)

(d)

3.2.7

DELIVERY OF THE COLON THROUGH THE ABDOMINAL WALL

The colon is delivered through the anterior abdominal wall. A colostomy needs to be able to 'travel'. Lying supine on the operating table, the colostomy may appear satisfactory, but in many (particularly elderly) people, on sitting up the abdomen may protrude quite some distance. If the intraperitoneal length of colon is short the colostomy finds itself tethered, leading to retraction and stoma care problems. To avoid this problem, the surgeon should consider the following:

- The colostomy site should be rather more distal in the sigmoid colon, therefore achieving a greater length of freely mobile intraperitoneal colon.
- Where length is at a premium, the lateral space probably should not be closed, as closure effectively shortens the intraperitoneal length and may reduce stoma travel.
- Mobilization of the descending colon (and if necessary the splenic flexure as well) (**Figure 3.2.8**).

Lateral space closure or an extraperitoneal tunnel both require an additional length of mobilized colon if 'travel' is not to be a problem. Where length is not an issue, either technique may be employed to reduce the theoretical risk of small bowel obstruction and parastomal herniation, respectively.

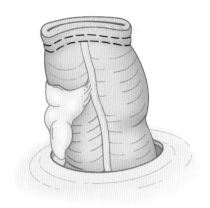

3.2.8

MUCOCUTANEOUS SUTURE

Before the main abdominal incision is closed, it is important to ensure, by adequate mobilization of the colon, that there will be no tension on the mucocutaneous suture line. Once the main abdominal incision has been closed and dressed, the colon is opened and a mucocutaneous suture is performed with 3-0 absorbable sutures. Given that the wafer of the stoma appliance has a certain thickness, a slight spout will help prevent stools getting underneath the wafer, leading to detachment. To achieve this, the suture is passed from the fat towards the epidermis, exiting through the subcuticular layer of the skin. This is followed by a bite through the bowel wall starting adjacent to the mucosal surface. The sutures are tied with the knot buried, which serves to raise a mucosal lip above the surface of the skin (**Figure 3.2.9**).

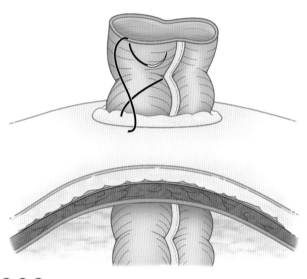

3.2.9

Minimally invasive colostomy

TREPHINE COLOSTOMY

A trephine incision is made over the marked stoma site as described above, and the peritoneum is opened. Two Langenbeck's retractors are used to pull the wound laterally and inferiorly. A pair of Babcock's forceps is introduced, and the sigmoid colon is grasped and delivered. The sigmoid may be distinguished from the transverse colon by:

- presence of appendices epiploicae;
- presence of left lateral peritoneal attachments;
- absence of omentum.

Scissors or a finger through the trephine wound may be used to divide lateral peritoneal attachments if required. The surgeon's fingers should be slid down the mesentery to ensure no twist exists. If an end colostomy is to be created and doubt exists as to which is the distal limb, air can be insufflated through the anus into the distal limb using either a rigid sigmoidoscope or a Foley catheter. Alternatively, a flexible sigmoidoscope can be employed (**Figure 3.2.10**).

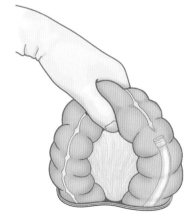

3.2.10

LAPAROSCOPIC COLOSTOMY

Patient position

The patient is placed in the Trendelenburg position with rotation of the table left side up. This helps to move the small bowel out of the pelvis and expose the desired segment of colon.

Port position

Port configuration for a laparoscopic sigmoid colostomy is shown in **Figure 3.2.11**. A 10 mm infraumbilical camera port is inserted, and abdominal contents and the site of intended colostomy formation are inspected. Two further 5 mm ports are inserted under direct vision in the right side of the abdomen as shown. A fourth port may be introduced into the left suprapubic region as required. This port configuration is identical to that used for laparoscopic left colon resection, and is preferred to colocating a port site with the stoma.

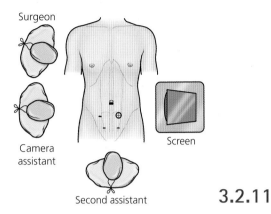

3.2.11

Assessment of mobility

Atraumatic graspers are introduced and an appendix epiploica of the sigmoid colon is identified and grasped. If the sigmoid colon is redundant and may be brought up to the abdominal wall easily with the pneumoperitoneum established, the colon may be delivered without further mobilization (**Figure 3.2.12**).

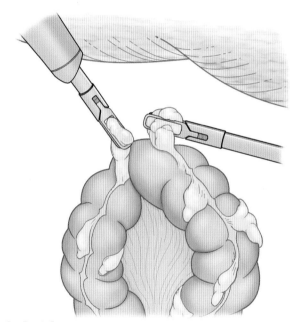

3.2.12

Mobilization of the colon

If adhesions or mesenteric attachments to the paracolic gutter are identified, these are dissected using coagulating scissors or a harmonic scalpel. An assessment of adequate mobility is again undertaken, then a window is made in the sigmoid mesentery, and a nylon tape passed through the defect. The stoma site is then fashioned as previously described (**Figure 3.2.13a,b**).

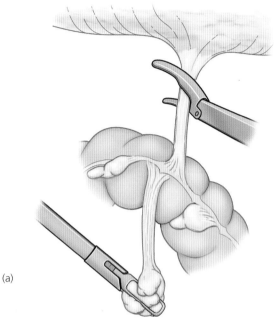

(a)

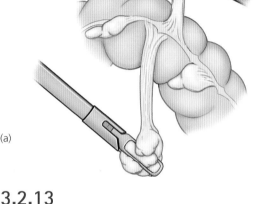

3.2.13

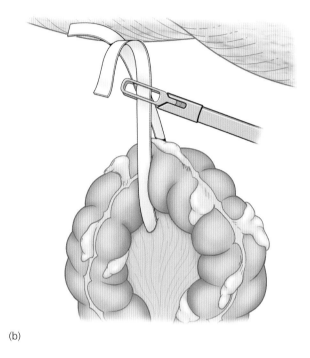

(b)

Delivery of the colon

The peritoneum is opened and the nylon tape brought through the stoma site to facilitate delivery of the colon. The pneumoperitoneum is re-established to inspect the intestine to ensure adequate hemostasis, the absence of tension or twisting of the mesentery, and the correct identification of the proximal and distal segments. The colon is then opened and secured using mucocutaneous sutures using the technique described above.

POSTOPERATIVE CARE

General management

The general care of the patient will largely be determined by the underlying surgical indication. In the elective situation, most patients are able to eat and drink immediately after surgery. It is important to check the viability of the intestine in the early postoperative period and to ensure that it has not retracted.

Care of the colostomy

An appliance is fitted as soon as the colostomy is constructed. As the effluent from a transverse colostomy may be liquid, loperamide, codeine phosphate, or other constipating agents may be required.

With a terminal colostomy, irrigation may be useful as an alternative to a permanent appliance in the young, well-motivated patient.

Early complications

LOSS OF VIABILITY

This will occur early in the postoperative course if the blood supply to the colostomy has been compromised. It necessitates reconstruction of the colostomy with viable colon. The terminal few centimeters of the intestine should be examined endoscopically prior to surgery, as occasionally only the last 1–2 cm of mucosa are ischemic, and this will heal without intervention.

SEPARATION OF THE COLOSTOMY

This usually arises as a consequence of tension on the mucocutaneous junction, and will require resuturing if circumferential. Partial separation may be caused by infection or excessive tension, and will usually heal spontaneously.

INFECTION

It is rare for sepsis to complicate construction of a colostomy, despite a potentially contaminated operative field. If it occurs, there may be some separation of the colostomy and surrounding cellulitis. A hematoma may be a predisposing factor, emphasizing the need for meticulous hemostasis in the colostomy wound. Providing drainage is adequate, the colostomy will heal, but there is a risk subsequent scarring might lead to some stenosis of the mucocutaneous junction.

Outcome

Long-term complications may arise in approximately half of patients with a permanent colostomy, with parastomal hernia by far the most frequent. Other reported complications include stomal prolapse, obstruction, retraction, and fistula formation.[1]

PARASTOMAL HERNIA

This is the most common long-term complication of permanent colostomy, and may arise in 30–40 percent of patients, with perhaps 10–20 percent of these cases requiring surgical intervention. Risk factors include obesity, increasing age, a history of previous hernia elsewhere, and increased intra-abdominal pressure. The incidence of parastomal hernia can be reduced by limiting the size of the trephine, by using an extraperitoneal technique, or by using a prophylactic mesh.

A lightweight sublay mesh has been most extensively reported, with a number of case series and randomized controlled trials demonstrating a significant reduction in parastomal hernia formation.[2, 3] However, patient numbers are small and very few emergencies or other patients at high risk of parastomal hernia were included in these trials. There is no apparent increase in the risk of septic complications associated with mesh placement. Routine use of prophylactic mesh cannot be recommended for all cases at present, although the outcome of further studies, including the multicentre PREVENT-trial[4] is awaited with interest.

REFERENCES

1. Londono-Schimmer EE, Leong AP, Phillips RKS. Life table analysis of stomal complications following colostomy. *Diseases of the Colon and Rectum* 1994; **37**: 916–20.
2. Serra-Aracil X, Bombardo-Junca J, Morena-Matias J *et al.* Randomised, controlled, prospective, trial of the use of a mesh to prevent parastomal hernia. *Annals of Surgery* 2009; **249**: 583–7.
3. Janes A, Cengiz Y, Israelsson LA. Preventing parastomal hernia with a prosthetic mesh: a 5-year follow-up of a randomized study. *World Journal of Surgery* 2009; **33**: 118–21.
4. Brandsma HT, Hansson BM, V-Haaren de Haan H, Aufenacker TJ, Rosman C, Bleichrodt RP. PREVENTion of a parastomal hernia with a prophylactic mesh in patients undergoing permanent end colostomy; the PREVENT trial: study protocol for a multicenter randomized controlled trial. *Trials* 2012; **13**: 226.

Stoma closure

JAMES SWEENEY

PRINCIPLES AND JUSTIFICATION

There are two forms of stoma, namely a loop and end stoma. Closure of end stomas will follow the general principles of resection and anastomosis, and are covered elsewhere in this text. This chapter will concentrate on closure of a loop stoma. Loop colostomy is now an uncommon stoma. Illustrations in this chapter show closure of loop ileostomy, but the technique for closure of loop colostomy is the same, although the author would strongly recommend that stapled closure be avoided in this setting.

PREOPERATIVE

Loop stomas will have been constructed to defunction the distal bowel, most frequently after resection and anastomosis, but also for fecal diversion when required for anorectal trauma and fistula management distal to the stoma. If there has been an anastomosis, the patency and integrity of that anastomosis should be evaluated prior to stoma closure. This can be either by contrast radiology with anteroposterior and lateral films or endoscopic assessment, which may also allow any stenosis to be dilated. The former modality is to be preferred as small defects may be overlooked with endoscopic assessment alone.

The timing of closure will depend in part on the reason for the loop stoma in the first instance and any postoperative treatment (i.e. adjuvant chemotherapy), however, the inflammatory reaction around the stoma makes the bowel friable to handling for a variable period.

As a general rule, it is advisable to wait about 12 weeks. While it is possible to close earlier provided the patient has recovered sufficiently from the previous surgery, the friability of the bowel prior to about 12 weeks does increase the risk of morbidity.

Bowel preparation

Bowel preparation is usually not necessary. A distal loop washout with normal saline may be indicated if the colon distal to the stoma contains a large amount of fecal matter that has been present for some time.

Preoperative antibiotics

Antibiotics against aerobic and anaerobic organisms should be administered intravenously 30 minutes to 1 hour prior to skin incision. A single dose only is required and continuation of antibiotics after surgery should be reserved for specific indications.

ANESTHESIA

The operation is usually performed under a general anesthetic. The procedure can be performed under local anesthesia, but there is moderate traction on the mesentery of the bowel, which causes pain and nausea and is not blocked by the local anesthesia within the wound.

OPERATION

Position of the patient

For most loop stoma closure procedures, the patient is placed supine. Preoperative antibiotics should have been administered by this stage and appropriate thromboembolic prophylaxis arranged.

Digital rectal examination should be performed at this stage to dilate a low anastomosis which can often be a little stenosed especially after double-stapled anastomosis.

Skin incision

The stoma can be mobilized using a circular incision at the mucocutaneous junction or via a transverse elliptical incision, which incorporates the stoma within its midpoint. Traction on the skin by the assistant facilitates this incision by stabilizing the area and everting the stoma. According to some, the former produces a more cosmetic scar, however, the wound cannot be completely closed and all patients require dressings until healed. In the author's opinion, the transverse elliptical incision is superior in that it allows better access for mobilization of the stoma from the anterior abdominal wall, can be closed with a subcuticular suture with an infection rate of less than 10 percent, and it is more convenient for the patient with ultimately good cosmetic results (**Figure 3.3.1**).

Tissue forceps (e.g. Allis) are applied to the rim of skin attached to the stoma and countertraction is applied with small right angle retractors in the subcutaneous space, repositioned and changed to deeper retractors as the dissection proceeds. With this traction on the stoma and countertraction, the dissection frees the stoma from the surrounding abdominal wall fat. The dissection can be conducted using sharp dissection with a size 15 scalpel blade, sharp dissecting scissors or diathermy. Whatever technique, it is important to remain in the correct plane (which is usually easy to recognize because of the contrasting color of the yellow fat of the abdominal wall and the small bowel mesentery) to avoid damage to the bowel or mesentery. If bleeding occurs, the surgeon is probably in the incorrect plane. Infiltration with local anesthesia may facilitate the demonstration of the correct plane. With

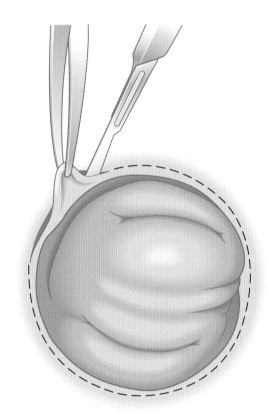

3.3.1

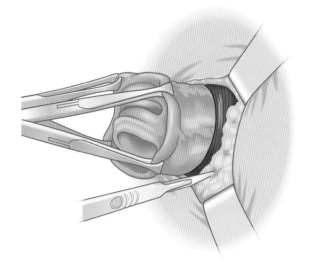

3.3.2

careful circumferential dissection, applying traction and countertraction, repositioning the retractors as required, the tissues of the anterior abdominal wall are freed from the bowel and the dissection continues to the anterior fascia, then through the abdominal wall musculature to enter the peritoneal cavity. If a parastomal hernia is present, this will be entered at this stage and facilitate entry into the abdominal cavity (**Figure 3.3.2**).

Once the peritoneal cavity is entered, the index finger is inserted through the opening to sweep around the anterior peritoneal surface to free filmy adhesions between the bowel and the peritoneum. Sometimes this is facilitated by hooking the finger under more fibrous adhesions and dividing adhesions by sharp dissection under direct vision. It is important that the intraperitoneal margins around the stoma opening are completely detached from the bowel prior to closure of the stoma and that sufficient length has been delivered to allow safe closure. After closure of the stoma, it is important to ensure that no loops of bowel are adherent to the intraperitoneal aspect of the wound so that they are not incorporated in the wound closure (**Figure 3.3.3**).

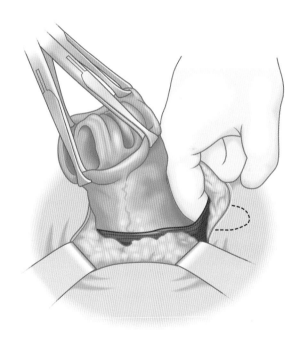

3.3.3

Once the stoma is fully mobilized, the everted aspect of the stoma is carefully dissected to unevert it. This is best done by inserting scissors between the two serosal aspects of the everted stoma to open the space and then dividing the adhesions between the two surfaces (**Figure 3.3.4**).

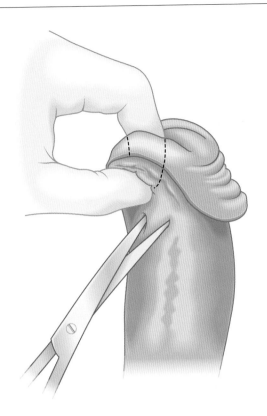

3.3.4

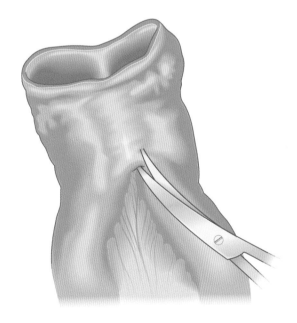

3.3.5

Adhesions between adjacent loops need to be divided to facilitate closure and minimize the chance of postoperative bowel obstruction. If continuity is being re-established by stapling, this step may not be required as the bowel may be lying in a configuration to facilitate stapling (**Figures 3.3.5** and **3.3.6**).

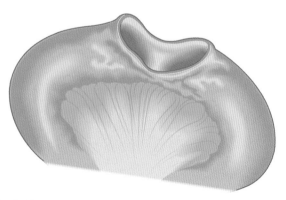

3.3.6

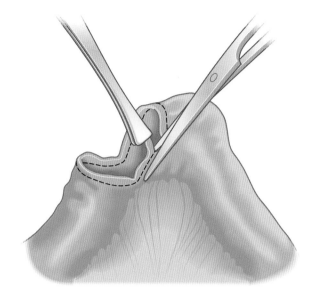

3.3.7

Once this has been performed, the rim of skin and scarring can be excised back to healthy bowel. Careful inspection of the bowel is required at this stage to identify any inadvertent enterotomy which should be repaired at this stage with interrupted absorbable sutures (**Figure 3.3.7**).

Technique of closure

The closure can be a simple closure, which involves half an anastomosis or excision of the stoma and reanastomosis with either a single layer sutured anastomosis or a stapled functional end-to-end anastomosis depending on individual preference.

HAND-SEWN CLOSURE

For a simple hand-sewn closure, this is best conducted with a single layer technique using seromuscular sutures, which helps invert the closure, placed as illustrated. This is definitely indicated if there is any doubt about sufficient length to allow safe stapled closure (**Figure 3.3.8**).

The bowel is closed transversely by initially placing sutures and tying at either end on the mesenteric aspect and applying lateral traction.

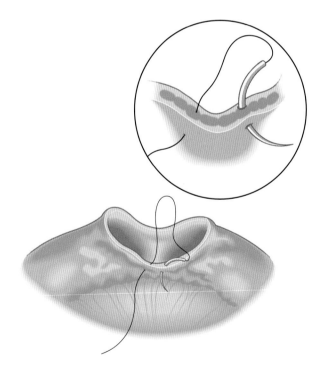

3.3.8

The midpoint on each is then defined and a suture placed, but untied. Any discrepancy in length can be adapted by repeating this process at the intervening two new midpoints (**Figure 3.3.9**).

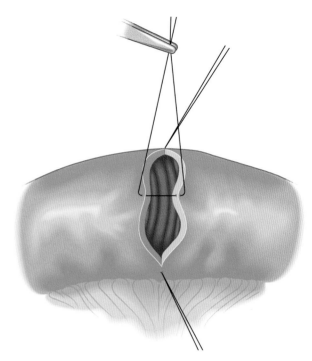

3.3.9

Commencing at each outer end, interrupted sutures are then placed and tied. The central four or five sutures are clipped and tied after all have been placed (**Figure 3.3.10**).

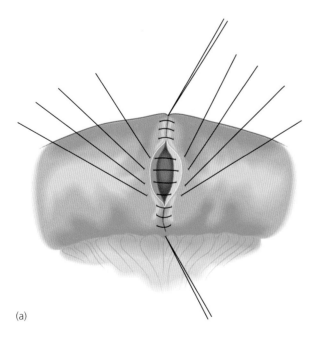

(a)

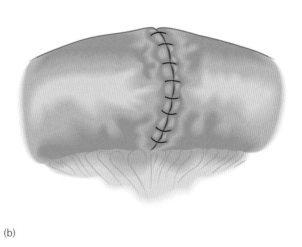

(b)

3.3.10

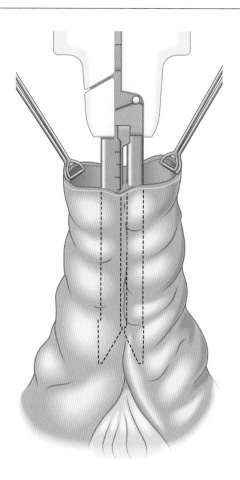

(a)

STAPLED CLOSURE

The bowel is prepared in the same manner, however, more length is required to perform this safely without the stapler entering the abdominal cavity. An open stapled anastomotic technique is recommended using a linear cutter (**Figure 3.3.11**a).

The mesenteric aspect of the bowel can be rotated out of the staple line by using De Bakey forceps to apply downward traction to it as the stapler is closed as shown. Usually a 55 mm endocutting stapler will be sufficient for closure of a loop ileostomy if the bowel has been adequately prepared, however, a 60- or 75 mm stapler may be needed. After the initial stapler application and firing, it is important that any bleeding from the staple line is

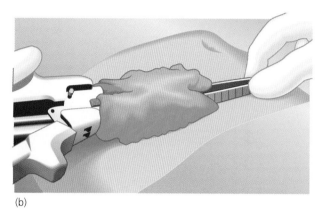

(b)

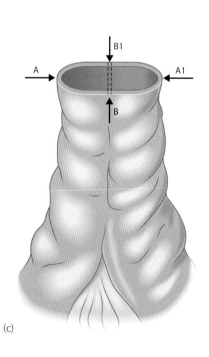

(c)

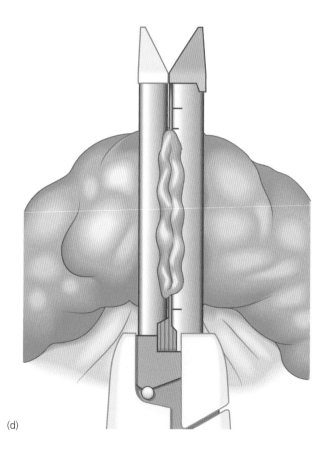

3.3.11

(d)

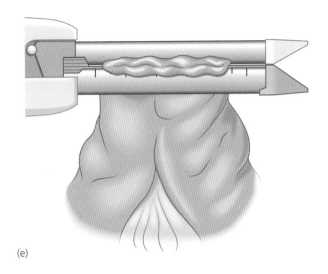

(e)

identified and secured. Applying Babcock forceps to the open bowel and then inserting sponge-holding forceps and spreading them open is a good technique for visualizing the staple line. Hemostasis can usually be achieved with a short application of the diathermy, but an under-running absorbable suture may be required.

The open ends of the bowel can then be closed by a second application of the linear cutter. With the linear cutter this can be achieved by orienting the bowel in two ways. The author's preference is to do this so that the second staple line is oriented parallel to the first (i.e. A to A1) rather than at 90° (i.e. B to B1) to it, as this facilitates oversewing it (**Figure 3.3.11c–e**).

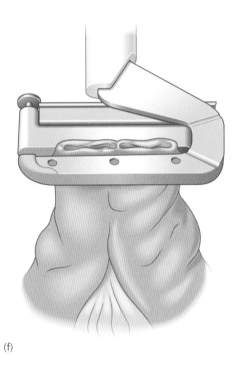

(f)

A linear stapler can be used with trimming of the excess bowel with a scalpel (**Figure 3.3.11f**).

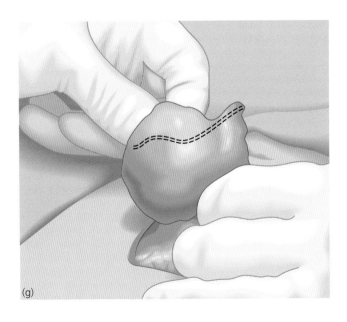

(g)

This second staple line can then be oversewn and inverted with 3-0 absorbable suture and a seromuscular crotch (trouser) stitch inserted (**Figure 3.3.11g–h**).

3.3.11 contd

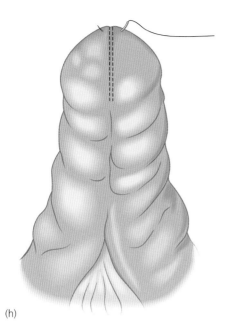

(h)

3.3.11 contd

Once the continuity of the bowel is re-established, it is reduced into the abdominal cavity. This requires careful handling of the sutured bowel. The anastomosis should be reduced first, if possible, to avoid pressure on the suture line. The stapled closure tends to be more bulky and some dilatation of the anterior abdominal wall defect may be required to facilitate this reduction. Ask the anesthetist to make sure the patient is relaxed prior to doing this (**Figure 3.3.12**).

It is important that any peritoneal sac, which may have developed in association with the loop stoma, is excised prior to closure of the wound. This allows for easier identification of the fascia and reduces the risk of seroma formation.

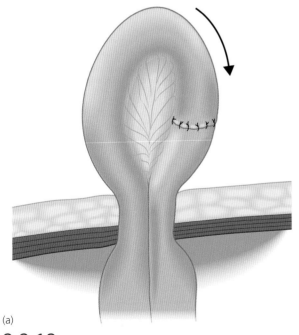

(a)

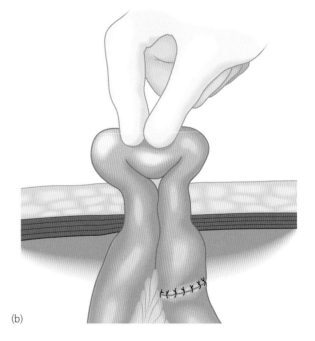

(b)

3.3.12

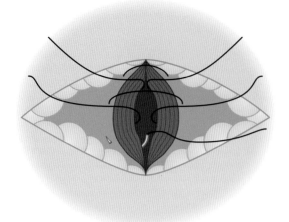

(a)

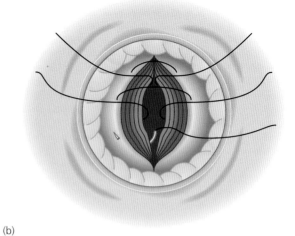

(b)

3.3.13

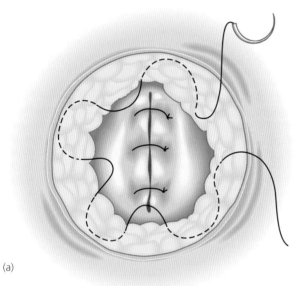

(a)

A mass closure of the fascial and muscle layers using strong monofilament absorbable or non-absorbable sutures is performed. If non-absorbable sutures are used, the knot should be placed deep to the posterior rectus sheath (especially in thin patients). Care should be taken to avoid the inferior epigastric vessels. Using interrupted sutures with placement of all sutures under direct vision to avoid incorporating bowel before tying usually ensures even placement of sutures and good closure. A warm saline wash should be utilized if there has been any wound contamination. Local anesthesia should be infiltrated into the wound at this stage. Drains are not required (**Figure 3.3.13a,b**).

Skin closure is then performed using a continuous subcuticular absorbable suture for the elliptical incision or a non-absorbable monofilament purse-string in the subcuticular layer for the circular wound (which then needs to be dressed until healed) (**Figure 3.3.14a–c**).

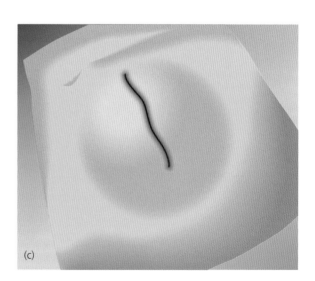

(c)

(b)

3.3.14

POSTOPERATIVE

Thromboembolic prophylaxis should be continued.

The patient can commence on free fluids after the usual appropriate interval following a general anesthetic. Simple regular analgesia (i.e. paracetamol) should be commenced.

The patient could commence a normal diet as tolerated the next day and be discharged when bowel function has returned.

COMPLICATIONS

Wound infection would be expected to occur in fewer than 10 percent of cases and normally occurs after discharge. Wound hernia can occur either early or late.

Anastomotic leak is uncommon after stoma closure. This is due to technical factors associated with the closure or forceful reduction of the closure into the abdominal cavity or distal obstruction. If peritonitis develops, then reoperation is mandatory.

Although uncommon, it is more likely that failure of the closure will result in a fistula through the wound, which treated conservatively can be expected to undergo spontaneous closure in most cases provided there is no distal obstruction. An alternative explanation is incorporation of an adjacent loop of bowel at abdominal wall closure or inadvertent enterotomy unrecognized at initial mobilization.

FURTHER READING

García-Botello SA, García-Armengol J, García-Granero E *et al.* A prospective audit of the complications of loop ileostomy construction and takedown. *Digestive Surgery* 2004; **21**: 440–6.

Giannakopoulos GF, Veenhof AA, van der Peet DL *et al.* Morbidity and complications of protective loop ileostomy. *Colorectal Disease* 2009; **11**: 609–12.

Hasegawa H, Radley S, Morton DG, Keighley MRB. Stapled versus sutured closure of loop ileostomy. A randomized controlled trial. *Annals of Surgery* 2000; **231**: 202–4.

van de Pavoordt HDWM, Fazio VW, Jagelman DG *et al.* The outcome of loop ileostomy closure in 293 cases. *International Journal of Colorectal Disease* 1987; **2**: 214–17.

Antegrade continence enema procedure in children

PADRAIG SJ MALONE

HISTORY

The ACE (antegrade continence enema) procedure is now accepted as an established treatment for intractable fecal incontinence secondary to conditions such as spinal dysraphism and anorectal malformation. The successful use of the ACE is described in numerous reports in thousands of patients with follow-up extending to 20 years, and it has also been demonstrated that a successful ACE significantly improves quality of life. Technical modifications have been introduced over the years and these are illustrated in this chapter. It is no longer recommended to disconnect the appendix from the cecum as previously described, and the *in situ* appendix is now the norm for the open ACE procedure. If no other procedure is required, a laparoscopic antegrade continence enema (LACE) approach is recommended. For patients in whom constipation is a major problem, it may be best to site the conduit in the left colon rather than the cecum.

In order to decide on a cecal or left colonic ACE, it can initially be performed colonoscopically as a trial, the percutaneous endoscopic colostomy (PEC), inserting a catheter as one would insert a percutaneous gastrostomy tube. This can then be replaced at a later date by a button or conduit, depending on the patient's wishes. If the appendix is absent or required for a simultaneous Mitrofanoff procedure, the Yang–Monti conduit is now the procedure of choice. The major ongoing complication associated with the ACE is stomal stenosis, which occurs in approximately 30 percent of patients, and this has led to a number of different techniques to construct the stoma.

PRINCIPLES AND JUSTIFICATION

The main indication for the procedure is fecal incontinence secondary to neuropathy and anorectal malformations, which has not responded to conventional therapy. Although the procedure has been used in patients with chronic constipation and complicated Hirschsprung's disease, the author is reluctant to recommend its use under these circumstances. However, if an ACE is used for chronic constipation, it may be best to site it in the left colon colonoscopically, as a clinical trial in the first instance. No child should have a colostomy without having the opportunity to consider the ACE as an alternative.

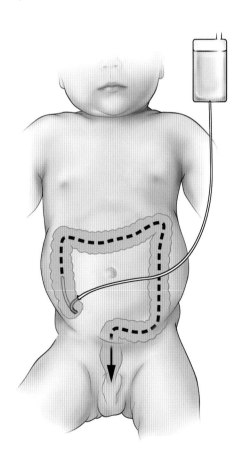

3.4.1

The ACE combines the principles of the Mitrofanoff continent, catheterizable conduit, and antegrade colonic washout to produce a continent, catheterizable colonic stoma through which washouts are delivered to produce complete colonic emptying and thus prevent soiling (Figure 3.4.1).

PREOPERATIVE

Assessment and preparation

Motivation of children and their carers is essential for a successful outcome. Intensive counseling is required and it must be stressed that the ACE is not a 'magic' cure. A rigid, time-consuming regimen is required postoperatively and this is a lifelong commitment. A successful ACE takes approximately 45 minutes every day or on alternate days. Many children being considered for an ACE will also have a neuropathic bladder, and it is vital that management of the bladder is assessed simultaneously. In many cases, a combined lower urinary tract reconstruction and ACE is appropriate, and double continence rates have been reported in 79 percent of children with this approach. It is vital, therefore, to have a pediatric urologist involved in the assessment of these children and in the planning of the operative procedure. Investigations may include ultrasonography, renography, and videourodynamics. In the case of an isolated ACE, usually no special investigations are required, but some authors recommend bowel transit studies to guide them as to where the conduit should be sited, in the cecum for isolated incontinence or in the left colon when performed for chronic constipation.

A preoperative full blood count is recommended, but crossmatch is only required when a simultaneous bladder reconstruction is to be performed. For children with a neuropathic bladder or renal scarring, metabolic renal function should be assessed preoperatively. The author favors a 48-hour bowel preparation program using sodium picosulfate and rectal washouts, together with a 5-day course of antibiotics, such as co-amoxiclav. As the child loses a great deal of fluid with the bowel preparation, an intravenous infusion is administered on the night prior to surgery.

ANESTHESIA

The operation is performed under general anesthesia, but there are no special requirements.

OPERATION

Incisions

When an isolated ACE is performed, a laparoscopic approach is now recommended, but if an antireflux valve is to be created, a right or left lower quadrant muscle-cutting incision is used. A midline incision is better if a simultaneous bladder reconstruction is being carried out. For a cecal ACE, it is usually possible to site the stoma in the umbilicus, but for a left-sided conduit, the stoma is usually sited in the left lower quadrant. For patients who are wheelchair-bound, it may be necessary to site the stoma on the upper abdomen for ease of access (Figure 3.4.2).

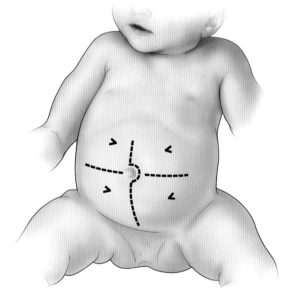

3.4.2

THE *IN SITU* APPENDIX ACE

Preparation of the appendix

The cecum is mobilized, the tip of the appendix is amputated, and a stay suture is inserted and the appendix stretched to reveal the mesentery. The mesentery is fenestrated between the vessels, as this allows the cecum to be wrapped around the appendix without compromising the blood supply. A 12Fr catheter is passed through the appendix into the cecum (**Figure 3.4.3**).

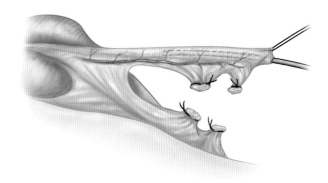

3.4.3

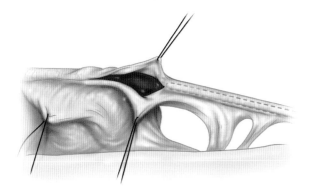

3.4.4

Creation of a cecal submucosal tunnel

A trough down to the submucosa is created along a tenia by a combination of sharp and blunt dissection. As the trough approaches the base of the appendix, a V-shaped incision is created around approximately 60 percent of its circumference; this allows the base of the appendix to be folded into the cecum without kinking. There is no need for a wide trough, as it is not planned to bury the appendix, it is simply there to fix the appendix when the cecum is wrapped around it (**Figure 3.4.4**).

Wrapping the cecum around the appendix

The appendix is folded over on to the exposed submucosa and the cecum is loosely wrapped around the appendix through the fenestrations in the mesentery using a 4-0 polyglycolic acid suture. The suture picks up the seromuscular layer on the cecum on each side and the appendix to anchor it in the tunnel. The wrap is continued until only a short length of appendix sticks out from the tunnel. The stoma is then ready to be created. It is important to anchor the cecum to the back of the anterior abdominal wall where the appendix emerges to prevent twisting and kinking of the conduit (**Figure 3.4.5**).

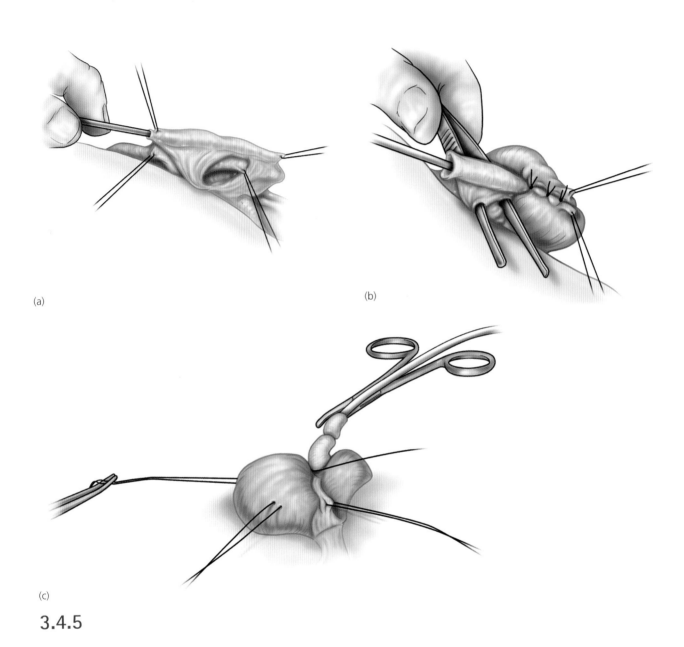

(a)

(b)

(c)

3.4.5

SIMULTANEOUS MITROFANOFF PROCEDURE/ ABSENT APPENDIX

Split appendix

When both a Mitrofanoff and ACE are required and the appendix is of sufficient length, it can be divided into two, provided the vascular anatomy is favorable. The ACE uses the *in situ* technique as described above, and the distal end of the appendix is available for the Mitrofanoff (**Figure 3.4.6**).

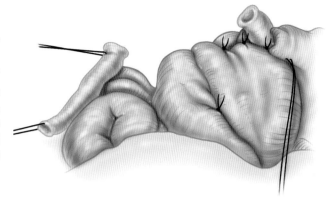

3.4.6

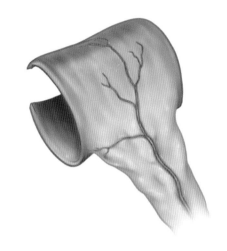

(a)

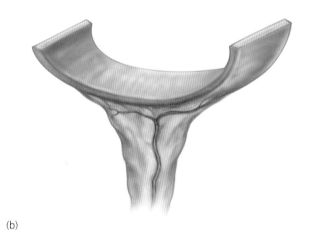

(b)

The Yang–Monti procedure

This technique can be used to create a conduit that can then be implanted into the colon at any site to create the ACE. It can be used when the appendix is absent and it is also used for a left-sided ACE. A 2 cm segment of ileum is isolated on its vascular pedicle. Bowel continuity is restored by a standard end-to-end anastomosis. The ileum is opened along the antimesenteric border. It can then be seen that the valvulae coniventes are now running in a longitudinal direction along the length of the bowel. The bowel is then tubularized over a 12Fr catheter by a single-layer, interrupted, extramucosal anastomosis using 6-0 PDS™ suture. One end is then implanted into a submucosal tenial tunnel in the colon and the other is brought to the skin as the stoma (**Figure 3.4.7**).

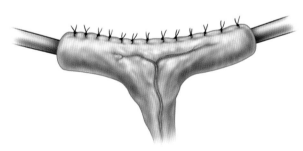

(c)

3.4.7

Creation of colonic submucosal tunnel

A tenia is stretched using proximal, distal, and two lateral stay sutures. The seromuscular layer of the tenia is incised with a scalpel down to the submucosa over a 5 cm length. The mucosa/submucosa is then freed from the overlying muscle using a combination of sharp and blunt dissection to leave an exposed strip of mucosa approximately 1 cm in width (**Figure 3.4.8**).

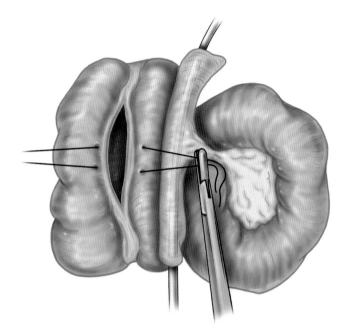

3.4.8

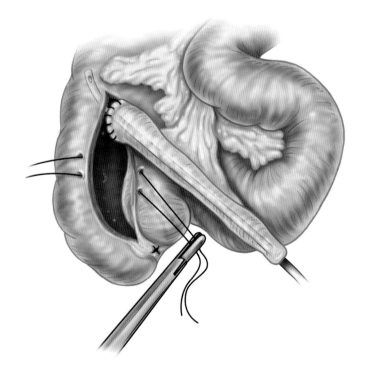

Monti-mucosal anastomosis

A small hole is punched in the mucosa of the colon using artery forceps. This is usually placed at the distal end of the mucosal tunnel. The mucosa is anastomosed to the full thickness of the Monti tube using a 5-0 polyglycolic acid suture over the catheter in the conduit (**Figure 3.4.9**).

3.4.9

Closure of the seromuscular tunnel

The seromuscular wall of the colon is closed over the Monti tube using interrupted 4-0 polyglycolic acid sutures, picking up partial thickness of the conduit wall to prevent it slipping out of the tunnel (**Figure 3.4.10**).

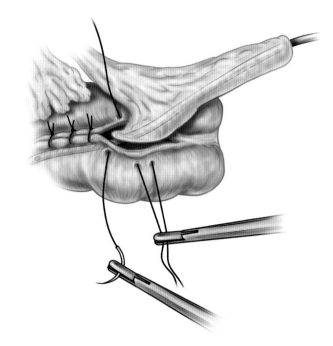

3.4.10

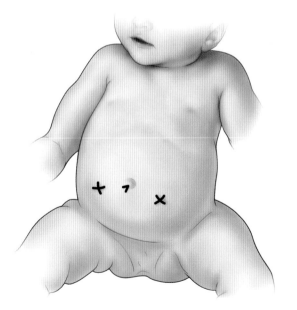

3.4.11

Laparoscopic antegrade continence enema

A 5 mm port is inserted at the umbilicus under direct vision. Two further 5 mm ports are inserted in both iliac fossae. The cecum is mobilized so the appendix can reach the umbilicus. The camera port is changed and the appendix is grasped with forceps and simply delivered through the umbilical port site, where a stoma is then created. The author does not usually create an antireflux valve during this procedure, and although leakage from the conduit is more common than when a valve is created, it is still not a common problem (**Figure 3.4.11**).

Percutaneous endoscopic colonic tube placement

Following bowel preparation and under general anesthesia, a colonoscope is passed to the distal descending colon and the light can be visualized in the flank. A needle and thread is passed into the colon, grasped, and delivered through the anus. This is attached to a gastrostomy tube, which is pulled up into the colon until the flange on the tube pulls the colon to the abdominal wall. The tube is fixed externally to the abdominal wall and washouts can be commenced the following day. After a trial, if the ACE works, the patient has a choice of keeping the tube, changing to a button, or having a conduit constructed (**Figure 3.4.12**).

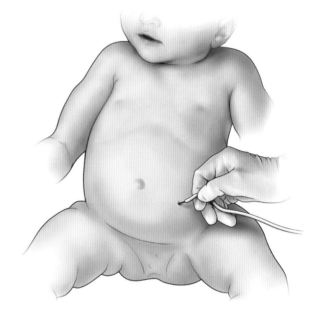

(a)

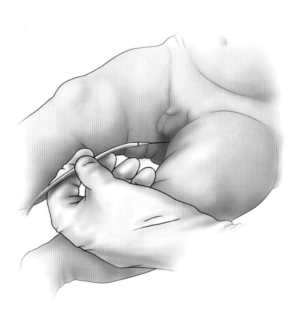

(b)

3.4.12

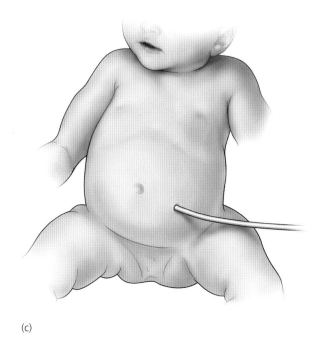

(c)

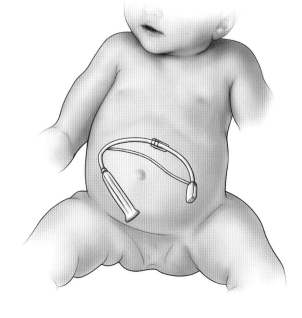

(d)

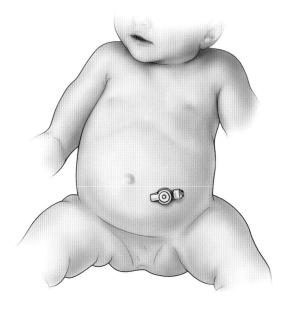

(e)

3.4.12 contd

FASHIONING THE STOMA

Abdominal VQC stoma

Two skin flaps (V and rectangular) are created at the site of the stoma. A hole is created in the abdominal wall that is sufficiently wide to allow the conduit to pass through freely. The cecum or colon is sutured to the anterior abdominal wall to prevent tension on the stoma or volvulus of the bowel on the conduit. The conduit is fish-mouthed and the apex of the V-flap is sutured into the defect using 5-0 Maxon™ sutures with the knots outside the catheterizing channel. The V-flap is gradually sutured into the defect until approximately 50 percent of the circumference of the conduit is complete. The rectangular flap is then sutured over the anterior circumference of the conduit until the anastomosis is complete. The resulting skin defect is closed in layers using 4-0 Maxon and 5-0 subcuticular polyglycolic acid sutures, resulting in a C-shaped wound (VQC stoma). A 12Fr silastic Foley catheter is left *in situ* for 4 weeks after the surgery prior to commencing catheterization (**Figure 3.4.13**).

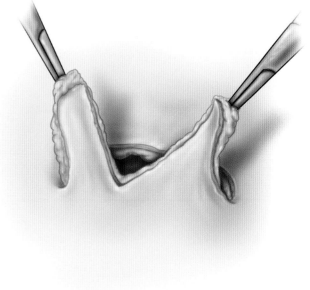

(b)

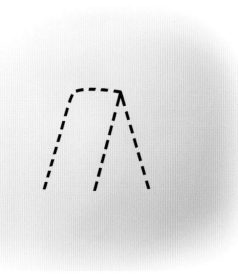

(a)

3.4.13

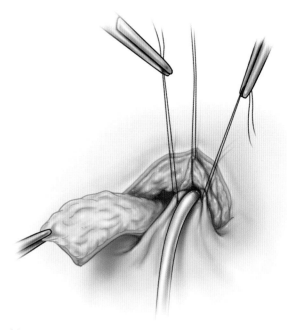

(c)

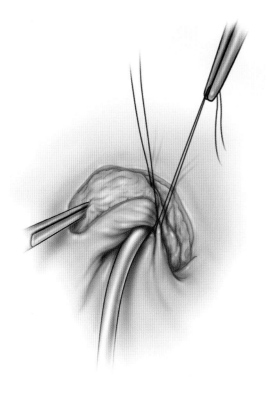

(d)

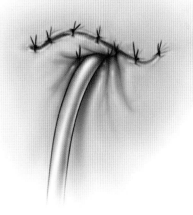

(f)

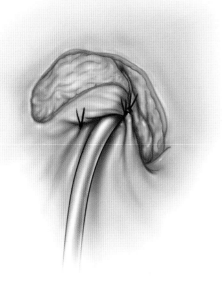

(e)

3.4.13 contd

Umbilical stoma

The umbilicus is everted and a V-flap is created from the everted skin. This is sutured into the conduit as described above, and the remainder of the anastomosis is completed by suturing the conduit to the umbilical rim (**Figure 3.4.14**).

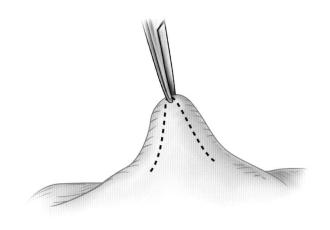

(a)

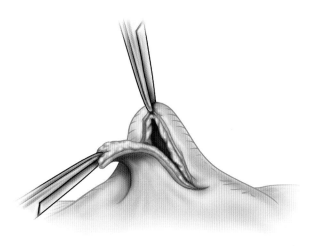

(b)

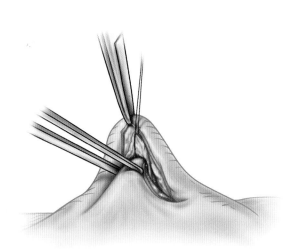

(c)

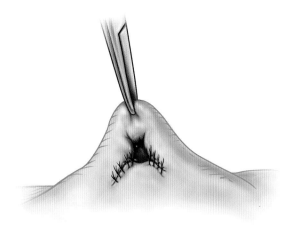

(d)

3.4.14

The ACE stopper

Despite the improvement in stoma stenosis rates with the operative modifications described above, stenosis remains the most common complication. This led to the development of the ACE stopper (**Figure 3.4.15**). ACE stoppers are now commercially available in varying sizes, 10–14 mm diameters and 15–100 mm lengths (Medicina, Bolton, UK), and these are very helpful for patients who experience ongoing catheterization problems. The author now leaves this *in situ* for three months following the creation of the ACE and it has produced a further significant reduction in stenosis rates.

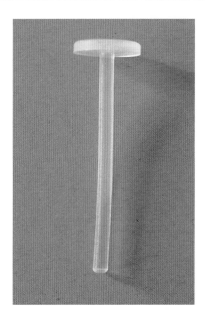

3.4.15 Medicina ACE stopper.

POSTOPERATIVE CARE

Following an isolated ACE, enteral feeding can commence the following day, and the first washout can be administered when the patient has recovered from the adynamic ileus. Once the child and carers are happy with the enema procedure, the child can be discharged with the indwelling catheter, to return 4 weeks later to learn intermittent catheterization, which seldom takes longer than 48 hours. An ACE stopper should be left *in situ* for a further three months. A standard 12Fr Nelaton catheter is used for washouts. The patient should be given some 8 and 10Fr catheters, because if catheterization becomes difficult, the smaller catheters can be used initially to help dilate the stoma. If severe stomal stenosis develops, dilatation under general anesthesia is recommended, following which a stopper can be left *in situ* for a period to reduce the risk of a further stenosis. Occasionally, stoma revision is required and this usually takes the form of a Y–V plasty.

ENEMA REGIMENS

There is no single correct enema regimen, and each patient develops an individual practice by trial and error. The author starts with 1 mL/kg of phosphate enema (Fletchers' phosphate, Fleet Pharmaceuticals, Zaragoza, Spain) diluted to half strength with an equal volume of tap water or normal saline. This is followed by a washout of tap water of between 10 and 20 mL/kg. A daily enema is given for the first few months, but after that about half the patients use the washouts on alternate days or, rarely, even less frequently than that.

Initially, many patients experience colicky abdominal pain, and this may be helped by reducing the concentration of the phosphate and the rate of enema infusion. If colic is persistent, the administration of mebeverine hydrochloride 30 minutes before the enema can help. Persistent pain may also be caused by constipation, and this can be managed by the administration of mineral oil via the ACE 4–6 hours prior to the washout.

If the enema does not produce a rapid result, the concentration of the phosphate can be increased in steps up to a full-strength enema, and in some patients this is used without a following washout. Most patients continue to use a washout, but if fecal leakage occurs between enemas, the volume can be reduced or increased and this usually resolves the problem.

Phosphate toxicity has been encountered, particularly in younger patients, and it is of vital importance that if there is no response from the enema after 6 hours, no further phosphate is administered until a result is obtained. Further washouts with tap water often help, but occasionally retrograde washouts are required.

Administering antegrade colonic enemas

Most patients use an infusion system such as a Kangaroo bag and pump set (Kendall, Tullamore, Ireland). The bag is filled with the required phosphate and infused over a 10-minute period. The bag is then refilled with water and infused over the next 15 minutes. Evacuation usually starts within 15 minutes and is complete 30 minutes later. As patients will spend a considerable time sitting on the toilet, the use of padded seat covers is recommended to reduce the risk of pressure sores.

COMPLICATIONS

The common complications and their management are discussed in the text. Uncommon complications include leakage of fecal fluid through the stoma, and if this occurs, the valve mechanism will need to be revised or a valve created, if this had not been done in the first instance.

OUTCOME

For patients with neuropathic conditions and anorectal malformations, the success rate of ACE procedures is 80–90 percent.

FURTHER READING

Chait PG, Shandling B, Richards HM. The cecostomy button. *Journal of Paediatric Surgery* 1997; **32**: 849–51.

Churchill BM, De Ugarte DA, Atkinson JB. Left-colon antegrade continence enema (LACE) procedure for fecal incontinence. *Journal of Paediatric Surgery* 2003; **38**: 1778–80.

Curry JL, Osborne A, Malone PS. How to achieve a successful Malone antegrade continence enema. *Journal of Paediatric Surgery* 1998; **33**: 138–41.

Gerharz EW, Vik V, Webb G, Woodhouse CRJ. The *in situ* appendix in the Malone antegrade continence enema procedure for faecal incontinence. *British Journal of Urology* 1997; **79**: 985–6.

Griffin SJ, Parkinson EJ, Malone PSJ. Bowel management for paediatric patients with faecal incontinence. *Journal of Pediatric Urology* 2008; **4**: 387–92.

Monti PR, Lara RC, Dutra MA *et al.* New techniques for construction of efferent conduits based on the Mitrofanoff principle. *Urology* 1997; **49**: 112–15.

Wedderburn A, Lee RS, Denny A *et al.* Synchronous bladder reconstruction and antegrade continence enema. *Journal of Urology* 2001; **165**: 2392–3.

Antegrade continence enema procedure in adults

JAMES HILL

PRINCIPLES AND JUSTIFICATION

Constipation

The antegrade continence enema (ACE) procedure was developed as a treatment for intractable fecal incontinence in the pediatric population and is established as a technique which significantly improves quality of life. The principle of the procedure is to establish a conduit from the anterior abdominal wall to the colon (usually the cecum). This conduit should be catheterizable and continent. The patient instils irrigation fluid via the conduit. The fluid acts as a mechanical flush and also stimulates colonic contraction. It has the advantage of being a relatively minor procedure and hence without major complications. This procedure has a role in the management of adult patients with severe constipation and can be used in patients with severe incontinence and for patients with mixed symptoms.[1, 2]

The technique has a long-term success rate of 50–60 percent; if unsuccessful, it does not compromise subsequent treatment options[2, 3] and if not used, the conduit will stenose and does not require excision. Reports indicate that the ACE can be used during pregnancy.

PREOPERATIVE ASSESSMENT

Prior to consideration for surgery, investigations should include colonic transit studies, defecation proctography, and anorectal physiology studies. Patients with pure slow transit constipation are uncommon; most have some degree of associated pelvic floor dysfunction. As such, most patients would not undergo an ACE procedure without a trial of biofeedback therapy. A trial of retrograde lavage is also worthwhile. It is invaluable for patients to have specialist nurse input and counseling; patient motivation is essential.

Patients most suitable for this procedure are those with slow transit constipation/severe incontinence and pelvic floor/anal sphincter dysfunction without any correctable anatomical abnormality.

Examination should confirm anal sphincter functional abnormalities, if present. Most patients perform irrigation on alternate days. The irrigation takes 30–40 minutes and is performed while sitting on the toilet (**Figure 3.5.1**). They need to be physically capable of performing the procedure.

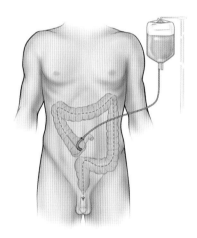

3.5.1 Irrigation procedure.

PREOPERATIVE MANAGEMENT

For an open appendicostomy, no specific bowel preparation is required for the procedure itself, but early postoperative washouts are aided if the colon is not overly loaded.

If the appendicostomy is brought out at the umbilicus, no marking is necessary. For a percutaneous endoscopic colostomy (PEC) tube or conduit elsewhere on the abdominal wall, consideration should be given to any previous scars and underwear.

Routine antibiotic and venous thromboembolism prophylaxis is given.

INCISION

A transverse incision is made at the level of the umbilicus. This should leave a gap of skin between the medial end of the incision and the umbilicus. This incision is deepened to the anterior rectus sheath, the rectus muscle divided and the peritoneum opened. The cecum is mobilized sufficiently for it to reach the umbilicus.

Mobilization of the appendix

The appendix is mobilized (**Figure 3.5.2**) to allow it to lie along one of the tenia coli on the antimesenteric border of the ascending colon. At this point, a small trephine incision is made at the umbilicus, the diameter of which should correspond to the diameter of the appendix. The relevant tenia coli is then stretched using lateral stay sutures and incised along its length and the muscle divided down to the mucosa to create a recess for the appendix. The mucosa is separated from the muscularis mucosae and muscularis propria by sharp and blunt dissection. A gap large enough to accommodate about two-thirds of the circumference of the appendix is achieved without too much difficulty.

Division of the tenia and creation of recess

The tenia is divided from close to the base of the appendix to a point that when the appendix lies in the recess, leaves sufficient length of appendix beyond the recess to reach the umbilical skin without difficulty (**Figure 3.5.3**). The distance from the skin to the peritoneal cavity at the umbilical cicatrix is short. The edges of the divided tenia coli are then sutured to the seromuscular layer of the wall of the appendix to secure the appendix in its recess.

Appendix sutured into the recess

Suturing the appendix into the recess acts as an antireflux mechanism (**Figure 3.5.4**). It is possible to close the tenia completely over the appendix, but care needs to be taken not to compromise the blood supply.[4]

It is advisable to amputate the tip of the appendix to ensure that it can be catheterized and measure the length of usable appendix.

The appendix is grasped gently with a Babcock's forceps and brought out to the umbilical skin. Prior to anastomosis to the skin, the appendix is catheterized with a size 12 Foley catheter to ensure that the catheter passes easily and in an orthograde direction into the ascending colon. Retrograde ileal irrigation is painful.

Once catherization is confirmed, the cecum is secured to the undersurface of the anterior abdominal wall.

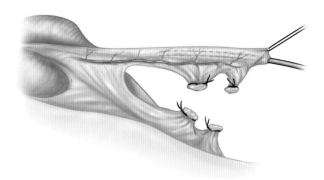

3.5.2 Mobilization of appendix.

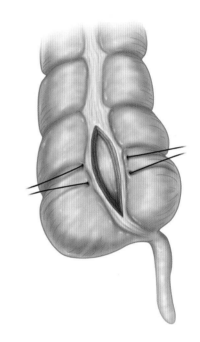

3.5.3 Creation of recess for appendix.

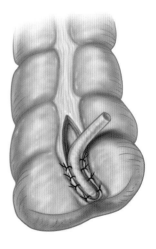

3.5.4 Suturing of appendix into its recess.

Creation of the V flap and suturing the conduit in place

The skin at the edge of the umbilicus is retracted vertically (**Figure 3.5.5**) and a V flap is created (**Figure 3.5.6**). The conduit is fish mouthed and sutured to the flap using 3-0 absorbable monofilament sutures (**Figure 3.5.7**). The catheter is left *in situ* and 10 mL of water inserted into the balloon. This is sufficient to keep the catheter in place. The abdominal wall is closed in layers with absorbable suture material (**Figure 3.5.8**).

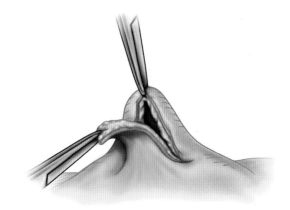

3.5.6 Creation of V flap.

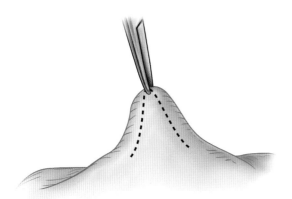

3.5.5 Markings for V-flap incision.

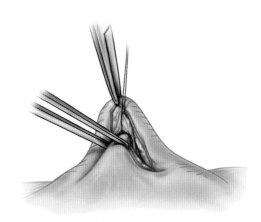

3.5.7 Suturing the conduit.

Laparoscopic procedure

A 5 mm port is inserted at the umbilicus and two 5 mm ports inserted, one in each iliac fossa. The cecum is mobilized such that the appendix will reach the umbilicus. The appendix is then delivered through the umbilical port site and then sutured to the skin, as described above. As no antireflux valve is created, the risk of reflux on to the skin is increased.

Percutaneous endoscopic colonic tube placement

Preoperative bowel preparation is required. It is the author's protocol to give two sachets of sodium picosulfate each day for the 3 days before the procedure. Retrograde lavage is administered on the day of surgery.

The colonoscope is passed to the cecum. The site of insertion is determined by transillumination and by digital

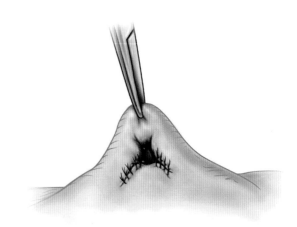

3.5.8 Closure.

indentation of the cecum lumen seen endoscopically (**Figure 3.5.9**). A standard gastrostomy kit is used. Distension of the cecum is maintained as tension of the colonic wall aids passage of the needle. A skinny needle is passed into the cecum to determine the correct path and is seen endoscopically to enter the right colon. The puncture cannula is then passed parallel to the skinny

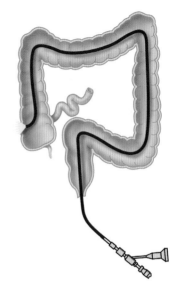

3.5.9 Colonoscope in cecum.

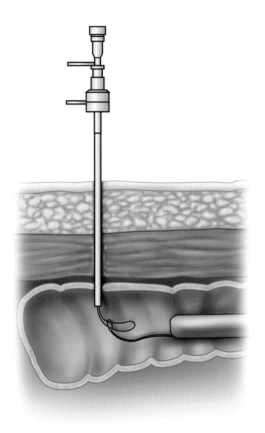

3.5.10 Puncture cannula in cecum.

needle along the same path. The double thread is passed down the trocar using the introducer device into the colon and grasped using a polypectomy snare (**Figure 3.5.10**). The colonoscope is withdrawn and the double thread connected to the tube. This tube is well lubricated and pulled into position (**Figure 3.5.11**). The trocar is removed when the tube reaches it. This is felt as resistance to the

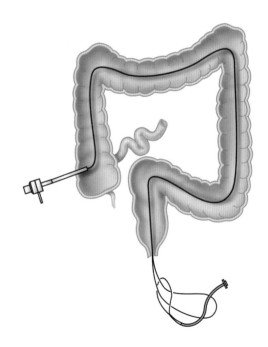

3.5.11 Colonoscope out, tube connected.

passage of the tube. The tube is then secured to the anterior abdominal wall (**Figure 3.5.12**).

If there is doubt or concern about the position of the tube, this should be checked endosocopically. Diet and fluids are taken the following day.

The advantages of the PEC technique are that it can be used as a trial of therapy, that reflux and stenosis are rare problems and that if successful, the patient has a choice of a button or conduit. After 6 weeks, the tube is replaced by a button device (**Figure 3.5.13**).

Button insertion can be impeded by a minor degree of skin level stenosis. If this occurs, the channel can be dilated using low friction catheters.

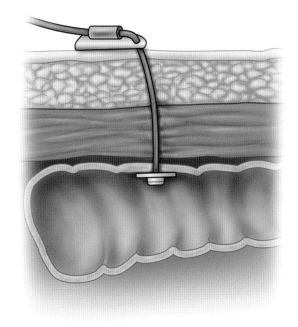

3.5.12 Fixation of the tube.

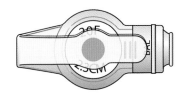

3.5.13 Button device.

Neo appendicostomy

In the event of previous appendectomy, a neo appendicostomy can be constructed using the terminal ileum. The terminal ileum is divided approximately 6 cm from the ileocecal valve. Bowel continuity is restored with an ileocolic anastomosis between the ileum proximal to the point of division and the ascending colon (**Figure 3.5.14**). A 12Fr urinary catheter is passed down the distal terminal ileum into the cecum and the balloon inflated. The lumen is reduced, using the catheter as a guide, by division along the antimesenteric border of the ileum (**Figure 3.5.14**). The redundant antimesenteric part of the terminal ileum is resected at the ileocecal junction preserving the ileocecal valve.[5] The conduit is brought out on to the abdominal wall and sutured to the skin with a V–Y plasty and the cecum sutured to the under-surface of the anterior abdominal wall.

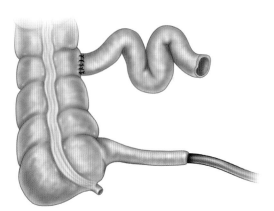

3.5.14 Neo appendicostomy.

POSTOPERATIVE CARE

Diet and fluids can be recommenced the following day. Irrigation with incremental volumes of 50 mL of water is performed until the fifth day when a full washout is performed. Patients perform the washout while sitting on the toilet. A colostomy irrigation set is filled with the appropriate volume of water and is positioned on a hook above shoulder level. The conduit is catheterized with a size 12 low friction disposable catheter (as used for intermittent urinary self-catheterization) and connected to the colostomy irrigation tubing. The fluid is instilled into the colon and the patient waits for evacuation of the fluid and colonic contents. This procedure takes about 30 minutes.

A standard regimen of between 500 mL and 1 liter of tap water is recommended. One teaspoon of salt per 500 mL of fluid is added. If this is insufficient to induce bowel evacuation, half a phosphate enema is used.

COMPLICATIONS

The most common complication is stomal stenosis. It will occur unless the appendicosotomy is regularly catheterized. If stenosis does occur, dilatation under general anesthetic is required. If it becomes a recurrent problem, an ACE stopper can be used (Medicina, Bolton, UK) (**Figure 3.5.15**). These can be left *is situ* for several months if required.

Reflux of irrigation fluid is an uncommon problem. Revision of the ACE to improve the antireflux mechanism is difficult and the problem is probably best managed with the stopper.

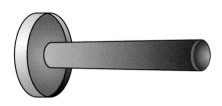

3.5.15 Stopper.

REFERENCES

1. Hill J, Stott S, MacLennan I. Antegrade enemas for the treatment of severe idiopathic constipation. *British Journal of Surgery* 1994; **81**: 1490–1.
2. Worsoe J, Christensen P, Krogh K *et al.* Long term functional results of antegrade colonic enema in adult patients: assessment of functional results. *Diseases of the Colon and Rectum* 2008; **51**: 1523–8.
3. Lees NP, Hodson P, Hill J *et al.* Long-term results of the antegrade continent enema procedure for constipation in adults. *Colorectal Disease* 2004; **6**: 362–8.
4. Poirier M, Abcarian H, Nelson R. Malone antegrade continent enema: an alternative to resection in severe defecation disorders. *Diseases of the Colon and Rectum* 2007; **50**: 22–8.
5. Christensen P, Buntzen S, Krogh K, Laurberg S. Ileal neoappendicostomy for antegrade colonic irrigation. *British Journal of Surgery* 2001; **88**: 1637–8.

4

Small intestine

Small bowel resection

CLARE-ELLEN MCNAUGHT AND JOHN MACFIE

PRINCIPLES AND JUSTIFICATION

The vast majority of small bowel resections are performed as an emergency due to bowel obstruction, vascular compromise, or perforation. Obstruction is typically caused by postoperative or congenital adhesions, hernias, inflammatory bowel disease, or tumors. Small bowel resection can be performed in a variety of ways but the technique of end-to-end, single layer anastomosis had been advocated by the UK Intercollegiate Surgical Training Committee.[1] This procedure is described in detail below. This chapter highlights the clinical and technical challenges of acute small bowel resection which must be overcome by the general surgeon on call.

PREOPERATIVE ASSESSMENT AND PREPARATION

A detailed medical history and examination is mandatory in every patient. Patients requiring small bowel resection are often dehydrated and have electrolyte abnormalities, particularly sodium, chloride, and potassium depletion. Initial management includes the establishment of intravenous access, aggressive fluid resuscitation, and urinary catheterization. Patients with hemodynamic instability and those with significant medical comorbidity should be transferred to a high dependency unit for invasive monitoring. In patients with small bowel obstruction, nasogastric aspiration reduces the risk of pulmonary aspiration and prevents further intestinal distension from swallowed air. There is no evidence for the routine use of broad-spectrum antibiotics. All patients should have deep vein thrombosis (DVT) prophylaxis in the form of low molecular weight heparin and compression stockings.

Plain abdominal x-rays will establish the diagnosis of small bowel obstruction in over 60 percent of patients, but further investigation may be required in the form of contrast computed tomography (CT) or gastrograffin studies. CT scans are helpful in determining the level and etiology of small bowel obstruction, but do not replace the need for careful, repeated clinical examination for the early signs of strangulation.

Indications for surgery

SMALL BOWEL OBSTRUCTION

The etiology of small bowel obstruction can be varied, but is most frequently seen in patients with adhesions from previous surgery. A proportion of these patients will settle with conservative management and not require laparotomy. A contrast CT scan may be helpful, but if there is no improvement within 48 hours, laparotomy should be considered. The presence of peritonitis, fever, tachycardia, and hypotension suggests infarcted or perforated bowel and the need for urgent investigation and intervention. Surgery should be performed immediately after fluid resuscitation in patients with obstructed hernias and those with no previous abdominal surgery, the so-called 'virgin abdomen'.

MALIGNANT DISEASE

The treatment of patients with a previous intra-abdominal malignancy and widespread carcinomatosis can be challenging. CT scanning may determine if there are one or multiple levels of obstruction. A frank discussion with the patient, oncologist, and palliative care team will often determine the most appropriate management. If surgery is performed, a simple bypass of an obstructing lesion may be preferable to radical resection. If no bypass is possible, the placement of a palliative 'venting' surgical gastrostomy tube will facilitate the drainage of gastric contents, allow removal of the nasogastic tube and improve patient comfort.

CROHN'S DISEASE

Patients with Crohn's disease (CD) can present with obstruction, perforation, or fistulation. Many will respond to treatment with steroids, immunosuppressant or immunomodulator drugs. Surgical intervention is indicated in those who fail to respond to medical management and in patients with obstruction related to fibrous strictures. The technical aspects of surgery relating to inflammatory bowel disease (IBD) are considered in detail in Chapters 4.4, 6.6, and 6.7. Patients with IBD are at increased risk of morbidity related to malnutrition and immunosuppression. A full nutritional assessment should be performed and any deficiencies corrected, if possible, prior to surgery. The risk of adrenal suppression must be considered and appropriate intravenous steroid cover given.

SUPERIOR MESENTERIC VASCULAR COMPROMISE

Acute small bowel ischemia can be caused by superior mesenteric artery thrombosis, arterial embolus, or venous thrombosis. The patient usually complains of severe pain, but the abdominal signs may be subtle. A high index of clinical suspicion is necessary, particularly in patients with atrial fibrillation or a past history of arterial disease. If the diagnosis is made preoperatively, a CT angiogram should be obtained and the opinion of a vascular consultant sought to determine the need for revascularization. An immediate laparotomy is usually required to resect necrotic bowel, with simultaneous revascularization in arterial ischemia or anticoagulation in patients with venous thrombosis.

ANESTHESIA

General anesthesia is required for small bowel resection. Combined thoracic epidural is recommended to reduce postoperative morbidity and analgesic requirements. Epidurals are contraindicated in patients with severe sepsis and coagulopathy. Prophylactic antibiotics should be given at the time of induction to reduce the incidence of wound infection. Pneumatic compression stockings should be used if the patient is at high risk of thromboembolism.

OPERATION

Position

The supine position is suitable for most patients. If an abdominal mass is palpable or Crohn's disease suspected, then the patient should be placed in a low lithotomy position to improve access to the pelvis and allow a second assistant to stand between the legs.

Incision

A midline incision is the usual choice in the acute situation, particularly where the underlying etiology is unknown. If preoperative scanning has shown an isolated pathology, then a transverse lower abdominal incision should be considered as this is associated with reduced postoperative pain, hernia formation and better cosmesis.

Extent of resection

The extent of resection is usually easy to judge, removing the obstructing lesion or the area of demarcated bowel completely. If there is any doubt over the viability of a segment of intestine, it should be wrapped in warm, saline-soaked packs and reinspected at 5–10-minute intervals. Any area of bowel with persistent loss of peristalsis and abnormal serosal discoloration should be excised.

There are two scenarios where the extent of resection may cause the surgeon concern, namely CD and mesenteric vascular injury. The surgeon must adopt a conservative approach in patients with CD, as extensive resection does not decrease the risk of recurrence and may result in short bowel syndrome. The bowel proximal to an obstructing Crohn's lesion is often thickened, but may not be significantly diseased. The extent of active disease can often be determined by the extent of mesenteric fat creeping. This characteristic feature of CD is fat encroachment of the antimesenteric surface of the bowel. A limited resection should always be the goal. In the majority of patients undergoing excisional surgery for CD it is usually possible to fashion an anastomosis. The exception to this would be those situations where there is significant sepsis or contamination.

A length of small bowel with multiple strictures is optimally dealt with by stricturoplasty, as discussed in Chapter 4.4.

In mesenteric vascular injury, there may be areas of intestine with unequivocal features of transmural infarction and other areas of dubious viability. Frankly ischemic bowel should be resected, but other areas should be left and reinspected at a 'second look' laparotomy the next day.

Technique

The diseased small bowel is fragile and care should be taken during mobilization to prevent serosal tears and unintentional enterotomy. The segment to be resected should be excluded from the abdominal cavity with large packs. The vascular arcade of the small bowel can be visualized by lifting the section and transilluminating the mesentery by shining the operative light behind it. This permits accurate ligation of the vessels and minimizes mesenteric hematoma formation. The mesentery should be divided close to the bowel. Wedge excision of the mesentery is not required unless a tumor is to be resected. The vessels should be isolated by pushing sharp-pointed forceps through the mesentery and applying straight artery clips. In CD and very friable mesentery, the mesentery should be transfixed with a 2-0 polyglactin (Vicryl™) suture. In other situations, 2-0 Vicryl ties suffice. A pair of crushing clamps is applied at each resection margin and the bowel transected with a scalpel blade. The small bowel content is 'milked' back and soft, non-crushing clamps are applied to the antimesenteric border 5 cm proximal to the cut ends. The crushing clamps are then removed. There is no need to trim the small bowel, unless the crushed area is more than 3 mm (**Figure 4.1.1**).

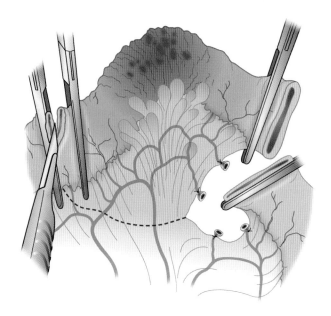

4.1.1

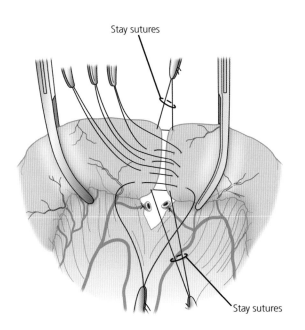

4.1.2

Interrupted serosubmucosal sutures are first placed at the apex of the mesenteric/antimesenteric borders and clipped to act as stay sutures. A 3-0 absorbable suture with an atraumatic round-bodied needle should be used. The authors prefer 3-0 PDS for anastomosis formation. Sutures are placed and tied at 4–5 mm intervals to complete the anterior wall of the anastomosis (**Figure 4.1.2**).

At this point, the positions of the stay sutures are exchanged by passing the antimesenteric stay through the mesenteric defect and pulling the mesenteric stay forward. This brings the posterior wall of the anastomosis into the anterior position. A further row of interrupted sutures are placed to finish the anastomosis. On completion, return the stay sutures to their original position (**Figure 4.1.3**).

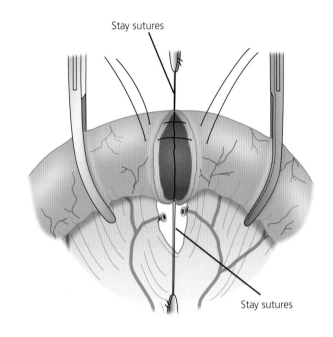

Stay sutures

Stay sutures

4.1.3

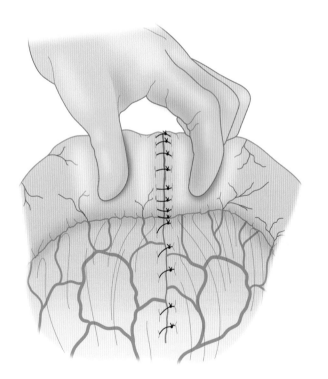

The soft clamps are removed and the patency of the anastomotic lumen confirmed by gentle palpation with the thumb and index finger. The mesenteric defect is then closed with interrupted 2-0 Vicryl, taking care not to devascularize the small bowel. Abdominal lavage with sterile, warm normal saline is performed only if there has been generalized contamination. There is no evidence for the routine use of abdominal drains. Mass closure of the abdomen is performed using a large, monofilament absorbable suture. The skin is closed with a subcuticular suture or wound clips, depending on the findings at laparotomy (**Figure 4.1.4**).

4.1.4

Alternative techniques

The technique described above can be used in most circumstances. In situations where the bowel is perforated or very friable, the authors often use gastrointestinal stapling guns to quickly resect the damaged segments and limit contamination. A two-layer, side-to-side anastomosis is useful when there is large size discrepancy between the two limbs of bowel to be anastomosed or when the bowel is very edematous. The role of laparoscopic surgery in acute small bowel obstruction is a subject of much debate but can be used safely in carefully selected patients by experienced laparoscopic surgeons.

POSTOPERATIVE CARE

The principles of enhanced recovery after surgery (ERAS) are well established in elective practice, but can also be adapted to the emergency setting.[2] Epidurals, intravenous paracetamol, and non-steroidal anti-inflammatory drugs should be used in appropriate patients to reduce the requirement for opiate analgesia. There is good evidence to suggest that the early introduction of oral fluids and diet is safe, even in patients with a very proximal anastomosis. Nasogastric tubes and urinary catheters should be removed as soon as the clinical recovery dictates. Patients should be actively mobilized, sitting out of bed on the day of surgery and walking with the physiotherapists on the first postoperative day.

REFERENCES

1. Thomas B, McCloy R. *Intercollegiate basic surgical skill course participant handbook.* London: Royal College of Surgeons, 2007.
2. Khan S, Gatt M, Horgan A *et al.* Guidelines for the implementation of enhanced recovery protocols. London: Association of Surgeons of Great Britain and Ireland, December 2009.

Meckel's diverticulum

DESMOND C WINTER

HISTORY

A diverticulum arising from the antimesenteric border of the ileum was first mentioned by Hildanus (1598), and later by Lavater (1672) and Ruysch (1701). Littre described the finding of an ileal diverticulum in a hernia sac (1742). Morgagni suggested it was a congenital remnant (1769). However, it was Johann Friedrich Meckel the younger (both his father and grandfather were anatomists of repute), who fully described the developmental anatomy and the congenital anomaly that went on to bear his name.[1]

PRINCIPLES AND JUSTIFICATION

During early development, the vitellointestinal (or omphalomesenteric) duct connects the midgut with the yolk sac. It obliterates by 10 weeks' gestation and the residual fibrous cord is usually absorbed. Failure to progress through this transition results in a number of anomalies of which the most common are Meckel's diverticulum in which no cord persists (>75 percent; **Figure 4.2.1**a), a residual fibrous cord from the abdominal wall to the ileal wall with or without a Meckel's diverticulum ('mesodiverticular band' 10–15 percent; **Figure 4.2.1**b), or a patent vitellointestinal duct that communicates with the umbilicus (5–10 percent; **Figure 4.2.1**c). There may be

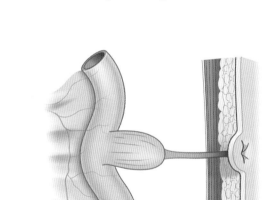

(b)

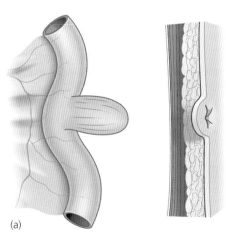

4.2.1   (a)

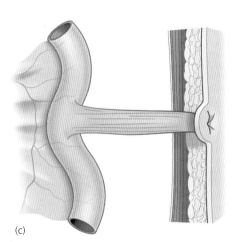

(c)

associated anomalies including a patent urachus, an umbilical sinus or polyp, or omphalomesenteric cysts. In keeping with its embryological origins, there may be a vascular mesentery (either partial or complete) running along the diverticulum at a right angle to the ileum.

Meckel's diverticulum has been deemed the anomaly of 2's based on the somewhat oversimplified (and erroneous) premise that it is present in 2 percent of the population with a 2:1 male to female ratio, is 2 inches long, found 2 feet from the ileocecal valve, may contain two types of heterotropic (gastric and pancreatic) tissue, and is subject to two main complications (bleeding and inflammation/perforation) 1:2 of which arise before the age of two years. However, there is far more heterogeneity in practice. Diverticula have been found within a couple of centimeters or more than 1 m from the ileocecal valve[2] and size varies from 1 to 26 cm, although the average is 3 cm long and 2 cm wide.[3] Heterotropic mucosa has been reported to be jejunal and colonic, in addition to the more common gastric (40–80 percent) and pancreatic (10–20 percent) ectopia. When present, the gastric tissue is mostly fundal gland (acid-secreting) in type and at the apex of the diverticulum.[4] Pancreatic tissue, if present, is usually in the subserosa or submucosa at the apex.

It is challenging to derive an accurate proportion of diverticula that present with clinical problems rather than incidental surgical or post-mortem findings. It is thought that approximately 20 percent become clinically apparent with the majority remaining asymptomatic. The most common childhood presentation is bleeding from ectopic gastric tissue, while in adults it is inflammation, perforation, or obstruction, the latter due to mechanical obstruction by the fibrous band or diverticulum (e.g. volvulus around the diverticular mesentery or inflammation causing local impingement). Occasionally, a Meckel's diverticulum is the site of a benign swelling (leiomyoma, fibroma, hemangioendothelioma, lipoma, neuroma, etc.) or malignant tumor (carcinoid, adenocarcinoma, or very rarely sarcoma).

Much has been made of the male preponderance of symptomatic Meckel's diverticula. This is as between 3:1 and 5:1.[5] Does this justify incidental removal in males? It is not possible to be prescriptive but, as a rule, incidentally detected Meckel's diverticula without adverse features should be left undisturbed. Relative indications include young males with long Meckel's diverticula (particularly where there is a large diverticular mesentery or attachment to other structures) and those with thickened bases suggesting ectopic tissue.[6]

PREOPERATIVE ASSESSMENT AND PREPARATION

Most patients who need surgery for a Meckel's diverticulum present as an emergency with the diagnosis usually made at operation. However, a careful history gives clues to the esoteric problem. Bleeding with a normal upper and lower endoscopy should alert the clinician to possible small bowel pathology. There may be a several-month history of grumbling midgut pain, erroneously labelled as an 'irritable bowel' by previous medical attendants. Some patients present to an emergency department with symptoms of central abdominal pain mimicking early appendicitis. However, they may be discharged when there is no progression to right iliac fossa peritonism only to represent 2 or 3 days later when the diverticulum perforates or causes full-blown obstruction. More commonly, the diagnosis is achieved only on cross-sectional abdominal imaging or at the time of surgery.

If presenting as an emergency, the patient should be resuscitated appropriately, maintained on intravenous fluids, and urethral catheter/nasogastric tube placed as needed. A urine sample, complete blood count, electrolyte profile, amylase, glucose, and blood grouping should be sent. Mechanical bowel preparation is not required. Deep venous thrombosis prophylaxis is administered according to local guidelines. The patient should be consented for laparoscopy and/or laparotomy with the usual discussion regarding the procedure, complications/risks, alternatives, anesthesia/antibiotic issues, and expected postoperative course. For those presenting as an emergency, it is helpful to explain to the patient in advance that he/she may experience some throat pressure as anesthesia commences (cricoid pressure with rapid sequence induction).

ANESTHESIA

General anesthesia is required and the additional benefit of epidural analgesia is at the discretion of the team. Prophylactic antibiotics should be administered intravenously prior to incision. The choice and scheduling should be appropriate for the pathology anticipated/found. In the elective setting, a single dose of coamoxiclav or first-/second-generation cephalosporin combined with metronidazole may be used. Alternatives are broader spectrum cephalosporin or to give metronidazole with gentamicin, bearing in mind the latter may prolong or potentiate neuromuscular blockade. More prolonged therapy may be appropriate in emergency cases. Urethral catheterization is not routinely used but may be appropriate for monitoring in patients with peritonitis or in whom there is anticipated difficulty with voiding.

OPERATION

Following skin preparation and antiseptic painting in the supine position, the patient is draped with exposure of the abdomen. The operative approach is dependent on whether it is performed by laparoscopy or by open access. Where there is a preoperative diagnosis or strong suspicion, a laparoscopic operation is begun with a periumbilical entry port inserted under direct vision (**Figure 4.2.2**). Pneumoperitoneum with carbon dioxide to a maximum pressure of 12 mm mercury is followed by insertion of two operating ports in the iliac fossa/flank positions. One is a 5 mm port, the other a 12 mm port to accommodate a laparoscopic stapler. Alternatively, if a 5 mm camera is used, then one 12 mm port and two 5 mm ports are sufficient (**Figure 4.2.2**).

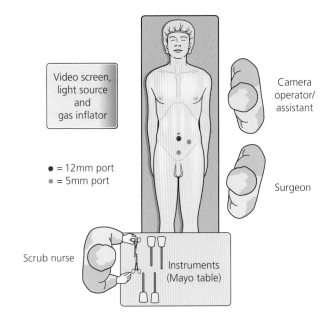

4.2.2

A thorough examination of the peritoneal cavity is performed and the Meckel's diverticulum identified. Resection is usually by simple diverticulectomy (wedge excision) at a 45–90° angle to the ileum to avoid narrowing the lumen. This can be performed with a laparoendoscopic stapler (**Figure 4.2.3**a,b). It is not necessary to undersew or oversew this staple line unless there are concerns regarding the integrity of the closure or risk of bleeding. Under these circumstances, 3-0 absorbable sutures are placed using laparoscopic needle holders. The specimen is easily extracted in an appropriate bag or laparoscopic retrieval device via the 12 mm port with extension as needed.

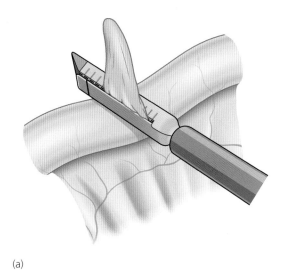

(a)

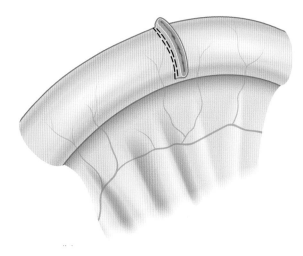

(b)

4.2.3

In the event that conversion is required or if the operation is determined to be open from the onset, a short midline laparotomy centered on the umbilicus is performed. A wound protector/retractor is inserted according to the surgeon's practice. The Meckel's diverticulum is identified and the ileal segment eviscerated for diverticulectomy (wedge excision) using a linear stapling/cutting instrument (**Figure 4.2.4**). Again, undersewing/oversewing is at the discretion of the operating surgeon, but is not routinely needed.

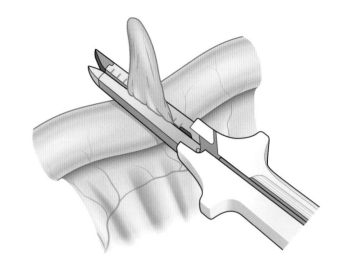

4.2.4

Alternatively, the diverticulum can be excised in a transverse direction using electrocautery/diathermy, as in **Figure 4.2.5**a. Closure of the resulting enterotomy is with 3-0 absorbable sutures (either interrupted or continuous) in a single layered anastomosis (**Figure 4.2.5**b). Segmental ileal resection may be required in patients with associated small bowel abnormality. This is performed as described in Chapter 4.1, following evisceration at a widened periumbilical port site. The fascia is closed using an appropriate absorbable suture (e.g. 0 or 1 polydioxanone sulfate). A subcuticular absorbable 4-0 suture achieves a neat cutaneous approximation, but alternatives (e.g. skin clips) are acceptable.

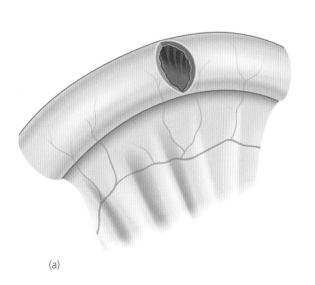

(a)

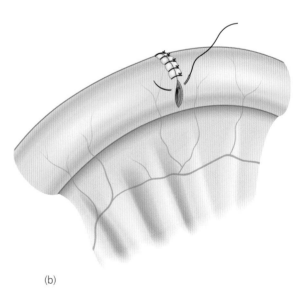

(b)

4.2.5

POSTOPERATIVE CARE

Intravenous fluids, parenteral analgesia and, if used, nasogastric tubes or urethral catheters are discontinued as soon as possible. Oral intake is usually tolerated within 24–48 hours of operation even where there has been obstruction. Patients with peritonitis may have a short-lived ileus, but parenteral nutrition is rarely required. The patient should be mobilized as soon as it is safe and comfortable to do so. Discharge is scheduled when the patient is able to eat normally with normal bowel and ambulatory function. An anastomotic leak should be suspected if there are signs of sepsis, especially in the absence of wound, pulmonary, or urinary infection.

OUTCOME

Most patients will have an uncomplicated postoperative course and benign histology, such that no follow-up will be needed other than a single clinic visit. The minority who have a complication requiring intervention or those in whom malignant histology is identified are followed as appropriate.

REFERENCES

1. Meckel JF. *Beitrage zur vergleichenden. Anatomie.* Leipzig: Carl Heinrich Reclam, 1808.
2. Jay GD III, Magulis RR, McGraw AB *et al.* Meckel's diverticulum: a survey of one hundred and three cases. *Archives of Surgery* 1950; **61**: 158–69.
3. Weinstein EC, Cain JC, Remive WH. Meckel's diverticulum: 55 years of clinical and surgical experience. *Journal of the American Medical Association* 1962; **182**: 251–3.
4. Stewart JH, Storey CF. Meckel's diverticulum: a study of 141 cases. *Southern Medical Journal* 1962; **55**: 16–28.
5. Veith FJ, Botsford TW. Disease of Meckel's diverticulum in adults. *American Surgeon* 1962; **28**: 674–7.
6. Park JJ, Wolff BG, Tollefson MK *et al.* Meckel diverticulum: the Mayo Clinic experience with 1476 patients (1950–2002). *Annals of Surgery* 2005; **241**: 521–3.

Malrotation

J CALVIN COFFEY

HISTORY

Concepts relating to mesenteric development have progressed significantly since WE Ladd first described the surgical management of congenital obstruction of the duodenum. As a result, understanding of abnormalities of rotation and fixation has evolved. In keeping with this it has been suggested that the term 'malrotation' is inaccurate and that 'non-rotation' or 'abnormalities' of rotation and fixation are more appropriate.[1]

Two points must be emphasized at the outset. First, the topography of the small and large intestinal mesenteries are intimately related, given continuity between both, and cannot be considered in isolation. Second, rotation and fixation are key events in intestinal mesenteric development. Thus, abnormalities of both will be included in this chapter.

DEFINITIONS

A brief description of the terminology used is justified in view of the nature of the embryologic processes involved and derangements in these.[1]

- **Rotation**: the process whereby both duodenocolic and cecocolic components of the gastrointestinal tract (together with associated mesenteric segments) turn counterclockwise first through 90° then through 270°.
- **Abnormality of rotation**: where rotation does not occur (i.e. non-rotation) or is incomplete (i.e. partial rotation). These have traditionally been grouped under the heading of malrotation.
- **Fixation**: the process whereby the small intestinal mesentery and/or colonic mesocolon become apposed to the posterior abdominal wall, then fixed in position or immobile. Importantly, fixation does not result in the loss or 'obliteration' of mesenteric structures as these are retained as discrete entities into adulthood.

- **Non-fixation**: where mesenteric fixation to the retroperitoneum is partial or absent in one or more locations.
- **Fusion**: following apposition of peritonealized mesenteric surfaces, the peritoneal surfaces coalesce to generate a fascial structure called the 'lamina mesenteria propria' or 'Toldt's fascia' of fusion. The interface between fascia and mesentery can be called the 'mesofascial plane', while that between the fascia and retroperitoneum can be called the 'retrofascial plane'.[2,3] This terminology is arbitrary, but is practical in the context of surgical techniques (see below under Operation).

NORMAL EMBRYOLOGIC DEVELOPMENT

> There is quite a variety of abnormalities found and they are apt to be extremely confusing unless the normal embryologic development is borne in mind.
>
> WE Ladd (1936)[2]

At the 8th week of development, the duodenojejunal and cecocolic components of the gastrointestinal tract are suspended within the dorsal mesentery and centered on the vitellointestinal duct. Shortly after herniation, these undergo a 90° counterclockwise rotation from the sagittal to the transverse plane. After return to an intraperitoneal position, both undergo a further 270° counterclockwise rotation. The mesocolon of the ascending and descending colon undergo fixation to the posterior abdominal wall. The mesocolon persists into adulthood continuous from the ileocecal to the mesorectal level. The small bowel mesentery finally takes up position medial to the right mesocolon. The fourth part of the duodenum is located caudal to the root of the transverse mesocolon with the left mesocolon positioned over the Toldt's fascia and retroperitoneum on the left.

PRINCIPLES AND JUSTIFICATION

The indications for surgical management of abnormalities of rotation relate to the complications that may arise or the future prevention of their development. The complications include intestinal ischemia or necrosis, obstruction, or recurrent cramping abdominal pain. Rotational anomalies account for 50 and 80 percent of emergency abdominal presentations in the first week and month of life, respectively. In adults, emergency presentation due to abnormalities of rotation is rare and abnormal rotation is mostly identified incidentally (see below under Disease status). Incomplete fixation of the ileocecal junction, or the right and left mesocolon is observed in 25 and 15 percent of all cases, respectively, and thus are far more frequently observed than rotational abnormalities.

PREOPERATIVE ASSESSMENT AND PREPARATION

Radiologic investigations

The surgical anatomy of the small intestinal mesentery and mesocolon are incompletely characterized in radiologic literature. While radiologic studies are of use in diagnosing an abnormality of rotation and/or fixation, they are imprecise in terms of accurate characterization of mesenteric topography. The advantage of preoperative radiologic diagnosis using either single, double, or triple contrast modalities facilitates intraoperative decision making and informs on port site placement when planning a laparoscopic approach.

Patient status

Given the risks of laparotomy alone, notwithstanding those associated with gastrointestinal resection and anastomosis (see Chapter 6.5), reversible morbidities such as electrolyte disturbances, anemia, malnutrition, and dehydration should be identified and corrected. Data relating to these, as well as chronic comorbidities, inform the surgeon on suitability for a restorative procedure should a major resection be required.

Disease status

Four broad categories of mesenteric topography are encountered depending on the point at which rotation and/or fixation halt (**Figure 4.3.1**). Note must be made of adhesions and the manner in which they effect the operative approach. The core topographic abnormality observed in complete non-rotation is illustrated in **Figure 4.3.1**. This mesenteric abnormality generates a folded appearance (inset) for the gastrointestinal tract as it

elongates following development. Adhesional abnormalities may be superimposed (**Figure 4.3.1**); however, once these are dealt with by adhesiolysis, the central mesenteric abnormality becomes apparent.

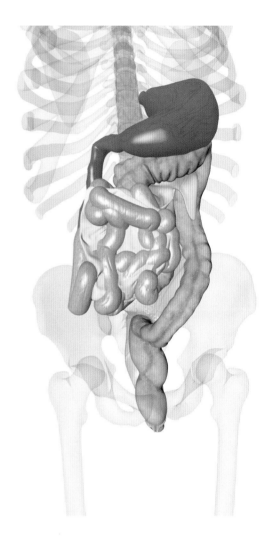

4.3.1 Digital sculpture demonstrating the conformation of the gastrointestinal tract and associated mesentery in the setting of non-rotation and non-fixation. The duodenojejunal flexure has not formed. The duodenum continues caudally into the right flank as the small bowel. The right colon and associated mesentery (i.e. contiguous with small intestinal mesentery) are positioned centrally with the transverse colon cephalad and the left colon in the normal location. The small bowel mesenteric pedicle is centered on the superior mesenteric pedicle and is thus narrowed. Of note, cessation of mesenteric and gastrointestinal rotation can occur at any stage such that a considerable variety of abnormalities intermediate between the normal and abnormal conformation (as depicted here) may arise. (Image created by Medical Illustration Department, University of Limerick, Ireland.)

- **Category one**: In this scenario, rotation proceeds through 90° then halts. At laparotomy, the following topography is observed. The second part of the duodenum continues caudad as the jejunum and the entire small bowel occupies a right-sided position with the ileocecal junction located medially (**Figure 4.3.1**). Hence a distinct duodenojejunal flexure of Treitz is not apparent as it did not form. In keeping with this, the right mesocolon is located medial to the small bowel mesentery and continues cephalad continuous with the transverse mesocolon. The latter is shortened in transverse extent (relative to that of the normal adult) and turns caudally at the splenic flexure to become contiguous with the left mesocolon. The left mesocolon is apposed to the posterior abdominal wall, and fixed in position. In this scenario, the entire small bowel is typically suspended from a narrow mesenteric pedicle containing the superior mesenteric artery. This, together with prominent duodenocolic adhesions, contribute to an increased risk of volvulus (**Figures 4.3.1** and **4.3.2**).
- **Category two**: Rotation continues through a further 270° and is followed by fixation. The normal adult mesenteric topography is observed in this setting (**Figure 4.3.1**). Although a detailed description of the resultant anatomic findings in the normal adult is beyond the scope of the current chapter, the key components should be described. The junction between the duodenum and jejunum forms the duodenojejunal flexure of Treitz. The small bowel mesentery is confluent with the right mesocolon around the ileocecal mesenteric confluence or flexure. The right and left mesocolon are apposed to the posterior abdominal wall and fixed in that position by Toldt's fascia. The mesosigmoid can be described as consisting of contiguous apposed and mobile components. The former is continuous with the left mesocolon (proximally). Both components converge to generate the mesorectum at the pelvic brim. In theory, rotation could halt at any point between 90° and 360° resulting in a broad range of possible mesenteric anomalies that are intermediate between categories one and two. Notwithstanding this, the left colon, sigmoid, and rectum invariably lie to the left and within the pelvis, respectively.
- **Category three**: Full rotation is not followed by mesenteric fixation. This occurs most frequently on the right side manifesting as a mobile ileocecal mesenteric confluence and right mesocolon. Incomplete fixation of the left mesocolon is less frequently observed. As a result of non-fixation, the ileocecal mesenteric confluence, which is normally located in the right iliac fossa, can occupy a more caudad or cephalad (sometimes subhepatic) position. Abnormalities of fixation can occur in isolation following normal rotational development. In fact, this is the most common manifestation of abnormalities of mesenteric development.
- **Category four**: This occurs when abnormal rotation is associated with incomplete fixation. These may coexist to variable degrees. As an example, the small bowel mesentery is observed located to the right side of a fully mobile right mesocolon. Immediately adjacent to the latter lies the left mesocolon which is also incompletely fixed and thus partially mobile. Increased mescolonic mobility and proximity is associated with prominent adhesion formation.

OBSERVATIONS RELATED TO ADHESIONS

A discussion related to congenital adhesions must be included at this point as these occur frequently in rotational abnormalities sometimes with disastrous sequelae. When two peritonealized structures come into frequent apposition, focal adhesions may develop that involve a condensation of peritoneum at these points. There are several normal variants of this in the healthy adult, the so-called 'congenital adhesions'. These should be listed to avoid interpretation as a developmental abnormality. They occur (1) in the left iliac fossa between the mesosigmoid and adjacent abdominal wall, (2) between the fourth part of the duodenum and the adjacent portions of the transverse and left mesocolon, (3) involving omentum and the cephalad aspect of the transverse mesocolon (thus semi-obliterating the lesser sac), and (4) involving omentum and appendices epiploicae. The process of adhesion development is problematic in the setting of rotational abnormalities given the proximity of mesenteric structures and serosal surfaces (see above under Disease status). A broad range of focal congenital adhesions can be observed between peritonealized omental, mesenteric, epiploical, mesocolonic, and somatic structures. In the setting of rotational abnormalities, the classic adhesions described include duodenocolic adhesions that extend from the second/third part of the duodenum to the ascending or transverse colon (**Figure 4.3.2**). These are divided in the Ladd's procedure (see below under Ladd's procedure).

ANESTHESIA

General anesthesia may be supplemented with an epidural catheter for narcotic and anxiolytic infusion during the postoperative interval.

OPERATION

The surgical management of rotational and/or fixation-related abnormalities may include gastrointestinal resection and anastomosis. As these are considered in detail elsewhere, technical strategies with specific relevance remain the focus here.

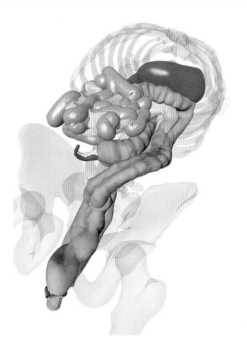

4.3.2 Digital sculpture demonstrating the conformational basis for possible sequelae in non-rotation. Proximity of the duodenum and colon facilitates the formation of duodenocolic adhesions that may constrict the duodenum. Once divided, the narrow small intestinal mesenteric pedicle is identified. This predisposes to volvulus and is addressed in the Ladd procedure through pexy and division of the peritoneum overlying the superior mesenteric artery. The stated aim is to 'broaden the mesenteric base' between small intestine and colon. Additional adhesions may occur between right and left colon that obscure the true mesenteric topography unless divided. (Image created by Medical Illustration Department, University of Limerick, Ireland.)

Surgical strategy

The primary aim is to delineate the true anatomic conformation of the intestine and associated mesenteries. The anatomic topography is dramatically different to that of the normal adult, such that a structured bottom-up approach is advocated firstly identifying anatomic constants. The proximity of peritonealized surfaces of the right, transverse, and left mesocolon is associated with adhesion formation. As a result, the non- or abnormally rotated topography of the cecocolic component of the gastrointestinal tract may remain unrecognized or obscured until these are divided. After identifying the appendix and ileocecal junction, one proceeds orally demonstrating the entirety of the small bowel, dividing adhesions between the latter and the lateral aspect of the right mesocolon. This process is repeated aborally to the rectosigmoid junction. Adhesion formation is generally prominent at the intersection between right, transverse, and left mesocolons. Fibrotic and adhesional processes can dramatically displace retroperitoneal fat and contained structures (i.e. ureters), such that these may be located on the lateral wall of the small bowel mesentery.

Thereafter, the surgical approach is predicted on managing the complications of abnormal rotation (i.e. torsion, intestinal ischemia/necrosis) and the prevention of future complications (i.e. broadening the mesenteric base, adhesiolysis, appendectomy, and pexy). Detorsion or reduction of the volvulus is performed in the counterclockwise direction, but requires that one firstly confirms oral and aboral anatomic constants as described above. The surgical management and techniques involved in dealing with ischemia/necrosis are dealt with elsewhere. In the absence of ischemia/necrosis, the operative strategy aims to reposition the small bowel and colon, as well as their respective mesenteric components with the least

likelihood of future volvulus. Some advocate repositioning mesenteric structures as near to normal as possible; however, this requires mesocolonic disruption. Included in the original Ladd procedure was a disruption of the peritoneum overlying the superior mesenteric artery. The aim was to broaden the base of the small intestinal mesentry in this location. An alternative that is reliable includes a pex procedure. Finally, most authors would also advocate an appendectomy.

Pex procedure

Unless a pex procedure is conducted, the risk of midgut volvulus is 24 percent.[1] Options for pexy include fixation of the cecum to either the right retroperitoneum or creation of a paravertebral gulley into which the right colon can be nested. Toldt's fascia is easily identified and provides a broad surface for pexy. Suture pexy is thus readily possible in that location. Estrada and Fitzgerald describe returning the duodenojejunal flexure to its normal anatomic location. This involves a disruption of mesocolon planes that is feasible but hazardous.[1] This approach has not been widely adopted.

Ladd's procedure

Ladd's bands represent 'abnormal peritoneal fixation bands'.[1] The classic Ladd's procedure involves lysis of duodenal, cecocolic, and small bowel adhesions to give the small intestinal mesentery a broad base (assisted by dividing the peritoneum overlying the small intestinal mesenteric pedicle) (**Figure 4.3.2**). The appendix is removed and the ascending colon is sutured alongside the descending and sigmoid colon, thereby securing the mesocolonic root and further volvulus.[4, 5] Cecopexy was not included in the original description.

LAPAROSCOPIC APPROACH

Laparoscopic appendectomy and duodenocolic dissociation (LADD) has been successfully used in the surgical management of abnormal rotation and fixation.[6,7] Laparoscopy provides a 20-fold magnified view of the gastrointestinal tract and mesentery. Magnification represents a drawback when diagnosing a non-rotation (more readily apparent on an overview) which is compounded by the proximity of the mesenteries and difficulty in ascertaining the position of the duodeno-jejunal juncture. When a rotational abnormality is diagnosed preoperatively, port site placement can be tailored to account for mesenteric proximity at the center of the peritoneal cavity. If conversion is anticipated, then port site incisions should be appropriately oriented.

DIVIDING THE FORESHORTENED MESENTERY

Both the right and transverse mesocolons are usually foreshortened in abnormal rotation. This presents problems in relation to hemostasis and adequate control of vascular pedicles. Dividing the mesentery between two clamps followed by overlapping suture ligation with a heavy and slowly absorbable suture (e.g. 1-0 chromic on a CTX needle) is a reliable means of ensuring hemostasis. This technique was initially popularized in hemostatic division of the difficult Crohn's mesentery.

ABNORMALITY OF ROTATION IDENTIFIED IN THE ONCOLOGIC SETTING

This is often the setting in which a rotational/fixation defect is encountered in the adult. Abnormalities of fixation facilitate mesenteric and mesocolonic mobilization according to oncologic principles. Non-rotation or partial rotation pose significant difficulties unless the true anatomic conformation is first confirmed. Conversion to an open procedure via a long midline laparotomy is likely the most appropriate approach in this circumstance. Given the topographic complexity of mesenteric structures, several anatomic points should be reiterated. As in the normal adult, the mesocolon is a continuous entity from small intestinal to mesorectal levels. It is separated from the retroperitoneum by Toldt's fascia. When a right hemicolectomy is planned, in the setting of abnormalities of rotation, a medial to lateral approach seems appropriate (there is no literature available that informs on this topic). Entry to the mesofascial or retrofascial planes is obtained by first freeing the right mesocolon from adhesions, then dividing the peritoneum where the mesocolon appears to become apposed to the retroperitoneum. Alternatively, access to the appropriate planes can be gained by dividing the peritoneum overlying the ileocecal mesenteric confluence. This anatomic constant is readily identified permitting rapid access to the appropriate plane for mesocolonic mobilization.

POSTOPERATIVE CARE

In the setting of an obstruction requiring resection, nasogastric aspiration should be maintained for an appropriate interval. Depending on the extent of adhesiolysis and mesenteric manipulation, this period can be quite variable. Supplemental nutrition may be considered if the postoperative ileus is prolonged. If gut viability was questionable, then a second-look laparotomy may be mandated. Clear liquids are reinstituted once the patient has passed flatus and has a soft, non-distended abdomen. The urinary catheter is normally removed on the second day, mobility permitting. Patients are usually suitable for surgical discharge 4–5 days after surgery.

REFERENCES

1. von Flue M, Herzog U, Ackermann C et al. Acute and chronic presentation of intestinal nonrotation in adults. *Diseases of the Colon and Rectum* 1994; **37**: 192–8.
2. Coffey JC. Surgical anatomy and anatomic surgery – clinical and scientific mutualism. *The Surgeon* 2013; 11(4): 177–82.
3. Culligan K, Walsh S, Dunne C, et al. The mesocolon: a histological and electron microscopic characterization of the mesenteric attachment of the colon prior to and after surgical mobilization. *Annals of Surgery* 2014; 260(6): 1048–56.
4. Ladd WE. Surgical diseases of the alimentary tract in adults. *New England Journal of Medicine* 1936; **215**: 705–8.
5. Ladd WE. Congenital obstruction of the duodenum in children. *New England Journal of Medicine* 1932; **206**: 273–83.
6. Fu T, Tong WD, He YJ et al. Surgical management of intestinal malrotation in adults. *World Journal of Surgery* 2007; **31**: 1797–803.
7. Lessin MS, Luks FI. Laparoscopic appendectomy and duodenocolonic dissociation (LADD) procedure for malrotation. *Pediatric Surgery International* 1998; **13**: 184–5.

Intestinal stricturoplasty

FEZA H REMZI

HISTORY

Between 50 and 70 percent of patients with Crohn's disease (CD) undergo surgery during their lifetime. Extensive surgical resection in these patients may result in development of short gut syndrome and associated nutritional deficiencies. After a successful report of stricturoplasty for multiple strictures involving the small intestine caused by tuberculosis,[1] stricturoplasty has become increasingly the preferred technique over extensive resection in patients affected by diffuse obstructive small bowel CD or in those with prior resections with impending short bowel syndrome.[2, 3, 4, 5, 6, 7, 8, 9]

PRINCIPLES AND JUSTIFICATION

When a stricture causes development of persistent bowel obstruction, treatment is necessary. Despite the successful reports after non-surgical treatment, surgery is warranted in most patients. Surgical procedures used for the treatment of strictures include dilatation, bypass, resection, and stricturoplasty. Stricturoplasty, a bowel-sparing surgery, should be considered in patients with aggressive disease, multiple short strictures, and those at risk of extensive loss of small bowel. The majority of studies showed comparable recurrence rates between stricturoplasty and bowel resection. Also, there have been many studies regarding safety and efficacy of stricturoplasty for CD.

Causes of strictures

Fibrostenotic CD is the most common cause of small bowel stricture. Other causes are ischemia following a bowel anastomosis, peptic ulcer disease, bilharzia, potassium salts, or non-steroidal anti-inflammatory drugs and tuberculosis.

INDICATIONS

CD patients presenting with severe recurrent symptoms of bowel obstruction along with weight loss or malnutrition need surgery. Stricturoplasty is not an option for all strictures. It can be considered for diffuse involvement of small bowel with multiple strictures, strictures in patients who had previous resections, anastomotic strictures that do not respond to dilatation, recurrent strictures causing bowel obstruction, strictures in patients with short bowel syndrome. Contraindications for stricturoplasty include short bowel segment affected by multiple strictures, phlegmon, internal or external fistula associated with the stricture site, small bowel perforation, colonic strictures, albumin level <2.0 g/dL, a stricture near resection site.

PREOPERATIVE ASSESSMENT AND PREPARATION

Although strictures can be detected on contrast radiographic studies and endoscopy, laparotomy is needed for definitive diagnosis. Hyperalimentation before surgery should be considered when the patient's nutritional status is compromised. Preoperative bowel preparation is avoided, because it may precipitate bowel obstruction. It is also prudent to mark patients preoperatively in case they may need a diverting stoma due to an associated phlegmon, need of multiple stricturoplasties, or suffer from severe malnutrition or anemia. Patients need to provide informed consent for a period of three to six months of hyperalimentation in the event of there being a need for a high jejunostomy in order to protect the suture lines resulting from multiple stricturoplasties.

OPERATION

The Heineke–Mikulicz procedure is the most preferred stricturoplasty for short-length strictures (<10 cm). Jaboulay stricturoplasty, side-to-side enteroenterostomy, can be performed for medium-length strictures. Finney stricturoplasty is performed with either the stapler or hand-sewn technique for 10–20 cm-long strictures. When the Finney procedure is not feasible or if bacterial overgrowth in the diverticulum created for the Finney procedure is a concern, Michelassi procedure, a side-to-side isoperistaltic enteroenterostomy, is an alternative for long-length strictures (≥20 cm).

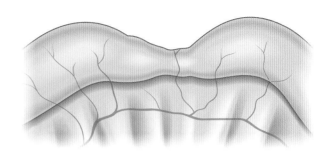

4.4.1

Heineke–Mikulicz procedure

A longitudinal enterotomy is made along the antimesenteric border of the stricture and two stay sutures are applied at the mid-point of the enterotomy.

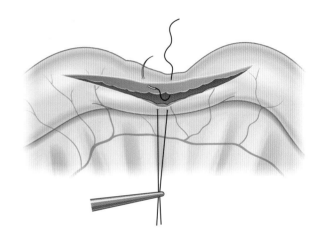

4.4.2

An ulcer may be seen at the site of the stricture. If so, a frozen-section biopsy should be performed to exclude malignancy and confirm the diagnosis.

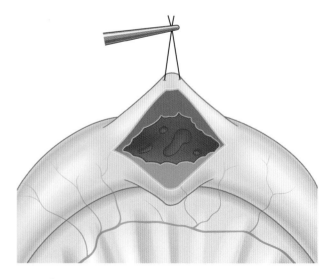

4.4.3

The index finger is used to detect other strictures.

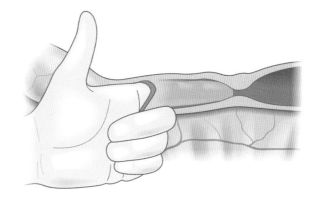

4.4.4

If another tight stricture is found, a new enterotomy is made.

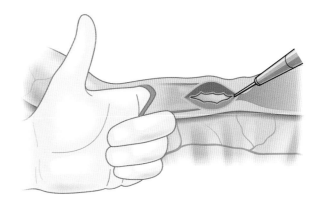

4.4.5

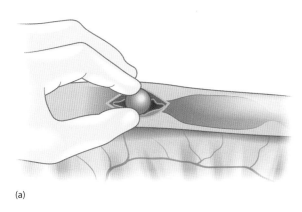

(a)

To look for more distant strictures, a 2.5 cm Bakelite ball can be inserted and passed through the small bowel up to the duodenum or down through the ileocecal valve.

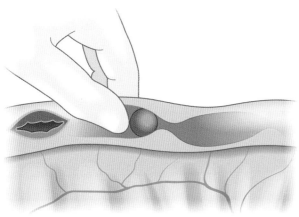

(b)

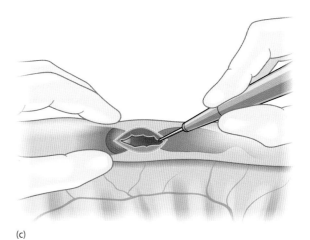

(c)

4.4.6

The procedure for closing the incision made for a short stricture using the Heineke–Mikulicz technique is to use two stay sutures to hold the edges together, while the anterior edges are anastomosed transversely using long-term absorbable sutures (2-0 or 3-0 polyglactin) in either a single or double layer in an interrupted fashion starting furthest away and working towards the surgeon.

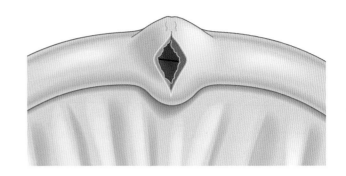

4.4.7

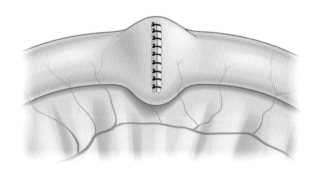

4.4.8

Stricturoplasty is then completed.

Finney procedure

In the hand-sewn Finney stricturoplasty, a stay suture is placed at the mid-point of the stricture. After the strictured area is folded over on to itself, a U-shaped enterotomy is created all the way through the stricture using a cautery. Another suture is applied on the normal side of the intestine to hold the U-shape in place. If there is a suspicion of malignancy, biopsy and frozen sections must be made.

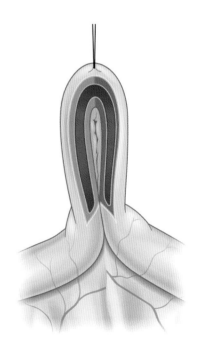

4.4.9

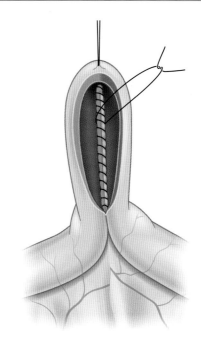

The posterior edges are sutured in a continuous fashion using long-term absorbable sutures.

4.4.10

To complete the procedure, anterior edges are sutured together using long-term absorbable sutures in one layer in an interrupted fashion.

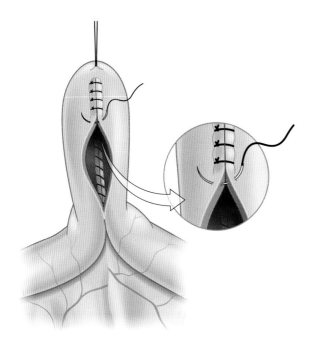

4.4.11

Michelassi procedure (the side-to-side isoperistaltic stricturoplasty)

The bowel segments affected by CD are approximated with a layer of interrupted seromuscular 3-0 polyglycolic acid sutures and then a longitudinal enterotomy is made on the antimesenteric border of each bowel segment.

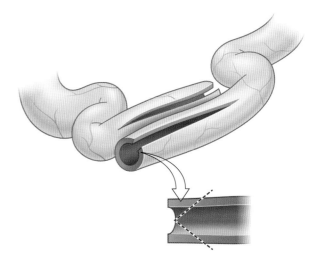

4.4.12

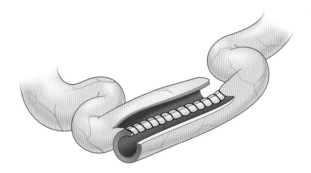

4.4.13

The inner suture line is then continued anteriorly and the outer suture line is closed. This layer is reinforced using interrupted seromuscular sutures and then the procedure is completed.

The inner layer of the posterior row is sutured using a continuous absorbable 3-0 polyglycolic acid suture material.

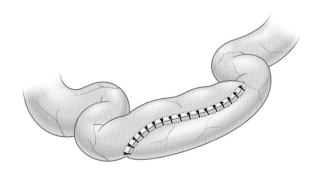

4.4.14

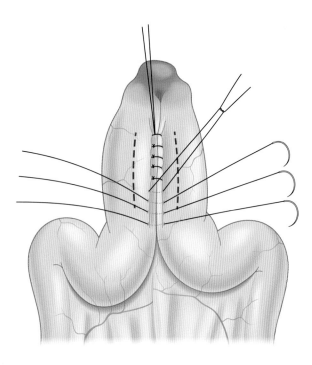

4.4.15

The inner layer of the posterior row of the stricturoplasty is sutured using a continuous absorbable 3-0 polyglycolic acid suture material.

Jaboulay procedure

In the hand-sewn technique, the strictured loop is first folded over on to itself. The posterior layer of stricturoplasty is created using interrupted 3-0 polyglycolic acid sutures. Incisions are made into small bowel loops using a cautery.

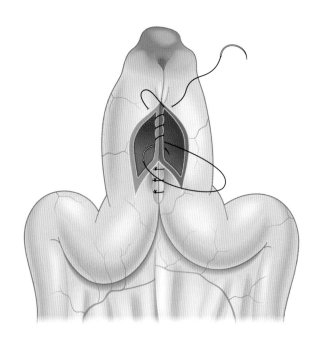

4.4.16

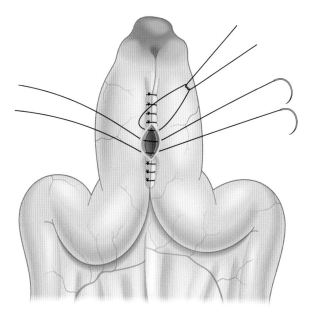

4.4.17

POSTOPERATIVE CARE

Complications

A meta-analysis of seven studies included 688 patients with CD undergoing stricturoplasty or bowel resection. The authors reported that patients undergoing stricturoplasty alone had a lower risk of development of the overall early postoperative complications than those undergoing resection, 12.7 percent in the stricturoplasty group and 19.1 percent in the resection group, although this difference was not statistically significant. Also, there was a similar trend in the development of bowel obstruction (2 versus 4.5 percent), intestinal hemorrhage (3 versus 6.7 percent), and septic complications (8.1 versus 11.2 percent) between the patients with stricturoplasty and those with bowel resection. Overall, postoperative mortality was 0.4 percent: one patient in the resection group and two in the stricturoplasty group.[7] In the meantime, it was reported that type of stricturoplasty was not predictive of postoperative complications.[8, 9]

OUTCOMES

Recurrence rate after stricturoplasty has been found to be comparable to that following bowel resection. In a recent study, Dietz et al.[8] reported 1124 stricturoplasties in 314 patients. With a median follow-up of 7.5 years, the recurrence rate was 34 percent which compares favorably with reported results of resective surgery. In the meantime, some studies reported that types of stricturoplasty performed did not influence recurrence[8,9] while others found a higher rate of recurrence following Finney or Jaboulay techniques compared to Heineke-Mikulicz

To complete the procedure, the anterior row is closed with a series of interrupted full-thickness non-absorbable sutures.

stricturoplasty.[4,6] However, a meta-analysis of 1825 stricturoplasties showed that the proportion of patients requiring additional surgery was decreased when a Finney stricturoplasty was used.[3]

CONCLUSION

Stricturoplasty can be safely performed in patients with fibrostenotic CD. It is associated with similar postoperative complication and recurrence rates compared with resective surgery.

REFERENCES

1. Katariya RN, Sood S, Rao PG, Rao PL. Stricture-plasty for tubercular strictures of the gastro-intestinal tract. *British Journal of Surgery* 1977; **64**: 496–8.
2. Michelassi F, Taschieri A, Tonelli F *et al.* An international, multicenter, prospective, observational study of the side-to-side isoperistaltic strictureplasty in Crohn's disease. *Diseases of the Colon and Rectum* 2007; **50**: 277–84.
3. Tichansky D, Cagir B, Yoo E *et al.* Strictureplasty for Crohn's disease: meta-analysis. *Diseases of the Colon and Rectum* 2000; **43**: 911–19.
4. Futami K, Arima S. Role of strictureplasty in surgical treatment of Crohn's disease. *Journal of Gastroenterology* 2005; **40** (Suppl. 16): 35–9.
5. Tonelli F, Ficari F. Strictureplasty in Crohn's disease: surgical option. *Diseases of the Colon and Rectum* 2000; **43**: 920–6.
6. Ayrizono M de L, Leal RF, Coy CS *et al.* Crohn's disease small bowel strictureplasties: early and late results. *Archives of Gastroenterology* 2007; **44**: 215–20.
7. Reese GE, Purkayastha S, Tilney HS *et al.* Strictureplasty vs resection in small bowel Crohn's disease: an evaluation of short-term outcomes and recurrence. *Colorectal Disease* 2007; **9**: 686–94.
8. Dietz DW, Laureti S, Strong SA *et al.* Safety and longterm efficacy of strictureplasty in 314 patients with obstructing small bowel Crohn's disease. *Journal of the American College of Surgeons* 2001; **192**: 330–7; discussion 337–8.
9. Dietz DW, Fazio VW, Laureti S *et al.* Strictureplasty in diffuse Crohn's jejunoileitis: safe and durable. *Diseases of the Colon and Rectum* 2002; **45**: 764–70.

Adhesiolysis

BRUCE P WAXMAN

DEFINITIONS AND SCOPE

Adhesiolysis refers to the operative procedure involving the division of adhesions. Adhesions form when a fibrous band or sheath of fibrosis develops between two mesothelial surfaces in the peritoneal cavity following injury and subsequent repair. The mesothelial injury may be either mechanical, usually caused by the surgeon, such as incisions, lacerations, contusion, abrasions, or tearing, or non-mechanical, such as that caused by heat (diathermy or laser), sepsis, ischemia, malignancy, foreign body reaction, inflammatory reaction, or irradiation. Adhesions may form anywhere in the peritoneal cavity, but our attention here will be focused on those involving the small bowel (**Figure 4.5.1**). A discussion of the pathogenesis of adhesions is outside the scope of this chapter.

In this chapter, the focus will be on those adhesions that have occurred after previous surgery, and the content will be confined to those related to the small bowel that may be encountered by general or colorectal surgeons rather than the pelvic adhesions involving the female reproductive organs, which are the subject of the vast majority of the literature on adhesiolysis.[1]

The operative procedure of adhesiolysis can be performed either by open surgery or laparoscopically. The majority of this chapter will focus on open adhesiolysis and the different techniques a surgeon can employ to deal with this challenging problem. Adhesions have been shown to develop in up to 93 percent of surgical patients, and the rate of complications related to adhesions is high with significant long-term consequences.[2] The volume of adhesions increases with the complexity and number of previous abdominal operations.

This chapter therefore outlines the general principles, and highlights some of the author's particular preferences of patient selection and operative techniques. The emphasis is on open adhesiolysis with some mention of laparoscopic techniques.

PREOPERATIVE

Disease status

Adhesiolysis is performed either in the emergency or elective setting determined by the clinical presentation. In the emergency setting, the diagnosis is usually small bowel obstruction where the patient has had previous abdominal surgery. Occasionally, adhesions may be encountered in patients with a 'virgin' abdomen. In the elective setting, adhesions will be encountered in any re-entry of the abdomen for procedures on the bowel or other organs, but there are two specific clinical scenarios which I refer to as the complex abdomen. One is the patient with chronic abdominal pain who has had multiple previous surgeries and, by definition, will have adhesions, and the objective of the surgery is to divide the adhesions in the hope that this

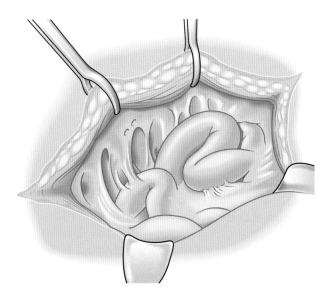

4.5.1

may improve the chronic abdominal pain. In this clinical setting, the operation should only be undertaken once the patient has been referred to and developed a professional relationship with a chronic pain management specialist as the key to managing this type of chronic abdominal pain is a combination of surgery, medication, and psychological support. The second clinical setting is the patient with recurrent episodes of small bowel obstruction where the objective of the operation is to divide the adhesions to prevent further obstruction. In this setting, a pre-operative CT enteroclysis is useful in establishing the presence of the dilated small bowel and the possibility of a line of transition between dilated and collapsed small bowel to allow a focused dissection of adhesions. More often is the case that a specific cut-off point is not demonstrated.[3]

It is preferable to thoroughly assess the disease status before proceeding with surgery as conservative measures can sometimes avoid the need for a lengthy and complex operation.

Patient status

Adhesiolysis remains a major undertaking and a major challenge, with the potential for significant morbidity, particularly if an inadvertent enterotomy should occur. The surgeon must assess each patient for reversible conditions such as anemia, dehydration, electrolyte imbalance, malnutrition, and medications that affect coagulation. Medical diseases such as diabetes, hypertension, cardiac and pulmonary disease should be well controlled and under the care of a medical physician or internist. A detailed history of pre-existing gastrointestinal dysfunction and/or a history of previous abdominal and bowel surgery is vital to ascertain the potential for any distal obstruction that may occur following adhesiolysis and/or bowel resection. Contacting and speaking with the surgeon, if possible, who has performed any previous surgery is helpful. Remember most of these are elective, and good preparation and obtaining as much information about the patient are the keys to success.

Surgeon status

Adhesiolysis in the complex abdomen is an operation that should be performed by experienced surgeons who have had formal training in general surgery and preferably colorectal surgery and have made a commitment to managing such patients not only in this operation but in the long term. Ideally, the operation should be performed by two surgeons with the above-mentioned qualifications, alternatively a senior and a junior surgeon, as often intraoperative decisions need to be made that benefit from the knowledge of another trained and experienced mind. The surgeon must also allocate sufficient time on the operating list as these cases may extend to more than 4 hours. It goes without saying that the surgeon should be well rested, aware of the principles of sleep hygiene, in good health, free of any prior engagements that day, and most importantly, free of any distractions, because this is tedious and challenging surgery that requires commitment and concentration. In addition, it is important to plan a break every 2 hours.

Infection

The presence of sepsis within the abdomen in combination with the operation for adhesiolysis adds an extra dimension to the complexity of the procedure and mandates the formation of a stoma in combination with adequate drainage, antibiotics, and peritoneal lavage.

Renal failure, diabetes, and immunosuppresion

Ideally, it is best for these medical issues to be under control before one proceeds with the operation of adhesiolysis. However, sometimes the situation is such that surgery becomes necessary. If such medical conditions pre-exist, then a conservative approach to the operation is best. Should an enterotomy or bowel resection be required, then a stoma is mandatory and abdominal wound management is best done either by fascia closure and leaving the skin open with a vacuum dressing or laparostomy.

Ureteric stents and female pelvic organs

When adhesions are predominantly in the pelvis following previous surgery, such as a Hartmann's resection, or in the context of previous complex pelvic surgery, performance of a cystoscopy and insertion of ureteric stents, with the aid of a urologist is recommended to aid in the identification of ureters and bladder. Adhesions of small bowel on to the uterus, Fallopian tubes, and ovaries encountered in the complex abdomen can be dealt with by an adequately trained general surgeon without the need for input from a gynecologist, unless there is gynecological malignancy when the advice and assistance of a gynecological oncologist is recommended.

Stomas

Having the patient assessed by an enterostomal therapy nurse preoperatively is recommended for siting of any stoma and postoperative management of a planned stoma or fistula. Enterostomal therapy nurses will also be involved in the management of the patient's abdominal wound or fistula following surgery. It is reassuring for the patient to develop a good relationship preoperatively, usually in the pre-anesthetic clinic.

Bowel preparation

This is not usually necessary.

ANESTHESIA AND INTENSIVE CARE (ICU/HDU)

Patients have a general anesthetic and muscle relaxation with or without an epidural, and as the operation is prolonged and the postoperative course may be complicated, ideally a central venous catheter and an arterial line should be inserted as well as an indwelling urinary catheter. Preoperative assessment by an anesthetist is essential with a planned admission to the ICU/HDU

postoperatively. The WHO Surgical Safety Checklist should be followed, which will include prophylactic antibiotics and deep vein thrombosis prophylaxis, the latter requiring chemoprophylaxis and the use of intermittent calf compression. Additional antibiotics will need to be given if the length of the operation exceeds 3 hours. Other factors relevant to reducing surgical site infection, such as maintenance of normothermia, adequate oxygenation, and control of blood pressure and blood sugar levels are mandatory. Because pain management is a common postoperative problem, these patients should be managed in consultation with the acute pain management team or the pain team that has been involved with their previous pain control regimen.

OPERATION

Patient position

The patient is placed in the modified Lloyd-Davies (lithotomy) position with the legs supported by Allen stirrups or similar leggings. The author finds that this position has many advantages, in particular for better access for all members of the operating team. The advantages are that it allows the scrub nurse, third assistant, or the surgeon to gain access to the patient between the legs, the last for dealing with difficult adhesions or dissection in the supracolic compartment particularly around the left upper quadrant, the region of the splenic flexure and/or spleen. Moreover, in some situations access to the anus and rectum is required and occasionally to the female genital tract. Needless to say, for a urologist to perform a cystoscopy and insertion of urinary catheters, this position is vital and for this reason the patient should also be placed on a table allowing for intraoperative radiology.

Preparation and draping

The author's preference is to palpate the abdomen with the patient asleep and relaxed to assess mass lesions or other intra-abdominal pathology. The incision is marked with an indelible pen identifying any old scars which will be excised and with cross-hatchings added to aid in skin closure, as well as clarifying the stoma sites identified by the stoma therapist. The author always wears a headlight to provide additional illumination which is particularly useful in the deep parts of the abdominal cavity. After skin preparation and draping, three irrigation bags are placed on each side and between the legs and a plastic incisive drape over the top encompassing the sterile drapes and the irrigation bags. Diathermy and suckers are attached and a two-way urology style giving set (Baxter® Cysto-Bladder irrigation

set) with warm Hartmann's solution set-up to aid in irrigation, which is a significant principle of the operative technique, hence the need for the irrigation bags.

Incision and re-entry

As all patients will have had previous surgery, the old scar is excised and the incision extended, preferably to the area of the abdominal skin above or occasionally below the extent of the previous scar. This will be the site used for entering the peritoneal cavity after dividing the fascia. The author prefers using diathermy throughout the dissection of abdominal skin subcutaneous fat and fascia. Skin flaps are developed at this stage on each side to aid in fascial closure at the end of the intraperitoneal part of the operation.

The abdomen is entered usually in the upper one-third of the abdomen which is often free of adhesions. If not, then careful dissection is undertaken. Once the fascia has been divided, the author reduces the level of the diathermy to 20 and continues dissection with diathermy into the peritoneal cavity. Use of artery forceps on the peritoneum and Morrison tissue forceps on the fascia aid in elevating the abdomen upwards, and the small bowel will fall away. Should small bowel be encountered stuck to the fascia, then one should move elsewhere in the line of the incision to gain entry to the peritoneal cavity free of small bowel. If this is not possible, then the dissection of the small bowel must commence at the level of the incision, by techniques as discussed below.

Exploration and adhesiolysis

The objective of the operation of adhesiolysis is to divide all adhesions from the duodenojejunal (DJ) flexure to the ileocecal valve (ICV). The reason is to divide all adhesions, but more importantly, that should an inadvertent enterotomy occur requiring repair, it is vital that there is no distal obstruction as the back pressure will inevitably lead to the breakdown of the repair and a leak and small bowel fistula.

Mesh and adhesions

In the complex case when mesh is encountered in the abdominal wound or elsewhere, it is the author's preference to remove all the mesh. Moreover, with small bowel stuck to the mesh then dissection is best done with the irrigation technique with sharp dissection (see below) 'shaving' the bowel from the mesh. The combination of an inadvertent enterotomy and mesh is a formula for fistula. This is less likely with all the mesh excised. The resultant fascial defect may require a component separation repair of the abdominal wound.

Techniques of adhesiolysis

SHARP DISSECTION WITH IRRIGATION

The author believes in the technique of sharp dissection[4] using a No. 10 scalpel blade in combination with irrigation and has developed an irrigating scalpel that combines an irrigating cannula attached to a No. 7 handle with a No. 10 blade that delivers warm Hartmann's solution over the cutting surface of the blade. Hartmann's solution is preferred as it is a buffered liquid and reduces rusting of the scalpel blade.

The irrigating scalpel is not vital to perform sharp dissection with irrigation. The alternative is to set-up the irrigating system as mentioned above with a mixing cannula at the end running warm Hartmann's solution over the area of dissection. This technique will require two assistants, one holding the irrigation system and retracting the wound and the second maintaining tension on the bowel (**Figure 4.5.2**). The advantages of the technique of sharp dissection with irrigation are:

- the operating field is kept clear from blood and other fluids providing good vision;
- creates an artificial edema which allows demarcation of tissue planes particularly between loops of small bowel;
- uses the principle of hydrodissection with gentle fluid pressure to aid in further dissection and separating tissues;[5]
- provides replacement of extra fluid losses during a lengthy abdominal surgery;
- potentially reduces the incidence of inadvertent enterotomy (the author's experience in 100 consecutive cases for re-entry surgery and division of adhesions using the irrigation technique is an enterotomy rate of 16 percent).[6,7]

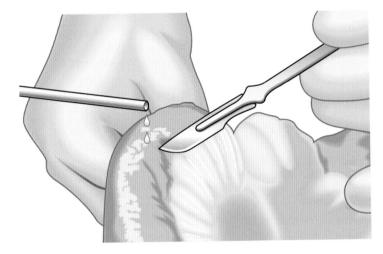

4.5.2

DISSECTION WITH SCISSORS OR DIATHERMY

Dissecting and dividing adhesions with scissors is the most popular technique with surgeons using Metzenbaum scissors, with some preferring the more robust curved Mayo scissors (**Figure 4.5.3**a). There is a potential for harm with the long-handled Metzenbaum when using the 'opening' technique to develop a plane as excessive traction forces may be applied to the tissues by virtue of the mechanical advantage effect created by the long handles and short blades with the fulcrum closer to the blades, which may result in tissues being torn, especially the friable bowel wall (**Figure 4.5.3**b). Using the scissors closed in a pushing manner may be as effective. The author uses scissors for dissection deep in the pelvis but, again, will use an irrigation technique with a pool sucker in close proximity. The author uses diathermy in preference to scissors for superficial easy accessible adhesions as the heat generated by the diathermy opens up tissue planes, with similar principles to irrigation, in that the gas can open up the planes between loops of small bowel and aid with better visualization of the serosa of the bowel in the dissection process.[4]

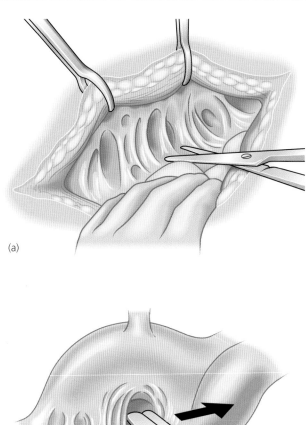

(a)

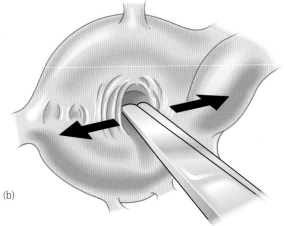

(b)

4.5.3

Assistance, traction and operative strategy

It is vital for the surgeon to have at least one trained assistant ideally a trained surgeon, and for there to be good exposure and adequate illumination. The author always wears a headlight which has significant advantages over the lights provided in the operating theater, particularly in the pelvis and in the left upper quadrant.

The importance of the assistant providing tension allows the use of traction and the development of vector forces in the identification of the adhesion and its division.

The author suggests a strategy of moving from one site to another when dissection becomes difficult, particularly when there has been previous infection or inflammation causing dense scarring. It is best to move away to an area where the adhesions are less difficult and later move back

to the difficult area as you may have been able to develop another plane or angle. Indeed, it is often useful to twist the bowel through 180° and dissect on the other side of the bowel, namely, on the mesenteric side rather than the anti-mesenteric side which will develop new planes and make the dissection easier. In addition, moving from one side of the operating table to the other not only gives the surgeon a break from the tedium of dissection, but provides a fresh approach and angle to the dissection.

The author is right handed and uses his left hand to help develop planes by blunt dissection and uses the index and thumb to finger dissect, 'pinching' the adhesions, sometimes called 'finger fracturing' the tissues, adjacent to the bowel to create a clear plane. He will often dissect down onto the left index finger using it as a solid background to dissect against, avoiding bowel injury.

Serosal tears, inadvertent enterotomy, and small bowel resection

The essential principle of adhesiolysis is getting in the correct plane and maintaining the intactness of the serosa. If small defects of the serosa occur these do not need repair, as they may create ischemic tissue and be the source of future adhesions. However, if what is often referred to as the 'stripe sign' is seen, this means that the inner circular muscle of the small bowel has been exposed and very soon the mucosa will appear leading to a full-thickness tear. Once the stripe sign is encountered, dissection should stop and restart at another site.

Should an inadvertent enterotomy occur, then this must be repaired at once, as it may be forgotten. The author's preference is interrupted 3-0 polydioxanone (PDS) sutures. Alternatively, the area is isolated with non-crushing bowel clamps and the rest of the dissection continues. Other inadvertent enterotomies may occur, and these can be encompassed in a small bowel resection including all enterotomies, always being aware to preserve as much small bowel as possible.

For small bowel resection and anatomosis, the author prefers an end-to-end anatomosis with a single-layer continuous technique using 3-0 PDS, 3-0 poly-propylene markers at each corner and Weck clips to identify the site of the anatomosis for subsequent identification radiologically. If multiple anastomoses are performed, then the number of Weck clips is increased with each anastomosis. When performing the anastomosis however, the author does use an irrigation technique with the same giving set and mixing cannula to improve the visualization of the layers of the bowel wall, and then just before completing the anastomosis performs intraluminal insufflation of the bowel, with soft bowel clamps on either side of the anastomosis, to test the integrity of the anastomosis.

Once adhesiolysis has been completed, it is vital to run the small bowel from the DJ flexure to the ICV to check that there are no inadvertent enterotomies or serosal tears. The author has not found any benefit of insufflating the small bowel with carbon dioxide or other techniques to test for inadvertent enterotomy. The length of the small bowel is measured with a sterile ruler to adequately document the length of small bowel remaining. Most patients will be able to maintain adequate nutrition with at least 100 cm of small bowel.

Barriers and solutions to prevent adhesions

Before abdominal closure and after extensive adhesiolysis, one should contemplate the use of a barrier or a solution to prevent further adhesions by reducing apposition of serosal surfaces for a period of time during which adhesions may form.[8] It is beyond the scope of this chapter to discuss the pathophysiology of adhesion formation. The most commonly used barrier is Seprafilm® and at least one study has shown that this reduces the incidence of adhesions and small bowel obstruction.[9] The author finds it difficult to use, particularly in abdominal closure, which is discussed later. Barrier sprays have been developed but have been withdrawn from the market. The use of solutions, e.g. Adept®, has gained in popularity recently, particularly as they are simple to use as they can be poured into the peritoneal cavity at the time of abdominal closure. The author's preference is not to use a barrier or solutions if an anastomosis has been performed. The topic of preventing adhesions is outside the scope of this chapter.

Abdominal closure

Following lavage of the peritoneal cavity with warm saline solution, the fascia and skin are closed. Drain tubes may be placed in the peritoneal cavity if there is an indication. They are best avoided. The author uses a bowel protector in the shape of a fish, made of a soft polymer, placed between loops of bowel and the fascia to protect the bowel while sutures are placed in the fascia. Should adhesive barriers be used unfortunately they stick to the 'fish' and may come out when the fish is removed. Should an adhesive barrier be used, then closure will require complete relaxation in the abdominal wall and cooperation with the anesthetist so that the fascia can be tented up away from the bowel to allow closure without interfering with the adhesive barrier. In the majority of cases, the author uses a continuous absorbable monofilament material (loop PDS). The subcutaneous tissues are then lavaged with saline and the skin closed with interrupted 3-0 nylon sutures and staples. The sutures are held up with artery forceps allowing easier placement of the staples and also maintenance of skin closure after the staples are removed. When it has been necessary to remove mesh and/or a significant fascial defect is present, then a components separation technique is preferred. Laparostomy is the last resort, and although the safest approach, it is a problem with exposed anastomoses with the potential for enterocutaneous fistulae.

POSTOPERATIVE CARE

Ideally, this will occur in the ICU/HDU. The author does not use nasogastric tubes but introduces a fluid diet early and believes in the philosophy of fast tracking (ERAS, early recovery after surgery). Should postoperative ileus develop, which is common, the early introduction, after 7 days, of total parenteral nutrition through a central venous line or peripherally inserted central catheter is recommended. Postoperative pain management is a significant problem and it is best to involve the acute pain service, intensivist, and/or the chronic pain management consultant who will be aware of the patient from preoperative counseling.

The surgeon must be vigilant during the postoperative period, always anticipating the possibility of an anastomotic leak or the breakdown of the small bowel at a serosal tear or repair of an enterotomy. Should the patient's condition deteriorate and require exploratory surgery, particularly in the context of a leaking anastomosis or a fistula, the author highly recommends the formation of a laparostomy and the application of an 'irrigating dressing' involving a large stoma or plastic bag, covering the whole wound with stoma adhesive around the wound edges with saline irrigation at one end of the bag and light pressure suction at the other. This is particularly useful for the management of enterocutaneous fistulae. Alternatively, one could use a vacuum dressing but it is the author's experience that, with a fistula, the canister becomes blocked and this makes the system inefficient.

LAPAROSCOPIC ADHESIOLYSIS

Laparoscopic surgery is now the accepted standard of practice in abdominal surgery and so has its uses in performing adhesiolysis. This is particularly the case in gynecological surgery where pelvic adhesiolysis is performed almost exclusively laparoscopically. The principles of laparoscopic surgery are discussed elsewhere.

There are significant risks of re-entering the abdominal cavity through an old scar to establish a pneumoperitoneum. Great care must be taken in Hasson cannula insertion to avoid injury to bowel adjacent to or adherent to the umbilicus (**Figure 4.5.4**). The other risk in laparoscopic surgery, in particular extensive adhesions, is that one cannot visualize all bowel loops and when dissecting with diathermy there is increased risk of inadvertent diathermy injury to the small bowel or other organs. It is always safer to open than persist with laparoscopic dissection in a maze of adhesions. The principles for laparoscopic adhesiolysis are similar to open adhesiolysis, in particular that the surgeon is well trained and has had significant experience with laparoscopic colorectal surgery and is accompanied by a well-trained assistant and nursing staff who are compliant and well trained in the use of laparoscopic equipment.[10]

It is beyond the scope of this chapter to provide a detailed description of laparoscopic adhesiolysis.

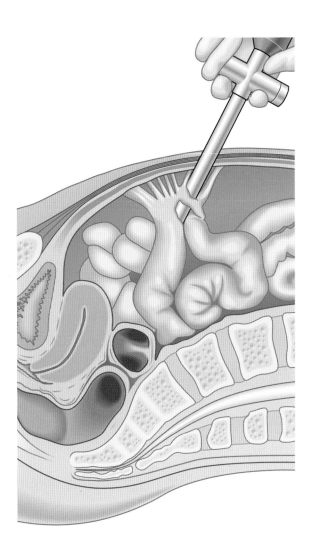

4.5.4

REFERENCES

1. www.adhesiolysis.org.

2. Ellis H, Moran BJ, Thompson JN *et al.* Adhesion-related hospital readmissions after abdominal and pelvic surgery: a retrospective cohort study. *Lancet* 1999; **353**: 1476–80.

3. Delabrousse E, Destrumelle N, Brunelle S *et al.* CT of small bowel obstruction in adults. *Abdominal Imaging* 2003; **28**: 257–66.

4. Fabri PJ, Rosemurgy A. Reoperation for small bowel obstruction. *Surgical Clinics of North America* 1991; **70**: 131–46.

5. Bokey EL, Keating JP, Zelas P. Hydro-dissection: an easy way to dissect anatomical planes and complex adhesions. *ANZ Journal of Surgery* 1997; **67**: 643–4.

6. Waxman BP, Carne P, Hensman C. Irrigation technique for division of adhesions and description of a modified scalpel. *Diseases of the Colon and Rectum* 1999; **42**: A19–20.

7. van der Krabben AA, Dijkstra FR, Nieuwenhuijzen M *et al.* Morbidity and mortality of inadvertent enterotomy during adhesiosiotomy. *British Journal of Surgery* 2000; **87**: 467–71.

8. Waxman BP. Can adhesions be prevented? *ANZ Journal of Surgery* 2000; **70**: 399–400.

9. Beck DE, Cohen Z, Fleshman JW. A prospective, randomised, multicenter, controlled study of the safety of Seprafilm® adhesion barrier in abdominopelvic surgery of the intestine. *Diseases of the Colon and Rectum* 2003; **46**: 1310–19.

10. Zerey M, Sechrist CW, Kercher KW. Laparoscopic management of adhesive small bowel obstruction. *American Journal of Surgery* 2007; **73**: 773–8.

Colon

Appendicectomy – open

GRAHAM L NEWSTEAD AND MARK D MUHLMANN

HISTORY

The first known case of surgical removal of the appendix occurred in 1735 by Claudius Amyand in London. It was not until 1886, however, after Reginald H Fitz read his paper to the first meeting of the Association of American Physicians in Washington DC, that the early surgical removal of the appendix became the standard treatment for appendiceal inflammation.[1] For over 100 years, the technique of open appendicectomy remained the gold standard. It allowed a safe, relatively simple way for removal of the appendix and it has been a procedure that new surgical trainees used to acquire basic surgical skills. In the 1990s, a laparoscopic approach to the appendix was popularized and is now often the preferred approach allowing some diagnostic and therapeutic benefits.[2] A recent Cochrane review[3] cited laparoscopic advantages to be decreased postoperative pain, decreased hospital stay, earlier return to work, and less wound infections, although at the expense of increased intra-abdominal abscesses. However, open appendicectomy remains a valid option especially in centers where laparoscopic expertise is unavailable and where the benefits would be minimal, such as in thin males where there is no diagnostic uncertainty and also possibly in children.[4]

PRINCIPLES AND JUSTIFICATION

Indications and contraindications

Appendicectomy should be carried out as soon as a clinical diagnosis of appendicitis is made. When the presentation is atypical, a computed tomography (CT) scan or ultrasound, or indeed diagnostic laparoscopy, may be helpful.

The differential diagnosis for appendicitis is wide, but most commonly includes mesenteric adenitis in children (which should delay surgery only if signs are minimal and hospitalization allows continuous reassessment), infective gastroenteritis, urinary tract infection, and gynecological pathology (which may warrant pelvic ultrasonography). In particular, pregnancy should be excluded in all cases to eliminate ectopic pregnancy.

There are no absolute contraindications to open appendicectomy, but consideration of a laparoscopic approach is relevant especially in women and the obese.

Masked diagnosis

Retrocecal appendicitis may be more severe than apparent on palpation due to the dilated cecum acting as a buffer between the inflamed appendix and the anterior abdominal wall.

Appendicitis in a long retrocecal appendix or with a cecum situated high in the right hypochondrium may mimic acute cholecystitis. A long intrapelvic appendix may present as a pelvic abscess and be confused with tubo-ovarian pathology in women.

Particular care must be taken in elderly and immunocompromised patients, in whom the clinical signs of appendicitis may be masked, as may the diagnosis.

Special situations

An appendiceal mass should usually be treated conservatively with antibiotics and bowel rest. Subsequent investigation with colonoscopy and CT scan is appropriate and possible interval appendicectomy carried out.

Appendicitis during pregnancy is managed best by early appendicectomy. Miscarriage and early onset labor are unusual with surgery which is safest in the second trimester.

Consent

Consent should be obtained with discussion of the general risks of surgery and anesthesia with specific mention of postoperative wound infection, intra-abdominal abscesses and the possibility of finding alternative pathology requiring extension of the incision or making a midline incision.

PREOPERATIVE ASSESSMENT AND PREPARATION

Intravenous fluid should be administered and the patient adequately rehydrated especially if vomiting has been a prominent feature. A single dose of preoperative broad-spectrum antibiotics is given to cover aerobic and anaerobic organisms and should be continued if significant peritonitis or perforation is found. The entire abdomen is shaved to allow for a midline incision in cases where it is required. Prevention of deep vein thrombosis is of paramount importance. Measures, including early mobilization and antiembolism stockings, are mandatory with use of subcutaneous sodium heparin or low molecular weight heparin used in appropriate patients. Indwelling urinary catheters and nasogastric tubes are not routinely used, but should be used in patients with generalized peritonitis.

ANESTHESIA

A fasting time of 6 hours for solids and 2 hours for fluids is preferred. General anesthesia is used with endotracheal intubation and muscle relaxation.

OPERATION

Position of the patient

The patient is placed in the supine position. Calf compressors are used, if available, in adults. An adhesive diathermy pad is applied to the patient's thigh.

Preparation of abdomen

The entire abdomen is prepared with a Betadine or chlorhexidine solution to allow extension or change of incision if required. The right lower quadrant is square draped to also allow access to the midline and the right flank above the anterior iliac crest.

Incision

The abdomen should be palpated before anesthesia to determine the point of maximal tenderness. The abdomen is palpated again following anesthesia and muscle relaxation to facilitate palpation of a mass. These factors, as well as concern for cosmesis, will determine the area over which the incision should be placed. The classic incision is the grid iron. This involves an oblique skin incision in the line of fibers of external oblique centered over McBurney's point. This is the point at the junction of the lateral third and medial two-thirds of a line passing from the anterosuperior iliac spine to the umbilicus, the classic surface marking for the base of the appendix. The preferred incision may be a transverse incision in the skin crease line starting approximately 2 cm medial to the iliac crest. A midline incision is appropriate for generalized peritonitis or when a large mass is palpated. If laparoscopy has been performed initially and a decision then made to convert to open surgery, the optimal position for the incision can be determined by palpating the abdominal wall over the position of the appendix, while observing the laparoscopic monitor (**Figure 5.1.1**).

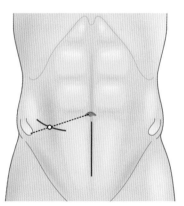

5.1.1

Incising the aponeurosis of the external oblique muscle

The skin is incised and the subcutaneous fatty tissue and Scarpa's fascia are incised. The superficial circumflex and superficial epigastric veins, if seen, can usually be dealt with by diathermy. The skin and fat are retracted, and a small incision is made in the lateral aspect of the fibers of the external oblique aponeurosis. A pair of scissors with the jaws opened a little is then pushed in the direction of the fibers, downwards and medially to their insertion into the anterior surface of the rectus sheath (**Figure 5.1.2**).

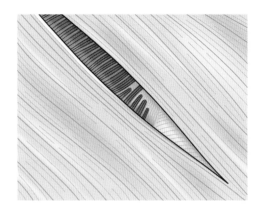

5.1.2

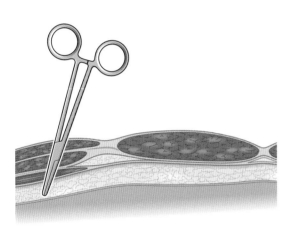

5.1.3

The internal oblique and transversus abdominis muscles

The fleshy muscle fibers of the internal oblique pass upwards and medially to insert into the anterior aspect of the lateral edge of the rectus sheath. An incision is made in the line of the most medial fibers, which are split by blunt dissection with scissors or artery forceps to separate them. Small intermuscular vessels can be secured by diathermy. Forceps are then used to split the transverse fibers of the transversus abdominis muscle, which insert into the lateral edge of the rectus sheath. These muscle fibers are similarly split. The wound retractors are replaced to include these muscle layers.

An alternative approach to the traditional muscle splitting is often used. Here the fibers of the lateral edge of the rectus sheath are incised. The fleshy body of rectus abdominis is then retracted medially and with lateral retraction; as well direct access into the preperitoneal space is achieved without splitting muscle (**Figure 5.1.3**).

Opening the peritoneum

The preperitoneal fat covering the peritoneum is gently cleared by blunt dissection and the peritoneum is grasped with an artery forceps. The tissue held by the forceps is inspected to ensure that no intestine has been trapped and a second pair of forceps is applied and further inspection made. The peritoneum between the forceps is incised along the line of skin incision for a small distance to allow inspection of the peritoneal cavity, again to ensure that no intestine has been inadvertently included. At this stage, turbid fluid may be seen. A sample may be taken for culture. It is a good idea to place a sump sucker into the peritoneal cavity to remove the fluid before major contamination of the wound edges occurs (**Figure 5.1.4**).

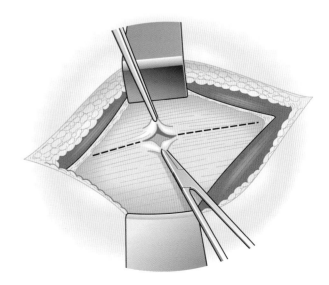

5.1.4

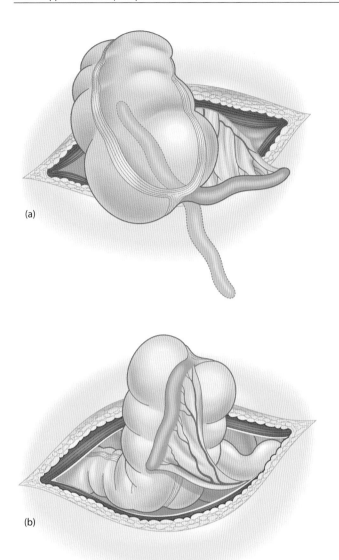

(a)

(b)

Identification and delivery of the appendix

The appendix has a highly variable location including being located in retrocecal, retroileal, or pelvic position. The index finger is placed in the peritoneal cavity to feel the inflamed appendix and to gently deliver it out of the wound. This is often difficult due to a retrocecal lie of the appendix and inflammatory adhesions. The key to finding the appendix is to locate the cecum and tracing a tenia to the point where the three teniae converge at the base of the appendix. Babcock's forceps can be placed on the tenia to allow traction to achieve delivery of the appendix; however, care should be taken to avoid serosal tears to the cecum. Serial placement of Babcock's forceps will allow the appendix to be delivered. Vascular adhesions will often need dividing to allow delivery. If this step remains difficult, do not be afraid to extend the wound to gain adequate exposure (**Figure 5.1.5**a,b). Retrograde appendicectomy may be required if access is still difficult (see below under Special circumstances).

5.1.5

Exploration of the peritoneal cavity

If the appendix is found to be normal, the index finger should be passed into the pelvis, particularly in women, to examine the right Fallopian tube and ovary. With wound retraction, it may be possible to place a Babcock's forceps on the round ligament to allow visual inspection. In smaller patients, the left Fallopian tube and ovary may be digitally assessed. The terminal ileum should be delivered, inspected, and returned segment by segment until the distal 60 cm of ileum have been assessed to exclude ileal disease and a Meckel's diverticulum. The mesentery should also be checked for lymphadenopathy as found in mesenteric adenitis (**Figure 5.1.6**).

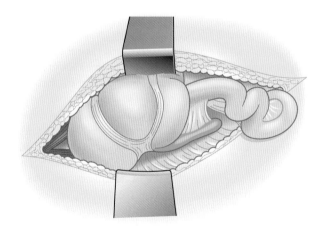

5.1.6

Division of the mesoappendix

The appendiceal artery arises from a posterior branch of the ileocolic artery. Branches of the appendiceal artery then run through the mesoappendix towards the appendix. To gain adequate exposure to it, the peritoneal fold beneath the cecum may need division to provide adequate mobilization. The appendix is displayed between one pair of Babcock's forceps at the tip and another near the base. Small windows are developed at the junction of the mesentery and the appendix using diathermy or artery forceps. The resultant pedicles containing the branches of the appendiceal vessels are ligated and divided. If the mesentery is thick, edematous, or short, stitch ties may be required (**Figure 5.1.7**).

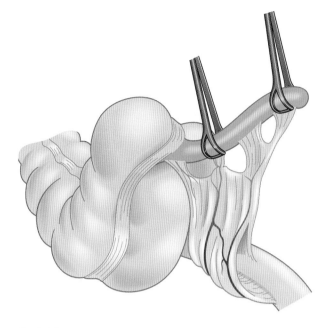

5.1.7

Insertion of purse-string suture

The classical purse-string used to bury the appendix stump is today considered unnecessary by many surgeons. If preferred, a circumferential purse-string using 3-0 Vicryl or PDS is placed 1 cm away from the base of the appendix, gathering small seromuscular bites of cecal wall and ensuring that the line of the now divided mesenteric attachment is not picked up, thus avoiding a small recurrent branch of the appendiceal artery. The purse-string is left loose (**Figure 5.1.8**).

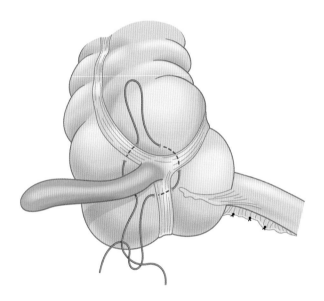

5.1.8

Ligation, division, and invagination of the appendix stump

The appendix is held vertically. An 0 Vicryl or PDS is used to ligate the appendix just above its base. The artery forceps is then applied to the appendix 5 mm above the ligature. The appendix is divided with a knife between the ligature and the artery forceps and the specimen handed with the knife and artery forceps to the scrub nurse. The small remaining amount of appendiceal mucosa visible outside the basal ligature can be lightly touched with diathermy and swabbed with Betadine or alternatively left alone, depending on the surgeon's preference (**Figure 5.1.9**).

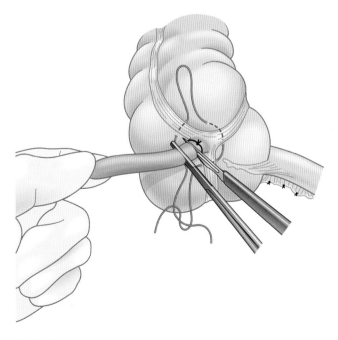

5.1.9

If one wishes to bury the appendix stump, then an assistant gently invaginates the stump with non-toothed forceps, while the purse-string is gently tightened and tied by the surgeon (**Figure 5.1.10**).

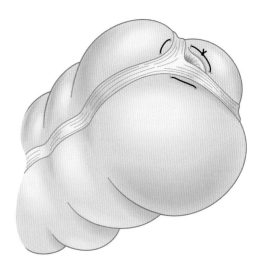

5.1.10

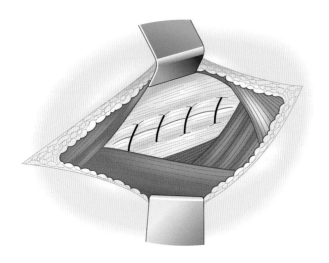

5.1.11

Wound closure

Free turbid fluid should be completely suctioned from the peritoneal cavity. If frankly purulent fluid is found, then warm normal saline should be poured into the right iliac fossa and aspirated until the return is clear. If no contamination of the peritoneal cavity is observed, no washout is necessary. An intraperitoneal drain is unnecessary in most cases. Wound retractors are placed deep to the muscles and outside the peritoneum. Small artery forceps are placed at either end of the peritoneal incision and in the middle of its upper and lower edges. A continuous 2-0 Vicryl suture is inserted, ensuring at all times that intestine is not inadvertently caught by the needle (**Figure 5.1.11**).

Further saline lavage is applied to the wound before muscle closure. If a muscle splitting incision has been done, the muscles of internal oblique and transversus abdominis are now approximated with interrupted 2-0 Vicryl sutures. The fascia of the internal oblique muscle rather than the muscle bundle should be picked up with minimal tension, thus avoiding ischemia (**Figure 5.1.12**).

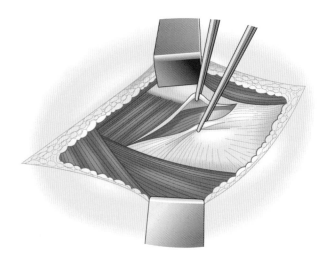

5.1.12

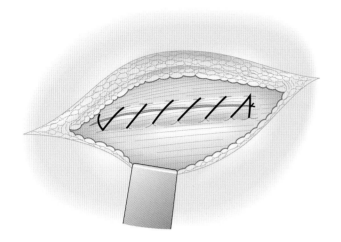

5.1.13

A continuous 1 Vicryl or PDS is used to close the external oblique muscle, preferably burying the knot in thin patients. Scarpa's fascia can be approximated with interrupted absorbable sutures and the skin closed with a 3-0 Monocryl subcuticular suture. If significant pus has been encountered, interrupted sutures are more appropriate and it may even be prudent to leave the wound partially or completely open or, alternatively, a small corrugated drain may be left in the subcutaneous space (**Figure 5.1.13**).

Special circumstances

MEDIAL WOUND EXTENSION

By incising the lateral edge of the rectus sheath, if not done so already, the rectus muscle is exposed allowing further medial retraction. Rectus muscle can be divided transversely with diathermy to further increase exposure. Care must be taken to avoid damaging the inferior epigastric vessels, which pass posterior to the rectus muscle (**Figure 5.1.14**).

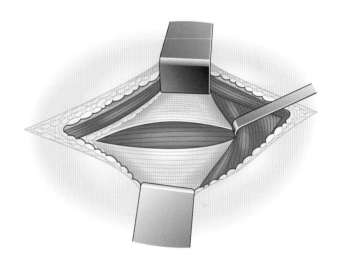

5.1.14

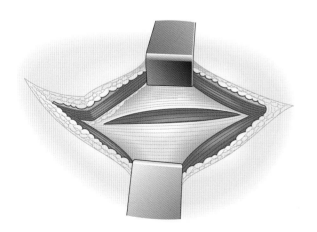

5.1.15

LATERAL WOUND EXTENSION

This is necessary to deal with a high retrocecal or subhepatic appendix. The skin incision should be extended above the iliac crest towards the lateral abdomen and flank. The muscle layers may be further split laterally, but fibers of the internal oblique and transversus abdominis muscles may need to be divided to gain optimum exposure. The use of a narrow retractor and laparoscopic instruments can also assist in this situation. An atraumatic laparoscopic bowel grasper can hold and retract a high cecum to aid division of adhesions and further mobilization can be achieved by use of an alternative energy source, such as a harmonic scalpel (**Figure 5.1.15**).

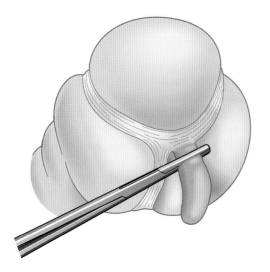

5.1.16

RETROGRADE APPENDICECTOMY

Having exposed the base of the appendix at its junction with the cecum, an artery forceps is passed through the mesentery and the appendix base is clamped, ligated, and divided as described above. The mesoappendix is then secured from the base of the appendix towards its tip by serial clamping, division, and ligation. At each stage, the cecum is gently pushed superiorly within the abdominal cavity to give exposure to the portion of mesoappendix being ligated (**Figure 5.1.16**).

When it is necessary to extend the incision laterally, incising the lateral peritoneum in the right paracolic gutter will allow the cecum and ascending colon to be gently pushed medially, thus exposing more of the elongated appendix (**Figure 5.1.17**).

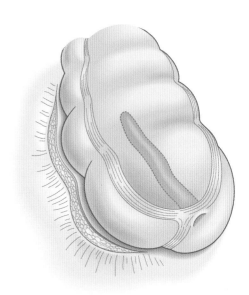

5.1.17

APPENDICEAL TUMOR

If the appendix contains a tumor less than 2 cm in diameter, confined to the appendix and involving neither the mesoappendix nor the base of the appendix, appendicectomy should include as much mesoappendix as possible. Most of these will be carcinoid tumors. Care must be taken to remove a mucin-filled appendix intact. Patients who have an obvious appendiceal adenocarcinoma, any neoplasm greater than 2 cm, or involvement of the base or mesoappendix should be considered for immediate right hemicolectomy to achieve optimal outcome (**Figure 5.1.18**).[5]

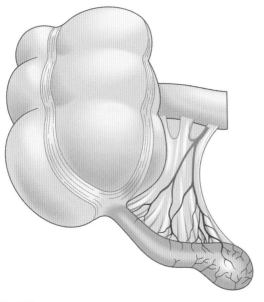

5.1.18

MASS IN THE RIGHT ILIAC FOSSA

The cecum and appendix are inspected to ascertain the underlying pathology. If omentum is adherent, it may be gently separated unless malignancy is suspected in which it should be taken *en bloc* with the specimen. The terminal ileum should be inspected for inflammation suggestive of Crohn's disease. If the inflammation is not causing obstruction and does not involve the cecum, appendicectomy may be carried out. In this case, care must be taken to ensure seromuscular apposition of the uninvolved cecum adjacent to the base of the divided appendix. If the Crohn's disease involves the adjacent cecum, a modified right hemicolectomy may be required. If such a resection is required, the surgeon can extend the excision in either a transverse or an oblique fashion. The use of a laparoscopic wound protector at this stage can greatly help with exposure. A midline incision is not often necessary, however the surgeon should not hesitate to make one if safe exposure cannot otherwise be achieved (**Figure 5.1.19**).

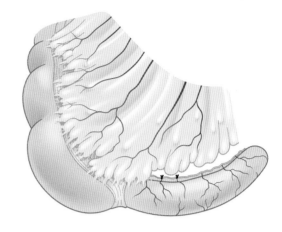

5.1.19

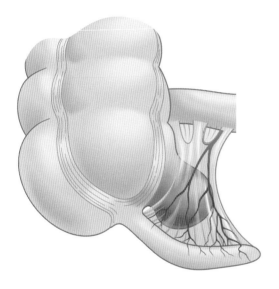

5.1.20

Local diverticulitis of the cecum may occur. If perforation has occurred, a limited right hemicolectomy must be performed. If diverticulitis without perforation has occurred, then this can be treated without resection. If the mass precludes a definitive diagnosis, it is reasonable to proceed as if dealing with a cecal tumor (**Figure 5.1.20**).

Tumors of the cecum may cause appendicitis. The cecum should be palpated carefully, and if an associated mucosal mass lesion is present, the wound may need to be closed and a midline incision made to allow an immediate right hemicolectomy to be undertaken (**Figure 5.1.21**).

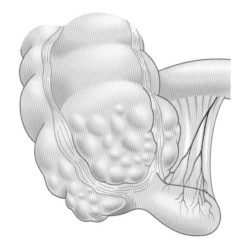

5.1.21

POSTOPERATIVE CARE

After reversal of muscle relaxation and extubation, the patient is transferred to the recovery room and kept under routine observation until awake and stable. Suitable analgesia and antiemetics are prescribed. Oral fluids can usually be tolerated early and the patient can progress quickly to a light diet, if there are no signs of ileus. Intravenous antibiotics are continued for 5 days in the case of generalized peritonitis. If non-absorbable sutures have been used for the wound, these are removed after 7 days.

Complications

WOUND INFECTION

The wound dressing may be removed after 24 hours to allow frequent inspection. Minor cellulitis may be treated with appropriate antibiotics. Wound collections are easily treated by removing a suture and probing to release accumulated pus.

INTRA-ABDOMINAL COLLECTION

Increasing abdominal or pelvic pain with diarrhea and fever heralds a peritoneal abscess. An abdominal CT scan should be performed with radiological drainage carried out and appropriate antibiotics commenced if a collection is found.

INTESTINAL FISTULA

This is a rare complication. Conservative treatment is appropriate initially, if there are no signs of peritonitis.

REFERENCES

1. Williams GR. Presidential address: a history of appendicitis. *Annals of Surgery* 1983; **197**: 495–506.
2. Faiz O, Clark J, Brown T *et al*. Traditional and laparoscopic appendectomy in adults: outcomes in English NHS hospitals between 1996 and 2006. *Annals of Surgery* 2008; **248**: 800–6.
3. Sauerland S, Lefering R, Neugebauer EAM. Laparoscopic versus open surgery for suspected appendicitis. *Cochrane Database of Systematic Reviews* 2009; (4): CD001546.
4. Aziz O, Athanasiou T, Tekkis P *et al*. Laparoscopic versus open appendectomy in children: a meta-analysis. *Annals of Surgery* 2006; **243**: 17–27.
5. Murphy EMA, Farquharson SM, Moran BJ. Management of an unexpected appendiceal neoplasm. *British Journal Surgery* 2006; **93**: 783–92.

Appendicectomy – laparoscopic

CONOR SHIELDS

HISTORY

In 1981, the first paper on laparoscopic appendicectomy by Kurt Semm was rejected on the grounds that the technique was unethical. From this rather inauspicious start, the laparoscopic approach to appendicectomy has evolved to become the standard approach in many institutions.

PRINCIPLES AND JUSTIFICATION

The indications for laparoscopic appendicectomy encompass those of open appendicectomy, but also extend to the patient who presents a diagnostic uncertainty, in whom a diagnostic laparoscopy and possible appendicectomy may obviate the need for multiple investigations. Furthermore, there are a number of patient groups in whom a laparoscopic approach may be preferable due to the anticipated difficulty of a traditional appendicectomy, including patients with suspected perforated appendicitis, obese patients, pregnant patients, and those undergoing interval appendicectomy.[1]

PREOPERATIVE ASSESSMENT

Prior to the induction of anesthesia, it is advisable to verify that the patient has an empty bladder, to minimize the risk of trocar injury if a suprapubic port is employed. If this is not practiced, passage of a Foley urethral catheter is indicated.

OPERATION

Position of the patient

Following induction of general anesthesia, the patient is placed in the supine position, with arms by the side. The surgeon is positioned on the patient's left side, while the operating monitor is situated on the right (**Figure 5.2.1**). During the establishment of pneumoperitoneum and placement of ports, the assistant stands opposite the surgeon, before joining the surgeon on the left side, standing in the cephalad position.

Port placement

The underlying principle of successful port placement in all laparoscopic procedures is that the operating instruments should be sufficiently 'triangulated', otherwise the surgeon will be impeded. A variety of port placement strategies has

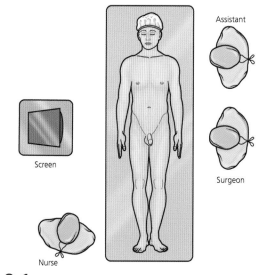

5.2.1

been described. The author's preference is for a 10 mm umbilical port, introduced via an open Hasson technique, a 5 mm suprapubic port, and a 10 mm left lower quadrant port, all placed under direct vision (**Figure 5.2.2**).

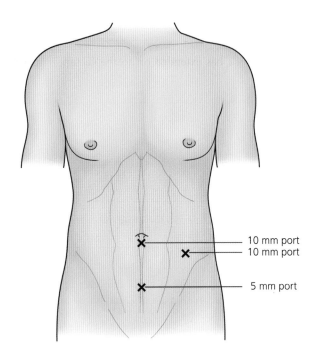

10 mm port
10 mm port

5 mm port

5.2.2 Port placement.

While other placement strategies have been described (left lower quadrant and right lower quadrant, left lower quadrant and right upper quadrant, and right lower quadrant and suprapubic), the advantage of operating ports in adjacent quarters as described here is that the assistant is simply required to direct the camera and is spared the task of retracting, rendering this approach feasible with an inexperienced assistant.

The exact placement of the operating ports is influenced by the patient's habitus, cosmetic considerations, and the need to avoid certain abdominal wall structures, such as the epigastric vessels. Ideally, the left lower quadrant port should be placed lateral to the rectus muscle. Transillumination using the camera is frequently useful to guide placement of this port. A single incision laparoscopic (SILS) approach has been described for treatment of appendicitis. The benefits of SILS are currently unproven, and the technique may simply represent an interim stage in the development of next generation instruments.

Instrumentation

While laparoscopic appendicectomy has been rendered more simple by the introduction of ultrasonic dissectors, bipolar electrothermal vessel sealing systems, and endoscopic stapling devices, there is rarely a need to employ

these technologies. Their introduction, not surprisingly, adds considerably to the cost of the procedure. While a concomitant reduction in operating time, conversion rate, and blood loss may render these instruments cost-effective, it is the author's view that this argument only holds true for more advanced laparoscopic procedures.

Standard laparoscopic equipment is almost always sufficient, comprising an atraumatic grasper, a dolphin-nosed dissector ('Maryland'), scissors, a suction/irrigation instrument, a retrieval bag, and Endoloops™. Where there is a significant degree of appendiceal necrosis, or a very bulky mesoappendix, endoclips, or an endoscopic stapler may be required.

Exploration

Before addressing the appendix, a diagnostic laparoscopy is performed, with particular attention to the pathologies of the female reproductive organs (ruptured ovarian cyst, salpingitis, ovarian torsion), sigmoid colon (diverticulitis), gall bladder (cholecystitis), and the terminal ileum (Crohn's disease, tuberculosis). The surgeon should now confirm the preoperative diagnosis of appendicitis by direct examination of the appendix.

Mobilization

Identification of the appendix is best achieved by placing the patient in the Trendelenburg position, tilted towards the surgeon ('right side up'), and identifying the cecum. The inflamed appendix will frequently be found adherent to the abdominal wall lateral to the cecum, or to the pelvic organs. In the majority of cases, it can simply be peeled free by coaxing with a closed instrument. It is imperative to identify the tip of the appendix, ensuring that it has not become detached and embedded in the abdominal wall. Once the appendix is freed, the atraumatic grasper, held in the surgeon's left hand, may be placed on the appendix, with care being taken not to crush or tear a friable and inflamed appendix. In this circumstance, grasping the thickened mesoappendix may be prudent. The aim is to skeletonize the base of the appendix, clearly exposing the interface between the appendix and the healthy cecum. Using the dolphin-nosed dissector (or scissors) in the right hand, the surgeon makes a window (**Figure 5.2.3**) between the appendix and mesoappendix.

A number of techniques have been described to ligate and divide the mesoappendix. The simplest approach is the sequential application of diathermy to the mesoappendix within the jaws of the dissector, using either the grasper or the scissors to divide the cauterized portion. Care must be taken to ensure that the mesoappendicular artery is adequately sealed before division, to avoid indiscriminate use of cautery within the mesentery in the search for a bleeding and retracted vessel. At all times, the active

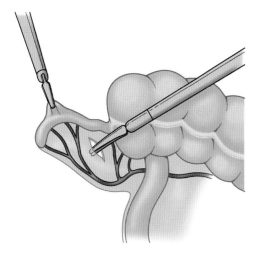

5.2.3 Window being created between cecum and appendix.

segment of each instrument must be kept within the visual field to prevent inadvertent injury to surrounding tissues.

An alternative approach is to deploy endoclips (**Figure 5.2.4**) across the mesoappendix, dividing between them. Otherwise an ultrasonic or bipolar instrument, or an endostapler, may be employed to ligate the mesoappendix.

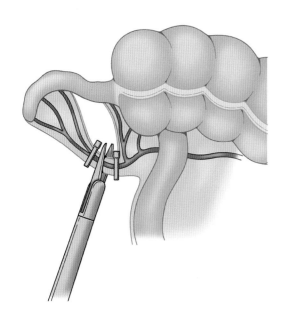

5.2.4 Endoclips placed across mesoappendix.

Ligation of the appendix

Once the appendix base has been completely exposed, the appendix may be transected at a level where it appears healthy. It is imperative that the appendiceal stump is left as short as possible, mimicking an open operation, following reports of recurrent appendicitis in patients with a long remnant. To avoid a long stump, the base of the appendix must be adequately visualized, necessitating a full and meticulous dissection.

The author's preference for appendiceal ligation is Endoloops; however, in the presence of appendiceal necrosis which has extended on to the cecum, it may be advisable to use an endostapler, incorporating a cuff of normal cecum within the stapler blades to ensure a healthy and viable transection line.

LIGATION OF THE APPENDIX – ENDOLOOPS

The Endoloop is introduced through the right hand port, and the grasper in the left hand port is 'lassooed'. The grasper is used to pick up the tip of the appendix, and using both hands, the surgeon maneuvers the Endoloop to the base of the appendix (**Figure 5.2.5**).

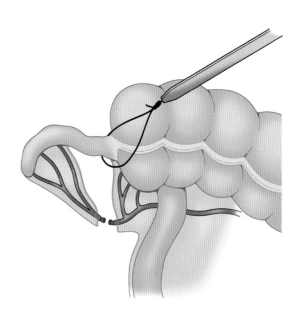

5.2.5 Endoloop being maneuvered to the base of the appendix.

To aid in placement, the appendix may be released and regrasped at its midpoint. Once a satisfactory position is achieved, the grasper should be handed to the assistant, who holds it in the left hand, maintaining the appendix in a vertical orientation. Tightening the Endoloop requires both the surgeon's hands. The tip of the Endoloop is moved into the visual field before tightening, as it is imperative that the tip does not become ensnared on any other structure prior to closure. The tip is used to guide final positioning of the loop (**Figure 5.2.6**).

alignment, the stapler is placed across the appendix base. The surgeon must ensure that the tissue within the stapler jaws is grossly normal (**Figure 5.2.8**).

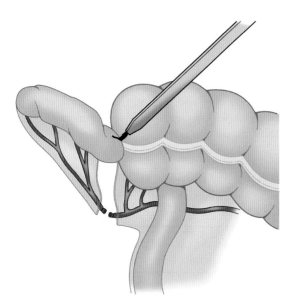

5.2.6 Endoloop being tightened at base of appendix.

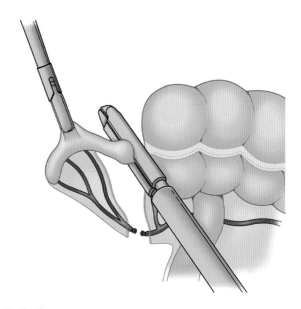

5.2.8 Stapler dividing appendix at base.

A minimum of two loops must be placed, approximately 1 cm apart, with scissors used to divide between them (**Figure 5.2.7**).

Specimen retrieval

Contamination of the abdomen and abdominal wall remains a risk following amputation of an appendicitis. Therefore, it is imperative that a firm grasp is maintained of the ligated appendix in the surgeon's left-hand instrument. A specimen retrieval bag may be passed via the 10 mm left lower quadrant port, deployed, and the appendix secured within, without any spillage of offensive material or loss of a fecalith. It may then be exteriorized through the left lower quadrant incision. Care should be taken to ensure that the retrieval bag is not breached during removal; a further fascial incision may be required to extract a bulky appendix.

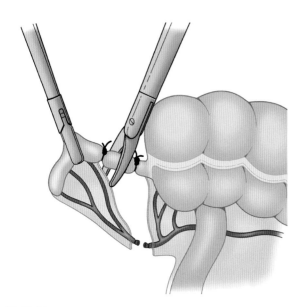

5.2.7 Dividing appendix between two tightened Endoloops.

Irrigation and washout

Given the purported increased incidence of pelvic abscess following laparoscopic appendicectomy, the role of irrigation and washout has assumed greater importance.[2] Despite the superb views afforded by modern optics, it still remains difficult to be certain that the pelvis has been adequately irrigated and cleared of infected material and debris, given the frustrating tendency of small bowel, omentum, and the pelvic organs to occlude the holes on the suction instrument. Nevertheless, the surgeon must be assiduous in irrigating the operative field (right lower quadrant) and the pelvis. It is the author's approach to fill the pelvis with irrigation fluid just before all instruments and ports are withdrawn, under vision. A standard, open

Current instrumentation mandates a 12 mm port for the deployment of an endostapler. This should replace the 10 mm operating port in the left lower quadrant. While the left hand grasper is used to hold the appendix in a vertical

pool suction instrument is then passed carefully via the umbilical incision to a position behind the bladder, with the suction tubing occluded during introduction to minimize the risk to other structures. Once the suction instrument is in the pelvis, the suction tubing is released, and the fluid in the pelvis, along with any associated debris and pus, is extracted. As this is performed in a 'blind' fashion, extreme caution must be exercised when passing the suction instrument not to traverse or damage any other structure. This ensures a more thorough pelvic lavage than with laparoscopic instruments.

The difficult appendix

An appendicectomy may be rendered challenging because of either its location (e.g. retrocecal) or the extent of the inflammatory process, which may have evolved to a phlegmonous mass involving omentum and terminal ileum. In these circumstances, a laparoscopic appendicectomy is a technically difficult operation, requiring an advanced laparoscopic skill set and an awareness of one's limitations. Difficulty in identifying the appendix may require mobilization of the cecum, as described in Chapter 5.4. If the appendix is still not satisfactorily identified, or separation of the small bowel from the inflammatory mass is proving hazardous, conversion to an open appendicectomy may be the most prudent option (Chapter 5.1). Reported conversion rates range from 0 to 27 percent.[3] It is the author's view that the Alexis® wound retractor (Applied Medical, Rancho Santa Margarita, CA, USA) is a useful adjunct in this situation, given that the traditional open appendicectomy will probably also prove challenging in this circumstance.

Port closure

To reduce the incidence of postoperative herniation, it is advisable to close all port sites greater than 5 mm. The author's preference is for a monofilament suture of polydioxanone (PDS™, Ethicon, Cornelia, GA, USA), or polytrimethylene carbonate (Maxon™, Syneture). The skin may be approximated by subcuticular sutures.

POSTOPERATIVE CARE

Nasogastric aspiration is usually not required following appendicectomy. Clear liquids can be begun almost immediately postoperatively. Intravenous fluids are usually discontinued on the first postoperative day, and a full transition to normal oral intake is usually achieved. Discharge may be contemplated on the first or second day postprocedure, unless there was significant contamination and pelvic sepsis requiring intravenous antibiotics. In this circumstance, the development of a postoperative ileus or diarrhea should raise suspicion of a pelvic collection. This may be adequately treated by radiological placement of a drain.

CONTROVERSIES

The normal appendix

With the increasing use of laparoscopy as a diagnostic tool, especially in females, the issue of management of the normal appendix occurs with some regularity. There are disparate views on this issue;[4] however, it is the author's preference to perform appendicectomy if no other pathology is encountered, unless precluded by the patient's general health. Furthermore, an apparently macroscopically normal appendix may harbor pathology on histological examination.

Pelvic abscess

Initial series of laparoscopic appendicectomy showed a pelvic abscess rate that was higher than that observed with traditional appendicectomy, raising doubts about the applicability of a laparoscopic approach to this disease. However, recent reports show equivalence in terms of outcome,[5] suggesting that as optic technology and instruments improve, and surgical experience evolves, complication rates have diminished.

The pregnant patient

Pregnancy is no longer considered a contraindication for laparoscopy.[6] Indeed, ascertaining the cause of an acute abdomen in pregnancy presents special difficulties and a diagnostic laparoscopy is frequently the ideal investigation. While there is no evidence favoring the Hasson technique over the Veress approach, the open approach seems intuitively safer. Port placement will also have to have regard for conformational changes in the abdominal wall and alterations in the position of abdominal viscera. Ideally, laparoscopy in pregnancy should be performed at a low inflation pressure and by an experienced surgeon.

REFERENCES

1. Kouwenhoven EA, Repelaer van Driel OJ, van Erp WF. Fear for the intraabdominal abscess after laparoscopic appendectomy: not realistic. *Surgical Endosccopy* 2005; **19**: 923–6.
2. Sauerland S, Lefering R, Neugebauer EA. Laparoscopic versus open surgery for suspected appendicitis. *Cochrane Database of Systematic Reviews* 2004; **(4)**: CD001546.
3. Fingerhut A, Millat B, Borrie F. Laparoscopic versus open appendectomy: time to decide. *World Journal of Surgery* 1999; **23**: 835–45.

4. Phillips AW, Jones AE, Sargen K. Should the macroscopically normal appendix be removed during laparoscopy for acute right iliac fossa pain when no other explanatory pathology is found? *Surgical Laparoscopy, Endoscopy and Percutaneous Techniques* 2009; **19**: 392–4.

5. Katkhouda N, Mason RJ, Towfigh S *et al*. Laparoscopic versus open appendectomy: a prospective randomized double-blind study. *Annals of Surgery* 2005; **242**: 439–48; discussion 448–50.

6. Sadot E, Telem DA, Arora M *et al*. Laparoscopy: a safe approach to appendicitis during pregnancy. *Surgical Endoscopy* 2010; **24**: 383–9.

Right colectomy – open

ROBERT R CIMA AND JOHN H PEMBERTON

PRINCIPLES AND JUSTIFICATION

A right colon resection is performed for a number of indications. However, the most common is for the treatment of a colonic malignancy. Other reasons include intestinal polyps not amenable to endoscopic removal, regional inflammatory conditions (e.g. Crohn's disease, perforated appendicitis), and rarely mechanical problems such as volvulus. Open resection represents the 'gold standard' comparison for other techniques, such as laparoscopic-assisted and hand-assisted right colectomy. Keys to the success of the operation, as for any intestinal operation, include adequate exposure, identification of the appropriate dissection planes, preservation of a blood supply, and a tension-free anastomosis.

In the majority of right colon malignancies, the patient is often asymptomatic from the lesion other than anemia which prompts colonic evaluation. Both the anatomy and physiology of the right colon contribute to the silent nature of right-sided malignancies. The large lumen and liquid character of the stool allows tumors to become quite large before they result in pain, obstruction, or a palpable mass. The elective nature of right colon resections for malignancy allows for a more thorough evaluation of both the patient and the disease. In nearly all cases of a right-sided malignancy, a computed tomography scan should be obtained to assist in the locoregional and distant staging of the disease. In particular, possible extraluminal invasion of retroperitoneal structures, namely the right ureter and duodenum, can be identified and appropriate contingencies made. When the index lesion is not diagnosed by colonoscopy, a colonoscopy should be performed to exclude synchronous pathology.

PREPARATION

Fortunately, most patients requiring an elective right colectomy can be medically optimized prior to surgery.

Important factors to consider prior to surgery are cardiopulmonary and nutritional status. The patient should be counseled to stop smoking prior to surgery. Ideally, as in the case of Crohn's disease, any septic foci should be adequately treated with a combination of systemic antibiotics and percutaneous drainage.

While still debated, the routine use of an oral bowel preparation prior to right colectomy is questionable. The data available suggest that omission of a bowel preparation does not lead to an increase in anastomotic or infectious complications.[1] Our personal preference is to omit an oral bowel preparation. Similarly, the use of oral antibiotics is questioned. Administration of appropriate intravenous antibiotics within 60 minutes of incision is adequate prophylaxis against a surgical site infection.[2]

OPERATION

Position of patient and preparation

After the induction of general anesthesia, the patient is placed supine on the operating table. To ensure the safety of the patient during possible changes in table position, we recommend the use of both chest and ankle straps. Pneumatic compression boots are applied as mechanical venous thromboembolism prophylaxis. An orogastric tube is placed as routine postoperative gastric drainage is not required. An indwelling urinary catheter is placed in a sterile fashion and the proposed area of the incision is prepared using an electric clipper. The entire abdomen is prepared using combination skin preparation that includes alcohol and either iodine or chlorhexidine. Use of a solely iodine-based preparation should be avoided as recent evidence suggests that it is an inadequate skin preparation and is associated with an increase in superficial surgical site infections.[3]

Incision

With rare exception, a periumbilical midline incision should be used for an open right colectomy. The advantages of this incision include the capability to extend it either cephalad or caudad to gain adequate exposure to the entire abdomen, it is based over the origin of the right colon blood supply (**Figure 5.3.1**), it does not interfere with the area over the rectus muscle in case an ostomy needs to be constructed either at the index operation or in the future, and finally it can be more easily used for future operations. Occasionally, a transverse incision may be used for a right colectomy, but this is usually when the original intent of the operation was for another indication such as acute appendicitis or a gynecologic problem.

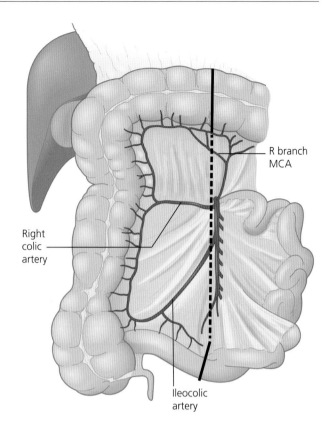

R branch MCA

Right colic artery

Ileocolic artery

5.3.1

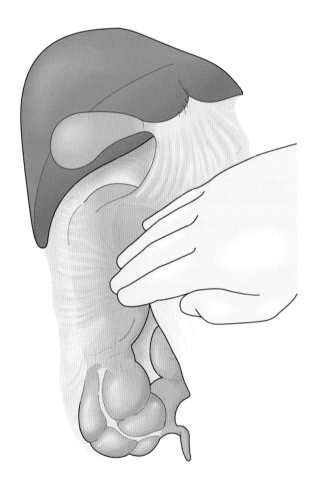

5.3.2

Exploration and mobilization

The surgeon stands on the patient's left side with the assistant on the right side. If an additional assistant is available, they should be positioned next to the first assistant to provide lateral retraction on the incision. Once the abdomen is entered, a thorough exploration of the entire abdomen is performed. In the case of a right colon malignancy, particular attention is directed toward the liver, the right lateral sidewall, and the peritoneal surfaces of the right colon and distal small intestine mesentery (**Figure 5.3.2**). Depending upon the patient's body habitus, retraction can be applied with either a hand-held abdominal wall retractor or a fixed retractor, such as a Balfour or Buckwalter.

The initial mobilization of the right colon begins near the ileal–cecal junction. The surgeon applies retraction cephalad and to the left upper quadrant at the base of the cecum and the terminal ileum (**Figure 5.3.3a**). This exposes the peritoneal fold that envelops the interface between the retroperitoneum and the cecum and the small bowel mesentery. This peritoneal covering is incised allowing entry into the embryologic fusion plane between the retroperitoneum and the small intestine mesentery. This relatively bloodless plane allows dissection up to the duodenum and exposes the retroperitoneal structures that

need to be avoided during a right colectomy: the right ureter, the gonadal vessels, and the vena cava (**Figure 5.3.4**).

Once the colon and small bowel mesentery are mobilized off the retroperitoneum, the lateral peritoneal attachments are incised. This is facilitated by having the surgeon retract the right colon toward the midline. The last step in the mobilization is to divide the peritoneal covering of the hepatic flexure (**Figure 5.3.3b**). The surgeon applies traction downwards and carefully exposes the second portion of the duodenum. The thin attachments of the colonic mesentery and the duodenum are divided with

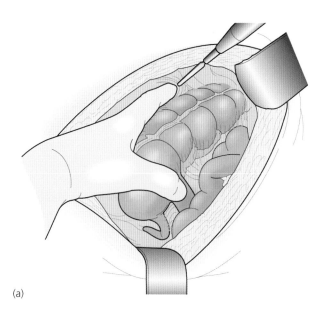

(a)

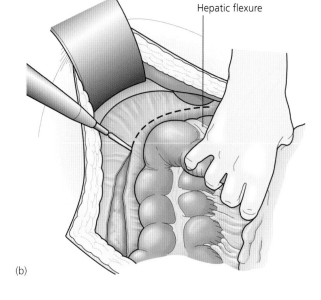

(b)

5.3.3

electrocautery freeing the entire right colon and mesentery to the midline. The greater omentum is usually dissected off the hepatic flexure and proximal transverse colon using the fusion plane where it attaches to the colon. However, in cases of hepatic flexure and proximal transverse colon cancers, the right half of the greater omentum is resected *en bloc* with the colon.

The length of bowel and mesentery that needs to be resected depends upon the indication for operation. In a right colectomy for cancer, the named vessels supplying the right colon are divided at their origin: ileocolic, right colic, and the right branch of the middle colic (see Fig. 5.3.1). Once the mesentery is divided, the bowel is prepared

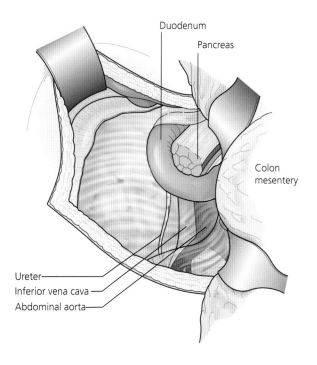

5.3.4

for an anastomosis (**Figure 5.3.5**). The right colectomy anastomosis can be performed either in a handsewn or stapled manner depending upon the surgeon's preference and condition of the bowel. In most routine cases, a side-to-side functional end-to-end stapled anastomosis is performed. The authors routinely use a 75 mm linear-cutting stapler to construct the enterocolotomy and then a 60 mm non-cutting stapler to close the end of the anastomosis. We then routinely oversew the cross staple

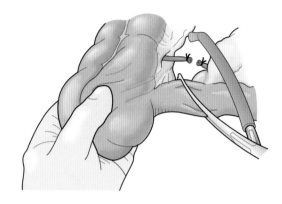

5.3.5

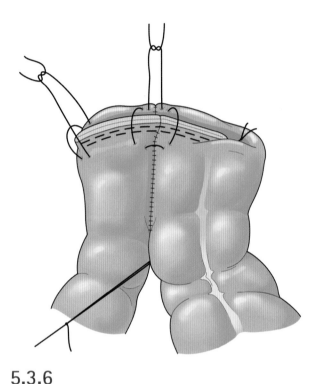

5.3.6

line with interrupted sutures. In cases where the bowel wall is thickened, a handsewn technique is preferred. We use a two-layer closure with an inner running absorbable suture and outer interrupted absorbable or permanent suture (**Figure 5.3.6**). For details of how to perform an intestinal anastomosis, please refer to Chapters 1.8 and 1.9. The surgeon has the option of closing the mesenteric defect. The bowel is placed back into its normal position and the omentum can be placed back over the region of the anastomosis. After the abdomen is inspected for any bleeding, the peritoneal cavity is irrigated with warm saline and the abdominal wall is closed in layers.

POSTOPERATIVE CARE

The authors' practice is to use a clinical pathway for colectomy patients.[4] The night of surgery the patient is permitted to start a liquid diet. Early mandatory ambulation is initiated that evening with the assistance of nursing staff. Minimal intravenous fluid is provided overnight. The patient receives two doses of intravenous antibiotics which are stopped within 24 hours of the incision time. The day after surgery the diet is advanced to a regular diet as tolerated. All intravenous fluid and the indwelling urinary catheter are discontinued at noon. The patient is transitioned to oral pain medication the day after surgery with a preference to scheduled non-narcotic pain medication including both acetaminophen and non-steroidal medications. Discharge criteria are passing flatus, tolerating a general diet, and adequate pain control. The patient is usually ready to leave on the second day after surgery.

REFERENCES

1. Guenaga KK, Matos D, Wille-Jørgensen P. Mechanical bowel preparation for elective colorectal surgery. *Cochrane Database of Systematic Reviews* 2009; (1): CD001544.
2. Darouiche RO, Wall MJ Jr, Itani KM *et al.* Chlorhexidine-alcohol versus povidone-iodine for surgical-site antisepsis. *New England Journal of Medicine* 2010; **362**: 18–26.
3. Nguyen N, Yegiyants S, Kaloostian C *et al.* The Surgical Care Improvement project (SCIP) initiative to reduce infection in elective colorectal surgery: which performance measures affect outcome? *American Journal of Surgery* 2008; **74**: 1012–16.
4. Eskicioglu C, Forbes SS, Aarts MA *et al.* Enhanced recovery after surgery (ERAS) programs for patients having colorectal surgery: a meta-analysis of randomized trials. *Journal of Gastrointestinal Surgery* 2009; **13**: 2321–9.

Right hemicolectomy – laparoscopic

HARRY L REYNOLDS JR AND CONOR P DELANEY

HISTORY

Laparoscopic colectomy is gaining acceptance as the literature expands and experience grows. Younger surgeons, who have been immersed in laparoscopic techniques throughout their training, are quickly adapting to laparoscopic colectomy as they move into practice. More experienced surgeons, trained in traditional open techniques, are eager to learn laparoscopic colectomy as the public continues to demand minimally invasive techniques. Since the publication of the COST (Clinical Outcomes of Surgical Therapy) trial, which demonstrated oncologic equivalence between open and laparoscopic segmental colectomy, interest in mastering laparoscopic techniques has escalated.[1]

Right hemicolectomy is a particularly attractive procedure to perform laparoscopically as it lends itself to a very standardized, reproducible technique which is relatively easily learned and is based on sound oncologic principles. Our approach to right colectomy emphasizes a structured, stepwise approach that works easily in most clinical situations.[2, 3]

PRINCIPLES AND JUSTIFICATION

Our standard procedure is designed to be performed safely by the operating surgeon even if a skilled assistant is not available. The operative procedure should move forward in an orderly fashion and the surgeon should remain cognizant of appropriate stepwise progression. If failure to progress is noted with any of the steps, then an alternative approach or conversion to an open procedure should be considered. This helps to ensure that operative morbidity is minimized and excessively long cases are avoided. Similar outcomes have been demonstrated in converted patients when compared to matched open controls utilizing this approach. The concept of standard algorithms is utilized through all aspects of patient care. Perioperative care paths are utilized from the clinic until hospital discharge. This standardization helps to decrease communication difficulties, reduce errors and ensure consistent and reproducible high-quality and efficient outcomes.

INDICATIONS

Right colectomy is usually performed for cancer or colonoscopically unresectable polyps. Patients with terminal ileal Crohn's disease may also be candidates for a laparoscopic approach. In general, most patients are deemed candidates for an attempted laparoscopic approach unless they have had multiple previous laparotomies with known extensive adhesions. A previous laparotomy is certainly not an absolute contraindication to proceeding and a careful open introduction of a Hasson trocar is reasonable to assess the extent of adhesions. Midline adhesions can often be lysed using a 5 mm camera and a 5 mm operating port placed laterally.

The minimally invasive nature of the technique is limited by the size of the incision necessary to withdraw the specimen. If the specimen is very bulky, a generous abdominal incision may be necessary, negating the advantages of a laparoscopic approach. A bulky tumor with known extension into the retroperitoneum or abdominal wall is a relative contraindication for all but the most experienced laparoscopic surgeons as the oncologic principles of *en bloc* resection of any adjacent structures must be applied. The use of a hand-assisted, hybrid approach may be considered in this situation. Introduction of the hand may permit further assessment of the extent of tumor and adequacy of resection by adding the surgeon's ability to feel the margin of the tumor in cases where this cannot be determined visually.

PREOPERATIVE ASSESSMENT AND PREPARATION

An oral polyethylene-based bowel preparation is given in case isolation of the pathology requires an intraoperative colonoscopic evaluation. Those in whom there is a large mass, or a well-documented location, receive no oral preparation, and simply take clear liquids the day before surgery. Lesions are generally tattooed preoperatively by colonoscopy if they are not well documented on preoperative imaging or previously tattooed. Preoperative subcutaneous heparin and sequential compression devices are used for deep venous thrombosis prophylaxis. A non-steroidal anti-inflammatory agent is typically given preoperatively (diclofenac suppository) and oral neomycin is prescribed for patients who underwent mechanical bowel preparation. Broad-spectrum intravenous antibiotics are administered within 1 hour before incision.

ANESTHESIA

General anesthesia is typically utilized. Abdominal wall relaxation is necessary for effective insufflation and laparoscopic visualization. Postoperative epidural anesthesia is unnecessary as postoperative pain is easily controlled with oral and intravenous analgesia, and in our hands, has not been found to improve short-term recovery over that seen with a perioperative care path and intravenous opiate.

OPERATION

Positioning

The patient is placed on a bean bag in a modified lithotomy position with the use of Yellofin™ stirrups. The arms are tucked and secured at the patient's side. In patients who are too obese to tuck both arms, the right arm is kept out. The bean bag and stirrup combination ensures patient security on the table with position changes throughout the case. Chest strapping is only used in the most obese to prevent a pannus rolling when in the lateral rotation. Shoulder supports are not used. A Foley catheter and orogastric tube are placed.

The legs are kept low to prevent interference with the instruments. The lithotomy position is utilized to facilitate handling of the flexures, particularly if mobilization of the splenic flexure is necessary with an extended right colectomy. This allows the surgeon to move between the legs if necessary. The assistant/camera operator begins on the patient's right for port placement then moves to the patient's left and caudad to the surgeon for dissection. The surgeon is cephalad to the assistant and also on the patient's left. The scrub nurse is typically positioned between the legs. The primary working monitor is on the patient's right side.

Port insertion

A standard equipment list is used, emphasizing limiting disposables to control cost. We favor reusable ports, and appropriate atraumatic bowel grasping instruments are needed. A 10 mm, 0° laparoscope is perfectly adequate for right colectomy and negates the need for an experienced camera operator who may have difficulty mastering a 30° scope. Alternatively, a 30° scope may be utilized, depending on the surgeon's preference. We place a 10 mm Hassan port at the umbilicus, eventually enlarging this port site to serve as the extraction site, making the need for a larger port for the 10 mm scope immaterial. Intracorporeal vascular ligation is performed. The choice of vascular ligation technique is the surgeon's choice. An energy source, clips, or staplers may be utilized. If a stapler is used, a 12 mm port is required in the left lower quadrant. If not, a 5 mm port can be used, negating the need for later port site fascial closure.

The procedure begins with the surgeon on the patient's left and the assistant/camera operator on the patient's right. Placement of a Hasson trocar is performed under direct visualization at the umbilicus. A small ~1 cm fascial incision is used and the peritoneal cavity is entered under direct visualization. This is facilitated by grasping the fascia with small Kocher clamps, incising the fascia then carefully opening the peritoneum. A purse-string suture of 0 polyglycolic acid suture is placed around the fascia and a Rommell tourniquet is used to facilitate securing the Hasson and prevent loss of pneumoperitoneum (**Figure 5.4.1**). The abdomen is insufflated, the laparoscope inserted, and the additional ports placed. Care is taken to avoid injury to the epigastric vessels. The left-sided ports should be at least 10 cm apart. A right upper quadrant port is occasionally used if the hepatic flexure is difficult. For the most morbidly obese patients, the left-sided ports are actually placed in the midline so that the instruments can reach the hepatic flexure and right side.

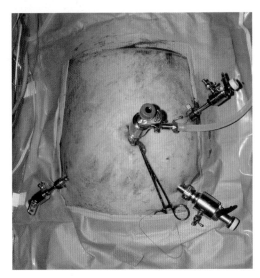

5.4.1

Laparoscopic assessment of resectability

The patient is placed left side down and in Trendelenburg of 10–15°. The left tilt is typically as far as the table will move to assist with positioning of the small bowel away from the ascending colon. The mild Trendelenburg permits some of the small bowel to remain in the pelvis, and the remainder to be distributed laterally and under the transverse colon. The assistant moves below the operating surgeon on the left side and takes control of the camera, which stays in the umbilical port. The surgeon works through both left-sided ports with atraumatic bowel graspers, reflecting the omentum over the transverse colon, thus facilitating visualization of the right colon (**Figure 5.4.2**). The tumor is assessed for size and fixation to the surrounding structures as an initial assessment of resectability is made.

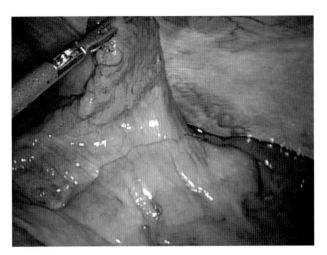

5.4.2

Isolation of ileocolic pedicle

The surgeon lifts the mesentery at the ileocecal junction, identifying the distal ileocolic pedicle which is handed to the assistant and retracted anteriorly, inferiorly, and laterally (**Figure 5.4.3a**). This is grasped with the assistant's left hand while working the camera with the right hand. The surgeon then addresses the proximal ileocolic pedicle, near the take-off from the superior mesenteric artery. The left hand is used to grasp the mesentery over the vessel which reveals a sulcus which is visible overlying the duodenum. The scissors cautery is used in the right hand to open the peritoneum posterior to the ileocolic and parallel to the superior mesenteric vessels. Care is taken to avoid injury to the underlying duodenum and to the adjacent superior mesenteric vessels (**Figure 5.4.3b**). The peritoneum is opened lateral to the pedicle as well and the ileocolic isolated completely near its base. The surgeon's right hand controls the pedicle while the left hand is used to divide the vessel with an energy device, stapler, or clips.

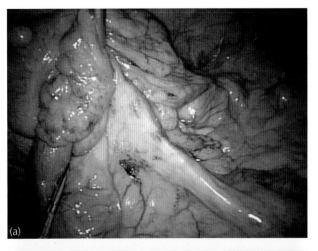

(a)

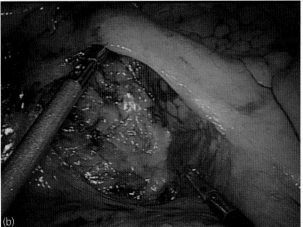

(b)

5.4.3

Mobilization of the ascending colon and hepatic flexure

The divided ileocolic pedicle is grasped and retracted anteriorly. Working in a medial to lateral fashion and preserving the retroperitoneal fascia overlying the kidney and ureter, the mesocolon is dissected from the retroperitoneum until fully mobilized, except for the most lateral attachments at the line of Toldt (**Figure 5.4.4**a). This mobilization continues up behind the hepatic flexure and down behind the cecum. The right branch of the middle colic may be visible at this point and may be isolated and divided in some patients. In those with a thicker mesentery, it is frequently divided later.

Then, retracting the colon inferiorly, the hepaticocolic ligament is divided (**Figure 5.4.4**b). For lesions at the cecum, the omentum may be mobilized off the flexure, but is taken *en bloc* for any pathology near the flexure. As mobilization of the hepatic flexure progresses, typically the previous medial dissection plane is entered, making takedown of the lateral attachments along the line of Toldt straightforward. The lateral attachments are further divided working laterally and heading inferiorly along the ascending colon (**Figure 5.4.4**c). Frequently, the entire colon can now be mobilized around the cecal base.

Although others have reported lateral to medial dissections, the medial to lateral approach has a number of advantages, including early isolation of the vascular pedicle, prior to colon mobilization. Colon mobilization prior to division can result in difficult visualization of the pedicle as the colon now has to be retracted to see the ileocolic vessels. The proper retroperitoneal plane is also immediately identified with this technique. In obese patients or patients with bulky tumors, this can be a little more challenging. Hand-assist approaches may be considered in this circumstance (see Chapter 5.5).

Mobilization of small bowel mesentery from the retroperitoneum

The cecum is retracted cephalad and anteriorly (**Figure 5.4.5**). The remaining small bowel mesenteric attachments and any lateral attachments of the colon are divided. We do not typically specifically seek to define the ureter, although it is generally seen during the dissection. The ureter is carefully defined, however, in patients with retroperitoneal sepsis from a psoas abscess, or with tumors which may be locally invasive posteriorly. In contrast, when in the proper dissection plane over the duodenum, the retroperitoneal fascial planes overlying the ureter are undisturbed. The ureter is, however, often visible coursing over the iliac vessels at the pelvic inlet and it is reassuring to note this. If there is any concern about proper dissection plane, certainly the ureter should be identified. At the conclusion of this dissection, the right colon should be fully mobilized from the retroperitoneum and can be moved into the left

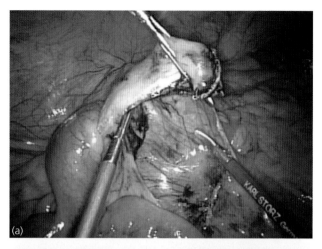

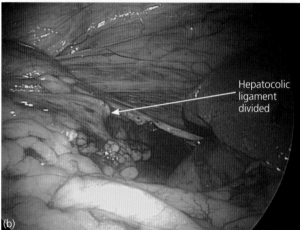

Hepatocolic ligament divided

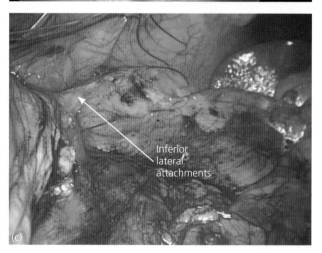

Inferior lateral attachments

5.4.4

abdomen exposing the complete retroperitoneum and c-loop of the duodenum. Care must be taken near the root of the mesentery to avoid injury to the third portion of the duodenum. Sharp dissection with the cold scissors may be prudent at this stage.

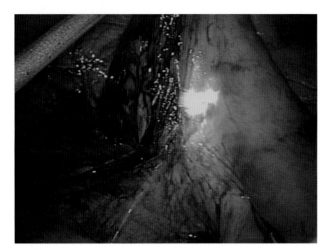

5.4.5

Division of right branch of the middle colic

In a thin patient, the right branch of the middle colic can be divided extracorporally or it can be divided prior to taking the lateral attachments of the colon. In most patients, particularly those who are obese, or have a lesion anywhere except the cecum, the vessel is divided intracorporally at this stage of the dissection. The hepatic flexure is lifted anteriorly and cephalad, holding the transverse colon much like the cape of a bullfighter. The assistant helps with this exposure. This reveals the inferior side of the transverse mesocolon and helps to visualize and isolate the middle colic vessels. Once the right branch is isolated, it is divided. An energy device facilitates this transection (**Figure 5.4.6**).

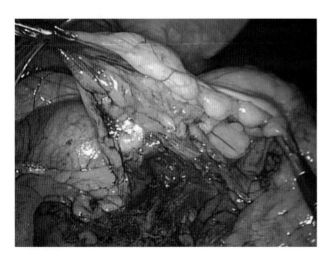

5.4.6

Dissection and intracorporal division of the middle colics can be very challenging. However, taking the right branch of the middle colic is essential for a proper oncologic resection in an ascending colon lesion. Likewise, intracorporal transection is essential for the patient with a foreshortened mesentery. If the vessels are not divided intracorporally, it can be difficult to extract the colon and to perform a safe resection and extracorporal anastomosis.

An extended right resection may be performed for more distal ascending or proximal transverse lesions, taking further branches of the middle colic vessels. This dissection may be facilitated by moving the surgeon between the patient's legs. The splenic flexure may also require mobilization for more distal lesions.

After transection of the right branch of the middle colic, the colon is now completely mobilized and the entire retroperitoneum is seen with the duodenum fully exposed (**Figure 5.4.7**).

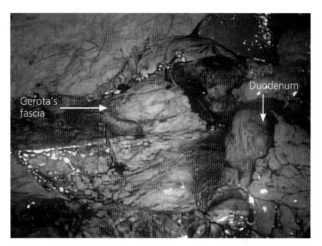

5.4.7

Closure of 12 mm port site left lower quadrant, if stapler used for vascular division

The left lower quadrant port site is closed with a figure-of-eight 0 polyglycolic acid suture, passed transfascially with a suture passer.

Umbilical incision and exteriorization of the right colon

The cecum or appendix is grasped through the right lower quadrant port and secured with an atraumatic grasper. All 5 mm ports are removed, the umbilical incision is enlarged to 4–6 cm, as needed, to safely extract the specimen. A wound protector is placed (**Figure 5.4.8**) and the right colon is passed with the previously placed grasper and extracted on to the abdomen. Care is taken not to twist the bowel.

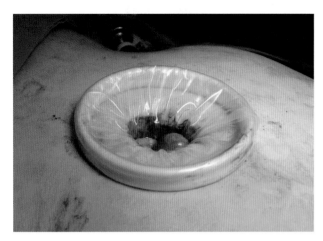

5.4.8

Standard extracorporal resection and anastomosis

After removal of the specimen, the terminal ileum is divided, typically with a GIA (gastrointestinal anastomosis) stapler. The marginal branches between middle colic branches are divided and the transverse colon is divided, just to the right of the left branch of the middle colic. An anastomosis is then completed. Typically, a side-to-side functional end-to-end stapled anastomosis is performed with the GIA stapler, closing the enterotomy with a TA (thoracoabdominal) stapler (**Figure 5.4.9**). Care is taken to ensure the mesenteric defect is straight and there is no twisting of the bowel ends prior to proceeding with anastomosis. A reinforcing crotch suture of 3-0 polyglycolic acid is used. Staple lines are oversewn if bleeding is noted. The mesenteric defect is not closed. The anastomosis is returned intra-abdominally. The midline fascia is closed with long-term absorbable suture (No. 1 polydioxanone). The skin is closed with an absorbable subcuticular closure.

POSTOPERATIVE CARE

A standardized perioperative care plan is in use which we have published previously. Orogastric tubes are removed before completion of the case. Intravenous fluids are minimized both intra- and postoperatively. Urinary catheters are discontinued on postoperative day 1. Patients are ambulated immediately postoperatively and an active walking program is encouraged. Intravenous opioids are limited and an oral regimen is encouraged as soon as liquids are tolerated. Non-steroidal anti-inflammatories are used in those without gastrointestinal or renal contraindications. Deep venous thrombosis prophylaxis is given pre- and postoperatively, typically with subcutaneous heparin. A liquid diet is offered immediately with advance to a soft diet as tolerated. Discharge criteria include tolerance of liquids, with passage of flatus or stool, adequate home support, and the patient wishing to be released from hospital.

SINGLE PORT APPROACH

Over the past several years, technology has improved so that a single laparoscopic port can be used. This permits identical steps of the procedure to be performed, using instruments passed through a port inserted into a 2.5 cm incision. For right colectomy, we place the single port in the midline at a short periumbilical incision. Straight laparoscopic instruments and a 5 mm energy source are used, and the procedure is performed exactly as described above, although with slightly more technical challenge. Short- and long-term outcomes of this less invasive procedure continue to be assessed (**Figure 5.4.10**).

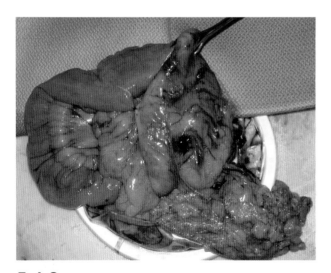

5.4.9

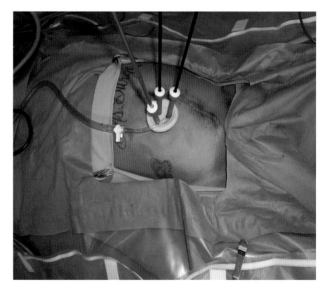

5.4.10

OUTCOME

If progress is not being made through the steps as outlined above, consideration is given to an alternate approach. Similarly, should adverse events occur, such as excessive bleeding, difficult anatomy, worries about adequacy of oncologic resection, or other concerns about ongoing safety of proceeding, the surgeon must be prepared to move to an alternative, or even open approach. Using this approach, our current conversion rate for right colectomies is less than 5 percent. Operative times are generally under 100 minutes, and mean length of stay is 3.7 days. Overall, good outcomes can be anticipated with careful attention to meticulous operative technique and perioperative care.[3, 4, 5, 6]

REFERENCES

1. Nelson H, Sargent DJ, COST Study Group. A comparison of laparoscopically assisted and open colectomy for colon cancer. *New England Journal of Medicine* 2004; **350**: 2050–92.

2. Delaney CP, Neary P, Heriot AG, Senagore AJ. *Operative techniques in laparoscopic colorectal surgery*. Philadelphia, PA: Lippincott Williams & Wilkins, 2006.

3. Senagore AJ, Delaney CP, Brady K, Fazio VW. A standardized approach to laparoscopic right colectomy: outcome in 70 consecutive cases. *Journal of the American College of Surgeons* 2004; **199**: 675–9.

4. Senagore AJ, Delaney CP. A critical analysis of laparoscopic colectomy at a single institution: lessons learned after 1000 cases. *American Journal of Surgery* 2006; **191**: 377–80.

5. Delaney CP, Chang E, Senagore AJ, Broder M. Clinical outcomes and resource utilization associated with laparoscopic and open colectomy using a large national database. *Annals of Surgery* 2008; **247**: 819–24.

6. Delaney CP. Outcome of discharge within 24–72 hours of colorectal surgery. *Diseases of the Colon and Rectum* 2008; **51**: 181–5.

Right hemicolectomy – hand-assisted laparoscopic surgery

KIRK A LUDWIG AND H DAVID VARGAS

HISTORY

Laparoscopic colorectal surgery has evolved rather slowly, primarily as the result of early difficulties in clearly showing patient advantages for the laparoscopic approach, oncologic concerns, and technical difficulties. To address oncologic concerns and the issues regarding whether there are benefits of minimally invasive colon surgery, multiple studies, including four major prospective, randomized, controlled trials were completed: each confirming that there are short-term, patient-related benefits for laparoscopic colon surgery, and these advantages do not come at the expense of a technique-related reduction in oncologic outcome.

There remains, however, the issue of technical difficulty in completing laparoscopic colorectal surgery which probably explains why the majority of colorectal surgery is still performed using open techniques. For laparoscopic right hemicolectomy, there are a number of technical options, including the hand-assisted laparoscopic approach illustrated here. A number of factors may favor choosing this approach over a standard laparoscopic operation. These factors include ease of operation in obese patients, excellent exposure of the middle colic vessels at the base of the transverse colon mesentery just over the pancreas, ease in managing bleeding, the ability to manage locally advanced or bulky tumors, the ability to do combined colon and liver resections for metastatic disease, the ease in managing reoperative abdomens, and the fact that this is a single surgeon operation that does not require a trained assistant. The entire operation flows in a single plane, it can be readily taught and adopted and even the laparoscopically naive surgeon can learn and use the technique as long as there is sufficient knowledge of the anatomy and proper planes of dissection. In addition, with hand-assisted laparoscopic colon surgery, the conversion rate is extraordinarily low. While conversion rates with standard laparoscopic right colon surgery are not reported

to be high, what is not known is how many patients are simply not offered a minimally invasive approach since due to obesity, tumor bulk, previous surgery, or other factors, they are simply not considered appropriate candidates for laparoscopy. Therefore the true 'conversion' rate remains unknown. With restoration of tactile sensation for the surgeon, enhanced operative exposure by manual retraction, three-dimensional perspective, and digital testing of adhesions and tissue planes, almost all patients can be offered a minimally invasive hand-assisted laparoscopic approach that has been shown to produce the same short-term, patient-related benefits as a standard laparoscopic technique.

Hand-assist laparoscopic colon surgery is a pragmatic, single surgeon alternative method associated with shorter operative times and decreased conversion rates while maintaining postoperative outcomes seen with standard laparoscopic colectomy.

PRINCIPLES AND JUSTIFICATION

Operative indications

The vast majority of right hemicolectomies are performed to manage neoplastic disease, either invasive cancer or large polyps that cannot be managed using colonoscopic techniques. As a general rule, since the likelihood that a polyp will harbor a cancer increases with the size of the polyp, when the indication for colectomy is a large adenoma, a formal resection should be performed. Another, not infrequent, indication for laparoscopic segmental colon resection is in the management of a malignant polyp that has been removed colonoscopically. If the polypectomy fails to meet one or more of the accepted criteria for a curative polypectomy, a formal resection is indicated. In these situations, the operation is conducted to remove the area of bowel involved so as to ensure that there is no cancer left within the bowel wall itself and to do a regional lymphadenectomy to remove potentially involved nodes. Again, a formal resection is recommended. Other much less common indications for a laparoscopic right colectomy might include management of right colonic bleeding from a vascular malformation or inflammatory disease due to right colon diverticulitis.

The formal right hemicolectomy for neoplasia involves the usual maneuvers that define an oncologic colon resection: (1) proximal lymphovascular pedicle ligation and complete lymphadenectomy, (2) wide *en-bloc* resection of tumor-bearing bowel segment with adjacent soft tissue and mesentery, (3) minimizing the possibility of tumor contamination to the abdominal cavity, the wounds or the bowel above or below the tumor.

The formal oncologic right hemicolectomy, then, involves proximal ligation of the ileocolic pedicle and the right branch of the middle colic artery for cecal tumors or the entire middle colic pedicle for tumors in the ascending colon up to the proximal transverse colon. The ileum is divided about 15–20 cm from the ileocecal valve which corresponds to a point on the small bowel at which the superior mesenteric artery ends. The transverse colon is divided at its midpoint.

As in any surgical setting, proper patient selection is critical. This is especially the case for laparoscopic colon surgery. Patient selection will vary based on the skill and the experience of the surgeon; however, there are certain situations that do not lend themselves well to a straight laparoscopic approach. These would include cases where there is significant small bowel dilatation or free perforation with peritonitis. In addition, obesity, or large bulky disease, whether malignant or benign, with adjacent organ fixation can also be difficult to manage. As stated previously, however, the hand-assisted approach may be advantageous in these situations. It is rare that any of the usual factors that might deter a surgeon from offering a standard laparoscopic right colectomy would exclude a patient from being offered a hand-assisted laparoscopic right colectomy.

PREOPERATIVE EVALUATION

For patients being prepared for surgery, a thorough preoperative assessment of cardiac, pulmonary, and nutritional status should be made. Appropriate diagnostic studies may include blood gasses, pulmonary function tests, electrocardiograms, and cardiac stress tests (pharmacologic or exercise-induced) and a chest x-ray.

For patients presenting with a non-obstructing, non-perforated colonic carcinoma, a preoperative colonoscopy is always performed to exclude synchronous benign polyps, which have been reported to occur in 12–62 percent of cases and synchronous cancers, which have been identified in 2–8 percent of cases. If the operative indication is a lesion that may not be well appreciated by manual palpation in the

operating room, such as a small cancer, a polyp that cannot be removed colonoscopically, or a malignant polyp, then the colonoscope should be used to mark the lesion with a permanent India ink tattoo. The tattoo should be placed in multiple quadrants near the lesion to avoid the situation in which a lone tattoo is placed on the retroperitoneal surface of the colon where it is not visible. Additionally, tumors can be marked with an endoscopic clip followed by an abdominal radiograph to precisely localize an anatomic segment and thus clarify the plan for resection preoperatively.

Also, as a general rule, all patients taken to the operating room for a laparoscopic right colectomy for neoplasia should have a staging computed tomography (CT) scan of the abdomen and pelvis. This is considered a standard staging study for patients with colorectal cancer and is of particular import when performing laparoscopic surgery due to the more limited ability to easily and readily evaluate the liver.

While there is now evidence to suggest that a full mechanical and oral antibiotic bowel preparation may not be needed for colon surgery, the authors generally continue this practice. The mechanical preparation makes intraoperative colonoscopy possible, should it be needed, and it facilitates palpation of lesions and manipulation of the colon. The mechanical preparation begins on the morning before operation, using 4 L of polyethylene glycol (GoLYTELY™) over 2–3 hours, and is followed by an oral antibiotic preparation with three doses of neomycin and either erythromycin or metronidizole taken later in the afternoon and evening. Intravenous antibiotics are administered in the preoperative holding area. In addition, most patients will be treated prophylactically with either heparin or a low molecular weight heparinoid.

OPERATION

Patient positioning and port placement

For the hand-assisted right colectomy illustrated, the patient is placed on the operating table in the supine position. Intermittent compression devices are placed, a general anesthetic is administered, and a urinary catheter and orogastric tube are inserted. Each elbow is padded with a sheet of foam and then both arms are tucked alongside the body. The arms are held in position by an encircling draw sheet. In addition, multiple pieces of 3-inch tape are used across the lower extremities and a piece is placed across the chest. These maneuvers are used to keep the patient on the operative table during the extremes of bed tilt that are often required to obtain exposure. Having both arms tucked is more secure for the patient and it also provides the surgeon and the assistant with maximal mobility around the operative table. The operative field should be lengthened by pushing the intravenous poles up towards the patient's head, and asking the anesthesia personnel to push the table away from their equipment. Again, this simply gives the operative team more room to maneuver around the table. The field is prepped from the nipples to the mid-thigh level and the towels are placed wide on the abdomen. The towels are held in position with an adhesive clear draping sheet. This is used to keep the towels in place, since when they are placed so widely on the abdomen, they can easily fall down the sides of the patient, exposing the unprepped table. This adhesive sheet also keeps instruments, cords, and cables from falling down alongside the patient outside the sterile field.

The camera cord, the fiberoptic light cord, and the insufflation tube are all brought onto the field at the patient's right shoulder. The tower at the patient's right shoulder will have a monitor, an insufflator, a light source, and the camera system. Additional monitors are really not needed for the illustrated procedure. At the patient's left shoulder, the energy sources are brought on to the field. This includes the electrocautery unit and the cutting/sealing energy device. A suction/irrigation unit can be brought onto the field at the foot of the bed.

For the hand-assisted laparoscopic right colectomy, the ports and the hand-assist device are placed as follows. The hand-assist device is placed in the midline, centered on the umbilicus. The midline wound is optimal based upon surgeon ergonomics, consideration of extracorporeal anastomosis, and maintenance of videoscopic perspective of the relevant anatomy for right colectomy. One should center this midline wound based upon palpable skeletal landmarks – the costal margin and iliac spine – given the variability in location of the umbilicus among different body habitus types. A rule of thumb is that the size of the incision for the device will be the size of the surgeon's glove in centimeters, but as a practical matter, one can usually obtain access with an incision that is 1 cm less. As a general rule, if one draws a line from the costal margin to the iliac crest, the middle of the hand-assist incision will be the midpoint of this line. There are currently two hand-assist devices on the market. The authors use the GelPort™ device. It is easy to use and it provides the advantage of being able to place ports, instruments, or staplers right through the device even with the hand in place. Also, the surgeon's hand can be brought in and out of the abdomen without losing pneumoperitoneum. This feature helps for teaching purposes, as it is easy to go from surgeon to assistant hand in the abdomen.

Pneumoperitoneum is established through a port placed through the hand-assist device. The laparoscope is passed into the abdomen through this port. Two 5 mm ports are then placed in the upper abdomen: one in the subxiphoid region and one in the left upper quadrant. The subxiphoid port will be for the laparoscope and the left upper quadrant port will be for a 5 mm sealing/cutting device.

The position of the subxiphoid port will vary depending on the patient and what is being done. It will usually be placed just to the left of midline. The further over on the transverse colon one plans to go, the further to the left one should place this port. Sometimes, the port will be placed through the falciform ligament. If the falciform ligament is large and obtrusive, it can be removed by grasping it with the left hand and excising it using the energy source through the left upper quadrant port. The left upper quadrant port should generally be placed in the midclavicular line, about halfway between the costal margin and the upper aspect of the hand-assist incision. If the port is placed too close to the costal margin, access to the right lower quadrant can be difficult; if it is placed too low, the hand and the energy source will interfere with each other during dissection in the right lower quadrant.

In the patient who has had previous abdominal surgery, adhesions at the midline should be lysed as the incision at the umbilicus is made. Once room is made, the hand-port can be placed and pneumoperitoneum can be established. If exposure is adequate, the subxiphoid and left upper quadrant ports can be placed and additional adhesiolysis can be conducted, as needed, If adhesions are such that the port can be placed, but there is no room to insert the hand, additional adhesiolysis can be carried out by simply pushing ports and instruments through the GelPort™ itself until sufficient room is created to place the hand and the supxiphoid and left upper quadrant ports.

For this operation, 5 mm ports can be used exclusively. If a stapling device is needed, it is inserted through a 12 mm port placed directly through the hand-assist device. A 5 mm, 30° laparoscope is used since this provides maximum flexibility as the scope can be moved to any port and the 30° degree angle allows the surgeon the best view in tight spaces.

There are a number of 5 mm energy sources that seal and cut well. With these tools, the surgeon has a 5 mm instrument that can be used to dissect bloodlessly and take any of the named mesenteric vessels.

OPERATIVE TECHNIQUE

This is a single surgeon operation. There is no need for a trained assistant to help with exposure. With the ports and the hand-assist device in position, the camera holder will be positioned at the patient's left shoulder and the surgeon will be on the patient's left side (**Figure 5.5.1**). Both focus their attention on the monitor on the patient's right. The patient is placed in strong reverse Trendelenburg position and is tilted to the left. This brings the hepatic flexure down. The abdomen is explored with the laparoscope and hand, and the liver is palpated (operative technique image).

The surgical dissection described is unique and proceeds in a counterclockwise, top-down, fashion beginning at the gastrocolic ligament. The authors recognize advantages and disadvantages to each right colectomy technique, and we would propose that among the strengths of this particular approach are the superior exposure and visualization of the middle colic vessels and the duodenum, both of which are critical anatomic elements of right colectomy.

The procedure can be viewed in five steps as follows:

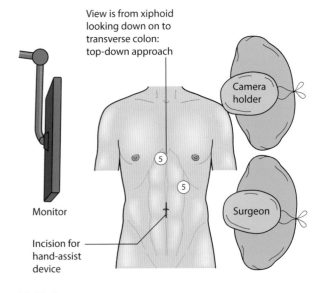

View is from xiphoid looking down on to transverse colon: top-down approach

Camera holder

Surgeon

Monitor

Incision for hand-assist device

5.5.1

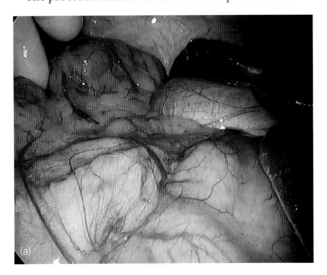

(a)

(b)

5.5.2

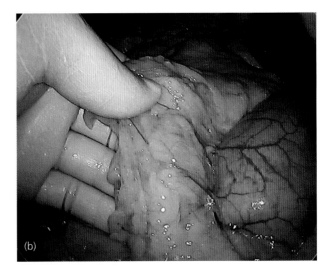

Step 1. The surgeon uses his left hand to grasp the greater omentum along the greater curve of the stomach and he makes a defect in it, just off of the gastroepiploic vessels (**Figure 5.5.2a**). This puts the surgeon into the lesser sac and the smooth, shiny ventral surface of the transverse mesocolon can be seen. Dissecting from either left to right or right to left, the surgeon develops the lesser sac by taking the greater omentum off the stomach (**Figure 5.5.2b**). The stomach has been elevated anteriorly, and one is looking into the lesser sac, with the transverse mesocolon below (**Figure 5.5.3**). As one moves to the right,

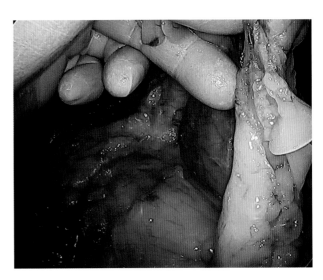

5.5.3

the anterior surface of the duodenum is exposed and the hepatic flexure comes into view. The hepatic flexure is taken down and Gerota's fascia is exposed (**Figures 5.5.4, 5.5.5** and **5.5.6**).

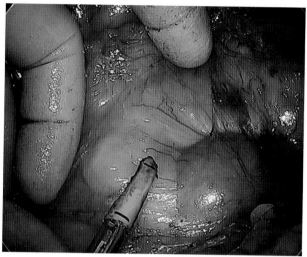

5.5.4

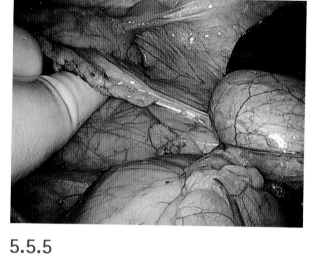

5.5.5

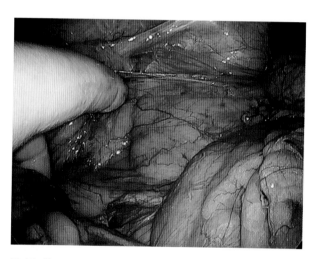

5.5.6

Step 2. The surgeon then mobilizes the right colon mesentery up off the retroperitoneum. Dissection is performed from medial to lateral, leaving the lateral attachments for later. The filmy attachments between the third part of the duodenum and the ileal and right colonic mesentery should be completely divided (**Figure 5.5.7**). This will expose the duodenum completely, essentially over to the ligament of Trietz. This extensive mobilization will help later when taking the mesentery and it will make extraction easy, even in the obese patient.

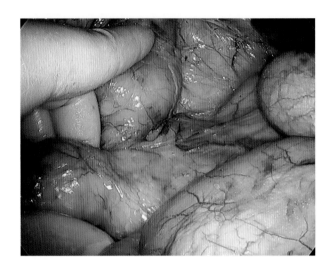

5.5.7

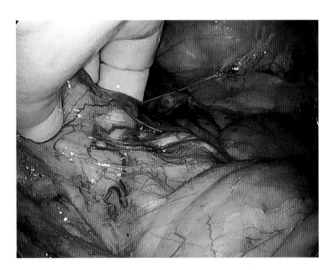

5.5.8

Step 3. With the right colon and ileal mesentery now completely freed from the retroperitoneum, the small bowel and right colon are flipped into the left lower quadrant. Now the ileal mesentery is draped over the palm of the surgeon's left hand (**Figure 5.5.8**) and the peritoneum at the base of the small bowel mesentery is taken from the base of the cecum in the right lower quadrant back up to the duodenum and on to the ligament of Treitz (**Figures 5.5.9, 5.5.10 and 5.5.11**). This is the embryologic fusion plane for the small bowel mesentery.

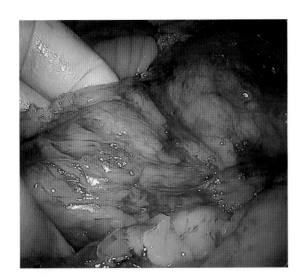

5.5.9

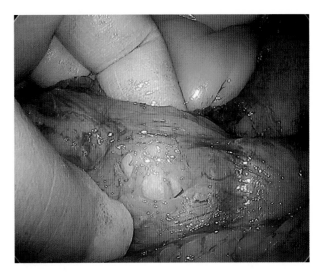

5.5.10

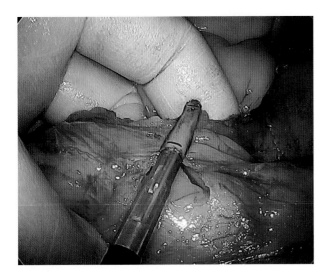

5.5.11

Once the small bowel mesentery has been released, the entire right retroperitoneum is now bare and the entire small bowel and proximal colon are suspended on the superior mesenteric artery and vein (**Figure 5.5.12**). The duodenum, the head of the pancreas, and Gerota's fascia are all in plain sight (**Figure 5.5.13**). The ureter and gonadal vessels will be beneath Toldt's fascia, which is covering the right retroperitoneum, and they should be identified as they cross the iliac vessels on their way to the pelvis (**Figure 5.5.14**).

With mobilization complete, it is now time to take the mesentery and vessels intracorporeally. This is recommended over extracorporeal ligation as they can be taken closer to their origin and division inside facilitates extraction, especially in an obese patient or when the mesentery is very thick. The larger the patient, the more important it is to do a complete mobilization and the more important it is to divide the vessels on the inside.

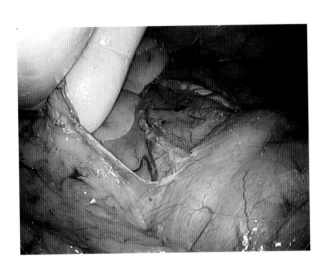

5.5.12

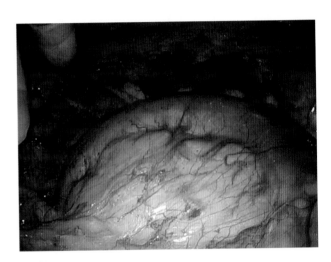

5.5.13

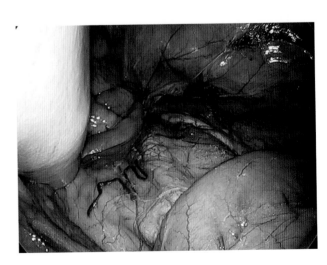

5.5.14

Step 4. The vessels and the mesentery are taken as follows: the surgeon grasps the transverse colon in his palm and then works his middle finger down to the base of the transverse mesocolon to the left of the middle colic vessels. A window is then developed in this area (**Figure 5.5.15**). This is the same window, to the left of the middle colic vessels, that one might create to perform a retrocolic gastrojejunostomy. It is very important

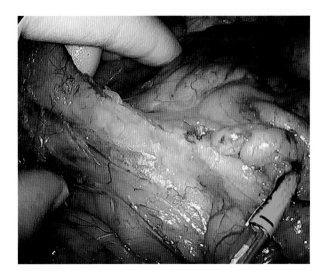

5.5.15

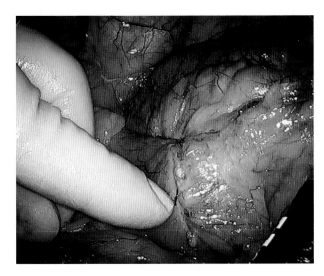

5.5.16

before taking the middle colic vessels, that the mesentery is cleared right down to its base of any omental or gastric attachments. The lesser sac should be very well developed. This makes taking the vessels near their origin feasible, and it facilitates control of bleeding, should this be encountered. The surgeon then moves across the base of the transverse mesocolon from left to right taking the middle colic vessels just over the pancreas (**Figure 5.5.16**). These vessels are clearly seen from above and from the side as they come up out of the retroperitoneum. One should move slowly through this area, as bleeding here can be difficult to control. Bleeding from large middle colic veins is the major risk. Too much traction on the mesentery of the proximal transverse colon can avulse these veins causing significant hemorrhage. This should obviously be avoided. A short stump of vessel should be left in case there is bleeding. This stump allows the surgeon room to control any bleeding with either a clip, a stapler passed through the hand-assist device, an Endoloop™ passed through the left upper quadrant port, or a stitch placed intracorporeally using the hand and a laparoscopic needle holder placed through the left upper quadrant port. Once the middle colic vessels are taken, there is usually a free space in the mesentery and the surgeon can sense the decrease in tension on the mesentery as the middle colic vessels are released. The surgeon then takes a sharp left turn and the ileocolic pedicle is identified (**Figure 5.5.17**), isolated (**Figure 5.5.18**), and divided (**Figure 5.5.19**). In about 90 percent of patients, the right colic artery is a branch of the ileocolic artery or the middle colic artery, so one should not routinely expect to find a right colic artery between the middle colic and ileocolic

vessels. If there is a right colic off the superior mesenteric artery, it is taken and the surgeon moves on to the ileocolic. The ileocolic should always be confirmed to be the ileocolic, and not the superior mesenteric artery. This can be easily accomplished by putting the hepatic flexure back in its place in the right upper quadrant and then grasping the cecum and pulling it down and to the right. This will 'tent' the ileocolic artery for anatomic confirmation. One can take the ileocolic vessel from its ventral surface with the hepatic flexure returned to the right upper quadrant, but it is better not to. Exposure is actually better, and problems are easier to manage with the hepatic

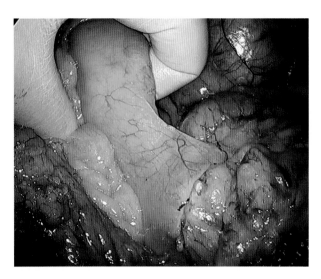

5.5.17

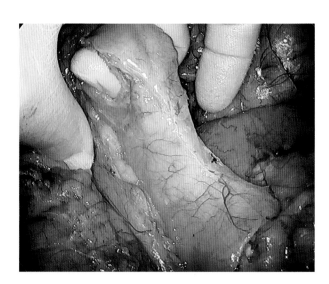

5.5.18

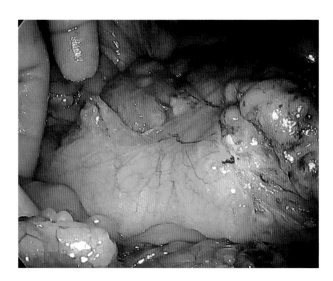

5.5.19

flexure pushed back down into the left abdomen as it is after the mobilization. Thus, if there is a problem with the ileocolic pedicle, the hepatic flexure does not interfere with exposure by falling into the field. Just as with the middle colic vessels, a stump of vessel approximately 2 cm long should be left on the superior mesenteric artery. This gives the surgeon room to maneuver should there be bleeding. If there is bleeding, it can be managed as described above for the middle colic artery. While the named mesenteric vessels are routinely taken with the cutting/sealing energy source, if the surgeon can feel with his fingers that they are highly calcified, they should be taken with a vascular load of the laparoscopic stapler passed through the hand-assist device alongside the surgeon's hand. Once the ileocolic artery is taken, the mesenteric window between the ileocolic and the superior mesenteric vessels is incised out to the marginal vessel along the ileum.

Step 5. Now that the bowel is completely mobilized and the major vessels have been taken, pneumoperitoneum is evacuated through the 5 mm ports, they are removed, and the bowel is extracted through the hand-assist device, which now acts as a wound protector (**Figure 5.5.20**). The marginal vessels along the ileum and the transverse colon are divided, the bowel is divided, and a hand-sewn or stapled ileocolic anastomosis is fashioned. The bowel is dropped back into the abdomen, the hand-assist device is removed, and the incision at the umbilicus is closed with a running absorbable suture and each of the wounds is closed with a subcuticular stitch and tissue adhesive. The mesenteric defect is generally not closed, but the surgeon should try to make sure that the anastomosis sits comfortably in the right upper quadrant and that the small bowel is returned to its proper anatomic position with no twist.

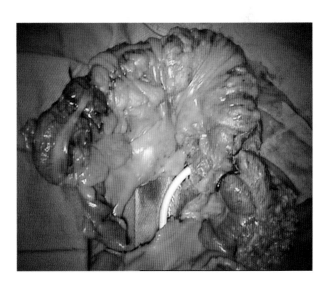

5.5.20

POSTOPERATIVE CARE

Standardized postoperative care includes early and frequent ambulation starting on the day of surgery, minimizing the use of narcotics and making use of oral and intravenous non-steroidal anti-inflammatory drugs (NSAIDs) or continuous local anesthesia delivered directly to the wound via a pump, and early resumption of oral intake. Discharge comes when the patient can tolerate a diet and there has been resumption of bowel function. This usually occurs on day 3, 4, or 5 depending on the patient's age, home situation, motivation, and/or anxiety level.

MANAGEMENT OF PROCEDURE-SPECIFIC COMPLICATIONS

The surgeon should be aware of several well-described complications from colon surgery. These include wound infection, intra-abdominal abscess formation, anastomotic leak and bleeding, and abdominal wound dehiscence. These are general complications of almost any colorectal operation and they are managed no differently after laparoscopic resection than after open operation.

RESULTS AND OUTCOME

When the literature is examined regarding the outcomes with hand-assisted laparoscopic hemicolectomy, there are few high quality data. This is especially the case for right colectomy. What data there are, however, indicate that the hand-assisted technique reduces operative time as compared to a straight laparoscopic approach, while maintaining the short-term advantages of straight laparoscopy. Cost analysis comparing hand-assist versus straight laparoscopic colectomy indicates similar overall expenditures and no significant differences. In addition, the conversion rate should be extremely low for hand-assisted procedures. Lastly, postoperative wound infection and hernia rates after hand-assisted laparoscopic colectomy are no different than after straight laparoscopic colectomy.

In conclusion, hand-assisted laparoscopic right hemicolectomy is a sound technique. While the authors would argue that the hand-assisted laparoscopic approach illustrated can be used to advantage for the vast majority of right colon resections, this operation is particularly well suited in managing the obese patient, the patient with a bulky tumor or mass and in situations where the surgeon is intent on a meticulous and thorough dissection of the middle colic vessels near their origin just over the pancreas. It is a technique that can be adopted well by the general or colorectal surgeon who has a good grasp of the anatomy, even if he or she has limited laparoscopic experience, and it is an operation that can be conducted by a single surgeon without the need for a trained assistant to provide exposure. Finally, operative times are decreased when comparing standard laparoscopic to hand-assisted laparoscopic approaches. All these advantages are gained without any apparent reduction in the short-term, patient-related benefits of minimally invasive colon surgery.

FURTHER READING

Aly EH. Laparoscopic colorectal surgery: summary of the current evidence. *Annals of the Royal College of Surgeons of England 2009*; **91**: 541–4.

Marcello PW, Fleshman JW, Milsom JW *et al.* Hand access vs 'pure' laparoscopic colectomy: a multicenter prospective randomized trial. *Diseases of the Colon and Rectum* 2008; **51**: 818–26.

Ozturk E, Kiran RP, Geisler DP *et al.* Hand-assisted laparoscopic colectomy: benefits of laparoscopic colectomy at no extra cost. *Journal of the American College of Surgeons* 2009; **209**: 242–7.

Sonoda T, Pandey S, Trencheva K *et al.* Longterm complications of hand-assisted versus laparoscopic colectomy. *Journal of the American College of Surgeons* 2009; **208**: 62–6.

Left colectomy – open

MARY R KWAAN AND DAVID A ROTHENBERGER

PRINCIPLES AND JUSTIFICATION

A left colectomy is typically performed for the treatment of a malignancy, diverticular disease, segmental Crohn's colitis, or ischemia.

This procedure poses unique technical challenges because of the variable blood supply to the left colon and the relationship of the left colon to adjacent structures. The arterial blood supply to the left transverse and descending colon segments is usually dependent on an arcade of vessels arising in a variable pattern from the superior and inferior mesenteric arteries. This arcade generally includes the left branch of the middle colic artery that merges near the splenic flexure into an arcade of vessels arising from the left colic artery to create the marginal artery of Drummond. Venous drainage of the mid-transverse colon may flow from the middle colic vein to the superior mesenteric vein, while the descending colon venous flow is to the left colic vein into the inferior mesenteric vein as it ascends over the psoas muscle in the retroperitoneum ultimately reaching the splenic vein. Intraoperative assessment of this anatomy is essential for the surgeon to plan an R0 resection of the colon and its adjacent lymph node-bearing mesentery and to preserve well-vascularized ends of colon to perform a safe anastomosis without tension. If this is not possible, extended resections of the proximal colon or sigmoid colon may be necessary. Pathology in the left transverse colon and descending colon may involve adjacent intra-abdominal viscera including the stomach, omentum, and spleen or retroperitoneal structures, such as the distal pancreas, left kidney, and ureter. Unplanned splenectomy is performed in up to 6 percent of left colon resections for a splenic flexure tumor because of inadvertent splenic injury.[1] Left colon cancers can invade the retroperitoneum requiring *en bloc* resection of involved distal pancreas or left kidney and ureter. Crohn's disease can cause retroperitoneal abscesses and fistulae.

A frequent complaint of patients after left colectomy is an alteration of bowel habits. This may include a transient increase in stool frequency, clustering of bowel movements, bloating, and constipation. Generally, this is self-limited and resolves within a few months of colectomy, although permanent alteration can occur, especially in patients with compromised anal sphincter function preoperatively.

PREOPERATIVE ASSESSMENT AND PREPARATION

As with any major abdominal procedure, attention should be given to medical optimization of the patient before the planned procedure. Preoperative colonoscopy and imaging studies are performed to assess the primary disease and exclude involvement of other sites and organs. If it appears extended, resections of other organs may be needed, and appropriate consultation with surgical colleagues is helpful. If a temporary or permanent stoma is a likely component of the procedure, the site for this should be marked before the patient is under anesthesia, with attention to skin creases and the patient's belt line. Ideally, this is done in consultation with an enterostomal therapist who can also provide teaching and counseling about stoma management.

Traditionally, patients undergoing left colectomy were given a full mechanical bowel preparation usually consisting of a clear liquid diet and a purgative bowel preparation, such as 4 liters of polyethylene glycol 1 day in advance of surgery. Clinical evidence is emerging that suggests no increased incidence of infectious events if a bowel preparation is omitted, but if there is the possible need for intraoperative colonoscopy, a bowel preparation is still advised.[2]

IMAGING

Frequently, imaging is obtained as part of the diagnostic evaluation. Cross-sectional imaging, for example computed tomography (CT) or magnetic resonance imaging (MRI), provides information about structures adjacent to the colon. Patients with colon adenocarcinoma should have a CT scan of the abdomen and pelvis to assess for metastatic disease in the liver. In the case of a locally advanced colon adenocarcinoma, proximity or invasion of the primary lesion to the spleen, pancreas, kidney, or ureter may prompt consideration and guide planning of an *en bloc* organ resection. In the case of a colectomy for Crohn's or diverticular disease, imaging may suggest inflammation near the left ureter. Preoperative planning of a left ureteral stent may facilitate the intraoperative dissection in this situation. Patients with Crohn's disease should have enteric contrast studies and/or endoscopy of the small and large intestine to assess for other sites of disease that may require concurrent resection or closer intraoperative examination.

PATIENT PREPARATION IN THE PERIOPERATIVE PHASE

A perioperative checklist or protocol can maintain consistency of process and promote safety in perioperative practices that will assure optimal surgical outcomes.

Patient positioning

Patients should be positioned in modified lithotomy to facilitate access to the anus for colonoscopy or proctoscopy. Such a maneuver may be unexpectedly required to identify intraluminal lesions or to perform and/or test a colonic anastomosis. An added advantage of this position is that the surgeon can stand between the patient's legs for optimal visualization of the left upper quadrant, while the assistant stands to the left side of the patient retracting the abdominal wall upward (see also Chapter 1.3).

OPERATION

Incision

A midline incision is performed to allow full access to the superior and inferior reaches of the left colon. Such an incision can be extended in either direction to maximize exposure. A midline incision preserves the integrity of the lateral abdominal wall for patients with inflammatory bowel disease, who frequently require reoperation over their lifetime and may require a stoma. For exposure of a difficult splenic flexure, the incision may extend to the xiphoid process. A self-retaining retractor, such as the Bookwalter or Omni-Track system, is placed to maintain exposure. These systems are flexible and can be changed as needed to facilitate exposure and dissection. Takedown of the splenic flexure is assisted by using an upward lift in the left upper quadrant.

Exploration

General exploration of the abdomen, including the colon, is done to confirm the presumed diagnosis and the appropriateness of the planned operative procedure. The operative plan is altered if unexpected pathology is identified or the location or extent of the pathology is other than anticipated. Large invasive lesions can be palpated and superficial or small tumors can be identified by a serosal tattoo that may have been placed previously during colonoscopy. Intraoperative colonoscopy can be performed if there is uncertainty about the location of the lesion of interest. The peritoneal surfaces and the solid organs of the abdomen are inspected by palpation and visualization. Unexpected nodules or masses may require biopsy, the results of which may change the operative plan. After abdominal exploration, the small intestine is packed with laparotomy pads into the right upper quadrant.

Extent of resection

Important considerations include the extent of colonic resection, for example in the case of inflammatory bowel disease, and the extent of mesocolic resection, as in the case of colon adenocarcinoma (**Figure 5.6.1**).

A cancer in the splenic flexure or proximal left colon requires a lymphadenectomy that includes ligation of the left branch of the middle colic artery near its origin and the left colic artery near its origin from the inferior mesenteric artery while preserving the sigmoidal arteries. The proximal transverse colon and sigmoid colon can be preserved for a colocolic anastomosis.

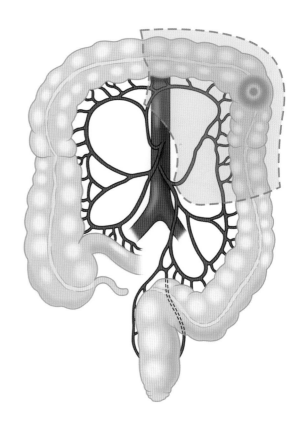

5.6.1

SPECIAL CIRCUMSTANCES

In cases where the blood supply to the remaining proximal transverse colon is inadequate or where the mobility of the right and transverse colon is not sufficient to support a tension-free anastomosis, a subtotal colectomy with ileocolic anastomosis should be performed. The distal aspect of this resection is at the junction of the left colon and the sigmoid colon (**Figure 5.6.2**). The resected mesenteric vessels include the right colic, middle colic, and left colic, with special attention paid to achieving a proximal ligation on the left colic and, in circumstances of a mid- to distal transverse colon lesion, the middle colic. The right colic need not be resected with a proximal ligation since the draining nodes of a left colon malignancy would not be expected in those vascular distributions.

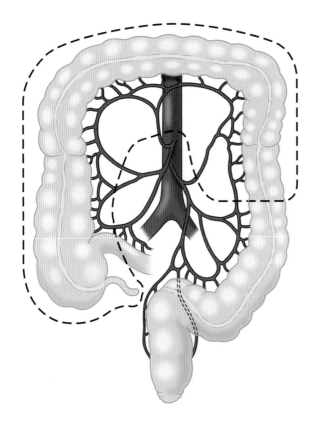

5.6.2

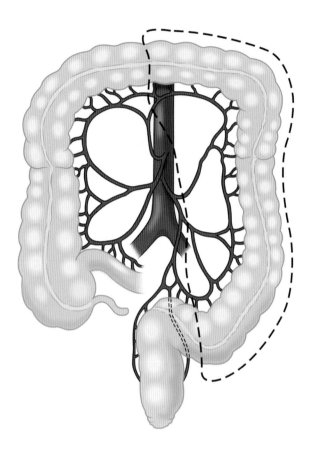

If the sigmoid colon is stiff and hypertrophied from incidental diverticular disease, it should not be used to support a colocolic or ileocolic anastomosis. It should be removed and a colorectal or ileorectal anastomosis should be performed (**Figure 5.6.3**).

5.6.3

Mobilization

For benign disease, mobilization of the colon provides access to proximal and distal margins of colonic transection, exposure of the mesocolon for safe transaction, and mobility for the subsequent anastomosis. The extent of mesocolic dissection is tailored to what is needed to achieve these goals and determined in part by the vascular anatomy. With a cancer resection, the colon and mesocolon require mobilization without cutting across tumor cells within the primary lesion or within metastatic lymph nodes. Resection of the primary tumor can usually be achieved without violating the cancer if it has not completely invaded the colonic wall ($\leq$T2). Tumors that invade through the colonic wall and into the pericolic fat require a wider dissection in the soft tissue and retroperitoneum. Subsequent mobilization of the mesocolon off the retroperitoneum is optimally achieved if dissection is performed sharply (either with electrocautery or scissors) and follows the embryologic fusion planes between the visceral and parietal tissue layers. This type of dissection, recently labeled as the 'complete mesocolic excision' is analogous to total mesorectal excision for rectal cancer. The goals of this dissection are to achieve complete excision of vessels, lymphatics, and lymph nodes that drain the primary tumor.[3]

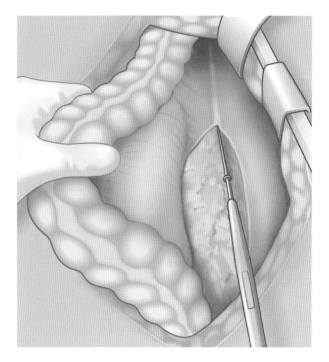

LEFT HEMICOLECTOMY

The left colon is pulled medially to expose the white line of Toldt. Electrocautery is used to incise the full thickness of peritoneum at this line, and the avascular plane between the left mesocolon and the left retroperitoneum is developed (**Figure 5.6.4**). The surgeon's fingers or a sponge stick can be used to gently wipe the retroperitoneum posteriorly and laterally so that the gonadal vessels and left ureter are displaced away from the mesocolon. If dissection proceeds too deeply, troublesome retroperitoneal venous bleeding occurs, and if too superficial, the colon and mesocolon will remain fixed to the retroperitoneum risking incomplete lymphadenectomy.

5.6.4

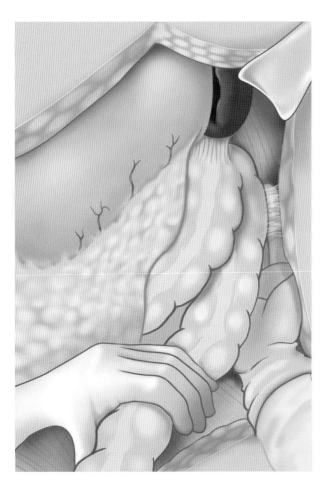

The surgeon can stand between the patient's legs as the dissection proceeds proximally and cephalad toward the spleen. The surgeon's right hand can be rolled out from under the left mesocolon, exposing the lateral peritoneal attachments for division by the assistant.

It is important not to pull down on the left colon because this can result in a splenic injury. Instead, the thrust of the dissection is upwards toward the splenic flexure (**Figure 5.6.5**).

5.6.5

As the mesocolon is elevated and rotated toward the midline, it serves as a fan-like retractor and may serve to keep the small intestine out of the operative field. As the mesocolon is dissected medially, retroperitoneal structures, such as the left ureter and left gonadal vessels, are exposed. However, caution must be used when applying electrocautery as defects through the mesocolon can be made, resulting in thermal injury to any small intestine on the medial aspect of the left mesocolon (**Figure 5.6.6**).

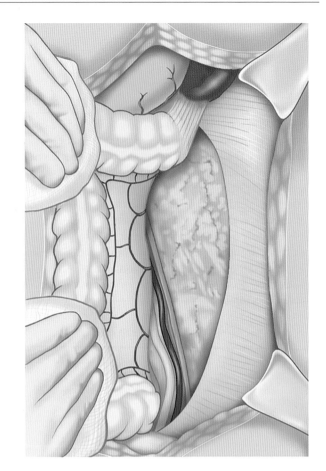

5.6.6

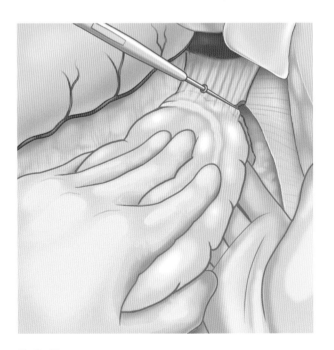

5.6.7

The splenic flexure is visualized with upward traction on the abdominal wall in the left upper quadrant. Any peritoneal bands to the spleen or attachments of the omentum to the spleen should be divided under direct view and using minimal tension (**Figure 5.6.7**). Once this is accomplished, the splenic flexure and distal transverse colon can be gently retracted inferiorly. Further blunt dissection of the retroperitoneum using a laterally directed wiping maneuver can aid in the mobilization of the splenic flexure. It is important to stay adjacent to the superolateral margin of the colon. The splenocolic ligament may contain vessels requiring ligation. A right angle or MD Anderson clamp can be used, and ties should be placed around the pedicles with passers. Alternatively, an energy device such as the Ligasure™ (Valleylab, Boulder, CO, USA) or the Harmonic Scalpel™ (Ethicon Endo-Surgery, Cincinnati, OH, USA) can be used.

If the splenic flexure is difficult to take down by only mobilizing the proximal descending colon, it is useful to turn attention to the distal transverse colon and enter the lesser sac by dividing the avascular attachments between the omentum and the colon. One can thus work to mobilize the splenic flexure along the left transverse colon from within the lesser sac by applying downward traction to the colon. The surgeon can then return to taking down the splenic flexure by further mobilizing along the proximal descending colon while applying right lateral traction to the colon. The surgeon may inadvertently enter the mesocolon either with the electrocautery or through fracture of the mesocolic tissues if proper care is not applied. The inferior mesenteric vein, as it courses toward the splenic vein, is sometimes responsible for a tightly adherent mesenteric–retroperitoneal interface in this location. If this is the case, it should be divided between clamps and ligated. In the circumstance of a splenic flexure malignancy, dissection in the proper plan is critical to provide the patient with tumor-free colonic and mesocolic margins.

SIGMOID COLECTOMY

When sigmoid colectomy is needed, the sigmoid colon is pulled medially to expose the white line of Toldt. Electrocautery is used to incise the full thickness of peritoneum at this line. Gentle blunt dissection can be used to wipe the retroperitoneum laterally and posteriorly. The dissection includes mobilization of the sigmoid colon and most of the descending colon up to the splenic flexure. If needed to allow a tension-free colorectal anastomosis, the entire splenic flexure is taken down and the inferior mesenteric vein is ligated. As this dissection proceeds distally, the left ureter can be exposed and protected as it courses over the iliac vessels. The dissection need not proceed this deep into the mesocolon if the resection is for benign disease, however, if the resection is for a sigmoid cancer, the ureter should be exposed to reassure the surgeon that the proximal extent of the mesocolic resection will include a proper lymphadenectomy. After mobilization of the descending and sigmoid colon is complete, the vascular supply can be visualized. Transillumination of the mesentery with a headlight can facilitate assessment of the vascular anatomy.

Division of the mesentery and resection

LEFT HEMICOLECTOMY

The mobilized left colon is retracted into the midline wound so that its mesentery can be exposed and transilluminated. The vessels selected for the appropriate mesocolic dissection are isolated by incising the overlying peritoneum and triply clamping, dividing, and double-tying the proximal stump (**Figure 5.6.8**). A 2-0 braided suture, such as polyglycolic acid or silk, can be used to secure mesenteric pedicles. For cancers, proximal ligation is standard. For a distal transverse colon or splenic flexure tumor, the left branch of the middle colic or the middle colic artery will need to be divided. In addition, the left colic will be divided, but the sigmoidal arteries are preserved. After proximal ligation is performed, the remaining mesocolon between the transected vessels and the bowel edge is divided serially between clamps and ligated.

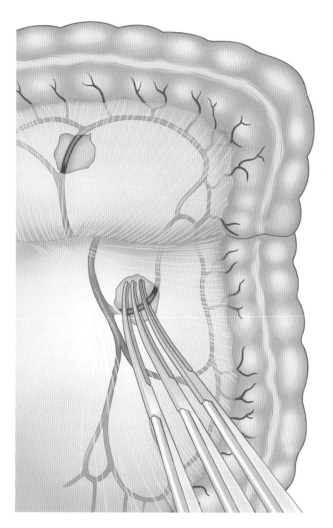

5.6.8

In the case of Crohn's colitis, there is no need to resect the mesocolon proximally. Generally, the safer approach would be to stay close to the colon when dividing the mesocolon. Fatty and inflamed mesentery in Crohn's disease can be addressed with serial figure-of-eight suture ligatures if discrete pedicles are difficult to dissect. Ligatures need to be tied down gently to prevent fracturing small friable vessels in the mesocolic fat. The diseased colon can be divided initially at the proximal or distal extent of resection to optimize exposure of and control over the mesentery. In this case, close attention should be paid to avoiding injury to the retroperitoneal structures.

Retroperitoneal structures, such as the pancreas, kidney, and especially the left ureter, should be kept in mind whenever the mesocolon is divided proximally. If mobilization was properly performed, injury to these structures is far less a concern.

The mesentery supplying the colon at the site of the proposed anastomosis is assessed to determine whether the blood supply supports healing. In addition, the bowel for the proposed anastomosis needs to be mobilized sufficiently so that there is no tension on the connection. For a splenic flexure adenocarcinoma, the sigmoid colon (if non-diseased and pliable) can usually be spared. Once the circumstances have been optimized for the anastomosis, a short distance of 1 cm or less is cleared along the mesenteric surface to allow accurate suture placement without compromising the vascularity of the anastomosis. The mesenteric flow at the proposed anastomotic sites should be pulsatile.

If a hand-sewn anastomosis is planned, a non-crushing (Dennis) clamp is placed across the intestine at the site for division, with a crushing (Kocher) clamp being placed in parallel on the 'specimen side' of the non-crushing clamp. The colon can be divided with a blade between bowel clamps, taking care not to spill fecal contents on

to the field. If a GIA stapler is chosen to divide the colon, the 'green' staple load (4.8 mm staple height) is preferred. Once both ends of the specimen are divided, the colon is sent off the field to be opened and examined by the pathology department while the procedure continues.

SIGMOID COLECTOMY

The inferior mesenteric artery is defined and transected proximally if cancer is present, or more distally if the sigmoid pathology is non-malignant. If a cancer is in the 'watershed' area between the proximal sigmoid and the distal descending colon, the inferior mesenteric artery is transected flush with the aorta (high ligation) and plans are made for a proximal descending colon or transverse colon to rectal anastomosis. If a cancer is present in the mid-sigmoid colon, the inferior mesenteric artery may be transected distal to the take off of the left colic artery (low ligation) and plans are made for a distal descending colon to rectal anastomosis. For a distal sigmoid colon cancer near the rectosigmoid junction, the dissection is that of a high anterior resection of the upper rectum discussed in Chapter 6.1. Regardless of the level of transaction, the left ureter is re-examined prior to division of the vascular pedicle. If the dissection of the mesocolon was difficult, or if there are any ambiguities about the anatomy, the right ureter should also be re-examined to ensure that it is not within the vascular pedicle. The inferior mesenteric artery is triply clamped, divided, and suture ligated. All the sigmoidal vessels will be included in the mesocolic resection, and the intervening soft tissue between the vascular pedicle and the proposed proximal and distal colonic transection lines is isolated and divided with clamps and ties. The proximal colon can be divided between bowel clamps as described above. An angled (Glassman) bowel clamp is easier to use for the distal transection at the rectosigmoid junction since the pelvis limits working space.

Mesenteric closure

When the mesenteric defect looks as if it will give rise to a problematic internal hernia, it is appropriate to consider closure of such defect. Frequently, this is not required after a sigmoid resection with anastomosis. It is a consideration after a left colectomy with a transverse colon to sigmoid colon anastomosis. In some situations, the cut edge of the mesentery may be tacked to the retroperitoneum to close portions of mesenteric edges that are impossible to bring together. After alignment, the mesocolon is closed with a continuous polyglycolic acid suture from its base near the proximal ligation point to within 5 cm of the site of anastomosis (**Figure 5.6.9**). Care is taken not to damage any vessels along the cut edges of the mesocolon which might diminish blood flow to the anastomosis. The mesocolic

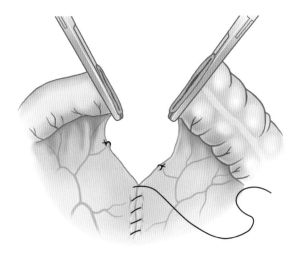

5.6.9

defect is most easily closed before the anastomosis is
created, but should not be completely closed so as to not
confine the space needed for manipulation of the bowel
ends during the anastomosis.

Anastomosis

LEFT HEMICOLECTOMY

Ideally, a primary anastomosis is performed following
colectomy. The surgeon's sound judgment is essential to
assure success. Factors that must be considered include
the patient's overall status, the condition of the peritoneal
cavity, the condition of the intestine and the completeness
of its preparation, and the assurance that the necessary
technical demands of an anastomosis, i.e. vascularity, lack
of tension, and accurate approximation, can be met. We
generally prefer a semi-closed, hand-sutured, minimally
inverting technique approximating the colon in an end-to-
end fashion.

The site of the anastomosis is isolated from the
surrounding field with laparotomy pads. The bowel clamps
are held parallel, approximately 3 cm apart by the assistant,
who directs the tips towards the surgeon's dominant hand.
The clamps are turned 90° upward to expose the posterior
wall, and interrupted 4-0 seromuscular sutures are placed
at approximately 1–1.5 cm intervals. The preferred stitch is
a 4-0 silk on an RB1 needle. The sutures at the mesenteric
and antimesenteric sides are left untied and tagged. The
intervening sutures are serially tied and trimmed as the
assistant holds the parallel Dennis clamps together (**Figure
5.6.10**).

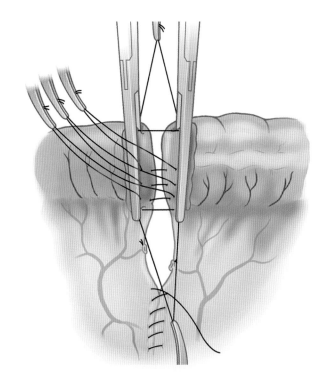

5.6.10

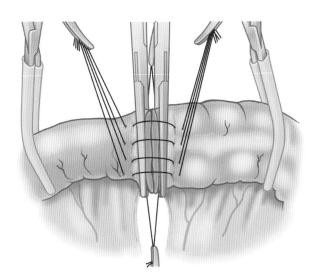

The Dennis clamps are rotated 180°, thus exposing the
anterior wall. A series of 4-0 seromuscular sutures are
placed about 1–1.5 cm apart and the ends tagged (**Figure
5.6.11**).

5.6.11

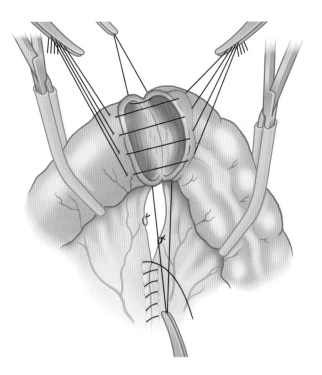

Occlusion of the intestine 3–4 cm from the ends is achieved by gentle digital compression or by a shod non-crushing clamp gently applied across the intestinal lumen only. The Dennis clamps are removed from first one cut end of the intestine and then the other. While the tagged sutures are held up to open the intestinal lumen, an assistant is ready to use suction if any stool begins to leak from the cut end (**Figure 5.6.12**).

5.6.12

After ensuring that none of the sutures have inadvertently picked up the opposite wall and that there are no major arterial bleeders, the surgeon ties all suture pairs. Proximal occluding pressure or shod clamps are removed. The anastomosis is completed by placing 4-0 interrupted full-thickness sutures between each of the previously placed sutures circumferentially. The surgeon must be certain that the anastomosis is well vascularized, widely patent, under no tension, and that the technique was not compromised in any way. The mesocolic suture is completed to close the mesenteric defect up to the wall of the intestine (**Figure 5.6.13**).

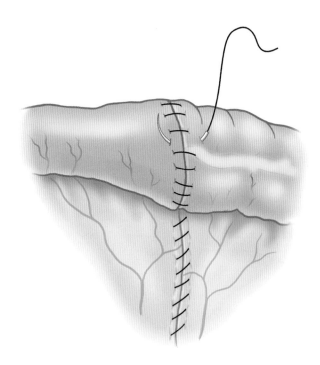

5.6.13

SIGMOID COLECTOMY

The preferred anastomosis after a sigmoid colectomy is a stapled end-to-end coloproctostomy (see Chapter 6.1). Upon occasion, the proximal rectum requires more extensive mobilization to facilitate easy placement of the EEA (end-to-end anastomosis) stapler flush with the transection line of the rectum. This dissection is more frequently required in colonic disease which may have resulted in inflammation and adhesions, such as diverticulitis or Crohn's colitis. If a circular stapler cannot be passed easily to the proposed site of the colorectal anastomosis, the surgeon should consider resecting an additional few centimeters of the proximal rectal stump as it may include diseased distal sigmoid or scarred proximal rectum, either of which could cause the anastomosis to fail.

Alternative anastomotic techniques

Unique problems demand flexibility on the part of the surgeon, and other anastomotic techniques may be preferred depending on circumstances and personal experience.

SIZE DISCREPANCY

Major size discrepancy in the two limbs of intestine does not usually pose a problem if the technique described above is used. The technique of continually halving the distance to guide suture placement on each end of the cut intestine can be used to easily accommodate a major size discrepancy. An acceptable alternative anastomotic technique is a side-to-side functional end-to-end stapled anastomosis. A total abdominal colectomy and ileorectal anastomosis may involve two limbs of intestine with major size discrepancy. If the rectum is large and the ileum small, the author's preferred approach is to use a double-staple technique.

DISTAL ANASTOMOSIS

Most colonic anastomoses are easily accessible and lend themselves to suturing. If a distal anastomosis to the upper- or middle-third of the rectum is required after a segmental or total colectomy, the circular stapled end-to-end anastomosis may be easier.

EDEMATOUS BOWEL

Obstruction often results in edematous bowel which can be hazardous to approximate because sutures or staples may pull out. A two-layer technique or reinforcement of a stapled anastomosis may be preferable in such situations. Alternatively, the edema may preclude a safe primary anastomosis, and a colostomy or ileostomy may be necessary as a first step.

Wound closure

After assuring a correct sponge and needle count and achieving hemostasis, the abdomen is irrigated, fluid is suctioned, and the fascia is closed with a running stitch, usually a slowly absorbable monofilament suture such as a number 1 looped or non-looped PDS (polydioxanone). The subcutaneous tissue is irrigated, and in most instances the skin is approximated by subcuticular sutures or skin staples. A pelvic or peritoneal drain is not routinely used.

POSTOPERATIVE CARE

Nasogastric aspiration is not required unless the patient had a pre-existing bowel obstruction. Clear liquids are begun when the patient is not nauseated or distended, as early as the first postoperative day. If tolerated, the diet is advanced to low residue solid food. Intravenous fluids are maintained until the patient is taking sufficient fluids orally. The urinary catheter is normally discontinued the day after surgery, if urine output is adequate. If there is evidence of infection or sepsis, the surgeon must suspect a leaked anastomosis. Generally, the patient has recovered sufficiently to be discharged 5 days after surgery.

REFERENCES

1. McGory ML, Zingmond DS, Sekeris E, Ko CY. The significance of inadvertent splenectomy during colorectal cancer resection. *Archives of Surgery* 2007; **142**: 668–74.
2. Slim K, Vicaut E, Launay-Savary M-V *et al.* Updated systematic review and meta-analysis of randomized clinical trials on the role of mechanical bowel preparation before colorectal surgery. *Annals of Surgery* 2009; **249**: 203–9.
3. Hohenberger W, Weber K, Matzel K *et al.* Standardized surgery for colonic cancer: complete mesocolic excision and central ligation – technical notes and outcome. *Colorectal Disease* 2009; **11**: 354–65.

Left hemicolectomy – laparoscopic

PAUL C NEARY

PRINCIPLES AND JUSTIFICATION

Laparoscopic resection is the most important technical development in colorectal surgery that has occurred over the last decade and offers patients considerable advantages compared to open resection. These include reduced incidence of postoperative wound infections, intra-abdominal adhesions, and postoperative ileus due to reduced handling of the small bowel, leading to shorter length of stay and potentially reduced hospital costs.[1,2] Initial concern regarding the oncological outcome after laparoscopic resection for colorectal cancer, including a possible increased incidence of port site metastases, initially delayed widespread acceptance of the technique; however, large randomized trials such as the Clinical Outcomes of Surgical Therapy (COST) Study Group[3] and the Conventional versus Laparoscopic Assisted Surgery in Colorectal Cancer (CLASICC) trial[4] have shown no differences in either local or distant recurrence rates or survival rates between laparoscopic and open resection.

There are fundamental differences in the skills required for laparoscopic compared to open resection and left-sided colonic resections should not be undertaken without the required training and experience. Tekkis et al.[5] assessed the learning curve for right- and left-sided resections and concluded that 55 cases were required for right-sided resections and 62 for left-sided resections. For surgeons at the beginning of the learning curve, resection for benign disease, such as for colonic polyps and uncomplicated diverticulitis, are the best options to start with in terms of case selection for laparoscopic left hemicolectomy.

CHOICE OF SURGICAL APPROACH AND TECHNIQUE

There are fundamental technical differences in undertaking either laparoscopic or open resection between benign and malignant disease. In benign cases, a full dissection based upon oncologic principles is not required. In malignant cases, a left hemicolectomy entails resection of the colon from the mid-transverse colon to the sigmoid colon. This involves take down of the splenic flexure and anastomosis of the transverse colon to the sigmoid colon with, in some cases, sigmoidectomy and anastomosis to the upper rectum. In this chapter, the operative techniques to perform left hemicolectomy alone or left hemicolectomy combined with proctosigmoidectomy in both benign and malignant disease are described. The operative steps and techniques are all based upon a standardized sequence that provides consistent results across a wide spectrum of colorectal pathology.[6,7]

PREOPERATIVE CARE

Assessment

The assessment of patients for major colonic surgery requires consideration of radiological contrast studies, colonoscopy, ultrasonography, and thoracoabdominal scanning (CT ± MRI ± PET), and tumor markers for those with colonic malignancy. Patients with colonic cancer are routinely discussed at a multidisciplinary meeting prior to surgery. The segment of colon to be excised must be localized prior to surgery. In those patients in whom a polyp or tumor is scheduled to be removed by laparoscopic segmental colectomy, the target lesion should be tattooed at colonoscopy prior to operation. It is prudent to ensure that in all cases of neoplasia the area of colonic lumen is tattooed 5 cm distal to the site of the tumor in order to reduce the chance of tumor seeding through inadvertent intraperitoneal injection of marking ink. In patients in whom a large tumor is visible on CT, the experienced operator may feel that preoperative tattooing is unnecessary; however, it is the author's view that such an approach can lead to unanticipated intraoperative difficulty. It is, therefore, a strong recommendation that in all cases where the surgeon is undertaking a segmental resection laparoscopically that the lesion is adequately localized preoperatively.

Patient education

Patients undergoing laparoscopic resection should be educated and counseled in full regarding the 'patient voyage' that they are undertaking. The risks of the surgery should be outlined and informed consent obtained. Those who may have a stoma postoperatively should undergo preoperative stoma education with a stoma therapist and, ideally, have had time to practice with the appliances preoperatively. It is important that those undergoing an enhanced recovery program should know what to expect and the patient-related goals that are to be expected on each postoperative day. The indoctrination of the patient into their expected care plan helps facilitate a smooth transition from postoperative stay to early discharge. In patients in whom prolonged convalescence and supportive care outside the hospital may be anticipated, preoperative education and planning are invaluable.

Preparation

Mechanical bowel preparation is undertaken for all patients undergoing laparoscopic left hemicolectomy in order to ease handling of the colon. The usual preparation consists of two sachets of Picolax® (sodium picosulphate) the day before surgery. High-volume preoperative bowel preparations that involve drinking over 4 liters of fluid preoperatively tend to result in small bowel dilatation and are therefore to be avoided. Unlike open surgery where bowel preparation may be avoided, manipulation of a stool-laden colon with laparoscopic instruments may be hazardous. Use of carbohydrate loading drinks preoperatively and minimizing preoperative fasting is to be recommended. In the perioperative period, prophylactic antibiotics are used against Gram-positive and Gram-negative aerobic and anaerobic organisms. Deep venous thrombosis prophylaxis is achieved using compression stockings and low molecular weight heparin injections are given subcutaneously.

LAPAROSCOPIC EQUIPMENT

The following laparoscopic equipment is required: 10 mm subumbilical Hasson port; one 12 mm trocar; three 5 mm trocars; three intestinal grasping clamps (35 cm, one bowel clamp should be long (40–45 cm shaft); a wound protector; a laparoscopic scissors (blunt tipped/square tipped scissors preferred); a laparoscopic Maryland forceps; a laparoscopic Alice forceps; an Endo-clip® (Covidien, Dublin, Ireland) applicator (or equivalent Ligaclip®, Ethicon Endo-Surgery, Cincinnati, OH, USA); 0° camera lens (30° lens is optional); an Endo-GIA®, Ethicon Endo-Surgery (or equivalent); an energy sealing device such as an ultrasonic dissector (Ultrasonic Harmonic scalpel®, Ethicon Endo-Surgery) or an advanced vessel sealing system (Ligasure®, Covidien). For external resection of the bowel and ligation of mesenteric vessels, a standard medium size laparotomy set is required. As a precaution a major laparotomy set should be available in case urgent conversion is required.

ANESTHESIA

General anesthesia with muscle relaxation is required. A Foley urinary catheter and orogastric tube are inserted. Patient-controlled analgesia is the preferred method of postoperative analgesia as it facilitates early postoperative mobilization.

OPERATION

Position of patient

The patient is placed supine on the operating table and cocooned on a beanbag. It is not the author's routine practice to use shoulder supports or strapping. Once general anesthesia has been induced, the legs are placed in Dan Allen or Yellowfin stirrups® (Allen Medical Systems, Ashby-de-la-Zouch, UK). The arms are tucked at the patient's side and the beanbag is aspirated. The abdomen is then prepared with betadine antiseptic solution and draped routinely. The patient is placed in the Trendelenburg (head down) position. The key elements of patient positioning are that the arms at tucked in by the patient's side and the hips positioned to permit slight extension when the stirrups are dropped below the horizontal. The anesthetic machine and intravenous giving set stands should all be placed above the patient's head line as the assistant holding the laparoscopic camera will otherwise find difficulty in achieving room while standing to the left of the surgeon (**Figure 5.7.1**).

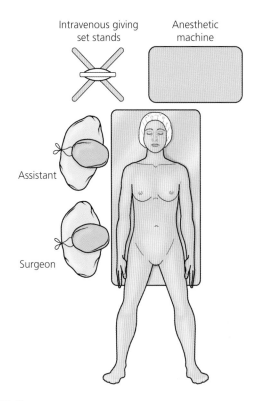

5.7.1

Instrument positioning

The main monitor is placed on the left side of the patient at approximately the level of the hip. The secondary monitor is placed on the right side of the patient at the knee level, and is primarily for the assistant during the early phase of the surgery and port insertion. The operating nurse's

instrument table is placed below and to the right of the patient's extended legs (**Figure 5.7.2**a). The surgeon stands on the right side of the patient at the level of the patient's hip, with the assistant standing on the patient's left. The assistant moves to the right side, at the level of the patient's shoulder, once the ports have been inserted (**Figure 5.7.2**b). If a second assistant is available, they

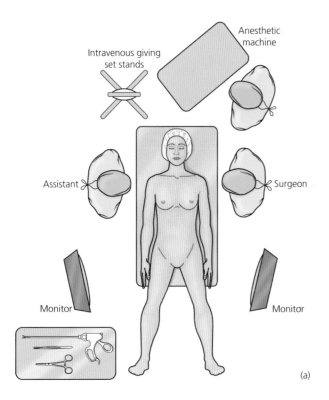

(a)

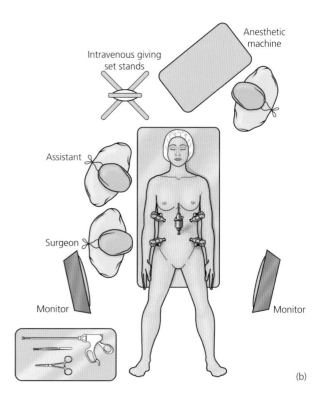

(b)

5.7.2

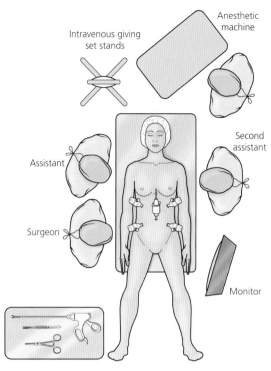

stand on the left side of the patient (**Figure 5.7.3**). An instrument holding bag (deep disposable plastic bag) is placed on each of the patient's hips to permit the operator to drop and change instruments at ease and a further supportive bag holding hand-held electrocautery as well as a thermos flask for cleaning or demisting the camera when required is placed opposite the surgeon on the patient's left side. In cases where a single lead laparoscopic camera is unavailable and dual light and camera sleeve is required then it is advantageous to tape both of these leads together to reduce line tangling intraoperatively.

5.7.3

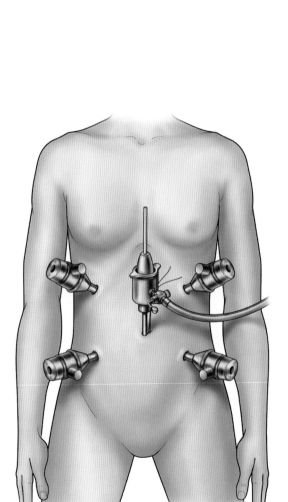

5.7.4

Trocar placement

The Hasson technique is used to gain the initial access to the peritoneal cavity (see Chapter 1.5). The 10 mm Hasson port is inserted and CO_2 is insufflated to a pressure of 12 mmHg. A 12 mm port is then inserted into the right lower quadrant 2–3 cm above and medial to the anterior superior iliac spine. This initial operating trocar location, 1 inch in and 1 inch up from the anterior superior iliac spine, may be placed more medially in an obese patient in those with a rotund (high/distensible) abdomen. This port site permits the entry of an Endo-GIA stapler. In very thin patients and when major vessel ligation is to be undertaken either extracorporeally or by using a 5 mm energy delivery device, then a 5 mm trocar port may be used. Specific care must be taken to avoid the inferior epigastric vessels by directing the trocar perpendicular to the abdominal wall during insertion. The laparoscope can also be used to transilluminate the abdominal wall so the surgeon can visualize any superficial vessels. A 5 mm port is then inserted in the right upper quadrant at least a hand's breadth superior to the right lower quadrant. A 5 mm left lower quadrant port is usually required to aid retraction of the colon, and for a difficult splenic flexure, a 5 mm left upper quadrant is sometimes required for extra retraction. All ports are inserted under direct vision. The port site insertions are mirror images of each other resulting in ports located right and left upper quadrants and right and left lower quadrants, respectively (**Figure 5.7.4**).

Preparation of the peritoneal cavity

The camera is inserted into the peritoneal cavity and an initial laparoscopy performed, looking for evidence of metastatic disease and carefully examining the small bowel and peritoneal surfaces. Adhesions to the abdominal wall are dissected and divided. Adhesions of the sigmoid colon that hold the often redundant sigmoid laterally and away from the midline should not be divided at this stage as these adhesions may effectively retract the sigmoid colon. The primary assistant stands on the patient's right side and on the left side of the surgeon (**Figure 5.7.5**). The surgeon inserts two bowel graspers through the two right-sided abdominal ports. The greater omentum and transverse colon are then reflected up over the stomach. If there is no space in the upper part of the abdomen, one must confirm that the orogastric tube has adequately decompressed the stomach. This creates additional space for the small bowel to move into, allowing easier exposure of the inferior mesenteric vessels. The patient is then placed in the Trendelenburg position. This helps to move the small bowel towards the head of the patient and away from the operative field.

In patients with malignancy, an unexpected finding of a fixed mass with involvement of contiguous organs is an indication for conversion to an open approach. If the operator is in any doubt that a complete oncological resection can be achieved laparoscopically then the case should be converted to an open approach. Preoperative CT imaging prevents such unexpected findings in up to 90 percent of patients.

In benign disease, there may be inflammatory attachments between the colon and small bowel. The first priority is to re-establish normal anatomy where possible. Inflammatory attachments of small bowel should be dissected off the sigmoid colon and particularly off the base of the inferior mesenteric vessels. A laparoscopic scissors with electrocautery is used and care taken not to injury the mesentery. A combination of sharp and blunt dissection is best. Where considerable dissection is required and a suspected small bowel iatrogenic injury is suspected, a marking suture can be placed on the affected segment in order to check it at the end of the procedure. This should be performed by direct inspection extracorporeally. Lateral adhesions are not routinely divided until later in the procedure unless it is necessary to visualize the inferior mesenteric pedicle. Similarly, in situations where a phlegmon is attached to the bladder, it is often better to perform the majority of the required dissection away from a potential colovesical fistula prior to directing the dissection to this area.

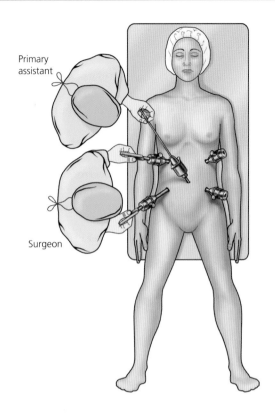

Primary assistant

Surgeon

5.7.5

OPERATIVE TECHNIQUES

There are several operative approaches that can be used in performing a left hemicolectomy. These are divided into a predominantly medial to lateral approach and a primarily lateral to medial approach. Proponents of each will argue that one approach is superior to the other, however the experienced operator will know both techniques and will adopt one or the other as demanded.

In a thin patient, lateral mobilization of the colon and extracorporeal ligation of the intra-abdominal vessels may be achieved. This approach is often faster and may be technically less challenging. In a thin patient, this approach can be used for both benign and malignant disease. As the patient's body mass index (BMI) increases however, the reliance on this approach will result in an ever increasing size of incision necessary for specimen extraction. This ultimately may result in an incision not objectively much different from that which a laparotomy incision would have entailed. These laparoscopically assisted laparotomies do not serve the patient well. To maintain a minimally invasive approach, mobilization and ligation of the mesenteric vessels should be completed intracorporeally, thereby permitting an average extraction incision of 5 cm.

Lateral approach for laparoscopic left hemicolectomy

This approach is suitable for patients with low BMIs and also in benign disease, such as a segmental Crohn's resection. The target is to perform a left hemicolectomy with resection of the distal transverse colon to the mid-sigmoid colon. The vascular ligation required in benign cases does not entail ligation of the inferior mesenteric artery or the left branch of the middle colic artery at their origin. Mobilization of the splenic flexure may be carried out by entry into the lesser sac and transection of the gastrocolic omentum or dissection of the gastrocolic omentum off the transverse colon as required. In suspected malignancy, the greater omentum that may be attached to the area of primary pathology should be mobilized *en bloc* with the specimen.

Lateral mobilization of the colon should be undertaken in a stepwise fashion. The steps involved in lateral approach to a laparoscopic left hemicolectomy are: (1) sigmoid colon mobilization; (2) left ureter identification; (3) descending colon mobilization; (4) entry into the lesser sac and transverse colon mobilization; (5) splenic flexure mobilization; (6) extraction and anastomosis.

SIGMOID COLON MOBILIZATION

The surgeon stands on the patient's right side with the first assistant as the camera operator on their left side. The second assistant should stand opposite the surgeon on the patient's left side (see **Figure 5.7.5**). The surgeon uses an atraumatic bowel grasper in the left hand and a scissors (or energy delivery device such as harmonic scalpel) in the right hand. The second assistant uses an atraumatic bowel grasper or a laparoscopic Maryland forceps to assist. The surgeon, using the grasper, pulls the sigmoid colon medially and cephalad. Dissection begins with sharp dissection along the line of attachment of the sigmoid colon to the lateral abdominal wall. Usually, this is superior to the line of attachment of the base of the mesentery to the retroperitoneum. Care must be taken to avoid penetrating the lateral parietal peritoneum lining the lateral abdominal wall. As the sigmoid is drawn medially, the surgeon will continue the dissection until the left ureter is identified. Sigmoid colon mobilization should be performed from the upper rectum to the distal aspect of the descending colon. Care must be taken in the amount of traction performed on the lateral aspect of the mesentery of the sigmoid colon as excessive force may result in the mesenteric vessels bleeding.

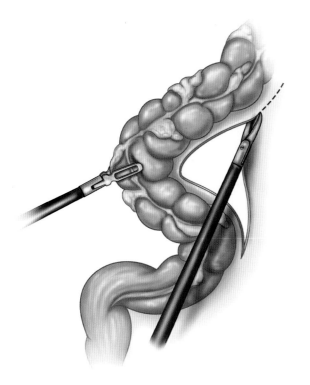

As the sigmoid is mobilized medially, the dissection continues until the line of Toldt becomes obvious (reflection of lateral peritoneum from the base of the mesentery of the descending colon) (**Figure 5.7.6**). The second assistant can aid the surgeon with countertraction of the peritoneum laterally using the left lower quadrant port site and an atraumatic grasper.

5.7.6

LEFT URETER IDENTIFICATION

Identification of the left ureter is a critical step and reduces the chance of ureteric injury. It should be performed as a matter of routine prior to consideration of ligation of any linear structure. The left ureter is retroperitoneal and is located medial to the psoas tendon and gonadal vessels. It tends to lie on the bifurcation of the common iliac artery. Following lateral mobilization of the sigmoid colon, the ureter can be tented medially or it can be drawn in medially by fibrosis secondary to diverticulitis or neoplasia. The ureter is identified by confirmation of vermiculation of the organ itself. Division of the peritoneum over the base of the sigmoid colon is often necessary to see the ureter. Care must be taken when elevating the peritoneum in order to avoid inadvertently dividing the ureter lying underneath. A Maryland grasper is used to pinch the ureter and confirmation of vermiculation is thereby achieved.

DESCENDING COLON MOBILIZATION

The surgeon now uses the left-handed grasper to lift the descending colon superiorly and somewhat medially. This permits continued identification of the line of Toldt. The action also allows the descending colon to act as a barrier to prevent the small bowel spilling over into the operating field. The second assistant may use a grasper to provide countertraction of the lateral attachments of the peritoneum. In cases where small bowel continually falls into the operative field, the second assistant may use a second bowel grasper placed through the left upper quadrant port site in order to hold back the wandering

small bowel. Tilting the operating table left side up may also be of benefit in these cases.

The perinephric fat and Gerota's fascia are left intact. The colon is lifted off the retroperitoneum by exerting traction with the left-handed instrument while the right-handed scissors is used to dissect along the line of Toldt. The operator will find that the right lower quadrant port will not allow completion of this line of dissection due to the distance or reach of the instrument. Once the maximum point of dissection is reached, the surgeon completes the dissection by moving the right-handed operating scissors to the left lower quadrant port site, and using a left-handed grasping instrument through the right lower quadrant port site. The assistants move to retract through the right and left upper quadrant port sites. It is not usually necessary for the surgeon to change their operating position from the patient's right side. The first assistant uses an atraumatic grasper to hold the transverse colon and distract the transverse colon medially in the line of the transverse colon towards the right side. The second assistant uses an atraumatic grasper to elevate the remaining aspect of the proximal descending colon or small bowel to aid the surgeon complete the lateral line of dissection as far as the spleen. Once the spleen has been seen and lateral aspect of splenic flexure reached, then this step of the dissection is complete. In cases where the final aspect of this step is difficult, then the patient may be placed reverse Trendelenburg to aid the dissection. In cases where the final aspects of lateral dissection remain difficult, then the surgeon may need to use the scissors through the left upper quadrant port site to complete this step.

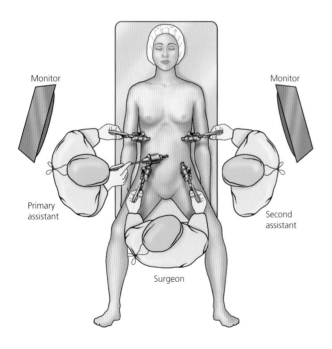

ENTRY INTO THE LESSER SAC AND TRANSVERSE COLON MOBILIZATION

The surgeon now moves to stand between the patient's legs and the patient is placed in the reverse Trendelenburg position (**Figure 5.7.7**). The first and second assistants move to stand further down the patient near the patient's hips and the video monitors should be adjusted to permit the surgeon direct vision of the screens. Two approaches may be used to dissect the gastrocolic omentum off the transverse colon and to gain entry into the lesser sac.

5.7.7

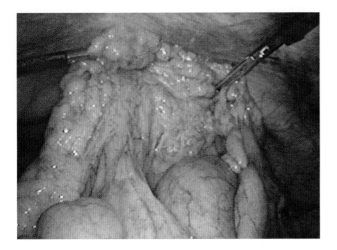

5.7.8

This involves either preservation of the greater omentum, which is easier in non-inflammatory conditions, such as a polyp or benign stricture, and resection of the greater omentum which is easier in Crohn's disease. In cases where preservation of the greater omentum is preferred, the assistants elevate the gastrocolic omentum from the transverse colon by lifting it from its attachment vertically and holding it like an 'open book' or wall of omentum (**Figure 5.7.8**). This exposes the undersurface of the greater omentum and the line of attachment to the transverse colon mesentery.

The surgeon, using a grasper in the left hand, distracts the colon inferomedially and dissects between the line of reflection (**Figure 5.7.9**). This permits entry to the lesser sac. The lesser sac may then be exposed by continuing the dissection between this line of reflection of the greater omentum and the mesentery of the transverse colon. In cases where this line of dissection is fused secondary to inflammation, or in very thin patients, it may be more advantageous to remove the greater omentum as part of the specimen. In these cases the assistant may distract the greater omentum caudad and the surgeon then dissects directly into the lesser sac through one of the avascular windows which are obvious in thin patients. The lesser sac is opened by continuing this line of dissection. Care must be taken in this case to avoid ligating the arterial arcade of the gastroepiploic vessels or injuring the stomach.

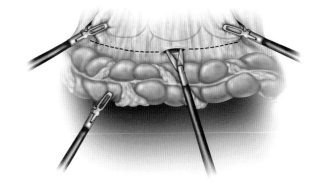

5.7.9

SPLENIC FLEXURE MOBILIZATION

The surgeon remains between the patient's legs and both assistants use graspers to elevate the greater omentum off the transverse colon. The surgeon then gradually moves along the line of dissection towards the spleen. The assistant's graspers should be repositioned one at a time in order to move along the line of reflection of the greater omentum maintaining traction towards the patient's right side. It is often useful if the surgeon uses a long-shafted instrument during this part of the dissection. As the dissection proceeds the lesser sac should become more obvious as it opens up (**Figure 5.7.10**). The pancreas is visualized and dissection continued until the spleen approached. At this stage, the previous plane of dissection of the descending colon is seen and dissection is continued until both planes are joined.

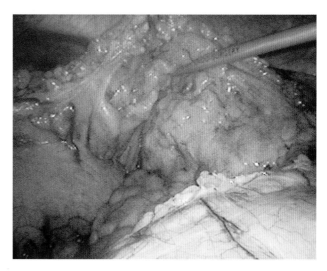

5.7.10

MESENTERIC VESSEL LIGATION

In cases where the pathology is benign, the patient is thin, and a full oncological dissection is not required then extracorporeal vessel ligation may suffice. In cases where intracorporeal vessel ligation is required, the descending colon mesentery can be ligated using an energy delivery device The surgeon stands on the patient's right side and the assistants in their original configuration (**Figure 5.7.2**). The mobilized colon is elevated by the assistants and the surgeon may progressively ligate the vessels starting from the sigmoid branches of the inferior mesenteric artery to the left branch of the middle colic vessels. The left ureter again must be identified prior to division of any vessels. In the case of a distal descending colonic tumor, the level of dissection will need to be continued down to the upper rectum, thereby combining a left hemicolectomy with a high anterior resection (proctosigmoidectomy).

EXTRACTION AND ANASTOMOSIS

The colon should now be mobilized from the distal sigmoid/upper rectum to the mid-transverse colon. In thin patients, extraction of the colon may permit extracorporeal ligation of mesenteric vessels. In cases where intracorporeal vessel ligation is required, energy delivery devices or laparoscopic stapling instruments are used. The extent of vessel ligation and level at which major vessels should be ligated is dependent on the underlying pathological process. Extraction of the specimen for a left hemicolectomy is through a midline incision. This permits externalization of the transverse, descending colon and proximal sigmoid colon and an extracorporeal resection to be performed. A wound protector is used in all cases. The transverse colon and sigmoid colon are externalized using Babcock graspers.

The choice of anastomosis is dependent on the surgeon. In all cases the principles remain the same: (1) adequate specimen resection; (2) tension-free apposition of anastomotic ends; (3) good marginal artery blood supply; (4) correct anatomical alignment of transverse and distal colon. See Chapters 1.8, 1.9, and 5.6.

Medial to lateral approach for laparoscopic left hemicolectomy

The medial to lateral approach with intracorporeal ligation of vessels allows preservation of minimally invasive techniques and a sound oncological approach to neoplastic disease. This remains the author's preferred approach in laparoscopic left-sided surgery. It is also useful in obese patients with benign disease. The medial to lateral approach is divided stepwise into: (1) identification of the inferior mesenteric artery; (2) identification of the left ureter; (3) vessel ligation; (4) medial mobilization; (5) lateral mobilization; (6) entry into the lesser sac; (7) transverse colon mobilization; (8) splenic flexure mobilization; (9) extraction and anastomosis.

The primary operator stands on the patient's right side and assistants to his left and opposite him (**Figure 5.7.3**). The port site positions are the same (**Figure 5.7.5**).

Identifying the inferior mesenteric pedicle

With the patient in the Trendelenburg position and the greater omentum reflected over the transverse colon the small bowel should drift away from the pelvic brim. The surgeon uses an atraumatic grasper to lift the sigmoid colon out of the pelvis and tents the medial aspect of the sigmoid colon mesentery superiorly (**Figure 5.7.11**). Using this approach, the inferior mesenteric artery is elevated off the retroperitoneum. The assistant's atraumatic grasping forceps may be used through the left lower quadrant port to tent the mesentery of the sigmoid colon at approximately the level of the sacral promontory. This demonstrates a groove between the right or medial side of the inferior mesenteric pedicle and the retroperitoneum. Incision along this sulcus permits diffusion of carbon dioxide gas along the tissue plane and helps to identify the correct line of dissection. A combination of sharp

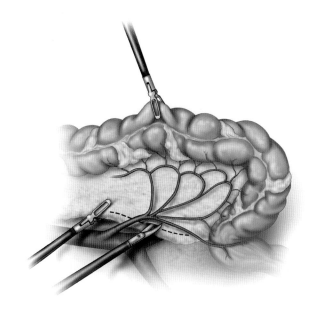

5.7.11

and blunt dissection is then used to define the inferior mesenteric vessels. Care must be taken to avoid injury to the presacral autonomic nerves which can be either tented up inadvertently or injured if the surgeon is in the incorrect plane of dissection. If there is difficulty getting into this plane, it is often useful to go slightly distal to the sacral promontory and elevate the mesorectum anteriorly, getting into the presacral space. Cautery is used to open the peritoneum behind the upper portion of the mesorectum. The temptation is to continue to dissect in towards the presacral plane as it tends to open up easily; however, dissection should be continued cephalad until the origin of the vessel is encountered.

Identification of the left ureter

It is critical to identify the left ureter before any major structures are divided. As ureteric stents are not routinely used, this is an essential operative caveat that reduces the chance of ureteric injury. The inferior mesenteric vessels are elevated superiorly from the retroperitoneum and the tissues on the posterior surface of the sigmoid mesocolon gently dissected down. This is achieved using the surgeon's left-handed atraumatic grasper to lift the inferior mesenteric artery and associated mesentery superiorly while gently pushing the attached retroperitoneal surface inferiorly with the back of the laparoscopic scissors in the right hand. This separation of the sigmoid mesocolon from the retroperitoneum should be relatively avascular. In the event that bleeding is encountered, then the selected tissue plane of dissection is incorrect (usually too high). As the dissection is carried laterally, the ureter should be visualized at this stage and be seen to vermiculate (**Figure 5.7.12**). Care must be taken not to dissect too deeply and injure the iliac vessels. If the ureter cannot be found, it has usually been elevated with the sigmoid mesocolon. The order of the structures encountered during this medial dissection is the left ureter, the gonadal vessels, and the psoas tendon. In the event the operator has reached the psoas tendon prior to seeing the ureter, then the dissection is too far lateral. If the left ureter cannot be identified, the lateral approach should be employed as described above under Lateral approach for laparoscopic left hemicolectomy. This combined approach is particularly useful in cases of complex diverticular disease or obesity. In the event that the ureter cannot be defined using these techniques, then consideration should be given to conversion to an open approach.

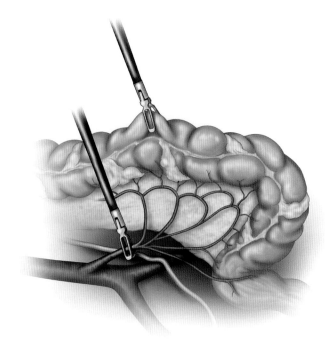

5.7.12

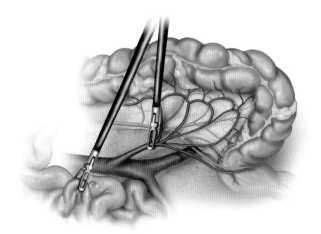

5.7.13

Vessel ligation

Attention is now turned to the origin of the inferior mesenteric vessels. The origin of the inferior mesenteric artery is dissected completely and the inferior mesenteric vein and left colic artery identified (**Figure 5.7.13**). This is achieved by the second assistant using two bowel graspers to first tent out the inferior mesenteric artery to provide tension (left lower quadrant port) and second to help keep the small bowel from encroaching into the operative field. The surgeon is then free to dissect out the named vessels prior to ligation.

In left hemicolectomy for cancer, the left colic artery and the inferior mesenteric vein are divided as close to their origin or insertion, respectively, as is possible. Where the tumor is located in the distal descending colon and the resection combines left hemicolectomy and sigmoid resection then both inferior mesenteric artery and vein are resected. In situations where the patient has severe athrosclerosis, the left colic artery may, on occasions, be preserved to facilitate a healthy anastomosis. For benign disease, such as diverticular disease, the inferior mesenteric artery and vein are divided together using a low ligation (distal to the left colic artery). For malignant disease, the vessels are taken separately and a high ligation is performed (proximal to the origin of the left colic artery).

A key point in division of major vascular pedicles is the concept of controlled division. The surgeon uses a grasper in the left hand to clamp the proximal aspect of the vessel to be divided. The vessel is then divided with the device of choice. This proximal control of the vessel with the left-hand grasper is essential as it permits ease of remedial action in the event of a spurting vessel or instrument vessel ligation failure. The subsequent division of the main vessels may be via a number of acceptable techniques. These may include formal vessel dissection to skeletonize the vessels and thereafter apply laparoscopic clips or to utilize an energy source. For the division of the inferior mesenteric artery, however, the author's preference is to use the Endo-GIA. The left colic artery and inferior mesenteric vein may similarly be divided using an energy delivery device or between clips as required. The operator must discipline

themselves to check for the ureter on each occasion prior to vessel ligation as the ureter may be drawn medially towards the origin of the inferior mesenteric artery (**Figure 5.7.14**).

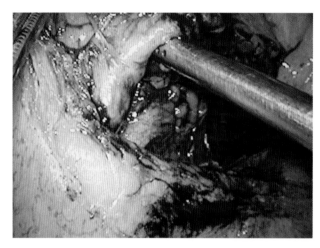

5.7.14

Medial mobilization

Having divided the left colic artery and inferior mesenteric vein distally the dissection is carried medially under the descending and sigmoid colon. The pedicle of the divided vessels is grasped and elevated away from the retroperitoneum using a grasper though the assistant's port in the left lower quadrant. The surgeon then uses the left-hand instrument to elevate the descending colon mesentery and dissect this away from the retroperitoneum using a combination of sharp and blunt dissection. This dissection is continued laterally towards the lateral attachment of the descending colon (medial view of line of Toldt), and superiorly, dissecting the bowel off the anterior surface of Gerota's fascia up towards the splenic flexure. The medial dissection may necessitate the sharp dissection of the proximal jejunum and fourth part of the duodenum from the base of the descending colon mesentery. As the apex of the medial mobilization is reached, the apex of the inferior mesenteric vein is seen (**Figure 5.7.15**). This may now be ligated to ensure a complete mesocolic excision. The only remaining vessel to be ligated is the left branch of the middle colic vessels. This is performed after the lesser sac is opened and transverse colon mobilized.

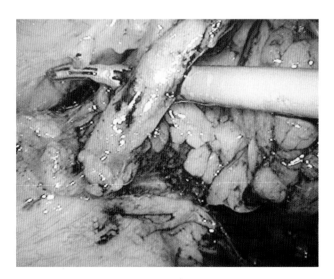

5.7.15

Lateral mobilization

The surgeon now grasps the rectosigmoid junction with an atraumatic bowel grasper in their left hand and draws the colon to the patient's right side. This allows the lateral attachments of the sigmoid colon to be seen and divided using electrocautery (**Figure 5.7.16**). Ecchymosis from the prior retroperitoneal mobilization of the colon can usually be seen in this area and once this layer of peritoneum is opened, the space opened by the retroperitoneal dissection is entered. Dissection now continues up along the white line of Toldt, towards the splenic flexure. As the dissection continues, the surgeon's left-hand instrument needs to be gradually moved up along the descending colon to keep the lateral attachments under tension. Elevating the descending colon and drawing it medially is a useful maneuver as it keeps the small bowel loops out of the operative field. As the dissection moves towards the splenic flexure, it is often necessary to move the dissecting instrument to the patient's left lower quadrant port and the atraumatic grasper (left hand) to the right lower quadrant port to facilitate completion of the lateral dissection. This allows the surgeon to reach up to the splenic flexure.

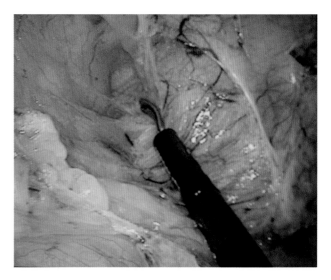

5.7.16

Entry into the lesser sac, transverse colon mobilization, splenic flexure mobilization

The technique for transverse colon mobilization and splenic flexure mobilization is as described for the lateral approach. Division of the left branch of the middle colic vessels may be performed at this stage. The transverse colon is elevated on the right and left side by the two assistants using the upper quadrant port sites. Care must be taken in dissecting in this area as the body of pancreas can inadvertently come into the operative field.

Extraction and anastomosis

In patients in whom a left hemicolectomy alone is required, extraction of the colon is through a midline incision. This is performed as described above. The choice of anastomotic technique depends upon the operator. The extracted specimen consists of the mid-transverse colon to the proximal sigmoid colon (**Figure 5.7.17**). In patients in whom a sigmoid resection is required, then a different sequence of concluding operative steps are employed. These entail: (1) mobilization of the upper rectum; (2 transection of the upper rectum; (3) ligation of superior rectal arteries; (4) extraction and resection of colon; (5) intracorporeal anastomosis.

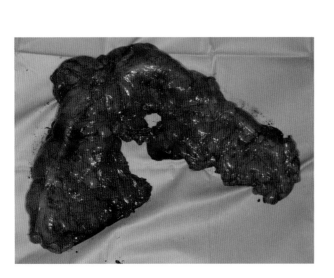

5.7.17

MOBILIZATION OF THE UPPER RECTUM

Mobiliztion of the remaining sigmoid colon and upper rectum is necessary in patients with sigmoid colon pathology. The divided inferior mesenteric pedicle is grasped and any residual lateral areolar adhesions are divided. The mesocolon and mesorectum are drawn medially displaying the left lateral pelvic sidewall. The final attachments are divided and the sigmoid is then drawn

up out of the pelvis. The upper part of the mesorectum is then mobilized adequately to allow the bowel to be divided just distal to the rectosigmoid junction. Great care is taken to stay in the correct plane in order to protect the ureter and the autonomic nerves. The sigmoid colon and rectum are then drawn to the left side to allow the dissection to continue on the right side of the rectum (see Chapter 6.4).

TRANSECTION OF THE UPPER RECTUM

The rectum is drawn up out of the pelvis using the assistant's port in the left lower quadrant. This brings the rectosigmoid junction up and above the sacral promontory. Cautery is now used to open the peritoneum on the right side of the rectum (**Figure 5.7.18**). An atraumatic bowel grasper is then used to open a plane between the rectum and mesorectum by advancing the instrument between the two structures and separating the jaws in an anteroposterior direction. An Endo-GIA stapler is then inserted through the right lower quadrant port and used to divide the rectum. Care is taken to ensure no other structures have been picked up by the stapler and that the stapler is perpendicular to the bowel. The stapler is introduced through the right lower quadrant 12 mm port site and the thinner inferior blade slipped through the window secured by the previous dissection. The tip of the stapler should be visible on the lateral 'far' side of the rectum prior to closing the instrument in order to reduce the chance of injury to the lateral pelvic sidewall structures. Once the rectum has been transected, the distal sigmoid colon and upper rectum remain connected only by the soft tissues of the mesorectum.

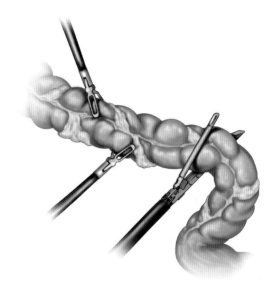

5.7.18

LIGATION OF SUPERIOR RECTAL ARTERIES

The proximal end of the specimen may now be elevated and this places the mesorectum under stretch. Electrocautery is used to divide the mesorectum with laparoscopic clips although other energy sources can also be used. The superior rectal arteries are divided, followed by the superior rectal vein. Before dividing the final piece of the mesorectum, the distal end is carefully inspected for hemostasis, as once the mesorectum is completely divided the rectum will retract into the pelvis. The surgeon then grasps the divided proximal end of the rectum in order to make a final check on mobility before the specimen extraction incision is performed.

SPECIMEN EXTRACTION AND RESECTION OF COLON

A 3–4 cm left lower quadrant muscle splitting incision is then made through the left lower quadrant port site (**Figure 5.7.19**). This can be enlarged, if necessary, to remove large tumor or phlegmon. It is the author's practice to use a small wound protector for all cases. The specimen should extend from the transverse colon to the transected upper rectal staple line. Remaining mesenteric vessels in the transverse colon are divided, confirming the

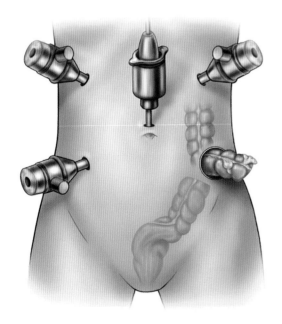

5.7.19

presence of pulsatile bleeding in the mesentery. The bowel is then divided using non-crushing bowel clamps and a Babcock is placed on the proximal end. The specimen is then examined to ensure adequacy of margins. A size 2-0 prolene purse-string suture is then inserted and the anvil of a size-29 circular stapler is inserted. There should be adequate reach of the proximal remaining bowel to enable a tension-free anastomosis. This can be confirmed by positioning the proximal colon over the symphysis pubis externally. In the event that the bowel does not reach easily, further mobilization of the transverse colon may be required. In this situation, the bowel is returned to the abdomen, the wound protector is removed, both the assistant and principal operating surgeon change their gloves and the wound is closed in layers. The usual culprit in the lack of sufficient length to facilitate an anastomosis is the incomplete mobilization of the transverse colon. In cases where a left hemicolectomy is combined with a proctosigmoidectomy the lesser sac must often be exposed back as far as the hepatic flexure to achieve adequate length. Following this added dissection, the proximal colon is again externalized and the marginal arterial blood supply confirmed as appropriate prior to proceeding. The wound is thereafter again closed as described.

INTRACORPOREAL ANASTOMOSIS

The abdomen is reinsufflated with gas and the proximal colon is located. Adequacy of reach is confirmed by placing the colon with anvil, into the pelvis. The proximal colon should lie comfortably without tension, otherwise further mobilization may be required. The correct orientation of the bowel is confirmed by checking the base of the mesentery.

The stapler is inserted into the rectal stump and the spike advanced through or close to the center of the transverse staple line. The anvil is now grasped using a laparoscopic Alice forceps and locked to the spike of the staple gun. Orientation is rechecked, then the staple gun is closed and the anastomosis fashioned. The staple gun is removed and the 'donuts' examined for completeness. The pelvis is irrigated and the anastomosis is tested by distending the rectum with air, using a rigid sigmoidoscope. Anastomotic tension is then checked by placing an instrument behind the mesentery, just above the sacral promontory, and elevating the colon away from the retroperitoenum. It is the author's practice to oversew the anterior part of the anastomosis laparoscopically with interrupted sutures in cases where there is no diverting stoma, though this is not evidence-based.

Closure

Hemostasis is confirmed and the abdomen is irrigated. All ports are removed under vision to ensure there is no bleeding from a port site. The fascia of the right lower quadrant port is then closed with 2-0 polyglactin, and the purse-string suture, which had been placed at the umbilical port site, is used to close the fascia at this site. Local anesthetic (Marcaine® 0.5 percent) is injected into all port sites and finally the skin is closed with subcuticular sutures. The patient is then woken up, extubated, and transferred to the recovery room where a standard postoperative care plan is followed.

POSTOPERATIVE CARE

The routine use of enhanced recovery programs has clearly reduced postoperative stay and morbidity. Pioneered by Kehlet[8] this approach has resulted in successful change for colorectal patients postoperatively. In the author's unit a more simplified postoperative recovery regime is in practice. Termed the RAPID protocol, it has achieved a significant reduction in the length of stay in both our open and laparoscopic cases.[9, 10]

SUMMARY

Laparoscopic left hemicolectomy is a technically challenging procedure due to the need to mobilize the splenic flexure, dissect the left colic and left branch of middle colic arteries and ligation of the inferior mesenteric vein. The anastomosis can be performed extracorporeally in the majority of cases. In patients in whom there is a distal colonic tumor, left hemicolectomy is combined with a sigmoid resection. This increases the extent of laparoscopic dissection and results in an anastomosis to the upper rectum.

With correct preoperative education, intraoperative technical proficiency, and use of enhanced postoperative care programs, colorectal patients can experience the benefits of minimally invasive surgery.

REFERENCES

1. Boyle E, Ridgway PF, Keane FB, Neary P. Laparoscopic colonic resection in inflammatory bowel disease: minimal surgery, minimal access and minimal hospital stay. *Colorectal Disease* 2008; **10**: 911–15.

2. Ridgway PF, Boyle E, Keane FB, Neary P. Laparoscopic colectomy is cheaper than conventional open resection. *Colorectal Disease* 2007; **9**: 819–24.

3. Clinical Outcomes of Surgical Therapy Study Group. A comparison of laparoscopically assisted and open colectomy for colon cancer. *New England Journal of Medicine* 2004; **350**: 2050–9.

4. Jayne DG, Guillou PJ, Thorpe H *et al*; UK MRC CLASICC Trial Group. Randomized trial of laparoscopic-assisted resection of colorectal carcinoma: 3-year results of the UK MRC CLASICC Trial Group. *Journal of Clinical Oncology* 2007; **25**: 3061–8.

5. Tekkis PP, Senagore AJ, Delaney CP, Fazio VW. Evaluation of the learning curve in laparoscopic colorectal surgery: comparison of right-sided and left-sided resections. *Annals of Surgery* 2005; **242**: 83–91.

6. Delaney C, Neary P, Heriot A, Senagore A. *Operative techniques in laparoscopic colorectal surgery*. Philadelphia, PA: Lippincott Williams and Wilkins, 2006.

7. Senagore AJ, Delaney CP. A critical analysis of laparoscopic colectomy at a single institution: lessons learned after 1000 cases. *American Journal of Surgery* 2006; **191**: 377–80.

8. Kehlet H. Multimodal approach to postoperative recovery. *Current Opinion in Critical Care* 2009; **15**: 355–8.

9. Lloyd GM, Kirby R, Hemingway DM *et al*. The RAPID protocol enhances patient recovery after both laparoscopic and open colorectal resections. *Surgical Endoscopy* 2010; **24**: 1434–9.

10. Al Chalabi H, Kavanagh DO, Hassan L *et al*. The benefit of an enhanced recovery programme following elective laparoscopic sigmoid colectomy. *International Journal of Colorectal Disease* 2010; **25**: 761–6.

Left hemicolectomy – hand-assisted laparoscopic surgery

CHRISTOPHER J YOUNG

PRINCIPLES AND JUSTIFICATION

Left hemicolectomy traditionally refers to resection of the descending colon, usually including the splenic flexure, resulting in an anastomosis between the transverse colon and the sigmoid colon. Many Western colons have diverticular disease and the sigmoid colon may be unsuitable due to muscular thickening and the presence of diverticular for anastomosis, necessitating anastomosis with the rectum. This is covered in Chapter 5.5. The majority of pure left hemicolectomies, when suitable to be performed, are done for polyps or malignancy in the elderly. Otherwise, in fit patients higher ligation than the colic artery by including the inferior mesenteric artery (IMA) and removal of its lymph nodes necessitates an anterior resection, and is preferred by many Western surgeons.

Indications and contraindications

Many surgeons have moved from pure or straight laparoscopic colorectal surgery to routine use of the hybrid hand-assisted laparoscopic surgery (HALS). This is due to the advantages of shorter operating time, increased spatial awareness and tactile feedback, direct surgical access to the region under the handport, a reduced conversion rate, and an expanded ability to deal with the transverse colon and more advanced pathology, without loss in measured pain levels or recovery time.

For those surgeons who selectively use HALS, indications include obese patients, cases where proximal pathology has not been able to be assessed preoperatively, and in bulky disease cases. If a handport is going to be used, its advantages should be used from the start of the case.

Consent

Consent should be obtained with discussion covering general risks of surgery and anesthesia, and specific complications of the entry wounds, risk of conversion to open procedure, and anastomotic and intra-abdominal complication risks.

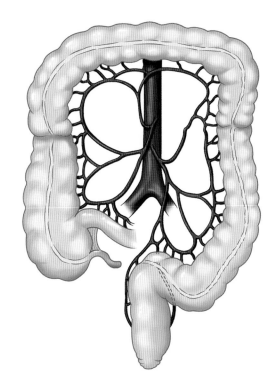

5.8.1

PREOPERATIVE ASSESSMENT AND PREPARATION

Patients routinely have colonoscopy and computed tomography (CT) scans performed. A mechanical bowel preparation with sodium phosphate or polyethylene glycol-based preparations is taken by the patient. Prophylactic antibiotics are used in the perioperative period covering Gram-positive and Gram-negative organisms. Deep vein thrombosis (DVT) prophylaxis is achieved with calf compressors and 5000 units subcutaneous heparin twice daily. Abdominal marking by enterostomal therapy should occur if there is the chance or intention of a temporary or permanent stoma.

ANESTHESIA

General anesthesia with endotracheal intubation and complete muscle relaxation.

OPERATION

For equipment, position of patient, preparation of abdomen, incisions, handport and port insertions see Chapter 5.5. For descending colon mobilization, see also Chapter 5.5.

Splenic flexure mobilization – peritoneal, splenic attachments, and left side

After the descending colon mobilization has reached near the curve of the splenic flexure, the patient will be placed in an additional 30° head-up position. Peritoneal bands between the splenic flexure and lateral peritoneal wall or to the spleen are divided (**Figure 5.8.2**). The splenic flexure approach is to then mobilize the left side of the splenic flexure, then the transverse colon, and then complete the splenic flexure mobilization.

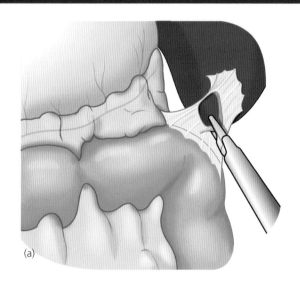

(a)

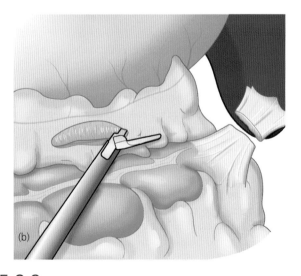

(b)

5.8.2

Splenic flexure transverse colon mobilization

The greater omentum is taken off the distal transverse colon, starting 6–10 cm away from splenic flexure and working towards the splenic flexure. The left hand is held flat, either fingers pushing transverse colon down towards the posterior abdominal wall, with a 5 mm DeBakey grasper holding the omentum up, or the left hand can be supinated and the thumb placed anteriorly. The omentum is dissected off from this point laterally, and as much towards the midtransverse colon medially as is required for adequate length.

During the transverse colon mobilization, the lesser sac will be entered, the stomach will be visualized, and any attachments from the stomach and the retroperitoneal structures to the transverse mesocolon can be divided.

With the left and transverse components of the splenic flexure mobilized and the lesser sac entered, the splenic flexure can be completed by bringing both parts together in an upturned U-shape with the palm and fingers of the left hand flat holding them together and down posteriorly, and dividing the splenocolic ligament and remaining retroperitoneal attachments (**Figure 5.8.3**).

Dissection and ligation of inferior mesenteric vein

For dissection and ligation of inferior mesenteric vein, see Chapter 5.5.

Sigmoid colon mobilization, if necessary

For sigmoid colon mobilization, see Chapter 5.5.

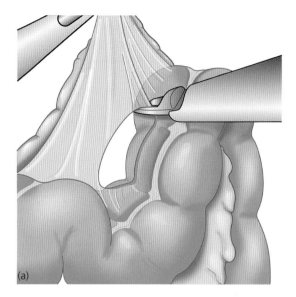

(a)

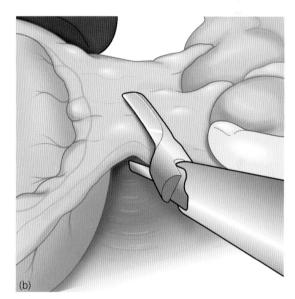

(b)

5.8.3

Vessel ligation

Following mobilization, the bowel will usually have enough length to be able to be removed through the wound retractor of the handport and allow mesenteric window formation, vessel ligation, bowel transection, and a functional end-to-end anastomosis (**Figure 5.8.4**). It may be necessary to mobilize more omentum off the transverse colon and to ensure there is no attachment to the stomach or retroperitoneal structures by the transverse mesocolon to bring the transverse colon down to the Pfannenstiel wound retractor. Likewise, a variable amount of sigmoid mobilization will need to occur if the bowel cannot be brought out via the Pfannenstiel incision. If not, following laparoscopic mesenteric window formation and vessel ligation, there will be sufficient length.

For a left hemicolectomy, this usually involves ligation of the left branch of middle colic artery near its origin from the middle colic artery, and ligation of the left colic artery near its origin from the IMA. Laparoscopic ligation of the left colic artery requires palpation and identification of the IMA, then the left colic artery, then creation of mesenteric windows either side of the vessel and ligation and transection with a linear stapler with vascular staples. Vascular ligation of bowel and mesentery brought out through the handport is performed with clamps and ties. The windows in the mesentery are then extended to the bowel wall.

Adjuncts to complete dissection and mobilization

If the colon mobilization has been completed laparoscopically, there is almost never an advantage with pelvic access from a midline extension, converting a transverse Pfannenstiel incision into an inverted T incision (Pfannenstiel and midline incision together). In the

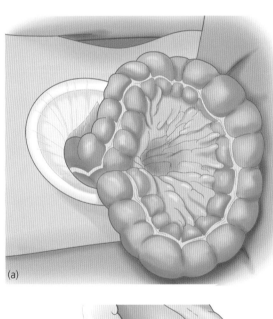

(a)

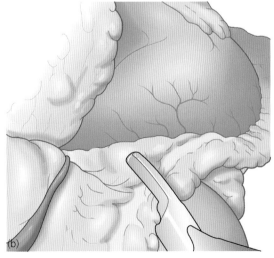

(b)

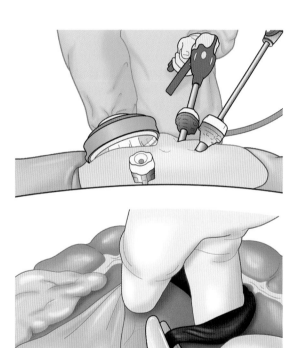

(c)

5.8.4

author's experience, this is a disadvantage with higher rates of pain, wound bleeding, and wound infection if there is any muscle cutting of the recti or conversion to open. A difficult sigmoid or difficult adhesions may need to be dealt with first and may be done directly through the open handport.

If mobilization becomes more difficult, the surgeon can progress from the laparoscopic approach with a hand through the handport, to the laparoscopic approach with instruments in the handport, to the open approach with instruments through the wound retractor of the handport, to the open approach with a non-muscle cutting extension of the Pfannenstiel incision and a circular self-retainer (Turner–Warwick with four small wound retractors) in the wound. The Pfannenstiel incision can be enlarged after removing the handport wound retractor. It is best to then lengthen the transverse skin incision and the vertical separation of the recti and the peritoneal incision.

Specimen resection and anastomosis

Following vessel ligation, the mid to distal transverse colon and the junction of the descending and sigmoid colon are transected with a linear cutting stapler, tapered more on the antimesenteric border towards the blood supply. The corners are cut off both ends of bowel to allow linear stapler insertion down the common limb of a functional end-to-end (side-to-side) anastomosis (**Figure 5.8.5**).

The remaining defect in the anastomosis is closed with a transverse linear stapler to limit how much bowel needs to be resected. The edges are held together by four Allis forceps to ensure no staple line is overlapping another staple line, to prevent the junction of three staple lines and potential weakness. The final staple line in under-run with a continuous 3-0 monocryl suture for hemostasis.

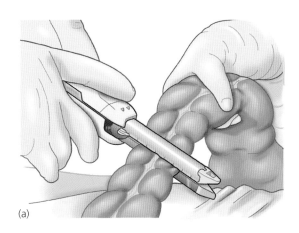

(a)

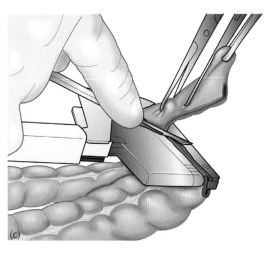

(c)

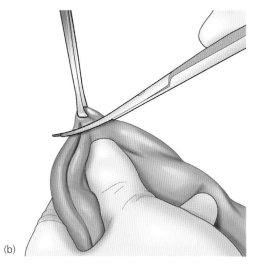

(b)

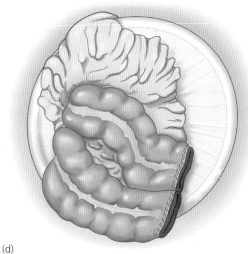

(d)

5.8.5

Wound closure

The Pfannenstiel incision is closed in layers initially with the posterior rectus sheath and peritoneum closed with a 1 Vicryl continuous suture, and then the rectus abdominis muscle bellies are closed with interrupted 0 Vicryl, just picking up the medial body. A continuous 1 PDS suture closes the anterior rectus sheath and the skin is closed with a 3-0 monocryl subcuticular suture. All port sites >5 mm are closed at the anterior rectus sheath level with 1 Biosyn on a J-shaped needle using S-shaped retractors for exposure.

POSTOPERATIVE CARE

Anesthesia will usually instill transversus abdominis plane (TAP) blocks and a patient-controlled analgesia (PCA) machine. Deep vein thrombosis (DVT) prophylaxis is maintained with TED (thromboembolic deterrent) stockings and subcutaneous heparin 5000 units twice daily. The nasogastric tube, if used intraoperatively, is removed, except in cases with large bowel obstruction.

Early mobilization is encouraged with fluids on day 1 postoperatively, as tolerated.

FURTHER READING

Kang JC, Chung MH, Chao PC *et al*. Hand-assisted laparoscopic colectomy vs open colectomy: a prospective randomized study. *Surgical Endoscopy* 2004; **18**: 577–81.

Marcello PW, Fleshman JW, Milsom JW *et al*. Hand-assisted laparoscopic vs. laparoscopic colorectal surgery: a multicenter, prospective, randomized trial. *Diseases of the Colon and Rectum* 2008; **51**: 818–26.

Nakajima K, Lee SW, Cocilovo C *et al*. Laparoscopic total colectomy: hand-assisted vs standard technique. *Surgical Endoscopy* 2004; **18**: 582–6.

Sarli L, Iusco DR, Regina G *et al*. Predicting conversion to open surgery in laparoscopic left hemicolectomy. *Surgical Laparoscopy, Endoscopy and Percutaneous Techniques* 2006; **16**: 212–16.

Sonoda T, Pandey S, Trencheva K *et al*. Longterm complications of hand-assisted versus laparoscopic colectomy. *Journal of the American College of Surgeons* 2009; **208**: 62–6.

Colectomy – complete mesocolic excision

WERNER HOHENBERGER

DEFINITION AND PRINCIPLES

Throughout the world, there are guidelines for the surgical management of colonic cancer, yet there are significant differences in reported five-year survival rates that vary in stage III disease between 44 and 85 percent. The explanation for such differences is multi-factorial, however one important element is the quality of surgical excision. Inadequate surgical technique leads to an inadequate resection specimen that may include the tumor but not the mesenteric package surrounding the tumor with preservation of the mesocolic planes of dissection including all potentially involved lymph nodes. These principles are respected in the technique of total mesocolic excision described by the author.

This procedure aims to address two main issues: (1) sharp dissection within embryologic planes: the parietal (somatic) plane (= prerenal fascia, Gerota's fascia) and the visceral plane, that covers intra-abdominal organs such as the colon (mesocolon), the rectum (mesorectum), but also the pancreas (mesopancreas) (**Figure 5.9.1**); (2) adequate dissection of the tumor draining lymph nodes with high ligation of the supplying arteries, because lymphatic spread follows in a reverse direction of the arterial blood supply of the respective site of the bowel involved by cancer (**Figure 5.9.2**).

Both principles have to be applied to any tumor of the large bowel.

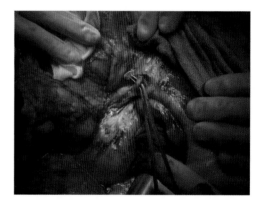

5.9.2 The mesocolon covering the central vessels is opened, the root of the superior mesenteric vein exposed and the root of the iliocolic artery which crosses the superior mesenteric vein (SMV) from below is dissected with a right angle instrument to be followed by its ligation.

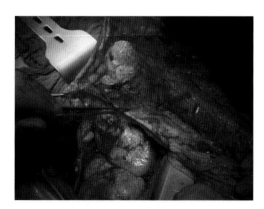

5.9.1 The parietal plane is completely exposed after mobilization of the ascending colon, the mesenteric root, and the duodenum, including the pancreatic head.

PREOPERATIVE IMAGING AND SURGICAL STRATEGY

In the past, preoperative imaging for colon cancer staging was mainly performed by computed tomography (CT) scan to detect potential liver metastases or invasion of neighboring organs. However, in the same way as the circumferential margin of clearance is important in the treatment of rectal cancer, the circumferential margin may play a similar important role in the resection of colon cancer. In this regard, preoperative magnetic resonance imaging (MRI) may be more suitable than CT scans in the staging of colon cancer, as MRI provides more detail regarding soft tissue planes and potential circumferential resection margins.

If a tumor is very close to the mesocolic plane of dissection, the dissection has to be extended to the next plane, with, for example, excision of the prerenal fat down to the anterior surface of the kidney. If any organ appears to be invaded by tumor on preoperative imaging, and this is confirmed by clinical examination at laparotomy, the organ must be included *en bloc* with the resection specimen. On occasion, this may include the pancreas whether or not the adherence may subsequently prove to be inflammatory adhesion and not malignant infiltration.

LYMPHATIC SPREAD OF COLON CANCER

Locoregional lymphatic spread mainly involves three compartments which are usually invaded consecutively. Skip lesions are very rare. The compartment consists of **pericolic nodes** along the colon. These are the first to be involved by tumor and are found at a maximum distance of 10 cm on each side of the primary tumor. The next compartment of lymph nodes consists of the **nodes along the named arteries** (ileocolic, middle colic, left colic, etc.), and the third compartments consists of the **central lymph nodes** along the superior and inferior mesenteric arteries.

For cancers of the transverse colon, including both flexures, lymphatic flow is more complex. Carcinomas of this part of the colon have a bidirectional outflow towards the middle colic artery and in addition in right-sided tumors to the ileocolic artery. Tumors distal to the middle colic vessels may also metastasize to the lymph nodes along the left ascending colonic artery and finally the inferior mesenteric artery. However, because of the close proximity of the pancreas and the gastroepiploic arcade, even more lymph node stations may be involved. This is particularly the case in cancer of the hepatic flexure, in which lymph nodes at the head of the pancreas may be involved and in left-sided tumors, nodes along the inferior aspect of the body and tail of the pancreas. In both situations, lymph nodes along the gastroepiploic vessels may be involved (**Figure 5.9.3**).

The lymphatic outflow of descending and sigmoid colon cancer follows a unidirectional pathway along the left colic and sigmoid arteries, respectively, towards the inferior mesenteric artery. The greater omentum needs only to be resected if it is attached to the tumor. In the vast majority of cases, however, it can be preserved and taken down from the transverse colon with full exposure of the lesser sac to allow transection of the transverse mesocolon at the inferior border of the pancreas. The middle colic artery can almost always be preserved. If adequate length

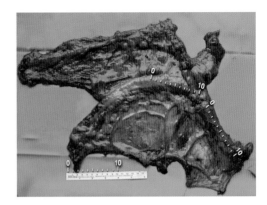

5.9.3 Pattern of potential lymphatic spread in a cancer of the splenic flexure. Because of the bidirectional lymphatic outflow at this site, the next arcade beyond a distance of 10 cm on both sides is included into the dissection. The pedicles include the high tie of the middle and left colic artery as well.

of the transverse colon cannot be achieved to bring it down to the rectum for the subsequent anastomosis, the middle colic artery and vein should be divided centrally to facilitate this.

PREOPERATIVE BOWEL PREPARATION

In many countries, following 'fast track principles', the bowel is no longer prepared preoperatively. It is the author's view that slight cleansing using 1–2 liters of saline solution is sufficient to clean the bowel adequately without obvious disadvantages to the patient or the danger of soiling the abdominal cavity after open transection of the bowel wall.

POSITION OF THE PATIENT AND INCISION OF THE ABDOMINAL WALL

For right-sided colon cancer, the patient is placed in a supine position. For cancers of the distal transverse colon, the descending and sigmoid colon, a combined lithotomy or 'rectal position' is used with the pelvis elevated and the legs spread and raised separately (see Chapter 1.6).

It is the author's preference to perform a midline abdominal incision for colonic cancer resections. For sigmoid and descending colon cancer, the incision starts in the suprapubic area and extends to the upper abdomen as for anterior resection. For right-sided hemicolectomy, the incision starts below the xiphoid process and extends just below the umbilicus on the right side.

MOBILIZATION OF THE COLON

The mobilization of the colon always starts with a paracolic incision of the peritoneum, and a lateral to medial dissection is performed. The parietal plane is exposed and the posterior mesocolic plane is dissected from the parietal plane in a sharp fashion using electrocautery with a long needle or scissors. The dissection plane follows the areolar tissue which can be well exposed by applying traction of the mesocolon and counter-traction putting pressure on to the parietal plane (**Figure 5.9.4**). It can be helpful to use a swab or a peanut to support blunt traction, strictly avoiding any tears, especially of the mesocolon.

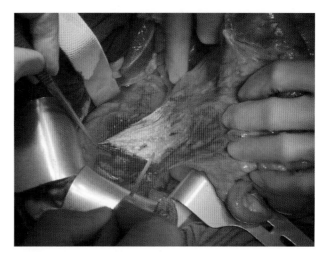

5.9.4 Full mobilization of the ascending colon by applying traction by the forceps and counter-traction by the assistant pushing apart the ascending mesocolon. The aerial tissue ('angel's hair') represents the dissection line to follow.

In sigmoid cancer, it is helpful to start with the exposure of the upper mesorectal plane first with dissection of the hypogastric nerves posteriorly and then opening the mesorectal plane superiorly, thereby exposing the mesosigmoid and the posterior plane of the descending mesocolon, as well as full mobilization of the splenic flexure (**Figure 5.9.5**).

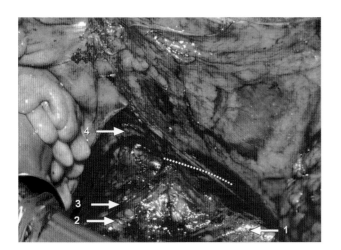

5.9.5 Aspect from the left into the peritoneal cavity. The upper mesorectum (covering the superior rectal vessels and the posterior aspect of the mesosigmoid and descending mesocolon) is dissected off the parietal plane (1), covering the gonadal vessels (2) and the ureter (3). Additional structures are the iliac vessels (dotted line) and left colic vessels (4).

On the right side, the entire mesenteric root including the cecum and ascending colon is mobilized, again starting with an incision of the peritoneum lateral to the colon.

The dissection plane now follows the areolar tissue between the ascending mesocolon and the retroperitoneal plane, which can be well exposed by proper traction applied with the flat hand of the assistant to the mesocolon and counter-traction with the surgeon's hand or using a sponge to the retroperitoneum. After this mobilization is complete, it is followed by a true Kocher maneuver (**Figure 5.9.6**).

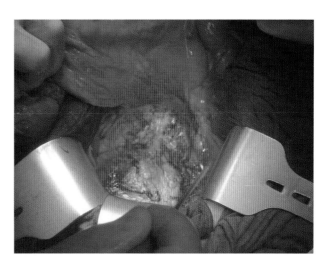

5.9.6 The right colon, the mesenteric root and the duodenum with the right pancreas are completely mobilized. The Treitz ligament is not yet divided. The intact parietal plane covers the vena cava and the right kidney with the surrounding retroperitoneal fat.

Now, the entire mesenteric root can be rotated clockwise so that the next step to take down the duodenum from the mesenteric route can be performed under direct vision. Then, the duodenum including the uncinate process of the pancreas is taken down off the ascending mesocolon (**Figure 5.9.7**), the mesocolon covering the superior mesenteric vein is incised to allow the following central lymph node dissection (**Figure 5.9.8**).

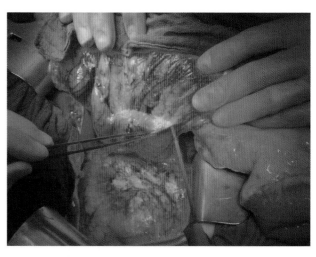

5.9.7 The attachments of the duodenum to the ascending mesocolon are incised by the needle of the diathermy following the 'angel's hair' next until the uncinate process (see Figure 5.9.8) is taken down from the mesocolon, too and the superior mesenteric vein is exposed, just covered by the mesocolon.

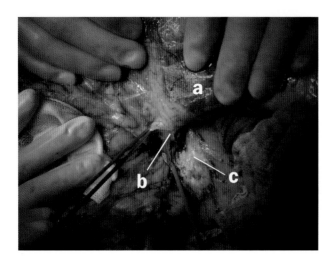

5.9.8 To gain access to the superior mesenteric vein and the artery behind, the mesocolon covering the vein (point a) needs to be divided (point b); (point c) uncinate process.

On the left side, the inferior mesenteric vein is divided just below the pancreas. Lymph node metastases are not found along the inferior mesenteric vein, confirming the observation that lymphatic drainage from the colon always follows the arterial blood supply. The pre-aortic superior hypogastric plexuses must be preserved when dividing the inferior mesenteric artery. The mesorectal plane covering the superior rectal artery ends right at this level. When dividing the inferior mesenteric artery, it should be realized that the superior hypogastric plexus encircles the root of the artery in a tent-like fashion. For that reason, the artery is fully exposed and divided without any surrounding tissue (**Figure 5.9.9**).

When following all these planes correctly, the ureter is always covered by the parietal plane and should be taped only in tumors invading the retroperitoneum or in recurrent disease.

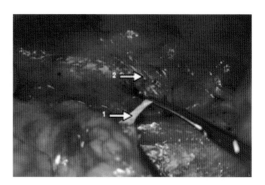

5.9.9 The inferior mesenteric artery (1) is completely freed from the surrounding autonomic nerve fibers (frequently called 'adventitia'); the superior hypogastric plexus covering the aorta is preserved including its tent-like portion (2) around the root of the inferior mesenteric artery (IMA).

'High tie' of the colic arteries

The high tie of the inferior mesenteric artery has been mentioned above under Definition and principles. The named branches of the superior mesenteric artery (middle colic, right colic, and ileocolic vessels) need more careful dissection and exposure compared to the left side.

Full access to the superior mesenteric vein as the first main vessel to be exposed is achieved only after the greater omentum is taken down from the right side of the transverse colon (see **Figure 5.9.1**), again following the embryologic planes. The right colic vein needs special attention during this dissection, because it frequently enters the right gastroepiploic vein and may cross the plane of dissection when taking down the omentum around the hepatic flexure. Uncontrolled blunt traction at the colon may lead to rupture of this vessel that is followed by significant bleeding (**Figure 5.9.10**).

The next step is to take down the duodenum from the mesenteric root, including the uncinate process of the pancreas (**Figure 5.9.7**). Now, the superior mesenteric vein with its two main branches, the middle and the ileocolic vein is fully exposed. They can be divided centrally but not before the covering mesocolon is incised right over the superior mesenteric vein (**Figure 5.9.8**).

Frequently, the ileocolic artery crosses the superior mesenteric vein from below (**Figure 5.9.2**). Sometimes, the ileocolic vein and the last branch draining the terminal ileum arise from a common trunk. It is important not to divide this trunk inadvertently assuming that just the iliocolic vein was ligated.

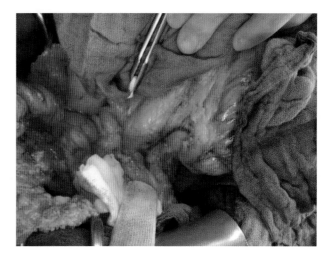

5.9.10 Frequently, the right colic vein joins the right gastroepiploic vein before running as a common trunk to the superior mesenteric vein. The uncinate process with the duodenum is retracted by a retractor.

After the anterior wall of the superior mesenteric vein is widely exposed, access to the superior mesenteric artery is achieved. This vessel, however, should never be stripped, instead the covering autonomous nerves must be strictly preserved with selective central ligation of the segmental mesenteric arteries. Otherwise intractable diarrhea may follow, which can completely be avoided if these nervous plexus are preserved.

EXTENT OF COLONIC RESECTION ACCORDING TO THE SITE OF CANCER

The 'arcade principle', mentioned above under Lymphatic spread of colon cancer, is very helpful to estimate which colonic arteries related to the lymphatic spread need to be divided. If one calculates a distance of 10 cm each side of the tumor border and include the next artery proximally, the complete field of potentially involved lymph nodes is included into the dissection.

For cancer of the cecum and the ascending colon, the main lymphatic route follows the ileocolic artery and much less frequently the right branch of the middle colic artery or the right colic artery (present in only about 10 percent of all cases). For that reason, the root of the middle colic artery can be preserved almost always and must be included only if there are obvious lymph node metastases. After exposure of the superior mesenteric vein, with central ligation of the corresponding colonic veins, the ileocolic artery and the right branches of the middle colic artery are divided followed by dissection of the root of the middle colic artery and vein down to their origin from the superior mesenteric vessels. This is now followed by sharp excision of the central mesenteric lymph nodes above and medially to the superior mesenteric artery (**Figure 5.9.11**).

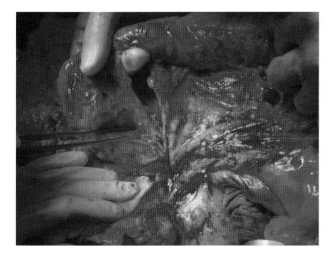

5.9.11 The superior mesenteric vein is fully exposed with the first jejunal vein running to the left crossing the superior mesenteric artery with the surrounding autonomous nerves preserved. The ileocolic vessels are tied centrally, the middle colic vein is also exposed left of the root of the middle colic artery. The branches running to the right will be divided centrally, next. The mesocolon next to the bowel is already divided.

This procedure results in a specimen demonstrated in **Figure 5.9.12** with long pedicles of the dissected vessels, no 'waisting' of the mesocolon in between, and intact mesocolic planes.

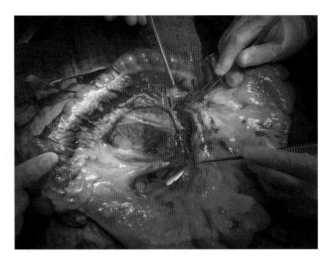

5.9.12 Intraoperative view immediately before transection of the transverse colon at the side demonstrated by the forceps. The index finger shows the site of the tumor. The supplying vessels, ileocolic artery and vein and the right branches of the middle colonic vessels, are divided centrally.

Cancer of the hepatic flexure

As described above, the blood supply and consequently the pattern of lymphatic spread of the transverse colon and the hepatic flexure is more complex. In larger series, lymph node metastases can be found over the head of the pancreas along the central part of the right gastroepiploic artery in about 5 percent of patients. However, metastatic lymph nodes are never found around the first branch of the gastroduodenal artery, the superior pancreaticoduodenal artery. Furthermore, either by direct invasion of the greater omentum or in advanced cases, lymph nodes in the greater omentum and along the right gastroepiploic arcade may be involved. However, there are almost no data in the literature on this subject. Consequently, and in keeping with personal experience, the lymph nodes over the head of the pancreas and the gastroepiploic arcade opposite to the site of the tumor in the transverse colon along a distance of about 10–15 cm, including the greater omentum, need to be resected to avoid local recurrence from lymph node metastases which are otherwise left behind.

The technical steps for resecting a colon cancer at the hepatic flexure begin as for resecting ascending colon cancer. However, the middle colic arteries are ligated centrally, finally leading to so-called extended right hemicolectomy. Moreover, the greater curvature of the distal gastric antrum is skeletonized. Then the dissection plane follows along the superior pancreaticoduodenal vessels which show many variations. The right gastroepiploic artery is divided, followed by the corresponding vein. Simultaneously, the infrapyloric nodes and those over the head and below the isthmus of the pancreas are included into the specimen with preservation of the mesopancreas covering the head and the uncinate process. As described, the right-sided greater omentum is divided with preservation of the left part, which is dissected off the middle and left transverse colon. The colon itself is divided about 10 cm distal to the root of the middle colic vessels.

Cancer of the left transverse colon and the splenic flexure

For surgery of tumors at this site, the patient is usually positioned supine. Only if the precise position of the cancer around the splenic flexure is uncertain and the descending colon may be involved is the combined lithotomy or 'rectal position' preferred.

The main draining lymph nodes are those along the root of the middle colic artery and, less frequently, of the left ascending colic artery. The lymph nodes along the ileocolic artery are never involved. For this reason, the ascending colon can be preserved.

The dissection starts in the same way as for cancer of the hepatic flexure, with mobilization of the right colon. The nodes over the pancreatic head are not, however, touched and the lymph nodes along the inferior aspect of the left pancreas including those caudal to the isthmus are dissected. There are usually only three to four lymph nodes in this area. If they are firmly attached to the pancreas due to earlier pancreatitis, dissection of these lymph nodes should not be continued because of the risk of postoperative pancreatitis and pancreatic necrosis (**Figure 5.9.13**).

The left part of the greater omentum opposite the tumor site over a distance of 10–15 cm is resected towards the specimen with dissection off the greater curvature of the stomach along the body and the proximal part of the antrum, with inclusion of the gastroepiploic vessels.

The middle colic vessels are then divided, centrally, followed by the left colonic artery right at its origin from the inferior mesenteric artery. According to the remaining vascular supply, the points of colonic transection are at the hepatic flexure and the proximal part of the sigmoid colon.

To restore continuity of the bowel, the author strongly recommends rotating the ascending colon anticlockwise which facilitates an end-to-end ascending to sigmoid colon anastomosis. The mesocolon is left widely open. If a direct anastomosis of the ascending colon with the sigmoid is performed, crossing the small intestine, postoperative anastomotic leaks are much more frequent, probably due to the tension induced on to the anastomosis by postoperative distension of the small bowel.

For cancer of the descending and sigmoid colon, the mesorectal plane of the upper rectal third is exposed first, followed by the sharp mobilization of the sigmoid and descending colon. Then the splenic flexure is taken down completely with dissection of the greater omentum off the transverse colon and central tie of the inferior mesenteric artery. The transection line distally is in the upper third

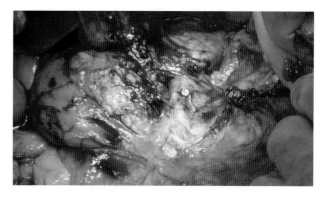

5.9.13 Dissection of the lymph nodes over the pancreatic head and along the inferior aspect of the left pancreas in cancer of the transverse colon, including the flexures; sup. Mesenteric vein with the central stump of the middle colic vein.

of the rectum and for sigmoid cancers in the distal part of the descending colon. For descending colon cancer, the proximal dissection depends on the arterial blood supply following the arcade principle with inclusion of the next proximal artery within a distance of 10 cm from the tumor.

In most cases of descending colon cancer, the mobilized transverse colon can be brought down to the upper rectum without tension. If this is not possible, the middle colic vessels have to be divided as described above to get adequate length. In this case, the proximal resection has to be extended to the hepatic flexure followed by an anticlockwise rotation of the ascending colon.

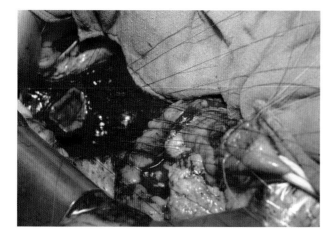

5.9.14 Interrupted extramucosal sutures of a descendo-rectostomy after sigmoid resection. The sutures of the posterior aspect of the anastomosis are all placed before the two ends of the bowel are approximated and knotted.

ANASTOMOTIC TECHNIQUE

Anastomosis to the upper rectal third is fashioned by single layer extramucosal interrupted sutures. The posterior half of the anastomotic sutures are placed without being tied, then the descending colon is brought down to the rectum and the sutures tied (**Figure 5.9.14**). The anterior half of the anastomosis is then completed, again with interrupted sutures. The retroperitoneum is subsequently closed medially by suturing the mesocolon to the mesenteric root.

All other anastomoses from small bowel to colon or right colon to left colon are performed using a running suture starting with a single internal stitch at the mesenteric site of the bowel, then placing two running sutures on both sides externally with a holding suture right at the antimesenteric side of the colon in between (**Figure 5.9.15**).

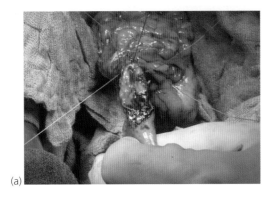 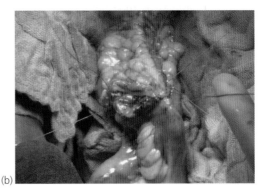

(a) (b)

5.9.15 The terminal ileum is anastomosed to the transverse colon after right hemicolectomy; the anastomosis is started by placing one internal single suture and two running sutures from outside (a). Next, both sides are completed by running extramucosal sutures (b).

MULTIVISCERAL RESECTION

In about 10 percent of colon cancers, neighboring structures or organs are attached to the tumor. It is important not to separate the adherent structures to test whether adhesions are benign or due to malignant infiltration. If the latter, the risk of later peritoneal carcinomatosis is significantly increased and survival reduced if the tumor plane is breached. For that reason, even if histopathological examination subsequently reveals inflammatory adhesions without malignant invasion, it is the author's view that all adherent organs must be resected *en bloc* extending the resection plane to the next plane beyond to the organ involved (**Figure 5.9.16**).

INTRA-ABDOMINAL DRAINS

In the author's personal practice, for all conventional colonic resections, no intra-abdominal drains are used. Only in perforated tumors, multivisceral resections, pre-existing ascites, due for example to concomitant liver cirrhosis or peritoneal carcinomatosis, is an intra-abdominal drain placed into the pouch of Douglas.

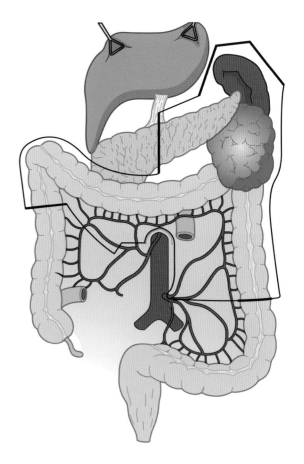

5.9.16 Cancer of splenic flexure invading the pancreatic tail and the abdominal wall. For local clearance, the resection had to be extended to the pancreas including the spleen and the abdominal wall. The lymph node dissection follows the same rules as for cancer of the respective site at the colon.

POSTOPERATIVE MANAGEMENT

In the majority of cases, the nasogastric tube is removed after the patient is fully awake and diet given the next morning. Some patients need a nasogastric tube reinserted, mainly after subtotal colectomy and resection of the gastroepiploic vascular arcade. Lymphorrhea is very uncommon and may develop after gross involvement of the central lymph nodes.

FURTHER READING

Havenga K, DeRuiter MC, Enker WE, Welvaart K. Anatomical basis of autonomic nerve-preserving total mesorectal excision for rectal cancer. *British Journal of Surgery* 1996; **83**: 384–8.

Heald RJ. The 'Holy Plane' of rectal surgery. *Journal of the Royal Society of Medicine* 1988; **81**: 503–8.

Hohenberger W, Weber K, Matzel K *et al*. Standardized surgery for colonic cancer: complete mesocolic excision and central ligation--technical notes and outcome. *Colorectal Diseases* 2009; **11**: 354–64.

Quirke P, Steele R, Monson J *et al*. MRC CR07/NCIC-CTG CO16 Trial Investigators; NCRI Colorectal Cancer Study Group. Effect of the plane of surgery achieved on local recurrence in patients with operable rectal cancer: a prospective study using data from the MRC CR07 and NCIC-CTG CO16 randomised clinical trial. *Lancet* 2009; **373**: 821–8.

West NP, Hohenberger W, Weber K *et al*. Complete mesocolic excision with central vascular ligation produces an oncologically superior specimen compared with standard surgery for carcinoma of the colon. *Journal of Clinical Oncology* 2010; **28**: 272–8.

Total colectomy – laparoscopic

RUSSELL STITZ

PRINCIPLES AND JUSTIFICATION

Laparoscopic colonic procedures were introduced in the early 1990s. By decreasing the size of the incision and operating within the closed abdominal cavity, laparoscopic colorectal surgery provides a method of performing colectomy which results in less postoperative pain, shorter hospital stay, fewer complications, and more rapid convalescence. The operative dissection must be equivalent to that performed in open surgery, particularly in cancer cases. It is important to realize that the laparoscope is a surgical tool and should be used where appropriate. Not all patients are suitable for a laparoscopic approach and limiting factors include obesity, tumor size and fixity, adhesions from previous surgery, low rectal cancer, and the male pelvis. As a general rule, patients should have a body mass index of less than 35. In morphologically challenging patients, it may be necessary to perform a hybrid procedure creating a larger incision, usually in the lower abdomen, to complete the procedure. Alternatively, a hand-assisted (HALS) approach can be considered. Timely conversion when progress falters is not a failure but shows good judgment.

Laparoscopic total colectomy (resection of the whole colon) requires the surgeon to be comfortable and competent with not only mobilizing the right and left colon but also the transverse which can be more challenging especially in larger patients.

Training

In addition to appropriate training in open colorectal procedures, the surgeon should have undergone additional training in advanced laparoscopic colorectal surgery, preferably with a period of preceptoring. Prior to attempting a total colectomy, the surgeon should already be practiced at segmental resection and comfortable mobilizing the splenic flexure. As first assistant (camera operator), the trainee surgeon not only learns the operative sequence but, importantly, is a co-surgeon, seamlessly moving with the surgeon to establish adequate exposure and provide correct tissue traction. For total colectomy, it is important to have an assistant experienced in laparoscopic colorectal surgery.

Indications

Total colectomy is usually performed as an elective procedure and the bowel is reconstituted by constructing an ileorectal anastomosis (IRA). However, in acute colitis which has not responded to medical treatment, the colectomy is associated with the creation of an end ileostomy and a distal 'mucous fistula'.

Indications for a total colectomy include synchronous carcinomas, familial adenomatous polyposis (FAP) where there is an appropriate genotype and phenotype, hereditary non-polyposis colorectal cancer (HNPCC), hyperplastic polyposis, Crohn's colitis, acute or fulminant colitis, and uncommonly, patients with marked colonic dysmotility (delayed transit).

PREOPERATIVE ASSESSMENT AND PREPARATION

Patients with medical comorbidities are stabilized preoperatively as much as possible. The patient has a bowel prep the evening before surgery and is given prophylactic antibiotics. Mechanical and chemical deep vein thrombosis prophylaxis are also part of the routine support measures. If a stoma is being considered, the patient is counseled by the stomal therapist who also marks the site of the stoma after preoperative examination in the sitting and standing positions.

ANESTHESIA

Nitrous oxide is avoided to minimize the occurrence of intestinal dilatation. During the procedure, the carbon dioxide pressure is maintained at 12 mmHg (or less in elderly people). It is not necessary to run the pressures at 15 mmHg (the capillary pressure). The anesthestist should be aware that both arms need to be by the side.

OPERATION

Planning

Because of the limited access and the dependence on technology, preoperative planning is important. The whole team needs to be familiar with the techniques and the technology. The following should be considered:

- The types of ports (trocars) that will be required. In our unit, we use 5 mm ports wherever possible as the defect does not need to be closed. The endoscopic linear stapling device requires a 12 mm port. If there has been previous surgery, particularly where there is a midline scar, the abdominal cavity is entered in the left upper quadrant using a direct optical insertion of a 5 mm port. Either disposable or reusable ports can be used. In the latter case, the port can be sutured to the skin in a way which allows full insertion of the shaft which is useful in larger patients.
- The position of the patient and the siting of the ports. The port sites may need to be adjusted to maximize exposure in a larger patient.
- What larger incision might be required if there is a need to convert or perform a hybrid operation.
- Where indicated, a stoma should be marked.

Instruments (Figure 5.10.1)

A 30° telescope is used routinely.

The harmonic scalpel is designed to divide tissues while simultaneously establishing hemostasis. It can be utilized for both sharp and blunt dissection and can safely divide vessels at least 3 mm in diameter. For larger vessels, it is safer to use clips as well. The harmonic is particularly useful when mobilizing the transverse colon and in the pelvis. Because it produces water vapor rather than smoke, better visibility can be obtained. It also has the advantage of being able to be used to grasp the tissues when repositioning although care needs to be taken that the active blade does not burn the bowel. It can be 'cooled' quickly by touching adjacent fat. The harmonic should not be used when dissecting on the bowel wall because of the

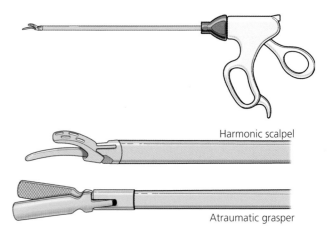

Harmonic scalpel

Atraumatic grasper

5.10.1

risk of thermal damage. For example, adhesions on the small intestine should be dissected with scissors.

Alternatively, endoscopic diathermy scissors, a diathermy hook or the LigaSure™ device can be used as dissecting tools and energy sources.

Bowel graspers with atraumatic jaws are mandatory. Typical alternatives include graspers with 3 cm jaws and atraumatic teeth or A-TRAC® graspers which have soft pad inserts.

In our unit, the ileorectal anastomosis is constructed by using an end-to-end stapling device. However, other options include an end-to-end sutured anastomosis, an end-to-side, and a functional end-to-end anastomosis, but these alternatives usually require a larger incision.

Locking clips (e.g. Hem-o-loks®) are more secure than open clips. An endoscopic linear stapling device is used to divide major vessels including the inferior mesenteric artery and vein and to transect the upper rectum.

Patient position

The patient is placed in the lithotomy position with both arms by the side. Adjustable Allen stirrups allow the thighs to be positioned so that the anterior aspect is in the same plane as the anterior abdominal wall (Figure 5.10.2a and b). This avoids interference with instrument movement particularly when dissecting the colon in the upper abdomen.

An electric table allows for rapid adjustment of the tilt of the table when head down, head up or lateral tilt is required to facilitate exposure.

The patient is placed on a 'jelly mat' or a bean bag to prevent slippage during the procedure. The latter is particularly useful if the patient is large.

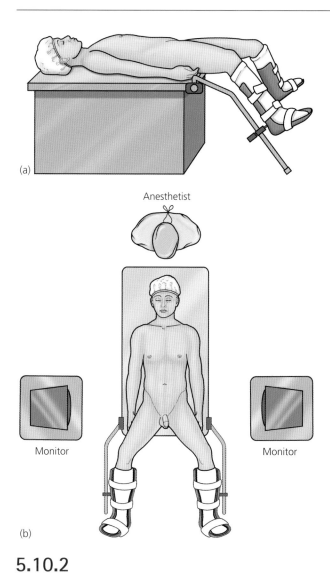

(a)

Anesthetist

Monitor

Monitor

(b)

5.10.2

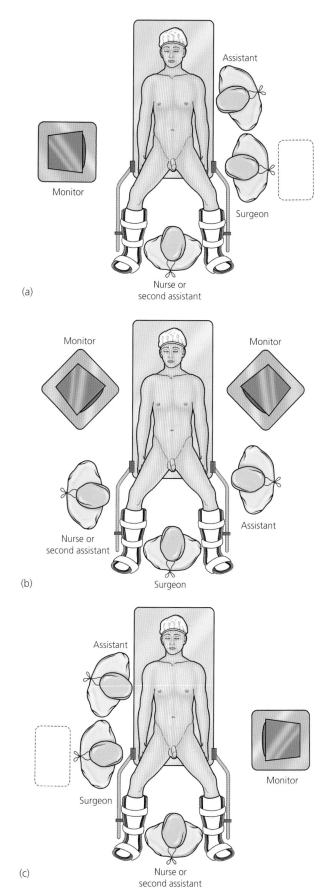

Assistant

Monitor

Surgeon

(a)

Nurse or
second assistant

Monitor

Monitor

Nurse or
second assistant

Assistant

(b)

Surgeon

Assistant

Monitor

Surgeon

(c)

Nurse or
second assistant

5.10.3

Position of the operating team and TV monitors (Figure 5.10.3)

As the operation requires the surgeon to stand on both sides of the patient (and between the legs), an additional screen is positioned on the side opposite to the camera/insufflator stack. Ideally, these screens should be able to be moved cephalad or caudally to facilitate the line of vision.

The dissection can commence on either side of the colon but it is usual to start on the right side and work distally. Initially, the surgeon and first assistant (camera operator) stand on the patient's left with the scrub nurse or a second assistant between the legs. The positions change as the operation proceeds.

Port sites (Figure 5.10.4)

As camera technology and telescopes have improved, it is now possible to eliminate the 10 mm umbilical Hasson port and replace it with a 5 mm port which does not require closure. A 5 mm port leaves minimal scarring and their position can be changed if the surgeon has problems accessing the dissection site. The 5 mm ports in the abdominal quadrants are inserted at the lateral rectus margin and the inferior epigastric vessels are visualized laparoscopically by reversing the 30° telescope as the lower abdominal trocars are inserted. Port defects of 10 mm (or greater) should be closed at the end of the procedure to minimize the risk of hernia formation. By placing the 12 mm port at the specimen extraction site, the need for separate closure of the 12 mm defect can be avoided.

Right colon dissection

The right colon can be mobilized using a lateral, medial, or retroperitoneal approach. The latter will be described as this approach optimizes accurate anatomical dissection by providing good access and exposure.

The patient is placed in the head down position and the table is rotated to the left so that the small intestine floats out of the pelvis and away from the site of dissection. It is not necessary to move all the small bowel out of the pelvis, the aim being to visualize the right pelvic brim in the region of the bifurcation of the common iliac artery. The surgeon and first assistant gain access via the left-sided ports as represented in **Figure 5.10.5**. The assistant operates the camera with the left hand and with the right hand uses a bowel grasper via the left upper quadrant (LUQ) port to retract the cecum in a cephalad and anterior direction. The surgeon completes the exposure of the base of the ileocolic mesentery with a bowel grasper in the left hand and inserted via the suprapubic port. The peritoneum can then be incised transversely at the pelvic brim using the harmonic shears or diathermy device (**Figure 5.10.6**). Hemostasis is established and with gentle blunt dissection, the plane anterior to the gonadal vessels is established. Progressively, the peritoneum is divided medially at the base of the ileal mesentery and laterally in the paracolic gutter as the dissection proceeds in a cephalad direction anterior to the gonadal vessels. A combination of sharp and blunt dissection is used ensuring that blood staining of the tissues is minimized; blood absorbs the

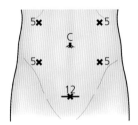

C - Camera port
5 - 5 mm ports
12 - 12 mm port
    - Pfannenstiel Incision

(a)

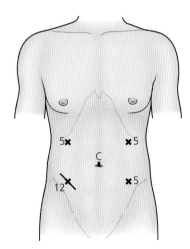

C - Camera port
5 - 5 mm ports
(b)   12 - 12 mm port and muscle splitting extraction site

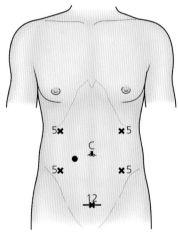

C - Camera port
5 - 5 mm ports
12 - 12 mm port
—— - Suprapubic extraction site plus mucous fistula
● - End Ileostomy

(c)

5.10.4

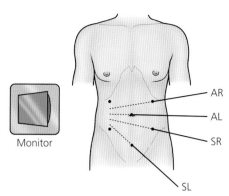

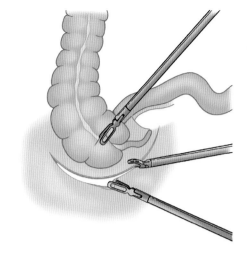

AR
AL
SR

SL

AR - Grasper in assistant's right hand
AL - Camera in assistant's left hand
SR - Dissector in surgeon's right hand
SL - Grasper in surgeon's left hand

Monitor

5.10.5

5.10.6

light and obscures the tissue planes. Provided the gonadal vessels are clearly visible, it is not necessary to formally expose the right ureter which lies further posteriorly. During this process, the surgeon and assistant change retraction points regularly to maintain exposure, but both operators should not release their graspers at the same time to avoid having to completely re-expose the operation site. As a general rule, the surgeon's left hand grasper retracts on the right side of the dissection (lateral) while the assistant's retraction is on the left side (medial) (**Figure 5.10.6**). The retroperitoneal plane is relatively avascular and the cephalad dissection usually reaches the duodenum expeditiously. The dissection then proceeds anterior to the duodenum to expose the head of the pancreas. By this time the lateral peritoneal division has usually reached the lateral aspect of the hepatic flexure.

The head down tilt is removed and the dissection moves to the anterior aspect of the hepatic flexure. The peritoneum between the duodenum and liver is incised and the cut extended laterally around the hepatic flexure to join the previously dissected lateral and retroperitoneal planes. This exposes the anterior aspect of the duodenum completely. If the hepatic flexure is high or adherent inferior to the liver, it is often helpful for the surgeon and assistant to temporarily change positions as this allows the harmonic in the surgeon's right hand to dissect proximally parallel to the colon along the inferior margin of the liver.

The assistant now pushes the cecum caudally and anteriorly into the right iliac fossa placing tension on the ileocolic mesentery. This causes the ileocolic vessels to come into relief as a clearly visible ridge and they can be fixed by the grasper in the surgeon's left hand. The peritoneum is incised on either side of the vessels near the junction with the superior mesenteric artery (SMA). This creates a window to the previous retroperitoneal

dissection where the duodenum can be visualized. The ileocolic vessels can now be divided using Hem-o-loks or the endoscopic linear stapling device. The latter is inserted via the suprapubic 12 mm port. The ileal mesentery is divided, lateral to the SMA, with the harmonic to reach the distal ileum approximately 10 cm proximal to the ileocecal junction. If the right colic is not a branch of the ileocolic, it is divided with the harmonic as the mesenteric division proceeds cephalad along the SMA to the middle colic vessels (**Figure 5.10.7**).

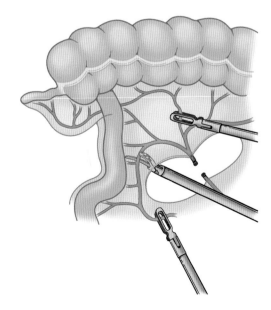

5.10.7

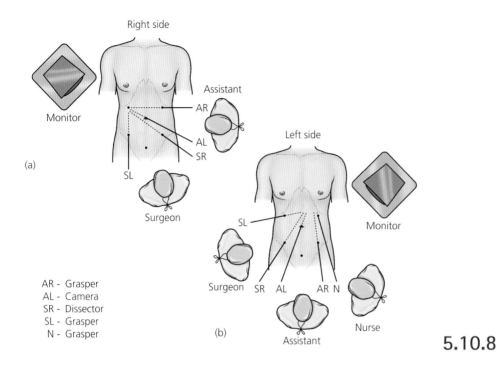

(a)

AR - Grasper
AL - Camera
SR - Dissector
SL - Grasper
N - Grasper

(b)

5.10.8

Transverse colon dissection

The surgeon moves to between the patient's legs accessing the peritoneal cavity via the lower abdominal ports (**Figure 5.10.8**a). The operating table is placed in the head up position.

The assistant uses the LUQ port to provide appropriate retraction with a grasper in the right hand as the right side of the transverse is mobilized across to the midline. If there is direct tumor infiltration of the adjacent omentum, this part of the omentum is included in the specimen. If not, the plane of dissection should be in the relatively bloodless embryological plane between the gastrocolic omentum and the transverse colon. Towards the middle aspect of the transverse, this dissection enters the lesser sac so it is often easier to enter the lesser sac in the midline initially and work proximally to separate the omentum from the colon and colonic mesentery, thus joining up with the previous dissection at the hepatic flexure. Exposure is enhanced by 'triangulation' particularly in more obese patients. That is, the surgeon, first assistant, and second assistant use their graspers to retract in three directions (**Figure 5.10.9**).

Once the omentum has been freed to the distal third of the transverse colon, attention can now focus on the middle colic vessels. With the transverse colon, or its mesentery, retracted anteriorly, the surgeon (standing between the legs) faces the mesentery on its inferior aspect. The middle colic artery common trunk or the right and left branches can now be identified and the peritoneum incised to expose the vessels. The vessels are then clipped and divided with the harmonic scapel. To accurately define

these vessels, it is often helpful to look both from the inferior mesocolic aspect and from the lesser sac surface. The latter displays the anterior surface of the pancreas and helps avoid dissecting too far posteriorly. As the dissection moves towards the splenic flexure, the surgeon moves to the right (**Figure 5.10.8**b).

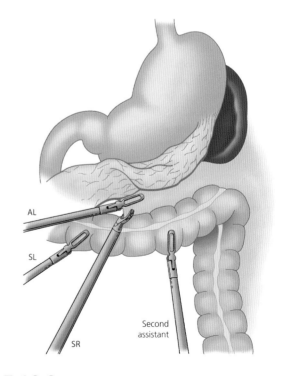

5.10.9

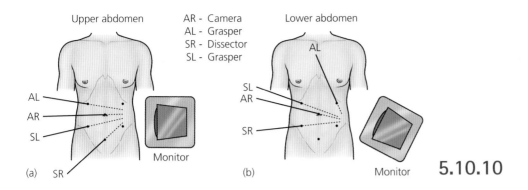

Upper abdomen

AR - Camera
AL - Grasper
SR - Dissector
SL - Grasper

Lower abdomen

AL
AR
SL

SL
AR
SR

Monitor

(a)   SR

(b)   Monitor

5.10.10

Splenic flexure

The table is tilted to the right with the head elevated. The surgeon and assistant now move to the right side (see **Figure 5.10.3**c) and face the TV monitor situated on the left side. The omentum is placed over the stomach to further expose the transverse colon and the assistant retracts the omentum by grasping it adjacent to the colon anteriorly and placing one jaw of the grasper in the lesser sac and the other in the peritoneal cavity. The second assistant, standing between the patient's legs, can use the left iliac fossa port to retract the transverse colon towards the left side. The surgeon retracts the colon at the dissection site to facilitate separation of the omentum in the direction of the splenic flexure thus exposing the lesser sac and the anterior surface of the pancreas (**Figure 5.10.9** and **5.10**a). The graspers are then moved progressively in a distal direction. Once dissection reaches the splenic flexure, the left lateral wall of the lesser sac is divided. Anatomically, it is usually easier at this stage to mobilize the left colon from the pelvic brim proximally to complete the splenic flexure mobilization.

Left colon

With the head down and the table tilted to the right, the congenital adhesions on the left side of the sigmoid mesentery are divided to facilitate exposure of the gutter at the base of the mesentery on the left. Directly behind this is the left ureter so the peritoneum is divided with care. The surgeon holds the colon with a grasper in the left hand and dissects proximally through the peritoneum in the paracolic gutter using the right hand and the suprapubic port. The first assistant uses the left hand to retract the peritoneum laterally through the right upper quadrant (RUQ) or LUQ ports (**Figure 5.10.10**a). Once the retroperitoneal tissues are exposed, the dissection proceeds medially as well as in a cephalad direction on the anterior surface of the perinephric fascia. When the descending

colon has been reached, the Trendelenburg tilt is removed. The surgeon now uses the left iliac fossa (LIF) port to dissect and the right iliac fossa (RIF) port to retract the colon while the assistant uses the RUQ port to retract the colon more proximally. The splenic flexure mobilization can now be completed.

Inferior mesenteric artery and vein

The peritoneum on the left side of the sigmoid mesentery is divided down to the pelvic brim and the left ureter identified.

Subsequently, attention focuses on the right side of the mesentery. The assistant retracts the sigmoid anteriorly to expose the right side of the mesentery using a grasper in the left hand and inserted via the LUQ port (**Figure 5.10.10**b). The landmarks include the right pelvic brim, the right ureter if visible through the peritoneum, and the inferior mesenteric artery. It is helpful to know that mesenteric fat is usually more prominent than retroperitoneal fat. The peritoneum is incised in a longitudinal fashion and is followed by gentle blunt dissection in the areolar plane posterior to the inferior mesenteric artery (IMA). When there is a suprapubic port, it is beneficial for the second assistant to insert a sucker via this port to lift the mesentery anteriorly. The surgeon can then complete the window behind the IMA which connects with the previous dissection on the left side. The hypogastric nerves are visible posteriorly at this point. The peritoneal division then proceeds proximally on the right side of the mesentery and across the anterior aspect of the origin of the IMA. The tissues posterior to the IMA are divided using blunt dissection. Hemostasis is established with the harmonic scapel and windows to the previous left-sided dissection are created. The origin of the left colic artery can now be identified and the IMA and inferior mesenteric vein (IMV) divided either proximal or distal to the left colic artery using the linear endoscopic stapling device and after confirming the position of the left ureter. The

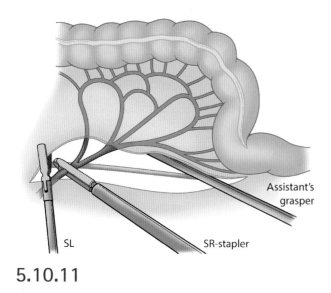

5.10.11

stapler is inserted via the 12 mm port (**Figure 5.10.11**). In a high ligation, the artery and vein are ligated separately. If there is bleeding from the staple line, the grasper in the surgeon's left hand is used to clamp the IMA pedicle and the pedicle can be clipped or ligated with an endoloop if necessary. The decision whether to perform a high or low ligation of the inferior mesenteric vessels is based on anatomical and pathological factors. In benign conditions, the mesenteric dissection can proceed closer to the colon with separate ligation of the left colic and sigmoid vessels and preservation of the inferior mesenteric vessels, as described below under Acute colectomy.

THE MEDIAL TO LATERAL APPROACH

An alternative method of dissecting the left side is to perform a medial to lateral approach, i.e. the medial dissection precedes that on the left side of the colon. This approach is particularly useful if adhesions, inflammation, or tumor obscure the anatomy on the left side of the sigmoid and descending colon. Again, the surgeon and assistant stand on the right side of the patient and the sigmoid is retracted anteriorly by the assistant using a grasper inserted via the LUQ port. This allows the surgeon to face and clearly visualize the base of the sigmoid mesentery on the right as described previously. After incising the peritoneum longitudinally, blunt dissection is used to display the IMA anteriorly and the bifurcation of the aorta and overlying hypogastric nerves posteriorly. Dissection behind the IMA defines the left ureter prior to extending the dissection in a cephalad direction. Hemostasis is important during this blunt dissection otherwise anatomical visualization is impaired. The origin of the left colic artery is identified and the IMV can be seen accompanying this artery superiorly. Once these structures have been defined satisfactorily, the surgeon performs the inferior mesenteric ligation as previously indicated. With the posterior dissection and vessel ligation completed, it is usually a straightforward

process to divide the lateral peritoneum and connect with the splenic flexure dissection. During this left-sided dissection and vessel ligation, the surgeon must constantly be aware of the position of the left ureter.

Upper rectum

With the patient in the Trendelenburg position and tilted to the right, the sigmoid is retracted out of the pelvis with the assistant's left hand operating a grasper in the LUQ port. The surgeon fine-tunes the exposure with the left hand and takes the posterior dissection into the bloodless plane behind the rectal mesenteric fascia and in front of the hypogastric nerves. The peritoneum at the junction of the right side of the rectal mesentery and the pelvic sidewall is divided carefully so that retroperitoneal structures are not damaged. The peritoneal incision is directed towards the anterior aspect of the rectum in its upper third (**Figure 5.10.12**). Similarly, with the surgeon retracting the sigmoid to the right and the assistant retracting the pelvic wall peritoneum to the left, the peritoneum is incised down the left side to join the previous dissection anterior to the rectum. The surgeon moves the dissection back to the right side of the rectal mesentery and the site of division in the upper third of the rectum (the teniae should have coalesced into a single longitudinal layer) is defined. The junction between the rectum and its mesentery can be identified by gentle blunt dissection. This is followed by division of the rectal mesentery using the harmonic shears on the variable setting. The rectum can now be divided at the same level as the mesentery using the endoscopic linear stapling device reloaded with a 'bowel' cartridge. The proximal staple line is grasped firmly with a ratcheted traumatic grasper to facilitate removal of the specimen.

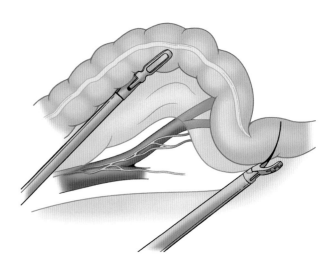

5.10.12

Specimen extraction

The suprapubic 12 mm port is removed and the specimen is extracted via a small Pfannenstiel incision (approximately 5 cm in length) using a wound protector. After delivering the colon, the distal ileum is divided and the anvil of a 29 mm end-to-end stapling device inserted into the ileum which is purse-stringed around the shaft of the anvil. The bowel is replaced inside the abdominal cavity and the wound closed.

Anastomosis

The pneumoperitoneum is restored, and the table tilted head down and to the left. The cut edge of the small intestinal mesentery is identified posteriorly at the level of the duodenum and the divided mesenteric edge followed downwards to ensure that there is no twisting of the mesentery. After cleaning the rectum with povidone-iodine, the end-to-end stapling device is inserted via the anus to the transverse upper rectal staple line. The shaft is advanced alongside the staple line and the ileal anvil docked with the rectal component. The orientation of the small bowel is checked once again prior to firing the staple gun. The integrity of the 'donuts' is confirmed and the anastomosis leak tested by instilling saline into the pelvis and insufflating air via a syringe in the anus. If there is a leak, this can be sutured laparoscopically and the anastomosis retested. A 28-Fr Foley catheter is inserted into the rectum and the balloon inflated to 15 mL.

POSTOPERATIVE CARE

Routine intravenous fluid and analgesia protocols are utilized and the full blood count and biochemistry monitored as indicated. The patient is commenced on free fluids postoperatively and graduated back to a low-fiber diet when the rectal catheter is ready to be removed. The latter is irrigated twice daily to prevent blockage and remains *in situ* until the small bowel activity stabilizes.

Early mobilization is encouraged with a view to discharging the patient from hospital on the fifth or sixth day postoperatively. The frequent, loose stool is managed with a bulking agent and loperamide.

ACUTE COLECTOMY

When laparoscopic colectomy is performed for acute colitis which fails to respond to medical management,

the operation is modified to accommodate the need to avoid an anastomosis. In addition, the surgeon should be cognizant of the requirement for subsequent restorative proctectomy. In principle, the aim is to perform the colectomy laparoscopically, constructing an end ileostomy and a closed 'mucous fistula'. Preserving the inferior mesenteric artery and vein also makes the subsequent dissection into the pelvis easier. If there is any doubt about the potential mobility of the small bowel mesentery, it is sensible to leave the ileocolic vessels intact as well.

The position of the patient is as described above. The site of the ileostomy is marked prior to surgery and the ports are positioned as shown in **Figure 5.10.4**c.

The operation proceeds as outlined previously commencing on the right and moving towards the left. The ileocolic vessels are ligated with Hem-o-loks or an endoscopic stapler. The mesenteric dissection and ligation of vessels can be performed synchronously, with the harmonic scapel, through the branches of the major colonic vessels rather than dividing the trunks separately. Locking clips are added for larger vessels where indicated. The sigmoid branches of the IMA are divided down to the distal sigmoid where the lower sigmoid branch or branches are preserved to ensure that the distal sigmoid reaches the suprapubic subcutaneous tissue without tension.

Once the colon has been mobilized, the distal ileum is divided with the endoscopic linear stapling device and the proximal and distal staple lines fixed with ratcheted toothed graspers inserted via the left-sided ports.

After creating the ileostomy trephine, the proximal ileal grasper delivers the small bowel to the ileostomy defect where it is grasped with a Babcock and brought to the surface for subsequent fashioning of the ileostomy. Direct visualization laparoscopically makes sure that the ileal mesentery is sitting satisfactorily.

A 5 cm Pfannenstiel incision is then made at the site of the 12 mm port and a small wound protector inserted prior to extracting the specimen. The extraction is facilitated by manipulating the grasper holding the distal limb of the ileum so that it can be delivered via the suprapubic incision. The lower sigmoid is then stapled with the reloaded endoscopic linear stapler. The sigmoid is secured with sutures between the sigmoid wall and the rectus sheath with the staple line lying without tension in the subcutaneous plane. The wound is closed using subcuticular sutures to the skin.

After dressing the wounds, the end ileostomy is matured.

Postoperatively, the patient is graduated rapidly back to a low-fiber diet which is an advantage in these patients who are often compromised nutritionally. Early mobilization is encouraged and this in turn facilitates early removal of the indwelling catheter.

Total colectomy – hand-assisted laparosopic surgery

THOMAS E READ

PRINCIPLES AND JUSTIFICATION

Published studies demonstrate that short-term outcomes after hand-assisted laparoscopic (HALS) colectomy are similar to those following conventional laparoscopic colectomy, with similar incision size, similar reduction in duration of ileus when compared to open colectomy, with the advantage of reduced operative times and conversion rates in the hand-assisted group as compared to the straight laparoscopy group.[1, 2, 3, 4, 5, 6, 7] HALS techniques are especially useful during total abdominal colectomy, given the need for performance of multiple complex maneuvers: mobilization of both flexures; separating the omentum from the transverse colon; and division of the transverse mesocolon. In a prospective randomized trial comparing straight laparoscopic versus hand-assisted laparoscopic total abdominal colectomy, HALS provided a 48 minute reduction in operative time ($p = 0.015$) with no difference in other outcomes.[4]

PREOPERATIVE ASSESSMENT AND PREPARATION

Although HALS total abdominal colectomy can be considered for patients with prior laparotomy and/ or complex intra-abdominal pathology, a detailed history should be obtained so as to assess the patient's appropriateness for laparoscopic management of their pathology. HALS total abdominal colectomy can be safely performed for patients with severe colitis.[8] However, patients with megacolon or septic shock may be better served by open operation. Potential intestinal stoma sites should be marked preoperatively. Although a trocar may be placed at the planned stoma site, other trocars and HALS incisions should not be placed within the anticipated boundaries of the stoma appliance, because the healing incisions will interfere with postoperative stoma management.

ANESTHESIA

General endotracheal anesthesia is used for HALS colectomy. Peak airway pressures should be assessed in the extremes of table position prior to draping to ensure that the patient can be adequately ventilated during the case.

OPERATION

Positioning

The patient should be secured to the operating table. My preference is to secure the patient by using a deflatable bean bag. The pads are removed from the thoracoabdominal portion of the table and wide strips of Velcro® are placed on the metal of the bed and the posterior aspect of the bean bag. This prevents the bean bag (and the patient) from slipping during the procedure. A large gel pad is placed inside the bean bag and the arms and shoulders padded. The arms are tucked at the sides and the bean bag wrapped around the torso and shoulders to cocoon the patient. The legs are typically placed in split leg position for access to the anus to perform intraoperative endoscopy or passage of a surgical stapling device. The bed is then tested in all the extremes of position to ensure that the patient does not slide and that access to the anus is maintained.

Choice of incision

The choice of incision is based on where the surgeon feels the incision will maximize safe completion of the procedure. It may be directly over the pathology (phlegmon, fistula, locally advanced tumor) or over the anticipated site of anastomosis. Typically, the HALS device is placed via a Pfannenstiel or lower midline incision for total abdominal colectomy (**Figure 5.11.1**). Transection of the rectum and mesorectum, one of the most difficult aspects

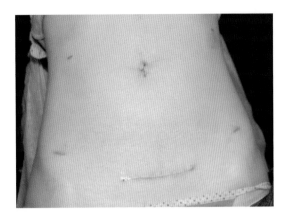

5.11.1 Skin incisions 2 weeks following hand-assisted laparoscopic total abdominal colectomy and ileorectal anastomosis.

of laparoscopic proctectomy, can be performed through this incision. Construction of ileorectal anastomosis can be performed under direct vision, and any anastomotic problems identified on leak testing can also be repaired directly. For patients with ulcerative colitis in whom restorative proctectomy will subsequently be considered, either a Pfannenstiel or lower midline incision will give access to the pelvis, although the Pfannenstiel tends to provide somewhat better access to the pelvis and seems to be associated with fewer wound complications than a midline incision. In addition, the Pfannenstiel incision is cosmetically appealing to many patients, especially to women.

However, if conversion to formal laparotomy will probably be required, a lower midline incision is preferable. Alternatively, if a Pfannenstiel incision was made at the outset of the case and formal laparotomy is subsequently required, the Pfannenstiel incision can simply be extended to allow greater direct access to the abdominal cavity.

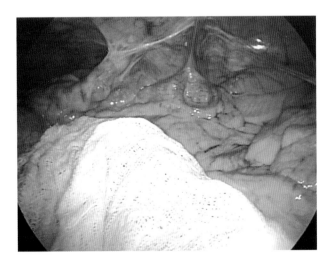

5.11.2 Laparotomy pad covering small bowel during hand-assisted laparoscopic total abdominal colectomy.

Mobilization of the colon

After making the HALS incision and placing the base of the HALS device, which functions as a retractor and wound protector, intra-abdominal conditions are assessed. As much mobilization as can be safely performed through the incision should be done at this point. Except in the morbidly obese, mobilization of the rectosigmoid can be performed through the HALS incision. The rectum can be divided at this point, as well as the mesocolon at the rectosigmoid junction. This maneuver allows direct end-on access to the left colon mesentery and facilitates laparoscopic manipulation of the sigmoid, as it is now disconnected from the rectum. In many patients, it is also possible to mobilize the cecum and ileal mesentery from their retroperitoneal attachments via the HALS incision. The ileum can be divided at this point if the anatomy is favorable. If the transverse colon is redundant, the omentum and transverse colon can be delivered through the incision and the omentum separated from the mid-transverse colon, and a small portion of the transverse mesocolon divided. These maneuvers help orient the surgeon to the anatomy of the omentum and transverse mesocolon later in the case, and accelerate laparoscopic mobilization of the transverse colon and division of the transverse mesocolon. While all of these maneuvers may be performed working directly through the HALS incision in some patients, obesity or disease pathology may dictate that the surgeon proceed directly with laparoscopic access after making the HALS incision.

After the limits of mobilization are reached through the small incision, laparoscopic access is established. It is often helpful to place a moist laparotomy pad in the abdomen prior to establishing pneumoperitoneum, to assist with small bowel retraction (**Figure 5.11.2**). It is imperative to keep an accurate account of the number of pads placed into and removed from the peritoneal cavity during the case. Care should be taken to avoid placing trocars too close to the skirt of the HALS device. The umbilical trocar can be placed under direct vision and the pneumoperitoneum established. Other trocars are then inserted. Mobilization of the colon can proceed in any sequence the surgeon prefers. However, it is advisable to begin the dissection at what is anticipated to be the most difficult part of the case, as if conversion to formal laparotomy is required, it is advantageous to convert early on, rather than to complete 90 percent of the operation only to convert to laparotomy near the conclusion of the procedure.

Mobilization of the left colon can proceed using a variety of techniques: medial-to-lateral; lateral-to-medial; or superior-to-inferior (after entering the lesser sac by separating the omentum from the distal transverse colon). The laparotomy pad should be opened and placed over the small intestine, with one corner at the ligament of Treitz and another corner at the pelvic inlet. It should be tucked gently around the left border of the small intestine (**Figure 5.11.2**). Throughout the case, the hand is used primarily as a retractor. Blunt dissection is discouraged, as it can lead to entrance into inappropriate tissue planes and cause unnecessary hemorrhage. Mesenteric vessels are divided using any secure method preferred by the surgeon. However, given that multiple vessels must be transected during total abdominal colectomy, it is more fiscally responsible to use an energy device or clip applier for vessel division rather than a stapler (**Figure 5.11.3**). The inferior mesenteric artery can be divided at its origin on the aorta for cases of malignancy, or more peripherally in the mesentery for benign disease. The inferior mesenteric vein can be divided adjacent to the ligament of Treitz or left *in situ* and the mesentery of the left colon divided anterior to the vein, as indicated by disease pathology and location.

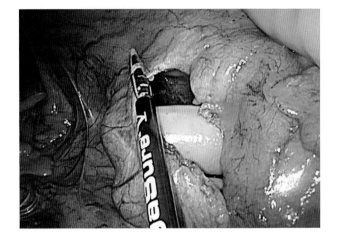

5.11.3 Division of transverse mesocolon.

The omentum can be separated from the transverse colon or resected with the colon (**Figure 5.11.4**). If the omentum is resected with the colon, it can be divided between the stomach and transverse colon using an energy device.

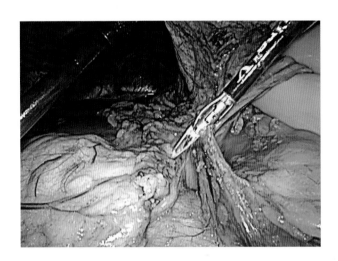

5.11.4 Separation of omentum from mid-transverse colon.

Using either method, the lesser sac is entered and the mobilization of the splenic flexure completed (**Figure 5.11.5**). It is helpful to have three-point retraction during the mobilization of the omentum; two graspers holding the omentum superiorly and anteriorly on the right and left, and the surgeon's hand retracting the transverse colon inferiorly. The surgeon's other hand can then utililize the energy device for dissection and vessel sealing. The fusion plane between the omentum and transverse mesocolon approaching the hepatic flexure is then opened and the right side of the omentum divided. Care should be taken to identify and preserve the duodenum and pancreas by staying anterior to these structures as the dissection is carried laterally around the hepatic flexure. Alternatively, mobilization of the hepatic flexure can be deferred until after mobilization of the right colon. The transverse

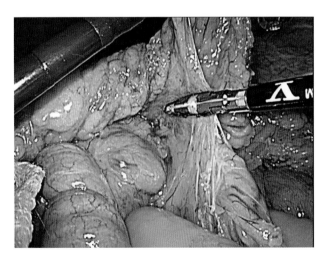

5.11.5 Mobilization of the omentum from the splenic flexure.

mesocolon can then be divided. It is often helpful to encircle the transverse mesocolon with the hand, so that relationships of the mesentery to the pancreas and root of the small bowel mesentery can be appreciated easily (**Figure 5.11.6**).

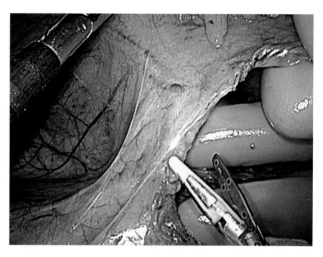

5.11.6 The surgeon's hand encircles the transverse mesocolon, so that relationships of the mesentery to the pancreas and root of the small bowel mesentery can be appreciated during transection of the middle colic vessels.

Mobilization of the right colon can proceed using a variety of techniques: medial-to-lateral; lateral-to-medial; inferior-to-superior, or superior-to-inferior (working retrograde around the hepatic flexure). If the hepatic flexure has not been mobilized previously, medial-to-lateral mobilization of the right colon mesentery extending anterior to the duodenum and pancreas, deep to the hepatic flexure, can be performed. This maneuver will define this plane clearly, so that when the surgeon returns to complete the retrograde mobilization of the hepatic flexure, the area of previous dissection anterior to the duodenum can be easily identified – it often appears purple in color – and the two planes of dissection can safely be connected (**Figure 5.11.7**). The ileocolic vessels are divided, leaving the terminal ileal mesentery as the only remaining connection of the colon specimen to the body.

Prior to exteriorization of the specimen, it is important to orient the small bowel and its mesentery. If ileorectal anastomosis is to be performed, my preference is to flip the entire small bowel and its mesentery into the right abdomen and line up the cut edges of the ileal mesentery and the sigmoid mesocolon in parallel. The hand can hold the intestine in correct orientation while pneumoperitoneum is released. The specimen is exteriorized and the ileal mesentery and ileum divided. Stay sutures are placed to maintain the alignment of the ileum and rectum for subsequent anastomosis. Anastomosis can then be performed under direct vision. If a small portion of distal sigmoid is preserved, a side-to-side anastomosis can be performed. Otherwise, an end-to-end anastomosis is constructed, either by stapled or handsewn method. It is important to perform air leak testing of the anastomosis and repair of any defect prior to closure, as this has been associated with lower clinical anastomotic leak rate than no testing.[9]

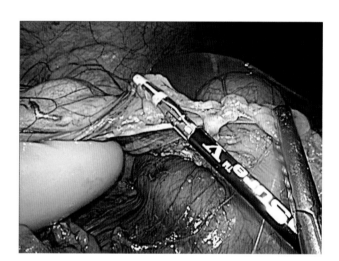

5.11.7 Mobilization of hepatic flexure.

If ileostomy is to be performed, it is important to remove the base of the HALS device and return the fascia of the HALS incision to its normal position prior to construction of the stoma opening. Otherwise, the fascia can impinge upon the ileostomy when it is pulled back to normal anatomic position during fascial closure.

If total abdominal colectomy is being performed for acute colitis, then the surgeon must make a decision regarding management of the rectosigmoid stump. The proximal rectum can be closed and left *in situ*, although this places the patient at risk for rectal stump blowout. Intraoperative endoscopic evaluation of the retained rectum, air leak testing the rectal stump closure with repair of any defect, suctioning out of residual rectal contents, and tube decompression of the rectal stump may be of benefit. Alternatively, a portion of distal sigmoid can be retained and brought to the skin as a mucus fistula. This will eliminate the risk of rectal stump blowout but has the disadvantage of giving the patient an extra stoma. An intermediate option is to bring the closed end of the distal sigmoid through the abdominal wall of the extraction incision, so that if there is a blowout, it will decompress through the wound (**Figure 5.11.8**).

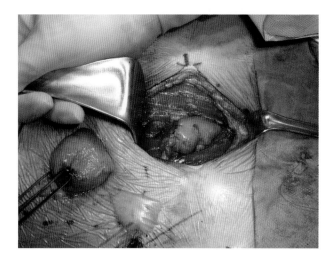

5.11.8 Closed end of distal sigmoid stump brought through abdominal wall of Pfannenstiel incision after colectomy for acute colitis.

POSTOPERATIVE CARE

Routine postoperative care is appropriate following HALS total abdominal colectomy.

OUTCOME

As noted above, prospective trials have demonstrated that short-term outcomes after HALS colectomy are similar to those following straight laparoscopic colectomy, with similar incision size, similar reduction in duration of ileus when compared to open colectomy, with the advantage of reduced operative times and conversion rates in the hand-assisted groups.[2, 4, 5, 6, 7] As expected given the magnitude of the procedure, the greatest reduction in operative times afforded by the HALS technique versus straight laparoscopic technique is seen during total abdominal colectomy.[4]

REFERENCES

1. Hand-assisted laparoscopic surgery vs standard laparoscopic surgery for colorectal disease: a prospective randomized trial. HALS Study Group. *Surgical Endoscopy* 2000; **14**: 896–901.
2. Kang JC, Chung MH, Chao PC *et al*. Hand-assisted laparoscopic colectomy vs open colectomy: a prospective randomized study. *Surgical Endoscopy* 2004; **18**: 577–81.
3. Litwin DE, Darzi A, Jakimowicz J *et al*. Hand-assisted laparoscopic surgery (HALS) with the HandPort system: initial experience with 68 patients. *Annals of Surgery* 2000; **231**: 715–23.
4. Marcello PW, Fleshman JW, Milsom JW *et al*. Hand-assisted laparoscopic vs. laparoscopic colorectal surgery: a multicenter, prospective, randomized trial. *Diseases of the Colon and Rectum* 2008; **51**: 818–26; discussion 826–8.
5. Martel G, Boushey RP, Marcello PW. Hand-assisted laparoscopic colorectal surgery: an evidence-based review. *Minerva Chirurgica* 2008; **63**: 373–83.
6. Rivadeneira DE, Marcello PW, Roberts PL *et al*. Benefits of hand-assisted laparoscopic restorative proctocolectomy: a comparative study. *Diseases of the Colon and Rectum* 2004; **47**: 1371–6.
7. Targarona EM, Gracia E, Garriga J *et al*. Prospective randomized trial comparing conventional laparoscopic colectomy with hand-assisted laparoscopic colectomy: applicability, immediate clinical outcome, inflammatory response, and cost. *Surgical Endoscopy* 2002; **16**: 234–9.
8. Chung TP, Fleshman JW, Birnbaum EH *et al*. Laparoscopic vs. open total abdominal colectomy for severe colitis: impact on recovery and subsequent completion restorative proctectomy. *Diseases of the Colon and Rectum* 2009; **52**: 4–10.
9. Ricciardi R, Roberts PL, Marcello PW *et al*. Anastomotic leak testing after colorectal resection: what are the data? *Archives of Surgery* 2009; **144**: 407–11; discussion 411–12.

Hartmann's procedure

PASCAL FRILEUX

HISTORY

In 1923, Henri Hartmann described an operation which is now defined as resection of the sigmoid colon with construction of a terminal colostomy and closure of the rectal stump (**Figure 5.12.1**). A variable length of rectum may also be resected. The indication was initially cancer of the upper or middle third of the rectum, at a time when anterior resection had not been developed. Today, Hartmann's operation is usually performed as an emergency procedure to treat the complications of various colorectal diseases.

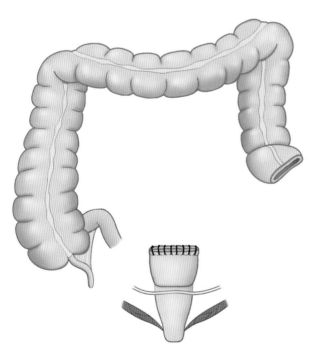

PRINCIPLES AND JUSTIFICATION

Indications and contraindications

Hartmann's operation is indicated when it is necessary to perform a resection of the sigmoid and when an immediate anastomosis appears unsafe. This operation allows resection of the sigmoid at the primary stage, but requires another major procedure for re-establishing the continuity.

BENIGN DISEASES

Hartmann's operation once represented the gold standard in perforated sigmoid diverticulitis that required urgent operation. There is now a debate between this procedure and primary anastomosis. Hartmann's operation is criticized for associated high morbidity and mortality rates and the difficulty of restoring intestinal continuity.[1] However, in the author's experience, Hartmann's operation is the safer procedure with a mortality close to zero and a permanent stoma rate of only 5 percent.[2] Selected patients with Hinchey grades II and III peritonitis from perforated diverticulitis may also be treated by laparoscopic lavage.[3]

Hartmann's operation is also indicated in acute ischemic colitis involving the sigmoid.

Acute colitis, in the form of toxic megacolon or fulminant colitis, may require an emergency colectomy, but it is generally agreed that primary coloproctectomy should be avoided in this situation, and total abdominal colectomy is favored. Some choose to close the rectal stump, while others (including the author) prefer a sigmoid mucous fistula to avoid the possible complications caused by leakage from the suture line in the rectum. If Hartmann's

5.12.1

procedure is selected, it is necessary to place a tube in the rectal remnant to drain the secretions produced by the inflamed mucosa.

Other indications include trauma with extensive destruction of the sigmoid or rectum, including iatrogenic perforation; volvulus of the sigmoid colon (see Chapter 5.13) with peritonitis and necrosis of the sigmoid colon; and postoperative sepsis after anterior resection in cases where the anastomosis cannot be conserved because of necrosis of the bowel or major disruption of the anastomosis

MALIGNANT DISEASES

While there was a place for Hartmann's operation in 1921 in the elective therapy of rectal cancer, this is no longer the case because re-establishment of continuity is often not carried out and the patient is left with a permanent colostomy. Malignant obstruction is now better treated by reconstruction after resection (see Chapter 6.1). The main indications for Hartmann's operation are in poor-risk patients and in some palliative cases associated with perforation of a rectal carcinoma.

OPERATION

The following description applies to cases of perforated diverticulitis.

Position of patient

The patient is placed in the lithotomy position with stirrups (see Chapter 1.3).

Incision

While some surgeons favor a left paramedian incision, most perform a midline incision from the pubis to midway between the umbilicus and xiphoid (**Figure 5.12.2**). The edges of the incision are protected with surgical drapes.

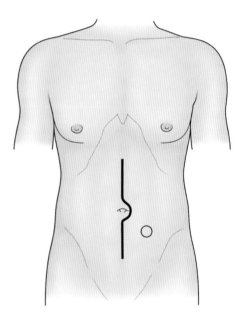

5.12.2

The peritoneal fluid is first sampled for bacterial analysis and is then aspirated. Full exploration of the peritoneal cavity is undertaken to identify the primary lesion and occasional associated diseases. In cases of perforated diverticulitis, the origin of the peritonitis is easily recognized.

Resection

The vessels in the mesocolon are ligated close to the colon, as in any benign disease. The first step is to mobilize the colon, starting from the descending colon where inflammation is minimal. The ureter is identified and the mobilization proceeds distally, using either sharp or blunt dissection according to the type of the inflammatory lesions. There is usually an easy plane of dissection between the sigmoid and the posterior elements (ureter and gonadal vessels), but adhesions may be dense at the level of the pelvic brim. The vessels and mesentery are ligated and divided (**Figure 5.12.3**).

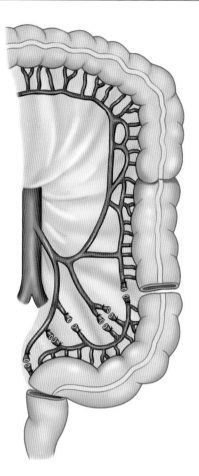

5.12.3

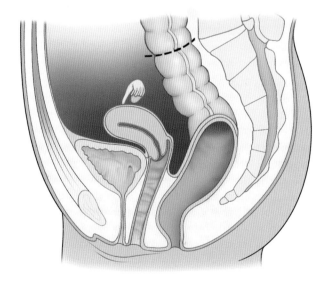

5.12.4

The site of proximal division of the colon varies with the extent of the inflammation; usually it is the limit between the descending and sigmoid colon. A GIA™ stapler or crushing clamps are used to divide the colon to avoid contamination.

The site of distal division is usually at the level of the sacral promontory because gross inflammatory lesions rarely extend beyond this point, and if this is the case, they are confined to the mesocolon and do not involve the bowel itself; a sigmoid resection extending down on to the rectum, at the level of the peritoneal reflection, would make the re-establishment of continuity significantly more difficult (**Figure 5.12.4**).

After the posterior aspect of the rectum at the level of the sacral promontory has been cleared, the rectum is closed using a TA-55™ stapler. A clamp is placed above the staple line and the rectum is divided. A suture line over the staples is not necessary, but the rectal stump may be sutured to the sacral promontory to keep it from folding over into the pelvis.

Peritoneal lavage

In the case of peritonitis, thorough peritoneal lavage using saline is indicated to remove fibrinous exudate and pus.

Construction of left iliac colostomy

A separate incision is made in the left iliac fossa at a point equidistant from the anterior iliac spine and the umbilicus. A circle of skin 3 cm in diameter is excised, followed by a cross-shaped incision in the fascia and peritoneal layer. The passage for the colostomy should admit two fingers. If possible, the site of the colostomy should be chosen before the operation, but in emergencies this is not always possible. This colostomy is temporary; therefore, it is not necessary to make a subperitoneal tunnel as for a permanent colostomy (see Chapter 3.2). The colon must be well vascularized and brought out without traction; this may require mobilization of the descending colon. The colostomy remains clamped until the abdominal wall has been closed.

Drainage

The main complications of Hartmann's operation for sigmoid diverticulitis are leakage from the rectal suture line and recurrent abdominal sepsis. In low-risk patients, drainage of the Douglas pouch may be achieved by a suction drain or any means of drainage; in high-risk patients with poor general condition and/or a heavy form of peritoneal inflammation, the author continues to use packing with a suction drain as described by Mikulicz (**Figure 5.12.5**). This gauze packing is made of a parachute-shape bag containing a 20-Fr silicone drain and long gauze swabs.[4] In addition to providing efficient drainage, particularly if a leak occurs on the rectal suture line, this form of drainage is associated with good restoration of the peritoneum in the lower abdomen that facilitates any subsequent operation for restoration of intestinal continuity.

Drainage of other abdominal spaces is not recommended.

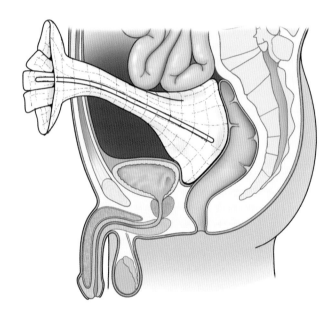

5.12.5

Closure of the abdominal wall

Conventional closure may suffice, but in poor-risk patients, a Vicryl® mesh may be placed over the viscera, the inferior part of which is placed between the bowel loops and the Mikulicz packing. This mesh reduces the incidence of abdominal wound dehiscence and protects the viscera in the event that dehiscence occurs.

EVACUATION AND DRAINAGE OF THE RECTUM

Gentle dilatation of the anus followed by evacuation and irrigation of the rectal contents is a useful precaution.

Postoperative care

Routine postoperative care is required, with special focus on the colostomy and the drains. If utilized, the Mikulicz packing is placed in a closed appliance and its tube is connected to a −100 mmHg suction; it produces 100–300 mL of discharge daily. From the 8th postoperative day onwards, the drain is irrigated via the tube by a daily infusion of 500 mL of saline + 50 mL of povidone-iodine; the gauze swabs are removed one by one from day 9 to day 11 and the bag itself is removed on day 13 at the bedside under mild analgesia. The rectal stump should be checked in case of signs of sepsis as it may contain a collection of pus.

Outcome

The outcome of Hartmann's operation is closely related to the condition of the patient and the severity of the initial disease. The remainder of this chapter relates to the outcomes of Hartmann's operation as used in the treatment of perforated diverticulitis.

Complications

The incidence of postoperative complications is high, especially in elderly patients and those with severe forms of sepsis.

- **Mortality**. The mortality after Hartmann's operation reported in the literature is an average of 15 percent;[1, 5] however, the author reported no deaths in a recent survey.[2]
- **Sepsis**. Rectal stump leak and/or intra-abdominal sepsis is reported to occur in 10 percent of patients,[2, 5] requiring local debridement or computed tomography (CT) scan-guided drainage.
- **Wound complications**. Wound infection and/or disruption may be observed, requiring local treatment; in extensive wound sepsis, reoperation or vacuum-assisted closure may be useful.
- **Stoma**. Stoma retraction, necrosis or infection may occur, but it rarely requires more than local care (see Chapter 3.15).
- **Reoperation**. An average of 10 percent of patients will need reoperation for sepsis, wound, or stoma complications.

RESTORATION OF CONTINUITY

The percentage of patients who eventually undergo restoration of intestinal continuity after Hartmann's operation for perforated diverticulitis varies in the literature around 80 percent, with groups reporting figures above 90 percent.[2, 6] Restoration of continuity should be considered in fit patients after good recuperation following the primary surgery; age is not a contraindication if the patient's general condition is suitable and the patient is well motivated. A full discussion on the risks and benefits is necessary. The patient should be aware that a temporary defunctioning stoma might be required. Operation is delayed for at least four months after the first surgery.

Preoperative assessment

Colonoscopy should be carried out to exclude neoplasia, diverticular disease or other focal abnormalities in the proximal colon. The rectal stump should be assessed by digital examination and radiography and any residual fecal material should be evacuated.

Preparation

The author uses routine preoperative bowel preparation. In the 'easy case', i.e. a long rectal stump with no local problems such as multiple previous operations or radiotherapy, the operation entails conventional dissection of the proximal colon, short excision of the upper part of the rectal stump, and a colorectal anastomosis. In selected patients, this may be performed laparoscopically. In more difficult cases, the surgeon must be prepared to undertake a low stapled or pull-through anastomosis.

Operative technique

THE EASY CASE

The patient is placed in the lithotomy position (see Chapter 1.6). A long midline incision is made and adhesions divided. The rectal stump is identified below the sacral promontory, where it may be adherent to bowel loops, the uterus, or the urinary bladder. This stage of the operation may be difficult, particularly in cases where the rectal stump has leaked, as dense adhesions may have formed. The rectal stump may also have retracted and be tightly adherent to presacral fibrous tissue. The ureters may be pulled medially by the scarring process and it is important to expose both ureters before completing the dissection. Identification of the rectal stump may be facilitated by placing a 30 mm bougie into the rectum through the anus and held in place by an assistant.

The mobilization of the rectal stump starts between the sacrum and the posterior aspect of the rectum and mesorectum; once the mesorectal plane is found and opened, dissection proceeds laterally and anteriorly. In women, identification of the vagina may also be facilitated by placing a bougie in the vagina. Once the apical 3–4 cm of rectal stump is dissected and an area is reached where the rectum is supple and the lumen adequate, it may be resected. The mesorectal remnant is divided first and the rectum itself is closed by a linear stapler and resected.

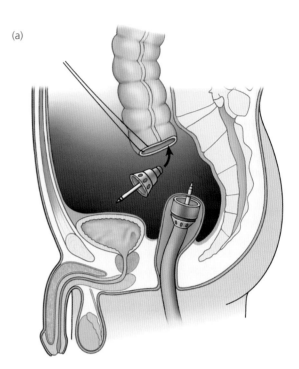

(a)

The proximal colon is dissected free from the stoma site, the descending colon and the splenic flexure are mobilized, and the anastomosis is carried out with a circular stapler (**Figure 5.12.6**).

In some cases, when the anterior aspect of the rectum is easy to dissect, it is easier and quicker not to resect the apex of the rectal stump and to make the anastomosis directly on to the anterior aspect of the rectum as an end colon to side rectum anastomosis. In this case, there should be no suspicion of leak from the top of the rectal stump and care should be taken to avoid including the bladder or the vagina in the anastomosis. An anterior rectal anastomosis is also recommended when after resection of the top of the rectal stump the stapler cannot reach the suture line due to fibrous adhesions and narrowing of the upper rectum; in this case, the anastomosis should be placed far enough from the rectal suture line to avoid ischemia of the bridge of rectal tissue.

(b)

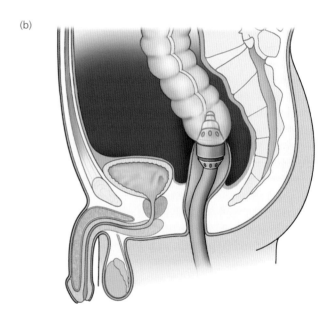

5.12.6 The stapler is passed transanally in the rectum and perforates either the staple line or the anterior aspect of the rectum (see text).

THE DIFFICULT CASE

When the rectal remnant is short, below the pouch of Douglas, dissection of the rectal stump is difficult. The bladder in men and the vagina in women are usually adherent to the sacrum and any effort of separation may lead to bleeding or perforation into the bladder or vagina. Opening the anterior aspect of the bladder and placing a bougie in the vagina may help. Dissection of both ureters down to the bladder trigone is necessary. Once a passage has been made on the midline, if the rectum may be dissected without too much difficulty, a stapled anastomosis may be constructed. If the rectum cannot be dissected safely, then a Soave pull-through anastomosis remains an option. The rectum is opened from above and a mucosal proctectomy is performed both from the abdominal and perineal approaches (**Figure 5.12.7**). A sutured coloanal anastomosis is then performed. In these difficult cases, a temporary defunctioning stoma is required.

(a)

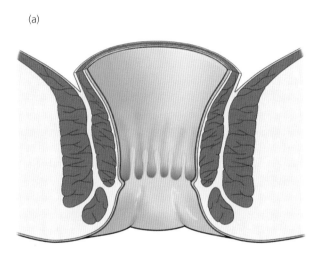

(b)

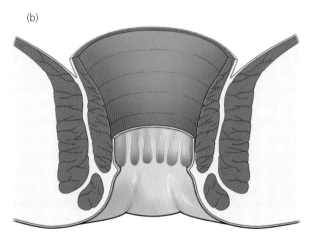

(c)

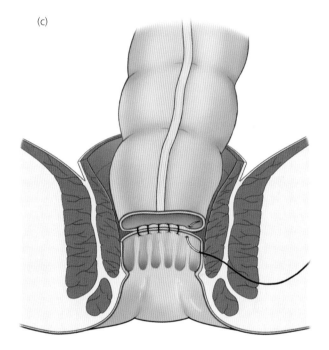

5.12.7

Outcome

After restoration of continuity, the mortality rate is low and the percentage of patients with a permanent stoma ranges from 0 to 5 percent.[1, 2, 5] Postoperative complications include pelvic sepsis, anastomotic leakage, wound difficulties, and urinary problems.

CONCLUSION

Hartmann's operation is a safe yet 'heavy' procedure in emergency colon surgery. Alternative procedures, such as immediate primary anastomosis, are suitable in selected patients only and Hartmann's operation should be the procedure of choice in high-risk, septic patients. The Mikulicz packing technique, albeit old-fashioned, provides remarkably efficient postoperative drainage of the pelvis.

REFERENCES

1. Constantinides VA, Heriot A, Remzi F *et al*. Operative strategies for diverticular peritonitis: a decision analysis between primary resection and anastomosis versus Hartmann's procedures. *Annals of Surgery* 2007; **245**: 94–103.
2. Frileux P, Dubrez J, Burdy G *et al*. Sigmoid diverticulitis. Longitudinal analysis of 222 patients with a minimal follow-up of 5 years. *Colorectal Disease* 2010; **12**: 674–80.
3. Myers E, Hurley M, O'Sullivan GC *et al*. Laparoscopic peritoneal lavage for generalized peritonitis due to perforated diverticulitis. *British Journal of Surgery* 2008; **95**: 97–101.
4. Frileux P, Quilichini MA, Cugnenc PH *et al*. Péritonites post-opératoires d'origine colique. A propos de 155 cas. *Annales de Chirurgie* 1985; **39**: 649–59.
5. Zingg U, Pasternak I, Dietrich M *et al*. Primary anastomosis vs Hartmann's procedure in patients undergoing emergency left colectomy for perforated peritonitis. *Colorectal Disease* 2010; **12**: 54–60.
6. Oomen JL, Engel AF, Cuesta MA. Mortality after acute surgery for complications of diverticular disease of the sigmoid colon is almost exclusively due to patient related factors. *Colorectal Disease* 2006; **8**: 112–19.

Emergency colectomy

SUSAN GALANDIUK

HISTORY

Emergency colectomy is performed less frequently today than in the past with improved medical management of inflammatory bowel and other intestinal disease, but is still required for a variety of indications. The need for emergency colectomy for severe *Clostridium difficile* colitis is rising. Emergency colectomy can be performed either laparoscopically, by a laparoscope-assisted procedure, or by an open technique. The type of surgical approach depends upon the patient's hemodynamic stability, the patient's prior surgical history, the comfort level of the surgeon, and the degree of bowel distention. With significant bowel distention and loss of intra-abdominal domain, laparoscopic open surgery may be safer and more expedient in skilled hands. The importance for the patient of well-performed emergency surgery is brought into perspective by a recent report on emergency surgery in hospitals participating in the American College of Surgeons National Surgical Quality Improvement Program. Nearly 26 000 patients undergoing elective colorectal resection in this program had a morbidity rate of 23.9 percent and a mortality rate of 1.9 percent compared to just over 5000 patients who underwent emergent colorectal resection with a morbidity of 48 percent and mortality of 15.3 percent – nearly eight-fold that of the elective patients![1] Regardless of surgical approach, the principles are the same with respect to surgical indications, optimizing the patient's condition for surgery, intraoperative patient management, technical tips to avoid complications following surgery, and postoperative patient care.

PREOPERATIVE ASSESSMENT AND PREPARATION

By the very nature of their disease, all patients in need of emergency colectomy will be ill and require more preoperative preparation than a typical elective surgery patient. Intravascular volume deficit is common to all these conditions. The extent of this deficit and any accompanying electrolyte and acid/base disturbance should be assessed and corrected as much as possible prior to surgery. The longer a patient has been ill, the longer preoperative preparation should be required. If the patient's condition permits, both left- and right-sided stoma sites should be marked depending upon the surgery anticipated. Complete laboratory evaluation including coagulation studies should be performed. Blood should be typed and cross-matched. A careful patient history should be obtained for the use of drugs, such as clopidogrel, non-steroidal anti-inflammatory medication, or anticoagulants. Patients treated with corticosteroids require intravenous stress dose coverage. All patients should receive broad-spectrum antibiotics preoperatively with good aerobic and anaerobic coverage. Depending upon the severity of the patient's illness, preoperative stabilization and monitoring in a critical care nursing unit may be warranted. This must be weighed against the urgency of the intervention required.

PRINCIPLES AND JUSTIFICATION

Colitis

Emergency colectomy for inflammatory bowel disease (IBD) not responding to maximal medical therapy is one of the most common indications for emergency colectomy. 'Toxic megacolon' is a descriptive term used to refer to a patient becoming septic from severe colitis. The patient exhibits signs of systemic sepsis, i.e. tachycardia, hypotension, and fever. In some cases, this is accompanied by a colonic ileus and dilatation of the colon (generally defined as >5 cm diameter of the transverse colon on a plain film of the abdomen). Colonic dilatation does not need to be present for a patient to have toxic megacolon. Other indications for emergency surgery in the presence of

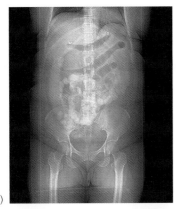

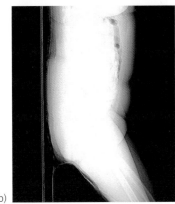

(a)

(b)

5.13.1 (a) Abdominal x-ray of a patient treated for 1 week for severe diarrhea of unknown etiology, presumed to have new onset of irritable bowel disease. The patient rapidly deteriorated despite intravenous steroid therapy and developed peritoneal signs. (b) By the time a general surgeon was consulted, perforation had already occurred as demonstrated by the large amounts of free air on the lateral film.

colonic IBD are perforation, massive bleeding (to follow in this chapter), and acute obstruction (**Figure 5.13.1**).

Emergent colectomy for *C. difficile* colitis is becoming more common due to a rising incidence of *C. difficile* colitis, an increasing awareness of its associated mortality, and the emergence of an especially toxic strain, known as B1/NAP1. Indications for surgery include toxic megacolon, organ failure, requirement for vasopressors, signs of peritonitis, or lack of response to medical therapy with worsening computed tomography (CT) findings within 24–72 hours (**Figure 5.13.2**).[2]

Diverticular disease

Emergency surgery for diverticulitis has undergone a significant change over the last 20 years. This has largely been brought about by the increased utilization of interventional radiology to drain intra-abdominal abscesses and to convert what were formerly emergent procedures into elective operations. Hinchey stage 1 and 2

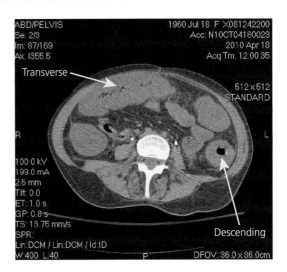

5.13.2 Computed tomography image showing view of transverse and descending colon in patient with fulminant *C. difficile* colitis, which was ultimately fatal. Note the tremendous bowel edema with near complete obliteration of the normal bowel lumen, especially in the transverse colon.

disease (pericolic and pelvic abscess, respectively) are now largely treated non-operatively. There is a growing school of thought that even such diverticular disease may not require subsequent surgery. Emergent surgery is currently usually performed for patients with Hinchey stage 3 and 4 disease, which includes patients with purulent peritonitis resulting from the rupture of a pericolic or pelvic abscess (Hinchey 3) or feculent peritonitis resulting from free perforation of a diverticulum (Hinchey 4).

The classification proposed by Hinchey is shown in **Figure 5.13.3**:

Stage 1: A pericolic abscess confined by the mesentery (**Figure 5.13.3**a).

Stage 2: A pelvic abscess caused by local perforation of a pericolic abscess (**Figure 5.13.3**b).

Stage 3: Peritonitis resulting from rupture of a pericolic or pelvic abscess into the general peritoneal cavity. There is no communication between the lumen of the bowel and the abscess cavity because of obliteration of the neck of the diverticulum by the inflammatory process. This is also known as acute non-communicating diverticulitis (**Figure 5.13.3**c).

Stage 4: Fecal peritonitis resulting from free perforation of the diverticulum. This usually develops rapidly and is also known as acute communicating diverticulitis (**Figure 5.13.3**d).

While Hartmann's procedure, with resection of the affected segment and end colostomy, remains the most common operation performed for perforated diverticular disease, some data suggest that primary resection and anastomosis with or without temporary diversion or intracolonic lavage may be preferable in selected cases.[3] The surgeon should select the most appropriate operation based upon the degree of contamination, patient comorbidities, and patient

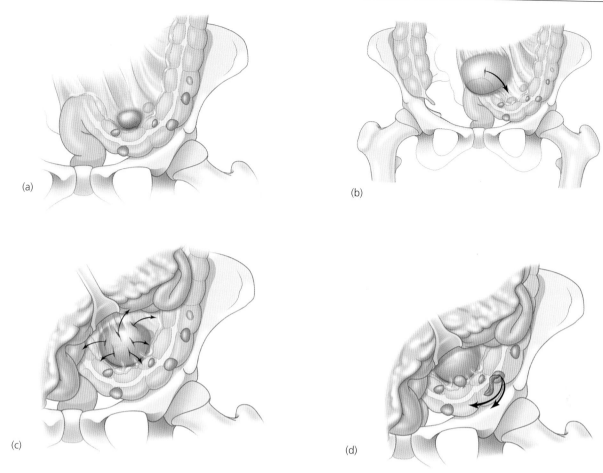

(a)

(b)

(c)

(d)

5.13.3

stability at the time of surgery. It is doubtless true that many patients treated by colostomy and Hartmann's procedure never undergo subsequent takedown of the colostomy. The emergence of reports of successful management of purulent peritonitis by laparoscopic lavage with or without repair of the perforation is intriguing. In a recent systematic review, only 38 percent of 231 patients treated in this manner underwent subsequent elective sigmoid resection, and of those who did not, recurrent diverticulitis developed in five of 128 patients.[4]

Colon cancer with obstruction and/or perforation

The frequency of performing emergency surgery for obstructing colon cancer has declined, since many patients with incompletely obstructing lesions are able to undergo semi-elective surgery and many patients with near-total obstruction are able to undergo endoscopic stenting, permitting surgery in the elective setting. The requirements for stenting are the availability of a skilled therapeutic colonoscopist and a lumen adequate to accomodate a guide-wire. Fluoroscopy is very useful. Most surgeons now recognize that primary resection for obstructing

cancer can be performed safely, provided the patient is hemodynamically stable. Primary anastomosis can be considered for carefully selected patients and favorable results have been reported for emergency resection of right- as well as left-sided lesions.

In the event of a perforation, one may assume that the patient has seeded their peritoneal cavity with cancer cells, and an aggressive approach with prompt resection and copious irrigation is warranted. If the cancer is adherent to any structure, this should be interpreted as invasion and failure to resect the involved structure will result in a local recurrence at this site. A preoperative carcinoembryonic antigen level should be obtained to facilitate postoperative patient follow-up. If the cancer is only diagnosed intraoperatively, this can be drawn in the operating room or in the recovery room.

Acute lower gastrointestinal bleeding

Emergency colectomy for lower gastrointestinal (GI) bleeding is occasionally necessary; however, it should only be undertaken if no bleeding source can be identified and in the presence of continued very high volume bleeding. Identification of the bleeding site and segmental colectomy is always preferable. The two most common causes of acute lower GI bleeding are diverticular disease and arteriovenous malformations.

In any patient with lower GI hemorrhage, one must obtain a history from the patient or a family member regarding use of anticoagulants, platelet inhibitors, or the presence of any bleeding dyscrasia or family history of such diatheses. This is especially important in view of the widespread use of anticoagulants and the patient's concept that aspirin is not a 'drug'.

Prior to proceeding with surgery, the following diagnostic studies/therapeutic measures will typically have been performed:

- Blood typed and cross-matched, as well as obtain serum blood urea nitrogen and creatinine (in the event that an angiogram is required), complete blood count with platelet count, prothrombin time, and partial thromboplastin time.
- Initial fluid resuscitation with lactated Ringer's solution then blood to stabilize the patient during the investigation of the bleeding source. Consider fresh-frozen plasma or platelets if the patient has been anticoagulated or on platelet aggregation inhibitors.
- Upper gastrointestinal endoscopy or insertion of a nasogastric tube to exclude upper GI bleeding, the former being much more accurate.
- Rigid proctoscopy to exclude hemorrhoidal bleeding or a rectal source of bleeding. This is superior to flexible endoscopic evaluation due to the large caliber suction utilized with rigid proctoscopy that can more completely excavate blood from the rectum for adequate visualization in cases of significant bleeding.

At this point, treatment will vary depending upon the stability of the patient and the activity of the bleeding:

1 Hemodynamically unstable (systolic blood pressure <100, heart rate >120), despite resuscitation: this patient needs to go immediately to the operating room for stabilization and treatment. The procedure of choice here if there is no evidence of blood in the small bowel is a total abdominal colectomy, ileostomy, and Hartmann's procedure.
2 Hemodynamically stable (systolic blood pressure >100, tachycardia <120), no continued bleeding: colonoscopy and further evaluation of small bowel if indicated with capsule endoscopy or other method on an elective basis.
3 Hemodynamically stable, slow ongoing bleeding: ^{99m}Tc-pertechnetate-labeled red blood cell nuclear medicine bleeding scans can detect bleeding rates of 0.1–0.5 mL/min and can be re-evaluated for up to 24 hours after the initial scan.
4 Hemodynamically stable, rapid ongoing bleeding: mesenteric angiograms detect bleeding rates >0.5–1.5 mL/min. In many cases, if a source of bleeding is identified, infusion of vasopressin, autologous clot or

a variety of beads or microcoils can be used to stop the bleeding.

Volvulus

Emergency surgery for volvulus is required when a cecal volvulus does not spontaneously reduce or when a sigmoid volvulus cannot be decompressed. Elective surgery for volvulus is usually performed following successful endoscopic decompression of sigmoid volvulus. Patients in whom sigmoid volvulus occurs are most commonly elderly and debilitated. The recurrence rate following decompression alone is high, and for this reason, elective resection is generally recommended. Initial endoscopic reduction can be performed with either a rigid or a flexible endoscope. In conducting the endoscopy, it is essential to inflate a minimum of additional air into the colonic lumen. Peritoneal signs mandate urgent surgical exploration.

Colon trauma

Colonic injuries without devascularization and involving less than 50 percent of the bowel wall can generally be closed primarily. There is less agreement and there are less prospective data regarding resection and primary anastomosis for destructive colon injuries (involving >50 percent of the bowel and/or with devascularization). While many feel that these too should be treated by resection and primary anastomosis regardless of risk factors, several studies suggest that patients receiving more than six units blood transfusion, those in whom operation is delayed by more than 6 hours from the time of injury, or associated with shock or a large amount of fecal contamination benefit from resection and diversion.[5]

ANESTHESIA AND PATIENT POSITIONING

Either an oro- or nasogastric tube should be inserted following endotracheal intubation, if one is not already present. Application of forced air blankets or circulating water warming systems will help prevent intraoperative hypothermia, and the anesthesiologist should have reliable methods of measuring core body temperature intraoperatively. One should ensure adequate intravenous access for rapid fluid administration should this become necessary, with at least two 14-gauge intravenous lines or their equivalent. In patients with significant cardiopulmonary morbidity, central venous access permits more accurate cardiopulmonary monitoring for the anesthesiologist and for the surgical team postoperatively. For all the indications for surgery mentioned above, Lloyd-Davies position (modified lithotomy position) is the most useful. This modified or low lithotomy position is important since it avoids impeding lower extremity venous return and subsequent reduction in lower extremity blood pressure which can be seen with 'high' lithotomy position. This position permits ready access to the anal canal for performing a stapled colorectal anastomosis and testing its patency, for performing a proctoscopy if needed to assess rectal mucosa, as well as permitting placement of rectal decompression tubes/drains, and providing space for an assistant to stand.

OPERATION

Colitis

Subtotal colectomy with Hartmann's procedure and end ileostomy should be the procedure of choice both for patients with IBD and for patients with *C. difficile* colitis requiring surgery. As techniques of total colectomy are illustrated elsewhere in this volume (see Chapters 5.9, 5.10 and 5.11), we will focus on those aspects unique to emergency colectomy.

Selection of open or laparoscopic procedure depends upon the degree of distention of the bowel (loss of intra-abdominal domain), comfort of the surgeon with either approach, ability of the surgeon to do the operation in a timely manner due to the illness of the patient, extent of prior abdominal procedures, and presence of intestinal perforation. In general, if there is a perforation in poorly controlled IBD, an open approach is preferred, since in these cases, the bowel can be extremely fragile and very intolerant of instrumentation.

IMPORTANT POINTS TO CONSIDER IN COLITIS

A common complication in these patients is pelvic abscess arising from 'non-healing' of the staple or suture line of the Hartmann's stump due to severe disease of the distal bowel. This complication can be avoided either by creating a mucous fistula or by leaving a long Hartmann's stump and incorporating it into the lower midline fascial closure with interrupted absorbable sutures of 1-0 polydiaxanone and closing the skin over it (**Figure 5.13.4**). In the event that the stump closure does not heal, it is easily treated by opening the lower portion of the wound. If a laparoscopic approach is utilized, the specimen retrieval site is used for this. If the proximal end of the remaining bowel cannot be brought to skin level, strong consideration should be given to rectal decompression with a soft catheter. The author prefers to use the 34-Fr straight catheters used to intubate continent ileostomies (Marlen Manufacturing, Bedford, OH, USA), since they have large side holes and drain more effectively than a Foley catheter, yet are soft. In patients with *C. difficile* colitis, this catheter can be used for postoperative antibiotic irrigation of the Hartmann's stump.

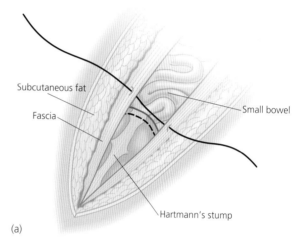

(a)

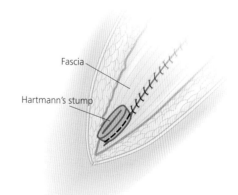

(b)

5.13.4 (a) Prior to closing abdominal wall. (b) Final version of the abdominal wall closing.

When the bowel is edematous, it can be hard to fashion a stoma. In these cases, the bowel can be made more pliable by performing a bidirectional myotomy using the diathermy. This amounts to scoring the serosa with the diathermy first in a longitudinal direction in parallel lines 1 cm apart and then performing the same procedure in horizontal lines 90° perpendicular to these to create a 'checkerboard' pattern (**Figure 5.13.5**).

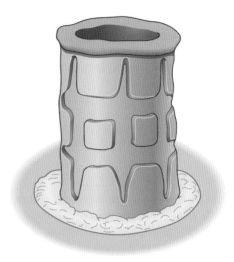

5.13.5

Also important is to create an ileostomy aperture that is large enough to permit easy passage through the abdominal wall. Although a two-finger aperture is usually sufficient, a larger aperture may be necessary if there is substantial bowel edema (**Figure 5.13.6**).

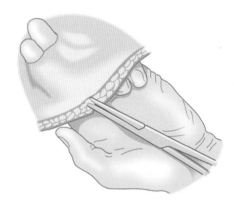

5.13.6

Perforated diverticular disease

Sigmoid colectomy with Hartmann's procedure and end colostomy is the procedure of choice for patients who are hemodynamically unstable, and in elderly patients with poor sphincter function or poor general health. The most common error seen when this operation is performed is to transect the rectum deep within the pelvis. Diverticulitis is a disease of the sigmoid colon. Resection of large portions of the rectum makes the subsequent surgery to restore intestinal continuity more difficult and should be avoided. The bowel in these cases is often thickened and does not easily staple. A 4.8 mm staple cartridge should be used if a linear stapling device is utilized and oversew the staple line or handsew if the bowel is too thickened. The line of proximal resection should be at the point of palpably normal bowel (**Figure 5.13.7**).

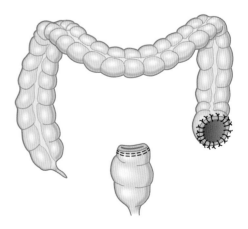

5.13.7

Resection, primary anastomosis, and loop ileostomy is the author's personal preference if there is significant fecal contamination in a stable patient. Here, standard resection is done and the anastomosis tested for patency by performing proctoscopy and checking for an air leak in a water-filled pelvis. After copious irrigation of the abdominal cavity with antibiotic solution, an omental flap is placed around the anastomosis. No pelvic drains are used since the anastomosis is above the peritoneal reflection. A carboxymethylcellulose/hyaluronic acid sheet is wrapped around the ileostomy to reduce adhesions and facilitate closure at 8 weeks postoperatively if a water-soluble contrast study confirms satisfactory healing of the anastomosis.

Resection, primary anastomosis, and intracolonic lavage can be utilized if there is purulent peritonitis and a resection is performed primarily, and in select cases of bowel perforation with localized peritonitis. A midline incision is performed. The point of proximal resection is chosen and the bowel at this point is divided with a linear stapler. A standard end-to-end colorectal anastomosis is constructed according to the surgeon's preference. Following this, colonic lavage is performed via a small enterotomy placed at the site of a planned loop ileostomy. An 18-Fr Foley catheter is inserted through the enterotomy and cannulated through the ileocecal valve into the cecum, and the balloon of the Foley inflated with 5 mL of water. The Foley can be further secured to the bowel using umbilical tape. The Foley catheter is connected to irrigation tubing such as used during cystoscopy, and this in turn is connected to a 3-L bag of normal saline, such as is used during cystoscopy. The fluid must be prewarmed to prevent patient hypothermia. A rigid proctoscope is inserted into the rectum and held over a refuse container and the irrigation clamp opened. The colon is irrigated until clear through the anastomosis. When the irrigation is completed, if desired, an additional 200 mL povodine iodine solution can be injected into the 3-L irrigating fluid bag and also rinsed through the colon

until this runs through the collecting evacuator tubing. Once the lavage is complete, the umbilical tapes are released, the Foley and irrigating tubing discarded, and the loop ileostomy constructed at the site of this enterotomy in standard fashion.

Laparoscopic lavage without resection for diverticular disease should not be undertaken in an unstable patient, if there is not opportunity for very close postoperative follow-up and if there is any suspicion that the perforation is associated with a diverticular stricture or distal obstruction. Different reports have described using from two to five trocars and irrigating volumes ranging from several to over 20 L. Most surgeons report using saline. If a perforation is found, it is sutured by imbricating the perforation with absorbable sutures. Surgeons differ regarding whether or not adhesions are taken down, but these often represent sealing of a perforation and should not be disrupted in many cases. Large bore closed suction drains should be placed liberally, both in the pelvis and in the left colic gutter.

Colon cancer with obstruction and/or perforation

These patients should have a nasogastric tube placed prior to induction of anesthesia. In cases where there is significant pulmonary comorbidity and signs of longstanding bowel obstruction, strong consideration should be given to placing a gastrostomy tube at the time of operation. If there has been perforation, insertion of a Poole-tip suction through the perforation site to evacuate as much stool as possible and then temporary suture closure of this site with a running 2-0 polyglycolic acid suture minimizes further contamination during the procedure. If there has not yet been perforation, the resection can be performed carefully with a non-decompressed bowel, or if the bowel is tense

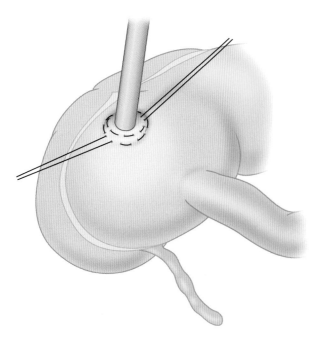

5.13.8

and difficult to handle, decompression can be performed using a Poole-tip suction through the cecum, through a double purse-string suture as illustrated (**Figure 5.13.8**).

As in the case of perforated diverticular disease, resection, Hartmann's procedure, and end colostomy is the most rapidly performed procedure and often the procedure of choice for patients who are hemodynamically unstable, have significant comorbidities, or have widespread fecal peritonitis. A high vascular ligation should be performed to obtain adequate lymph node clearance, although in the case of cancers with perforation, the prognosis is already of concern.

If the patient is hemodynamically stable during surgery and there is localized contamination, but there is still concern regarding anastomotic healing due to patient malnutrition or tissue factors at the time of surgery (edema, friability, gross mismatch of bowel caliber of proximal and distal bowel ends), resection can be performed either with primary anastomosis and proximal diverting loop ileostomy (as previously described for diverticular disease) or with exteriorization of the anastomosis as a loop stoma. Both of these procedures allow for subsequent re-establishment of intestinal continuity, in most cases without a formal laparotomy.

In cases where a right or extended right hemicolectomy is necessary, exteriorization of the anastomosis as a loop stoma is easily performed. Here, the back wall of the ileocolic anastomosis is first constructed, and the two end stay sutures left long to help with traction (**Figure 5.13.9**). A standard ileostomy aperture is made in the abdominal wall at the stoma site closest to the anastomosis. The bowel may have to be additionally mobilized to permit the bowel to be moved to this area. The two lateral stay sutures are then used together with a Babcock clamp to

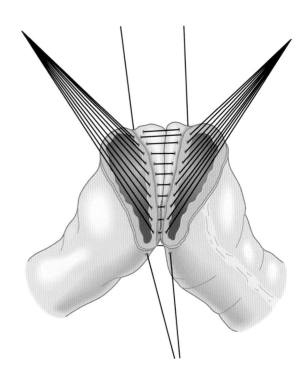

5.13.9

pull this loop of bowel through the ostomy aperture. The colon and ileum are tacked to the subcutaneous tissue of the stoma site using two 3-0 chromic catgut sutures on the antimesenteric aspect of the bowel (**Figure 5.13.10**a). The

stoma is matured as a loop, keeping the colonic lumen as the skin level efferent limb and everting the ileal proximal limb as the afferent limb, using 3-0 chromic catgut suture (**Figure 5.13.10**b).

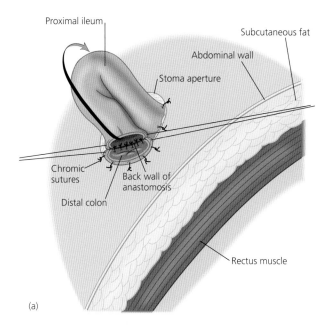

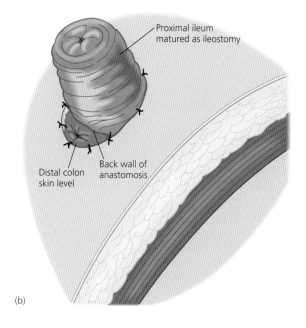

5.13.10

Acute lower gastrointestinal bleeding

If the source of bleeding is known, a segmental colectomy should be undertaken (see the corresponding chapters regarding right [Chapters 5.3 and 5.4] or left [Chapters 5.6, 5.7 and 5.8] colectomy). Total abdominal colectomy with or without ileorectal anastomosis should be performed only when the precise source of colonic bleeding cannot be identified. Otherwise, a more limited resection is preferable (see Chapters 5.10 and 5.11).

Volvulus

Most sigmoid volvuli are initially managed with endoscopic decompression followed by interval surgery. If emergency surgery is necessary, it is performed by midline laparotomy secondary to the tremendous distention of the sigmoid colon. Typically, the mesenteric base of the volvulus is very narrow. The redundant loop of sigmoid is resected to permit a tension-free anastomosis. The decision on whether or not to divert is made upon bowel viability, the

presence of bowel perforation, or necrotic bowel and the degree of bowel distention present at the time of surgery, as well as the patient's stability and general medical condition. If the patient is not diverted, consideration should be given to a transrectal drainage tube for colonic decompression.

As with sigmoid volvulus, the decision whether or not to resect a cecal volvulus depends upon viability of the colon. Here, the operation is also performed through a midline laparotomy. In the event that there is non-viable bowel, an ileocecal resection must be performed. If the patient is hemodynamically stable and there is no contamination, a primary anastomosis may be performed. This is the procedure with the lowest recurrence. However, if the patient is in shock, or if there is significant contamination, an ileostomy and 'long Hartmann's' (stapled closure of the proximal transverse colon) or mucous fistula, or exteriorization of the anastomosis as previously described in this chapter should be considered.

If there is cecal distention, but no sign of non-viable bowel, the patient can, in some cases, be treated using a cecostomy tube, which also functions as a cecopexy. A 32-Fr Malecot catheter can be utilized for this. The tube is placed into the cecum through a double purse-string suture of 2-0 polyglycolic acid suture. Prior to placing this tube, the fecal contents of the bowel can be aspirated through this same site with Poole-tip suction. The Malecot tube is passed through the abdominal wall, then through the greater omentum, and finally into the cecum, so the purse-string sutures can be tied. These sutures are then led alongside the tube through the omentum and used to anchor the cecum to the anterior abdominal wall (**Figure 5.13.11**). When the tube is removed, which is not done less than 2 weeks postoperatively, the omentum acts as a buttress to seal off the site. This approach is occasionally useful in high-risk patients where there is concern regarding anastomotic healing.

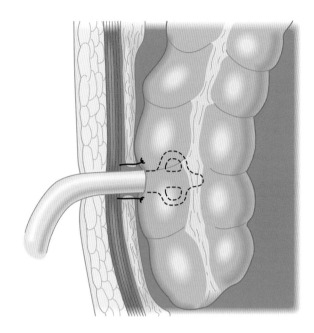

5.13.11 Malecot catheter passing through abdominal wall and omentum into cecum.

Colon trauma

Indications for surgery will have been established by focused abdominal sonography for trauma (FAST), helical CT scan, or clinical indications (wound to abdomen penetrating fascia with hypotension). Access is via midline laparotomy incision. Initially, rapid inspection of the abdomen with placement of packs is done to ascertain the extent of visceral injury. Injuries are addressed in order or their impact on the blood loss/hemodynamic stability. The extent of fecal contamination is assessed. If present, bowel clamps or surgical staplers are used to minimize further contamination. Colonic injuries affecting <50 percent of the bowel circumference are debrided and closed primarily in one or two layers with suture according to surgeon preference. With injuries such as shown in **Figure 5.13.12**a,c, where there is significant destruction and devascularization, the affected segment is resected and if

no significant risk factors are present, primary anastomosis is performed according to the surgeon's method of choice. The author favors a hand-sewn, two-layer anastomosis. If, however, there has been a delay of >6 hours from the time of injury to surgery, >6 units of blood transfused, significant fecal contamination, or accompanying shock, a stoma should be considered (**Figure 5.13.12**b,d). If the point of resection is proximal to the mid-descending colon, the surgeon should also perform either a mucus fistula or exteriorize the distal end, after sewing the back row of the anastomosis, as described earlier in this chapter.

If the patient is in shock and has multiple other injuries, the best procedure for destructive injuries with devascularization is to perform a resection and staple off both ends of bowel. The anastomosis is performed at a later date when the patient has stabilized and issues such as coagulopathy, hypothermia, and hemodynamic instability have largely resolved.

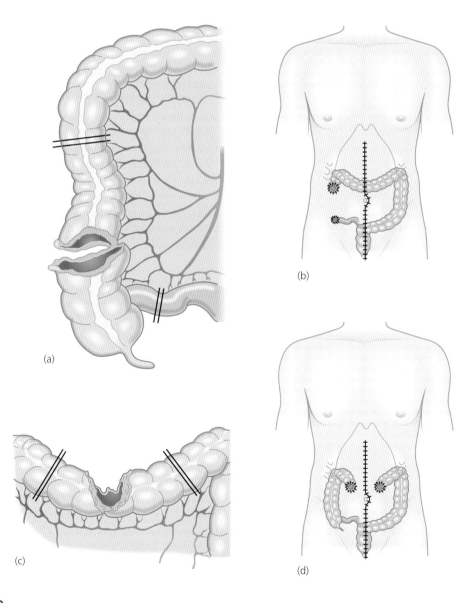

(a)

(b)

(c)

(d)

5.13.12

POSTOPERATIVE CARE

For IBD patients undergoing surgery, since the most severe disease has been removed, intravenous steroid therapy can be carefully tapered. Patients with *C. difficile* colitis undergoing emergency surgery will require more support postoperatively. Multiorgan system failure is common and prolonged intensive care unit stays are the norm. Nutritional support with enteral or parenteral nutrition and irrigation of the rectal stump with vancomycin continue postoperatively.

In managing a cecostomy, it is essential to irrigate the tube with 30-mL normal saline every 2 hours (scheduled, not as needed) to prevent it from becoming occluded with fecal matter. Postoperative care and outcome mainly depend upon whether or not there was perforation or necrotic bowel present at the time of laparotomy.

For patients with perforation of any cause or significant intra-abdominal contamination, broad-spectrum antibiotics should be continued for 3 days postoperatively and the patient's white blood cell count then carefully monitored. These patients are at high risk of inter-loop, pelvic, and subphrenic abscesses. The latter two are easily treated by CT-guided drainage, whereas inter-loop abscesses may be difficult to access for the interventional radiologist and require intravenous antibiotic treatment or even reoperation.

For patients with lower gastrointestinal hemorrhage, postoperative care is largely focused on continuing patient resuscitation, correction of clotting abnormalities by administration of fresh frozen plasma, or cryoprecipitate as needed. Packed red blood cells are administered to restore blood volume to normal levels.

Postoperative care after laparotomy for trauma is directed towards the usual care of the injured patient, addressing treatment of all their associated organ injuries.

OUTCOME

Short-term outcomes for patients requiring emergency colorectal surgery depend both upon the severity of the patient's acute illness and the extent of underlying comorbidities. Long-term outcomes depend both upon the patient's general health and also the underlying primary diagnosis. Several disease entities require specific comment:

- *Colitis.* Unless granulomata are present, differentiation between Crohn's disease and ulcerative colitis cannot be made in most patients operated on for toxic or fulminant colitis. Extensive counseling with the patient is necessary prior to proceeding with a planned completion proctectomy and ileal pouch-anal anastomosis, completion proctectomy, or continued observation. No intervention should be undertaken until the patient's nutritional and performance status have been restored to normal and no sooner than two months after the initial colectomy.

- In patients with *C. difficile* colitis undergoing emergency surgery, mortality rates of >30 percent have been reported. These patients typically require lengthy intensive care unit stays and often have multiorgan system failure. Consideration to takedown of the ileostomy should only be done as with IBD patients when the patient's nutritional and performance status have been restored to normal. If the patient is elderly, has decreased sphincter tone, and/or decreased mobility, the ileostomy should not be closed.

- *Cancer.* Perforation and obstruction are independent prognostic variables associated with poor long-term outcome, as are tumor factors such as advanced T-stage, poor differentiation, mucin production, neural and vascular invasion.[6]

- *Lower gastrointestinal hemorrhage.* Rebleeding is uncommon, if the source has been correctly identified. It is crucial that a rectal source be excluded prior to proceeding to a laparotomy, since one of the most common causes of 'rebleeding' is an overlooked distal source.

- *Trauma.* Multiple studies have shown the safety of performing primary colonic anastomosis in a variety of settings and the most recent have even shown this to be safe for the treatment of wounds with significant tissue destruction and devascularization. In the presence of significant delay from the time of injury, significant transfusion requirement, significant fecal contamination or shock, proximal diversion is still warranted. In these cases, in view of the associated injuries which often include serious head injury, in many cases, intestinal continuity will not be re-established sooner than six months postoperatively and the patient and family should be so informed.

REFERENCES

1. Ingraham AM, Cohen ME, Bilimoria KY *et al.* Comparison of hospital performance in non-emergency versus emergency colorectal operations at 142 hospitals. *Journal of the American College of Surgeons* 2010; **210**: 155–65.

2. Jaber MR, Olafsson S, Fung WL, Reeves ME. Clinical review of the management of fulminant clostridium difficile infection. *American Journal of Gastroenterology* 2008; **103**: 3195–203.

3. Constantinides VA, Tekkis PP, Athanasiou T *et al.* Primary resection with anastomosis vs. Hartmann's procedure in nonelective surgery for acute colonic diverticulitis: a systematic review. *Diseases of the Colon and Rectum* 2006; **49**: 966–81.

4. Toorenvliet BR, Swank H, Schoones JW *et al.* Laparoscopic peritoneal lavage for perforated colonic diverticulitis: a systematic review. *Colorectal Diseases* 2010; **12**: 862–7.

5. Demetriades D. Colon injuires: new perspectives. *Injury* 2004; **35**: 217–22.

6. Mulcahy HE, Skelly MM, Husain A, O'Donoghue DP. Long-term outcome following curative surgery for malignant large bowel obstruction. *British Journal of Surgery* 1996; **83**: 46–50.

Colonic stenting

RAKESH BHARDWAJ AND MIKE C PARKER

INTRODUCTION

Surgical intervention for colonic obstruction carries significant risks to the patient compounded by the risk of colonic perforation as the colon proximal to the point of obstruction distends. In the presence of a competent ileocecal valve, a 'closed loop' may lead eventually to gross cecal distension and, in extreme circumstances, cecal perforation. In patients with localized obstructing disease, the choice of surgical procedure is dependent on the position of the lesion. For right-sided colonic lesions, resection and construction of an ileocolic anastomosis is usual, whereas management of left-sided colonic lesions is more complex and often necessitates formation of an end colostomy after resection. Stamatakis et al.[1] showed that 59 percent of patients who present with left-sided colonic obstruction had a successful one-stage surgical resection, while 41 percent underwent a Hartmann procedure. The reversibility of this stoma was variable. Patients with advanced malignant disease are often frail and surgical management may involve either a colonic bypass procedure, resection with stoma formation, formation of a stoma alone, or no procedure at all.

HISTORY OF COLONIC STENTS

Early attempts at colonic decompression with a nasogastric tube or chest tube were unsuccessful as the tubes were of small caliber and were prone to obstruction. Dohmoto[2] first described the use of a metal stent to relieve malignant rectal obstruction. This was followed by sporadic similar reports predominantly for the palliation of obstructing lesions. Two further cases of stenting of inoperable rectosigmoid carcinoma were described by Itabashi et al.[3] The stents described were those used originally for relief of esophageal obstruction. The use of the Wallstent® enteral endoprosthesis (Boston Scientific, Natick, MA, USA), designed specifically for colonic use, was first reported by

Soonawalla et al.[4] Seven patients underwent stenting, with successful stent deployment in five. The two failures were due to inability to negotiate the stricture. Of the five cases, all proceeded to have subsequent uncomplicated surgical resection of the obstructing lesions.

A systematic review of the literature by Khot et al.[5] on the use of self-expanding metal stents (SEMS) from 1990 to January 2001 revealed 58 publications. Analysis of outcomes was possible in 29 papers and, of 598 patients selected, the intended treatment was palliative for 336 (56 percent) and 262 (44 percent) were treated with the intention of surgical intervention at a later date. The overall clinical success was reported in 525 (88 percent) patients; however, of 233 patients selected for surgery and successfully stented, 212 (95 percent) went on to have a successful one-stage surgical resection of the colonic segment.

INDICATIONS AND PROPERTIES OF COLONIC STENTS

Colonic stents enable a minimally invasive method of managing complete large bowel obstruction. While stents are used in the vast majority of cases for malignant obstructing lesions, on occasions benign strictures are encountered. These can be quite challenging as there may be an associated inflammatory component within the stricture. There are two different circumstances in which a stent is placed across an obstructing lesion.

First, it can be used as a 'bridge to surgery'. In this setting, a colonic stent is placed with a view to subsequent physiological optimization of the patient. After an appropriate interval, definitive surgery can then be undertaken. If definitive elective surgery is undertaken and circumstances are favorable, a laparoscopic approach also has the advantage of further reducing the physiological insult to the patient. Second, a stent could be used in the palliative setting for an obstructing colonic lesion where it is paramount to maintain a quality of life for the patient.

There are no absolute contraindications to stenting apart from peritonitis. They are particularly useful in managing colonic obstruction in frail patients or in patients in whom immediate surgery is too hazardous. However, there are some instances where colonic stents are not ideal. They are not usually used for low rectal (<6 cm from the anal verge) lesions as the patient can often complain of considerable discomfort after stent deployment or the stent may be extruded through the anus. Right colonic obstructing lesions are not usually stented, as a limited colectomy may usually be carried out effectively in the emergency setting. Furthermore, stenting in the right colon can be quite a technical challenge, in some circumstances an antegrade approach may be useful.[6]

An ideal colonic stent is one that can be inserted easily transanally, can negotiate the colonic folds, be comfortably deployed, allow a sufficient channel for fecal material to pass, and remain in position. There are two types of metallic stent systems: expandable and self-expanding. The former needs to be manually expanded, while in the latter the radial force generated after deployment allows a sufficient channel for the passage of feces. Self-expanding stents have to be of the correct diameter; if too narrow, they may migrate and if too wide may cause colonic erosions leading to perforation.

There are a number of colonic stents commercially available; most have a mesh design and are constructed from steel or nitinol. Nitinol stents are constructed from a nickel and titanium alloy. They have 'shape memory' reverting to a predetermined configuration after deployment, usually after 2–5 days. The inherent flexibility of nitinol affords some colonic peristalsis. The reader is directed to Stoeckel et al.[7] for details of material and design considerations of self-expanding nitinol stents. In the United States, the FDA (Food and Drug Administration) have approved several stents for use in malignant colonic obstruction. Boston Scientific (Natick, MA, USA) produce the Wallflex®, Wallstent®, and more recently, the Ultraflex™ stent. Bard (R Bard, Murray Hill, NJ, USA) manufacture the Memotherm™ stent and Wilson-Cook

Medical (Bloomington, IN, USA) the Z-stent®. They differ in their construction, diameter, and offer varying lengths. The stents from Boston Scientific have the advantage of permitting 'through-the-scope', as well as 'over-the wire' delivery systems. Various designs for the stents are shown in **Figure 5.14.1**.

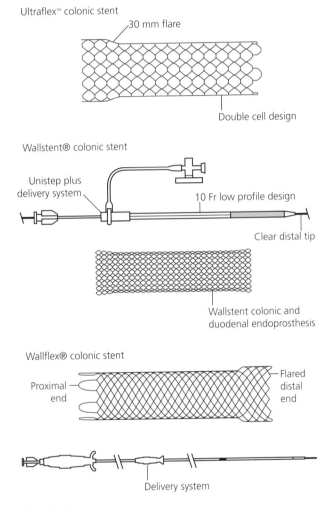

5.14.1 Design of various colonic stents.

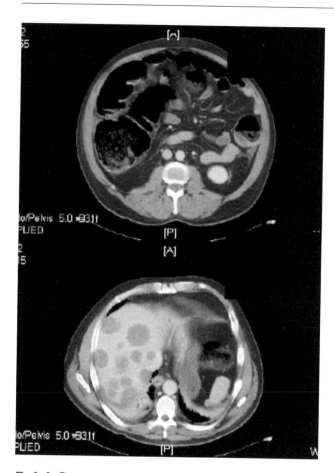

5.14.2 (a) Computed tomography (CT) scan with axial image demonstrating marked cecal distension (from an obstructing rectosigmoid tumor). (b) CT scan with axial image in the same patient demonstrating widespread liver metastases.

OPERATION

Assessment

Patients who present with colonic obstruction need urgent clinical assessment. Treatment starts with resuscitation of the patient, while therapeutic options are considered. Computed tomography (CT) is the investigation of choice as it allows assessment of the site of the colonic lesion and concomitant disease. This often guides treatment into either a curative or palliative direction (**Figure 5.14.2**).

If access to a CT scanner is not readily available, retrograde administration of a water-soluble contrast agent usually confirms the presence of complete obstruction (**Figure 5.14.3**). Although this is a useful technique, it is only possible if the patient can retain the contrast and can tolerate the procedure.

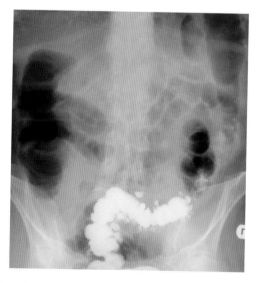

5.14.3 Single-contrast radiological study identifying point of left colonic obstruction.

Preparation

Prior to insertion of a colonic stent, resuscitation of the patient involves administration of intravenous fluids and restriction of oral intake. A nasogastric tube is often necessary to decompress dilated small and large bowel. Analgesia and antibiotics are given at the discretion of the admitting physician. A phosphate enema is usually given to facilitate the passage of an endoscope. Optimization of these patients may have to be undertaken in a dedicated high-dependency unit.

The insertion of a colonic stent should ideally be undertaken by a multidisciplinary team as advocated by Soonawalla et al.[4] This combined approach includes an endoscopist, radiologist, radiographer, and nurse. Rarely, for distally placed rectal lesions, laser ablation prior to stent deployment may be employed to facilitate a passage through the obstructing lesion. However, this is most unusual as the purpose of the laser is to recanalize the rectal lumen and therefore a stent may not be warranted.

Anesthesia

Patients usually require intravenous sedation and analgesia. Common agents used may include midazolam and pethidine. Colonic muscle relaxants, such as buscopan, may be employed on occasions.

Position of patient

The patient is initially placed in the left lateral position on an x-ray screening table. However, the patient may have to be rotated to facilitate the procedure. It is essential a nurse accompany the patient to ensure the patient's anxiety is minimized. Patients require oxygen saturation, pulse rate, and blood pressure monitoring throughout the procedure.

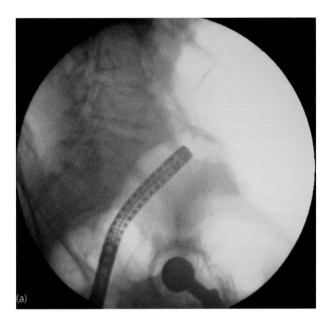

(a)

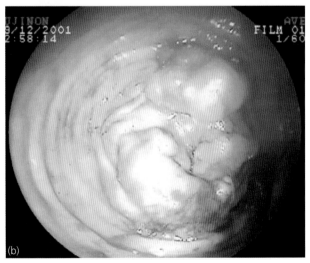

(b)

5.14.4 (a, b) Endoscopic and fluoroscopic view of endoscope in position distal to the obstructing colonic lesion.

Procedure stages

COLONOSCOPY IS PERFORMED TO THE LEVEL OF THE OBSTRUCTING LESION

The endoscopy should be undertaken by an experienced endoscopist to minimize patient discomfort. Attention should be paid to reducing colonic looping during intubation, especially if per endoscopic stents are used. Caution should also be exhibited with the use of air insufflation as this could exacerbate proximal colonic distension and result in cecal perforation. If the 'through-the-scope' approach is indicated, a wider diameter channel on the colonoscope is required for the passage of the colonic stent. Once the colonoscope is near the obstructing lesion, contrast is injected through the irrigation channel to highlight the proximal and distal margins of the lesion. It also enables visualization of the stricture (**Figure 5.14.4**).

Guidewire placement is more likely to be successful if contrast is seen to pass across the obstruction; conversely if no contrast appears proximal to the lesion, guidewire placement may be less successful.

GUIDEWIRES ARE PASSED THROUGH THE STRICTURE

Once the stricture is identified an initial (usually hydrophillic) guidewire is placed across the stricture. A Van Andel catheter is placed over the initial guidewire to allow a second safety wire to be placed through the Van Andel catheter (**Figure 5.14.5**). The initial guidewire is then replaced with a stiffer guidewire (e.g. Zebra guidewire) through the Van Andel catheter to allow the insertion of the stent over this stiffer wire. The Van Andel catheter is then removed and the safety wire is secured to the patient. The purpose of the second safety wire is to ensure that the stricture is traversed should the primary guidewire retract in a caudal direction beyond the stricture.

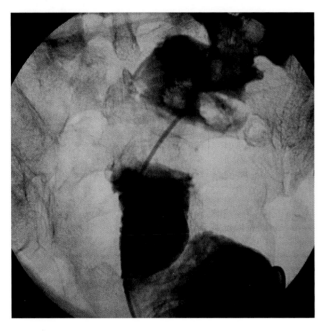

5.14.5 Guidewire placed across stricture.

INSERTION OF STENT OVER GUIDEWIRE

Once the catheter is removed, the stent is passed over the guidewire across the stricture. It is essential that the guidewire and the stent are kept taut to enable adequate passage of the stent (**Figure 5.14.6**).

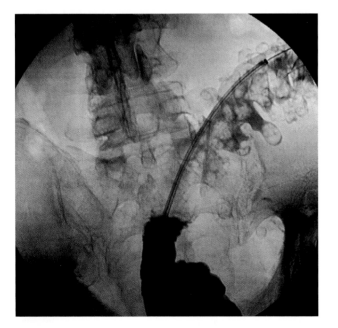

5.14.6 Stent in place over guidewire across stricture.

Significant resistance may be encountered as the undeployed stent passes through the stricture. Radiological screening facilitates this passage. The proximal and distal markers on the stent should straddle the lesion to ensure correct placement (**Figure 5.14.7**).

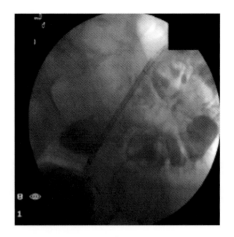

5.14.7 Proximal and distal markers noted on the stent to facilitate stent position.

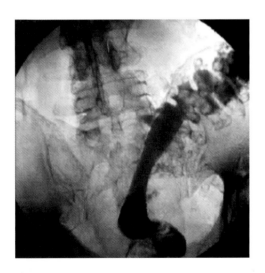

5.14.8 Stent deployment across obstructing colonic lesion.

DEPLOYING THE STENT

Once the position of the undeployed stent is deemed to be satisfactory, the stent is ready to be deployed. Whichever system is deployed, whether trigger or retraction, there are several maneuvers that help correct positioning. First, the stent system must be taut to allow correct transmission of the deploying mechanism. Second, as the stent is deployed, there is a tendency for the cephalad aspect of the deployed stent to migrate proximally in the colon. It is essential that some caudal force is provided. Although the proximal and distal markers are noted fluoroscopically, in some stents there is a 'point of no return' beyond which deployment of the stent is not reversible. This point may be noted fluoroscopically or on the deployment device. It is essential that the physician is satisfied that the stent is deploying correctly before this point of no return. The stent can then be fully deployed (**Figure 5.14.8**).

POSITION AFTER DEPLOYMENT

Once the position is satisfactory, the stent is deployed. The stent position is checked fluoroscopically and endoscopically. Colonic decompression usually occurs quickly, with passage of flatus and stool. Characteristic features of correct placement include 'flaring' of the ends and the appearance of a central 'waist' (**Figure 5.14.9**).

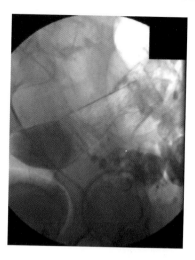

5.14.9 Flaring and waisting noted immediately after stent deployment.

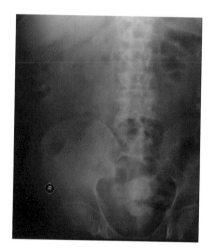

5.14.10 Check radiograph showing that the colorectal stent placed across a rectosigmoid lesion has not migrated and that there is expansion of the central portion of the stent.

To ensure stent position is maintained and the central part of the stent is expanding, the authors recommend a plain abdominal radiograph at 24 hours post-deployment (**Figure 5.14.10**). The stents may also be checked using CT scans, particularly when used for staging patients with malignant disease (**Figure 5.14.11**).

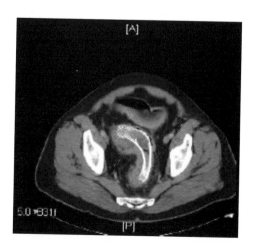

5.14.11 Computed tomography axial image demonstrating colorectal stent *in situ*.

'Through-the-endoscope' placement

The nature and position of the obstructing lesion may permit non-fluoroscopically guided SEMS placement, where the endoscope first traverses the lesion. Pre-stent dilatation of the stricture is associated with a high risk of perforation and is not to be encouraged. The SEMS may then be deployed either using a stent delivered through the working channel of the endoscope or with a guidewire placed across the lesion to assist SEMS placement. It is essential that the physician ensures that the correct stent system and endoscope are selected if a 'through-the-scope' system is chosen.

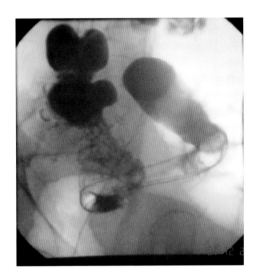

5.14.12 Multiple stent usage in a patient with a large obstructing sigmoid tumor.

Multiple stent use

On occasions, several stents may be required to relieve the obstruction. These may be used to negotiate difficult lesions where either the lesion is long or the stent has immediately migrated during deployment and the expansion of the stent is not sufficient to relieve the obstruction. However, the major theoretical limitation of multiple stent use is that colonic peristalsis can be hindered. **Figure 5.14.12** shows three stents *in situ* across a large obstructing sigmoid tumor in a patient with widespread metastatic disease. This patient was successfully palliated at our institution and was discharged within 24 hours. The patient subsequently died about three months later of metastatic disease without further colonic obstruction.

COMPLICATIONS OF COLORECTAL STENTS

Stent migration occurs in approximately 10 percent of cases, usually several days post-deployment.[5] Most migrated stents cause no symptoms. In such cases, further stents can be inserted, particularly in those patients being treated palliatively. In some cases, stents that dislodge through the anal canal require manual or endoscopic removal. Factors that predispose to stent migration include laser pretreatment, chemotherapy, or the presence of benign tumors. Perforation of the colonic wall as a complication can be immediate, at the time of insertion, or post-deployment. It has the potential disadvantage of shedding malignant cells into the peritoneal cavity. It occurs in approximately 4 percent of cases and previous balloon dilatation is a contributing factor.[5] Clinical reobstruction after placement of a SEMS may be due to tumor ingrowth or overgrowth of the stent, stent migration, or fecal impaction. Persisting pain occurs in 5 percent of patients after SEMS deployment. This is often related to the stent expanding and simple analgesics can often help. The symptoms usually settle. However, if a stent is placed in the low rectum, patients may experience significant discomfort and tenesmus. In some cases, where the stent is placed in a low rectal lesion, the stent can be extruded through the anus. Bleeding is uncommon and usually occurs from friable aspects of the tumor and is self-limiting. Blood transfusion is rarely required. Occasionally, the stent may cause some mucosal damage leading to ulceration, but this is not often of clinical concern.

Postoperative care

Close observation of the patient is essential. Resuscitation, if still required, is continued. Once the physician is satisfied that there is a satisfactory colonic lumen, the patient can be encouraged to take food as soon as is practical. Patients are encouraged to ambulate and venous thromboprophylaxis is given. A plain abdominal radiograph is taken 24 hours after insertion to ensure continued correct positioning of the stent (**Figure 5.14.10**).

CONCLUSION

SEMS are an effective way of dealing with a challenging emergency surgical condition. Their use either as definitive therapy in advanced disease or as a bridge to resection (**Figure 5.14.13**) seems to have been widely clinically incorporated. Its continued use depends on a multidisciplinary approach and the benefits to the patients are being explored in national randomized trials. However, there have been problems in national trials. The Dutch Stent-in I was prematurely closed as a result of several late non-procedure-related perforations near the proximal stent end. Concern was also raised within the national French trial, which was also stopped prematurely. Within this, there was a poor success rate and two stent-related perforations were noted. The CReST trial is a randomized national UK-based trial comparing SEMS and surgery for obstructing colonic lesion.[8] Due to the early cessation of the above two European trials, the UK trial was inspected, but this analysis did not require the trial protocol to be amended. There are three primary end points of the CReST trial: 30-day mortality, length of hospital stay, and presence of a stoma. Many centres in the UK are now participating in the CReST trial. The collated results would clarify some of the issues that are of concern.

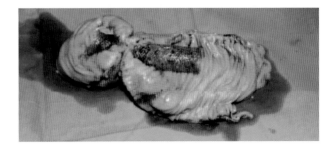

5.14.13 Stent noted in the colonic lumen after successful placement. The patient went on to have an elective surgical resection of the initially obstructing lesion.

REFERENCES

1. Stamatakis J, Thompson M, Chave H. *National audit of bowel obstruction due to colorectal cancer, April 1998–March 1999.* London: Association of Coloproctology of Great Britain and Ireland, July 2000.
2. Dohmoto M. New method: endoscopic implantation of rectal stent in palliative treatment of malignant stenosis. *Endoscopica Digestiva* 1991; **3**: 1507–12.
3. Itabashi M, Hamano K, Kameoka S, Asahina K. Self-expanding stainless steel stent application in rectosigmoid stricture. *Diseases of the Colon and Rectum* 1993; **36**: 508–11.
4. Soonawalla Z, Thakur K, Boorman P *et al.* Use of self-expanding metallic stents in the management of obstruction of the sigmoid colon. *AJR American Journal of Roentgenology* 1998; **171**: 633–6.
5. Khot U, Wenk Lang A, Murali K, Parker MC. Systematic review of the clinical evidence on colorectal self-expanding metal stents. *British Journal of Surgery* 2002; **89**: 1096–102.
6. Gandhi P, Osman HS, Rashid HI *et al.* Palliative on-table antegrade stenting of proximal colon cancer. *Colorectal Disease* 2000; **2**: 281–7.
7. Stoeckel D, Pelton A, Duerig T. Self-expanding nitinol stents – material and design considerations. *European Radiology* 2004; **14**: 292–301.
8. CreST. The role of endoluminal stenting in the acute management of obstructing colorectal cancer. Available from www.crest.bham.ac.uk/investigations/CReST_Protocol_v2.1_16072009.pdf.

6

Rectum

Anterior resection of the rectum

BRENDAN J MORAN

INTRODUCTION

The main indication for anterior resection is treatment of rectal adenocarcinoma. It entails removal of some or all of the rectum with restoration of intestinal continuity. The term anterior resection is, by definition, only applicable if the superior rectal artery has been ligated and an anastomosis constructed at least to the top of the rectum (**Figure 6.1.1**).

This chapter focuses on anterior resection for rectal cancer, though the principles are applicable to other less common diseases in which some or all of the rectum is excised. Rectal cancer accounts for approximately 30 percent of all colorectal cancers and is defined as an adenocarcinoma with its lower edge at, or within,

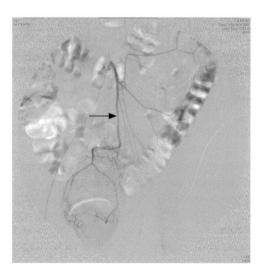

6.1.1 Inferior mesenteric angiogram outlining the blood supply to the rectum and left colon. The main vessel continues caudally as the superior rectal (arrow) having given off the left colic and sigmoid branches.

15 cm of the anal verge. It is treated predominantly by surgical excision, with the addition of neoadjuvant therapy (preoperative radiotherapy or chemoradiotherapy) in selected individuals, as this can reduce local recurrence and may facilitate surgical excision in advanced disease.[1]

Anterior resection is not required for all patients with rectal cancer. Early tumors, perhaps 5–10 percent of all with rectal cancer (although this percentage may increase with screening), can be treated by local excision alone (see Chapters 6.13 and 6.14). Tumors that involve the anal sphincter complex or levator ani muscle (approximately 10–15 percent) require excision of the anal sphincter complex through abdominoperineal excision with the creation of a permanent stoma (see Chapter 6.10). For each patient the feasibility of restorative resection ultimately depends on the tumor, the patient, and to a lesser extent, the surgeon. The tumor factors concerned are the distance of the lower tumor margin from the anal verge, fixity of the tumor to surrounding tissues and the presence or absence of metastatic disease. Patient factors include body habitus, size and depth of the pelvis, and both anal sphincter integrity and function. Surgeon-dependent factors include experience and training, availability of resources (such as stapling instruments, adequate tissue retractors, etc.) and availability of a suitably experienced surgical assistant and operating room team.

The planning and execution of anterior resection for rectal cancer currently revolves around what has been described as 'circumferential awareness' that incorporates circumferential staging, circumferential down-staging, circumferential surgery, and circumferential pathology.[1] Circumferential staging incorporates clinical examination and, more recently, cross-sectional imaging, particularly pelvic CT and MRI (**Figure 6.1.2**).[2]

In advanced tumors, that either involve or threaten the margins, circumferential down-staging and/or 'downsizing' may be achieved by preoperative radiotherapy or chemoradiotherapy (called neoadjuvant therapy). The concept of circumferential surgery has emanated

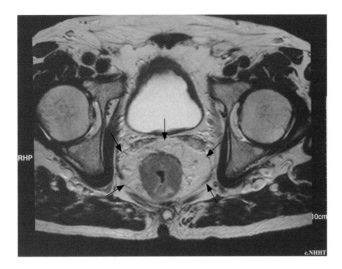

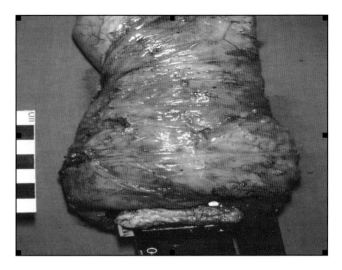

6.1.2 Pelvic MRI showing a circumferential rectal cancer surrounded by the mesorectum (arrows). The mesorectal fascia is clearly visible and a total mesorectal excision in the mesorectal fascial plane will have a clear circumferential resection margin (CRM). The radiological stage is mrT3 with predicted clear CRM.

6.1.3 A total mesorectal excision specimen, illustrating the shiny mesorectal fascia surrounding the fatty mesorectum and sealed at the distal end with a linear stapler as utilized in the Moran triple stapling technique.[5]

from the description of total mesorectal excision (TME) popularized by Heald et al.[3, 4] with 'specimen-orientated surgery' (**Figure 6.1.3**).

The principles of optimal surgery for rectal cancer revolve around the embryology and anatomy of the rectum whereby the lymphatic drainage (which is associated with the arterial blood supply) is almost exclusively proximal and is generally confined within the mesorectal fascia. While the palpable luminal distal edge almost always corresponds to the histological distal extent of a rectal cancer, distal spread in the mesorectum is common and it is this feature that underlies the rationale for TME. However, distal mesorectal spread rarely extends more than 2–3 cm beyond the lower palpable luminal edge of the tumor, although for safety reasons a distal mesorectal clearance of 5 cm, where feasible, is recommended.[4, 6] For tumors of the upper rectum, the rectum and mesorectum can be divided 5 cm distal to the lower edge of the tumor and a mesorectal transection rather than TME performed. Mesorectal transection rather than TME may reduce the incidence of postoperative surgical complications, particularly anastomotic leakage, and is associated with better postoperative functional outcomes (e.g. evacuation and stool frequency).

One of the major technical advances that facilitates safe restoration of intestinal continuity after TME, has been the development of anastomotic stapling instruments;[5] this, coupled with the recognition that adenocarcinoma rarely spreads distally in the muscle tube and that a 2 cm clearance beyond the macroscopic tumor in low tumors provides a safe distal margin. A distal margin of less than 1 cm may be adequate for ultra-low tumors.[6]

PREOPERATIVE PREPARATION

Preoperative preparation is essential and to 'fail to plan is to plan to fail'. A rectal neoplasm should be assessed by an experienced clinician who should perform a rectal examination and rigid proctosigmoidoscopy. The height of the lower edge of the tumor should be measured in centimeters from the anal verge using a rigid proctosigmoidoscope with the patient awake and recumbent in the left lateral position. The surgeon should assess the integrity of the anal canal and, if possible, assess the mobility, or otherwise, of a palpable tumor. The tumor should be biopsied to confirm the diagnosis and to exclude other rare lesions such as squamous carcinoma, infiltrating prostatic carcinoma, or lymphoma, whose management differs from that of adenocarcinoma. The author has found it very helpful to re-examine the patient, particularly a patient with a low rectal cancer 'under sedation' at colonoscopy. Occasionally, an EUA (examination under anesthetic) is required and may be a useful addition, particularly in a patient with an ultra-low rectal cancer.

The remainder of the colon should be assessed to identify synchronous neoplasia (present in 3–4 percent) by either colonoscopy, computed tomography (CT) colonography, or a barium enema. Colonoscopy has the advantage of allowing biopsy or removal of synchronous lesions. The benefits of CT colonography are the facility to stage the abdominal cavity for metastatic disease and to outline the proximal bowel in patients with stenotic lesions in whom colonoscopy may not be feasible. Current best practice also incorporates staging for systemic disease by chest and abdominal CT scan and local pelvic staging of the rectal tumor, ideally by magnetic resonance imaging (MRI), to assess the relationship of the tumor to the mesorectal fascia (**Figure 6.1.2**).[2] MRI also provides details of relevant pelvic pathology, such as ovarian or uterine in the female or prostatic enlargement in the male, all of which may limit surgical access or require synchronous treatment.[2]

The clinical details and radiological investigations of all patients with rectal cancer should be discussed at a colorectal multidisciplinary team (MDT) meeting to optimize the management strategy.

PATIENT CONSENT AND IMMEDIATE PREOPERATIVE CARE

Medical diseases such as diabetes, hypertension, cardiac and pulmonary diseases should be optimized. Arrangements should be in place for postoperative critical care if required. The patient should be consented by the surgeon and optimal stoma sites marked on both sides in case a stoma is required. It is prudent to consent for a permanent stoma in addition to temporary defunctioning stoma should an unexpected event render this necessary. In addition to the complications after any intestinal resection, such as leakage, hemorrhage, etc., the possibility of sexual and bladder dysfunction after rectal cancer surgery needs to be outlined. This is usually as a result of injury to the pelvic autonomic nerves during rectal mobilization. In females, the possible need for oophorectomy should be discussed. It is the author's policy to also consent patients for appendicectomy to treat synchronous, or avoid metachronous, appendiceal pathology.

In contrast to surgery for colon cancer, an empty large intestine is desirable for restorative rectal cancer surgery, particularly if there is a need for a defunctioning stoma. An ileostomy proximal to a full colon may not reduce the consequences of an anastomotic leak. Optimal bowel preparation can be achieved by combining clear fluids by mouth for 48 hours before surgery with oral laxatives.

Systemic antibacterial agents, including anerobic cover are given at induction of anesthesia and continued for at most 24 hours postoperatively.

Prophylaxis against deep venous thrombosis is commenced by a combination of heparin or its analogs (depending on the usage of epidural anesthesia) and mechanical calf compression devices, once the patient is positioned on the operating table.

OPERATION

Patient positioning

The lithotomy-Trendelenburg position is optimal as it allows per anal palpation and inspection, washout of the lumen, and insertion of the circular stapling instrument to complete the anastomosis. An additional advantage is that a second assistant can stand between the patient's legs. It is essential to ensure that the patient is well down on the table such that the anal canal is readily accessible. The patient is kept horizontal during the abdominal phase of the operation and can then be tilted head down by 15–20°, or more, to facilitate the pelvic dissection. It is important not to maintain steep Trendelenburg positioning for extended periods to reduce the risk of lower limb compartment syndrome, and if a steep position is required the tilt should be temporarily reverted every 20–30 minutes for a period of 3–5 minutes.

Good lighting is essential. Optimal lighting can be obtained by readjusting the movable operating lights during different phases, use of a headlight, and by retractors with integrated lighting.

On-table examination, skin incision and abdominal exploration

A rectal examination should always be performed prior to painting and draping with the mandatory addition of a vaginal examination in females.

A long vertical midline incision provides optimal access to the abdomen and pelvis (**Figure 6.1.4**). While some surgeons advocate a long transverse incision, or even a modified extended Pfannenstiel incision, access to the splenic flexure and pelvis is, in the author's opinion, inferior compared with that available through a midline incision, particularly in overweight patients with a low rectal cancer.

The abdominal cavity is fully palpated with particular attention directed to the liver and spleen, greater omentum, stomach, and small bowel, and the entire colorectum including the appendix. The surgical procedure is then planned, including the sequence. For example, if a low anterior resection is planned, mobilization of the splenic flexure is almost always needed. It is the author's personal preference to complete splenic flexure mobilization at the beginning of the operation, thus avoiding the temptation to omit this at the end of a long operation with the potential to compromise on anastomotic tension and blood supply to the neorectum.

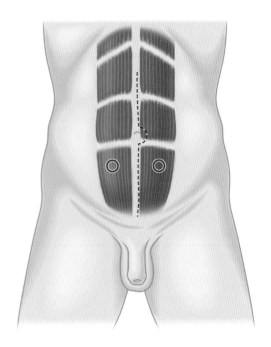

6.1.4 A midline incision extending upwards from the symphysis pubis and which may need extension to the xiphisternum. The optimal site for a defunctioning stoma has been marked preoperatively by an enterostomal therapist.

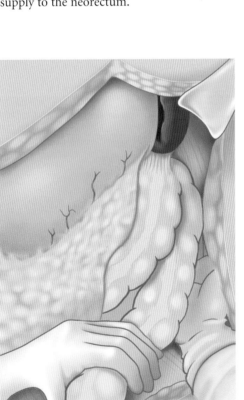

6.1.5 Incision of the peritoneum to mobilize the splenic flexure.

Commencing the dissection and splenic flexure mobilization

The operating surgeon stands on the left side of the patient with the first assistant on the patient's right. The assistant lifts the sigmoid colon anteriorly and to the right. The peritoneal reflection on the lateral side of the left colon (identified by the white line of Toldt) is divided by scissors or diathermy and followed cranially towards the splenic flexure. The plane of dissection in the left upper quadrant is developed between the colon and the urogenital structures (Gerota's fascia surrounding the kidney and the gonadal vessels). At this juncture, if the spleen is mobile on the diaphragm, a large moist swab placed gently between the spleen and diaphragm helps to push the spleen into view and facilitates splenic flexure mobilization (**Figure 6.1.5**).

The greater omentum is now retracted anteriorly and to the patient's left and the 'bloodless' plane between the transverse colon and omentum is developed by sharp scissors dissection or by diathermy incision. The apex of the splenic flexure attachments (lienocolic ligament) is visualized by downwards colonic traction from the patient's right with countertraction by a retractor under the left rib cage. The assistant standing on the patient's right side maintains colonic traction and also insinuates the index finger of the right hand behind the colon on the left. This facilitates division of the apical lateral attachments by the operator who stands either on the patient's left side or temporarily between the patient's legs.

Ligation and division of the inferior mesenteric vessels

The left-sided colonic mobilization is continued inferiorly by the left-sided operator with identification of the ureter (usually positioned medial to the gonadal vessels and crossing the bifurcation of the common iliac artery) and the fascial covering of the uppermost part of the 'mesorectal package'. This maneuver is facilitated by the right-sided assistant applying traction on the sigmoid, anteriorly and to the right, taking care not to damage the mesentery of the colon. Once the plane has been developed at the pelvic brim to just beyond the midline, it is the author's practice to insert a small swab behind the mesentery at the level of the pelvic brim. The sigmoid traction is now reversed and the assistant surgeon on the patient's right can identify the correct point to incise the right-sided peritoneum by a combination of air in the tissues and anterior displacement of the mesentery by the small swab. The swab helps to protect the autonomic nerves at the level of the pelvic brim. The right-sided peritoneum is incised caudally to the pelvic brim and cranially towards the root of the inferior mesenteric artery (IMA). At this point the surgeon on the patient's left places the left index finger behind the pedicle and with left thumb anteriorly can palpate the IMA between index finger and thumb. The peritoneal attachments are divided and superior hypogastric plexus structures mobilized away from the right side of the pedicle by sharp dissection. The index finger is then advanced cranially on the left side, parallel to the midline where a 'window' in the mesocolon will be identified above the origin of the IMA between the aorta and the inferior mesenteric vein (IMV) and ascending left colic artery running side by side at this point (**Figure 6.1.6**). This window is opened, the autonomic nerves are again freed until the root of the IMA is clearly identified. It is important to check that the left ureter has not been elevated in this maneuver by visualizing the structures to the left of the pedicle. Once the IMA pedicle has been isolated it is clamped, divided, and ligated approximately 2 cm from the aorta to reduce risk of injury to the preaortic nerves and to achieve a 'high' but not 'flush' tie of the IMA.

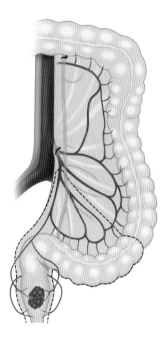

6.1.6 Mobilization, ligation, and division of the inferior mesenteric vessels.

The IMV should next be divided above its last branch, at the inferior border of the pancreas where is disappears cranially to join the splenic vein. This ensures maximum length and mobility of the left colon for later anastomosis. In 5–10 percent of patients, a substantial branch of the superior mesenteric artery lies near the IMV at this point and provides a significant portion of arterial blood supply to the left colon. Judgment is required to determine whether this vessel should be divided to facilitate colonic mobilization or preserved if division is likely to compromise colonic viability.

Mobilization of the mesorectum and rectum

This is oncologically one of the most important stages of the operation. The surgeon must develop a mental picture of the position and extent of the tumor, based on the prior clinical and radiological assessment. The circumferential concepts of TME surgery are applied to ensure clear margins on the resected specimen. It is helpful to divide the descending colon at this stage, a so-called 'division of convenience' using a linear cutting stapler. This particularly facilitates the posterior pelvic dissection (**Figure 6.1.7**).

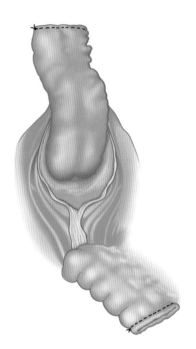

6.1.7 Mobilization of the rectum and mesorectum. The colon has been divided using a linear cutting stapler and the posterior plane is being developed anterior to the superior hypogastric plexus and hypogastric (presacral) nerves.

Posterior dissection

The avascular areolar tissue plane (mesorectal fascia) which surrounds the mesorectum is identified, and it is worth remembering that the mesorectum resembles a bilobed lipoma. The rectum is lifted gently forwards from the bifurcation of the hypogastric nerves and dissection commences in the midline using diathermy, aiming to minimize direct or collateral heat damage to the nerves. Dissection is extended downwards anterior to the curve of the sacrum on the surface of the mesorectal fascia. When there is sufficient space, a St Mark's rectal retractor (with integral illumination if available) is introduced behind the specimen. This helps to spread and 'tent' the hypogastric nerves and aids identification. It is important to gently position the retractor and apply firm but gentle pressure to expose the mesorectal fascia and the layer of areolar tissue or what has been called 'angel hair' where dissection should proceed. In this maneuver the operator (standing on the patient's left) and the first assistant on the right have to position and control the angulation and force of retraction, aided by the second assistant between the legs when more forceful retraction is needed. The angulation and degree of retraction are vital and are a dynamic activity that can only be controlled by direct vision such that an assistant between the legs can help but not position or alter the angle of traction.

It is important to note that all four hands of the operator and assistant are needed for retraction, countertraction, and dissection. A sucker can be a useful retractor, in addition to its role in removing diathermy smoke and fluid. It is useful to wash out the pelvis on a regular basis; the author's preference is to use sterile water with dilute proflavine which is hypotonic and therefore cytocidal, as this helps to visualize the tissue planes. Others use povidone iodine but colour distortion may interfere with visualization of the tissue planes.

Dissection proceeds in the angel hair areolar tissue and should be predominantly from medial to lateral and from below upwards in an anterolateral direction allowing the hypogastric nerves to drop away posterolaterally. It is important to focus on circumferential mobilization rather than try to proceed too far posteriorly at this stage. Dissection in the lateral and anterior planes should be commenced at this juncture.

Lateral dissection

The lateral attachments are mobilized by extending the dissection plane forwards from the midline posteriorly around the side walls of the pelvis. It is important to remember that the inferior hypogastric plexuses (formed by the hypogastric nerves and the pelvic parasympathetic nerves) curve forwards tangentially around the surface of the mesorectum in close proximity to it. The nervi erigentes (pelvic parasympathetic nerves) lie more posteriorly in the same plane as the hypogastric nerves and should be visualized and preserved as they may be easily 'tented up' and damaged at this point. The nervi erigentes then curve forwards and converge like the base of a fan to join the hypogastric nerves and form the neurovascular bundles of Walsh (**Figure 6.1.8**).[7, 8] Thus the nerves lie at the outer edges of Denonvilliers' fascia and are in danger of injury at the 10 o'clock and 2 o'clock anterolateral positions just behind the lateral edges of the seminal vesicles in the male. More distally, they curve forwards and are less vulnerable to injury.

As the lateral dissection moves deeper into the pelvis, one or two middle rectal vessels may be encountered and occasionally may require to be occluded by precise diathermy or ligation after application of a slender curved artery forceps. There are almost always some slender nerve branches at this point as well and it is usually these branches which form the so-called 'lateral ligament'. When medial traction is applied these branches will 'tent' the plexus and it is important to divide them by sharp diathermy or scissors dissection on the mesorectal surface. The previously described clamping of the lateral ligaments is unnecessary and potentially injurious to the pelvic nerves.

If bleeding is encountered it is often wise to place a pack gently on the area (personal preference is to use an adrenaline-soaked swab) and move the dissection to another area, perhaps the other side or anteriorly.

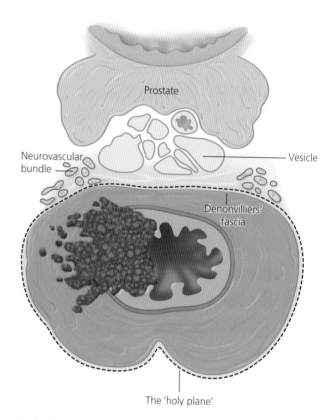

Prostate

Neurovascular bundle

Vesicle

Denonvilliers' fascia

The 'holy plane'

6.1.8 Schematic outline of mesorectal fascia with the neurovascular bundles anterolaterally in the male pelvis.

Anterior dissection

In males, the traditional teaching has been to incise the peritoneal reflection anteriorly but a more satisfactory approach is to follow the plane forwards from behind anterolaterally on both sides until the seminal vesicles are visualized (**Figure 6.1.9**).

A small swab may be placed on the anterior surface of the rectum and the plane immediately in front of Denonvilliers' fascia is developed by sharp dissection in the midline anteriorly. Dissection is then carefully extended laterally to meet the lateral dissection, remembering that the autonomic nerves converge to form the neurovascular bundles at the lateral edge of Denonvilliers' fascia. Denonvilliers' fascia also marks the anterior extent of the 'tumor package' and lies like an apron anterior to the anterior mesorectum, behind the vesicles, until it fuses inferiorly with the posterior fascia of the prostate. For this reason, Denonvilliers' fascia must eventually be divided by scissors or diathermy to access the lowest few centimeters of anterior rectum. This should be well beyond the distal edge of the cancer except in ultra-low resection for a distal rectal cancer.

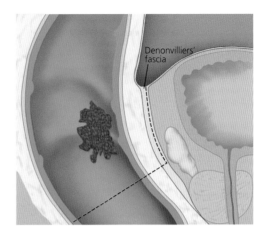

6.1.9 Schematic view of prostate and vesicles with rectum posteriorly. The author's preference is to dissect along the dotted line anterior to Denonvilliers' fascia.

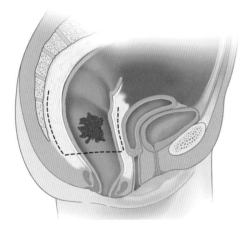

6.1.10 The plane of dissection in total mesorectal excision in the female for a mid or low rectal cancer.

Anterior dissection in females

In females, the uterus, if present, should be lifted forward (**Figure 6.1.10**). There is a similar condensation of fibrous fascia anteriorly, analogous to Denonvilliers' fascia in the male. It is often difficult to access the plane anterior to the rectovaginal septum behind the cervix and posterior fornix and this plane is best approached, as in the male, by continuation of the anterolateral dissection from the side wall. Troublesome bleeding may be encountered from the vaginal venous plexus. Attempts to control the bleeding may be futile until the vagina has been fully mobilized off the anterior rectum allowing the stretched venous plexus to collapse down. The peritoneal reflection may be adherent to the posterior fornix and require to be dissected off by diathermy dissection.

Anterolateral dissection

Connecting the lateral to the anterior dissection is a critical point in the dissection. It is usually best to continue the dissection from posterior to anterior as the autonomic nerves will usually be visible and the correct plane is just medial to the autonomic bundles. There is a tendency to stay too far laterally with attendant risks of injury to the autonomic nerves or troublesome bleeding from the lateral pelvic sidewall. Careful assessment and reassessment is essential at this point to access the correct operative plane. The anterolateral peritoneal and subperitoneal incisions are curved medially towards the midline in the front to preserve the autonomic nerve structures.

Extended resection in special cases

With current optimal preoperative staging, it should be uncommon to unexpectedly find a rectal tumor that extends into adjacent organs. It is important to be aware that while adhesion to an adjacent organ may be inflammatory, in approximately half of the cases it is malignant and rupture of a malignant adhesion will almost certainly result in tumor spillage and dissemination, with a high risk of local recurrence. For this reason it is prudent to resect an adherent organ rather than gamble on the adhesion being benign.

UTERUS AND VAGINA

Involvement of the vagina and uterus is usually detected at preoperative imaging and during vaginal examination prior to surgery. A large fixed cancer, even with neoadjuvant chemoradiotherapy, is best removed by *en bloc* resection of the uterus and rectum and as much of the posterior vaginal wall as is needed to clear the tumor safely. The vagina may be closed primarily in most patients but if the defect is large, particularly in a sexually active patient, reconstruction using a musculocutaneous flap may be needed (see Chapter 7.1). The need for this should be anticipated and appropriate assistance and resources should be available.

SEMINAL VESICLES

Involvement of the vesicles on one or both sides may be managed by dissection anterior to the vesicles removing them *en bloc* with the rectum. The ureters must be carefully identified and preserved. It may be prudent in such cases to consider stenting the ureters preoperatively to facilitate identification. The neurovascular bundles are at particular risk in such a dissection.

PROSTATE

It is possible, though technically difficult, to remove a part of the prostate with an adherent rectal cancer. However, gross prostatic involvement may require pelvic exenteration or in selected cases a nerve preserving prostatectomy *en bloc* with the rectum. Modern MRI imaging should predict this eventuality and the assistance of an experienced urologist is required.

URETERS

The ureters may be involved in rectosigmoid or colonic cancers, but are seldom in danger of injury during the dissection for mid or low rectal cancer. However, in complex pelvic surgery it is always prudent to visualize and in most cases mobilize the ureters. It is always safe to divide the tissues anterior to the ureteric tunnels in both sexes as they are anterior to the pelvic plexuses and are crossed only by the vas deferens in the male and the uterine vessels in the female. A locally advanced tumor may invade the distal ureter and require *en bloc* resection. Depending on the size of the defect and height of the ureteric resection, it may be possible to perform a scalloped end-to-end anastomosis over a ureteric stent or, alternatively, to reimplant the proximal end into the bladder or the opposite ureter. Again, urological assistance is strongly recommended.

BLADDER

Rectal cancer involving the bladder would usually have been predicted by pelvic MRI imaging. Neoadjuvant chemoradiotherapy is generally indicated. Cystocopy should be performed to determine the site of bladder invasion relative to the ureters. The operative strategy for a rectal cancer invading the bladder requires consultation with a urologist and varies from partial cystectomy, excising a disk of the involved bladder, *en bloc* with the rectal tumor, to pelvic exenteration particularly if the trigone is involved. Bladder involvement is much more common in males, as in females the uterus and vagina intervene between the rectum and bladder acting as a barrier to bladder invasion.

INFERIOR HYPOGASTRIC AND PELVIC PLEXUSES

Although the focus of this chapter has been on identification and preservation of these nerves, a locally advanced tumor, adherent to the pelvic sidewall, may require nerve resection. The prevascular plane outside the nerves along the aorta and major vessels may be developed and followed. It may be possible to limit dissection in this plane, and nerve removal, to one side. Bladder and sexual function will be affected depending on the particular nerves excised.[8]

INTERNAL ILIAC AND PELVIC SIDEWALL NODES

There is a wide variation in the reported incidence of pelvic sidewall nodal involvement. There is, however, general agreement that involvement is mainly associated with low rectal cancer and can often be predicted by pelvic imaging. The surgical management of involved pelvic sidewall nodes is complex with attendant risks (see Chapter 6.12).

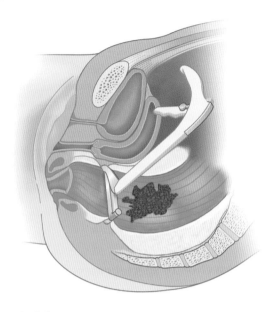

6.1.11 Schematic drawing of a linear stapler being applied across the anorectal muscle tube below the cancer.

Distal washout and anastomosis

Following mobilization, the rectum, with its surrounding mesorectum, remains attached to the pelvic floor by the anorectal muscle tube. It is the author's practice to now occlude the muscular tube below the tumor and a useful technique, particularly for low rectal cancer, is to use a 45 or 30 mm linear stapler.[5] The rectal tumor is palpated between finger and thumb and the linear stapler applied distally and fired (**Figure 6.1.11**). A proctoscope is then introduced into the anal canal and the lumen below the staple line should be irrigated with repeated infusions using a 50 mL syringe or through a catheter irrigation system. Sterile water, povidone iodine, or dilute proflavine solutions, are recommended (**Figure 6.1.12**).

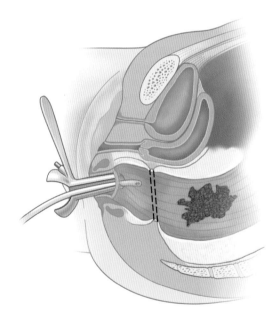

6.1.12 The anal canal and distal rectum are washed out below an occlusive staple line.

Once the washout is complete, a second linear stapler is applied distal to the occlusive staple line and fired across the washed muscle tube. It is often difficult to safely get below the staple line for very low tumors and a useful modification is to place and fire the proximal stapler, leave it in position during washout and then place a further stapler (usually 30 mm diameter) distal to the first instrument and apply the staples. The muscle tube is sectioned with a scalpel on the upper edge of the distal stapler as shown (**Figure 6.1.13**).

The specimen is now removed. Prior to removal of the distal stapler, the proximal resection margin should be carefully inspected and palpated, to ensure it is clear of tumor. If there is doubt the staples may be removed and the lumen inspected directly. In the occasional case where clearance is marginal, another linear stapler can be positioned below the second one and further clearance obtained. If the resection margin is adequate, the distal linear stapler is removed leaving a transverse staple line across the anorectal tube.

The pelvic cavity is washed copiously and inspected for bleeding. Hemostasis is secured with carefully applied diathermy or suturing on occasions. For troublesome presacral, pelvic sidewall, or other bothersome bleeding a hemostatic agent, such as Tachosil™, may be very helpful. Rather than repeated futile attempts at diathermy or suturing, packing the pelvis will usually arrest bleeding if left in place for 10–15 minutes.

Where a TME has been performed and a coloanal anastomosis required, a 'neorectal' reservoir provides better functional outcome than a straight colonic anastomosis.[1]

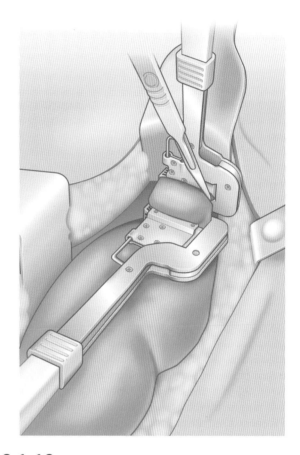

6.1.13 The muscle tube is sectioned between two 30 mm linear staplers in the Moran triple stapling technique for low rectal cancer.

A side (colon) to end (anorectum) anastomosis provides an adequate reservoir and is the easiest to construct (**Figure 6.1.14**). Alternatives include construction of a colonic J-pouch and a transverse coloplasty. To facilitate side to end anastomosis, approximately half of the staple line on the distal end of the colon is excised and the lumen washed out. This allows assessment of the distal colonic blood supply and inspection of the mucosa. An appropriately sized circular stapler is selected (28–31 mm is optimal) and the head detached. The detached head of the gun is inserted into the lumen, spike first, and the spike brought out through the anterior mesenteric border approximately halfway between the tenia coli, approximately 4 cm from the colonic end. The defect in the staple line is closed with interrupted absorbable sutures. The author also prefers to invert the remaining staple line with interrupted sutures. This technique provides a flat surface for the proximal part of the anastomosis and leaves room in the anvil for the thicker proximal bowel (**Figure 6.1.14**).

Circular stapled anastomosis

The anorectal remnant is palpated from between the legs. The anal canal may have to be dilated gently to accommodate the lubricated circular stapler. Relaxation of the sphincter by perianal application of glyceryl trinitrate (GTN) (cream applied 30–60 minutes, or alternatively sublingual GTN spray 5 minutes beforehand) may facilitate introduction of the stapler. Care must be taken not to disrupt the transverse staple line and the abdominal surgeon may have to bimanually assist in this step to ensure safe placement. A St Mark's retractor helps to visualize the anorectal stump and retract vesicles and prostate in the male, or vagina in the female, anteriorly. Once the circular ring of the gun is visible clearly through the bowel wall the gun is opened and the protruding spike guided through the bowel, ideally just behind the linear staple line. The head of the gun is brought down and engaged with the shaft. The gun is slowly closed until the tissues are in apposition as seen on the tissue indicator mechanism on the circular gun (**Figure 6.1.14**).

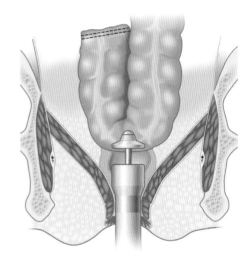

6.1.14 Side to end stapled anastomosis.

At this point, it is mandatory to check the alignment of the proximal colon (including the transverse colon) to ensure that there is not a 360° twist of the colonic mesentery prior to firing the stapling instrument.

The circular stapler is fired according to the specific manufacturer's instructions. Generally after firing, the position should be maintained for 1–2 minutes which may reduce the risk of anastomotic bleeding. The gun is then opened as per instructions and removed.

The donuts are inspected and the excised tissue donuts are checked to be intact. Following anastomosis of a low rectal cancer the distal donut should be sent for histology. The anastomosis is gently palpated for integrity and can be air-tested by filling the pelvis with water and insufflating air via the anal canal, using a syringe or proctoscope. If an air leak is identified, this should be repaired with interrupted sutures, if necessary using a transanal approach.

Defunctioning a low anastomosis after TME

Even if the anastomosis is airtight, consideration should be given to temporarily defunctioning all coloanal anastomoses after TME. A recent randomized trial reported a 28 percent leak rate in patients after TME without a defunctioning stoma compared to 10 percent in those with a loop stoma.[9] Factors which have been shown to increase the risks are height of the anastomosis from the anal verge (particularly below 5 cm, which includes all patients after a TME), male patients, preoperative chemoradiotherapy, intraoperative technical difficulties such as major bleeding and absence of a defunctioning stoma. A defunctioning stoma also reduces the consequences of an anastomotic leak and the need for emergency reoperation.[10] It is the author's preference to place a defunctioning loop ileostomy which may be closed 6–8 weeks later.

If a temporary stoma has not been placed and there are concerns in the postoperative period, an anastomotic leak should be sought by a rectal contrast study (commonly now performed in combination with an abdominal CT). If detected, emergency reoperation surgery is usually required and may entail anastomotic excision with end colostomy. In selected patients, the anastomosis can be preserved with use of broad-spectrum antibiotics, adequate drainage of any collections, and defunctioning by a proximal loop stoma.

High anterior resection and mesorectal transection

Tumors of the upper rectum (lower edge 11–15 cm from the anal verge) may be considered suitable for mesorectal transection 5 cm below the palpable edge of the tumor. The mobilization is the same although the lowest and most difficult part of the rectal and mesorectal mobilization

can be omitted provided it is possible to get safely 5 cm tangentially below the lower edge of the tumor.

The rectum is irrigated below a clamp or linear stapler as described above under Distal washout and anastomosis, page 454. The washed rectum is then stapled with a linear stapler prior to perianal circular stapling as described. An end to end anastomosis is usually constructed as a 'neorectal reservoir' may not evacuate as well when anastomosed above the anorectal junction. The risk of leakage from such an anastomosis (once found to be airtight) is much less than after a coloanal anastomosis as the remaining rectum and mesorectum fill the pelvis. Therefore a defunctioning stoma can be omitted.

The use of drains following large bowel anastomosis is questionable and there is evidence that following colonic anastomosis use is unnecessary, even deleterious. After low anterior resection, however, presacral collections are common and may become infected contributing to anastomotic leak. It remains the author's preference to insert two low pressure closed suction drains placed in the presacral cavity and removed at about 48 hours. Irrigation fluid, either proflavine solution or sterile water is poured into the pelvis prior to abdominal closure and allowed to flow freely through the drains as the abdomen is closed to prevent early drain blockage.

POSTOPERATIVE MANAGEMENT

Postoperative recovery may be complicated by ileus such that accelerated or enhanced recovery may not be successful after a low anterior resection and care should be taken to recognize the symptoms and sign of ileus. Some patients require reinsertion of a nasogastric tube, intravenous fluids and intravenous nutrition, on occasions, until normal bowel function returns.

Anastomotic leakage

As outlined above, leakage is a major risk after any rectal anastomosis, particularly a low rectal or coloanal anastomosis.[9] Etiological factors may include the large cavity created by rectal and mesorectal excision with the risk of a presacral hematoma and/or increased pressure above a closed sphincter. As outlined above, the consequences of leakage are diminished if the bowel has been cleansed and is defunctioned.

Management of the stoma

Expert stoma care is essential to optimize recovery and speed up hospital discharge to home. The stoma may be closed 6–8 weeks later provided a water-soluble contrast study of the anastomosis has not demonstrated a leak. If a leak is detected the contrast enema is repeated two months later until resolution of the leak is documented prior to stoma closure. Prior to stoma reversal it is mandatory to digitally examine the anastomosis under anesthetic as a narrowing to 1–2 cm is common and the anastomosis can be safely dilated by the examining finger. Persistent symptomatic anastomotic stricturing is rare unless there has been colonic ischemia, inadequate colonic length, or gross pelvic sepsis, usually a consequence of a leak.

Anorectal function after low anterior resection

If anorectal function was satisfactory prior to the diagnosis of cancer and the patient did not receive neoadjuvant therapy, postoperative evacuation and continence should be acceptable, even after a low anastomosis. In the early postoperative months, most patients will have increased stool frequency, urgency, and often soiling after an anterior resection or following reversal of a defunctioning stoma. This will normally improve over time but can take a year or more to optimize. Reassurance, use of mild constipating agents, and dietary advice may be helpful in many. Neoadjuvant or adjuvant radiotherapy may have additional adverse effects on anorectal function and function may deteriorate over ensuing years. The author's preference is to limit the use of neoadjuvant therapy to patients in whom preoperative clinical and image-predicted resection margins are threatened or involved.

CONCLUSION

Rectal adenocarcinoma is a common cancer and is curable by surgery alone in most cases.[1] Recent advances in pelvic imaging by MRI,[2] adoption of the surgical concepts of total mesorectal excision,[3, 4] and current excellent mechanical stapling instruments[5] have revolutionized the management and outcome of this technically challenging but eminently curable cancer.

REFERENCES

1. Daniels IR, Fisher SE, Heald RJ, Moran BJ. Accurate staging, selective pre-operative therapy and optimal surgery improves outcome in rectal cancer: a review of the recent evidence. *Colorectal Disease* 2007; **9**: 290–301.
2. Mercury Study Group. Diagnostic accuracy of preoperative magnetic resonance imaging in predicting curative resection of rectal cancer: prospective observational study. *BMJ* 2006; **333**: 779–84.
3. Heald RJ, Husband EM, Ryall RDH The mesorectum in rectal cancer surgery – the clue to pelvic recurrence? *British Journal of Surgery* 1982; **69**: 613–16.
4. Heald RJ, Moran BJ, Ryall RDH *et al.* Rectal cancer. The Basingstoke experience of total mesorectal excision, 1978–1997. *Archives of Surgery* 1998; **133**: 894–8.
5. Moran BJ. Stapling instruments for intestinal anastomosis in colorectal surgery. *British Journal of Surgery* 1996; **83**: 902–9.
6. Karanjia ND, Schache DJ, North WRS, Heald RJ. 'Close shave' in anterior resection. *British Journal of Surgery* 1990; **77**: 510–12.
7. Walsh PC, Schlegel PN. Radical pelvic surgery with preservation of sexual function. *Annals of Surgery* 1988; **208**: 391–400.
8. Quinlan DM, Epstein JI, Carter BS, Walsh PC. Sexual function following radical prostatectomy: influence of preservation of neurovascular bundles. *Journal of Urology* 1991; **145**: 998–1002.
9. Mathieson P, Hollbook O, Rutegard J *et al.* Defunctioning stoma reduces symptomatic anastomotic leakage after low anterior resection of the rectum for cancer. A multicentre randomized trial. *Annals of Surgery* 2007; **246**: 207–14.

Anterior resection – laparoscopic

HESTER YS CHEUNG AND MICHAEL KW LI

PRINCIPLES AND JUSTIFICATION

Laparoscopic anterior resection of the rectum is performed for a variety of conditions, with malignancy being one of the most common indications. For this reason, the operations described in this chapter are focused on rectal cancers; oncological principles are followed in the same manner as in open surgery.

While laparoscopic rectal cancer excision is increasingly performed worldwide, the procedure is by no means easy. The learning curve is steep – it is estimated on average a surgeon needs to perform at least 30 such resections in order to surpass the learning curve. As a beginner it is desirable to pick up small and mobile lesions in the rectosigmoid or upper rectum as starting points; tumors in mid or low rectum necessitate both dissection deep down in the true pelvis and, in many cases, splenic flexure mobilization, both of which require considerable skill and experience to ensure a smooth procedure. The following operations are thus described in this ascending order of complexity.

INDICATIONS AND CONTRAINDICATIONS

The clinical indications for laparoscopic anterior resection are the same as those for traditional open operations. Patient factors, such as obesity and previous operations, could make the laparoscopic procedure more difficult; on the other hand, if successfully performed, the laparoscopic approach is associated with increased short-term benefits in obese patients. Patients with compromised cardiopulmonary function require special attention as they tolerate prolonged pneumoperitoneum poorly; close liaison with an experienced anesthetist is essential.

As far as disease factors are concerned, one important contraindication is the presence of locally advanced disease with significant perirectal soft tissue involvement, especially those tumors with contiguous organ involvement (e.g.

invasion to uterus and urinary bladder), which in our experience often precludes a total laparoscopic approach. While a hand-assisted laparoscopic approach might be feasible under these circumstances, these bulky tumors are often better managed through a conventional laparotomy. A laparoscopic approach is also difficult and not routinely recommended in obstructed rectal tumors or tumors with perforation.

PREOPERATIVE PREPARATION AND ASSESSMENT

This is essentially the same as for open surgery. A routine staging computed tomography helps to exclude locally advanced tumors and allows better patient selection especially for the novice. Preoperation pulmonary function should be assessed in patients with chronic pulmonary disease. Stoma siting is performed preoperatively if a low resection is anticipated, or when a covering ileostomy is deemed necessary. Patients should undergo standard mechanical bowel preparation, and receive perioperative antibiotics and prophylaxis against deep vein thrombosis in the usual manner. However, in patients with subacute obstruction or endoscopically obstructed tumors, a vigorous bowel preparation may precipitate acute obstruction and hinder laparoscopic dissection. In these circumstances, a formal preparation with standard oral agents is not recommended; rather, emphasis should be placed on dietary restriction (e.g. low residue diet for 2–3 days before surgery).

OPERATING TEAM AND THEATRE SET-UP

Laparoscopic rectal cancer surgery is never a single-surgeon operation. A dedicated team consisting of at least two experienced surgeons and one camera assistant are essential. Experienced anesthetists, nurses, and technicians who are familiar with the procedures, the handling of various laparoscopic instruments and function of the ancillary technology also form an integral part of the team.

Like other advanced laparoscopic procedures, laparoscopic rectal cancer surgery is best carried out in an integrated endolaparoscopic operating suite, where there is a universal plug and play system for various endoscopes and laparoscopes. Recommended instruments include: (1) a 30° telescope; (2) four atraumatic forceps for handling of bowel and other fine tissues; (3) three grasping forceps for holding sutures or cotton tapes; (4) ultrasonic dissection device, 5 or 10 mm in size, or Ligasure™ device (Tyco Healthcare Group LP, Boulder, CO, USA), 5 or 10 mm in size; (5) laparoscopic bipolar coagulating forceps (Gyrus Medical Limited, Cardiff, UK), 5 mm in size; (6) endoscopic clip applicators and clips; (7) endostaplers of various size, used for bowel transection (blue, gold, or green cartridge) and vascular division (white cartridge); (8) a circular stapler for bowel anastomosis; and (9) a sterile plastic zip-lock bag or Alexis® wound retractor (Applied Medical, Rancho Santa Margarita, CA, USA), acting as a parietal protective drape during specimen retrieval.

OPERATION

This is indicated for tumors in the rectosigmoid junction or upper rectum. Mobile rectosigmoid tumors are particularly easy to operate on and are ideal cases for the novice. A 5 cm distal mural and mesorectal margin is obtained for operations performed with curative intent.

Position of the patient and trocar placement

The positions of the patient and the surgical team are shown in **Figure 6.2.1**. In positioning the patient, it is important that hip flexion be kept to a minimum; otherwise, the patient's thigh will be in the way of the chief surgeon's right hand. Throughout the procedure the patient is predominantly put in a 20° Trendelenburg position with a right-side down tilt. This position helps to clear the small bowel loops off the lower abdomen and pelvis. The port sites are shown in **Figure 6.2.2**. The two ports on the right iliac fossa are created for use by the chief surgeon, whereas the assistant surgeon operates via 5 mm ports over the left iliac fossa, i.e. both surgeons operate with two hands.

Pneumoperitoneum is first established via a subumbilical blunt trocar using an open technique. The abdominal cavity is then visually explored in a systematic manner; emphasis is placed in the detection of possible liver secondaries, pelvic deposits, and peritoneal seedlings. If liver secondaries are suspected, laparoscopic ultrasound examination is carried out through laparoscopy ports. The lesion in the upper rectum is next identified. Other trocars are then inserted under direct vision. Tattooing the site of the tumor may need to be done if not done previously.

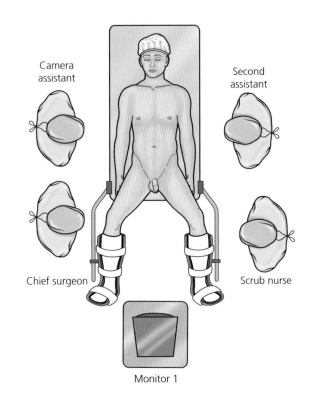

Camera assistant

Second assistant

Chief surgeon

Scrub nurse

Monitor 1

6.2.1

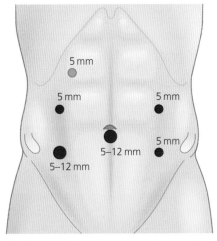

5 mm

5 mm   5 mm

5 mm

5–12 mm

5–12 mm

● Port site for laparoscopic anterior resection
● Additional port site for laparoscopic TME

6.2.2

Exposure of the pelvis

In the case of a female patient, for better pelvic exposure the uterus is first hitched up by passing sutures (00 prolene on a straight needle) underneath the two Fallopian tubes near the uterine cornu and tying them to the lower anterior abdominal wall (**Figure 6.2.3**). The stitch should pass through the skin and be tied over a piece of gauge as a reminder to the surgeon to replace the uterus at the end of the procedure.

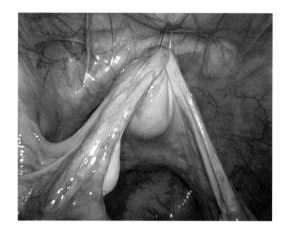

6.2.3

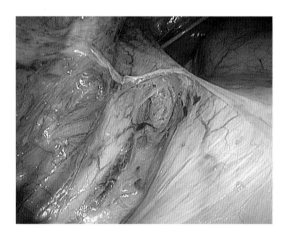

6.2.4

Sigmoid mobilization and vascular control

For sigmoid mobilization, discussion continues as to whether lateral-first or medial-first approach should be used. While the individual approach is purely a matter of personal preference, we favor the lateral-first approach because this is what we normally do in open surgery. Besides, in our experience the left ureter is more easily identified in the left lateral peritoneal space (**Figure 6.2.4**), especially during the learning phase. However, sometimes the presence of complex inflammatory conditions (abscess, fistula, severe diverticular disease, etc.) in the sigmoid colon mandates the medial-first approach.

For simplicity the lateral-first approach is described here. The lateral peritoneal attachment of the sigmoid (Toldt's fascia) is first divided (**Figure 6.2.5**). This is continued upwards to as high as is comfortable. Following this, a mesenteric window is created at the sigmoid mesentery at the level of rectosigmoid junction. The window should be created in an avascular region near the sigmoid colon just beneath the mesenteric epiploic appendix. A cotton tape, cut to 15–20 cm long, is then tied around the bowel

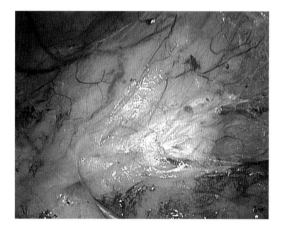

6.2.5

through the window. By grasping the cotton tape and moving it to and fro, the assistant surgeon can provide the necessary countertraction and exposure for subsequent mesenteric division and rectal mobilization (**Figure 6.2.6**). On the left lateral peritoneal space, the left gonadal vessels and medially the left ureter are identified under the retroperitoneum (i.e. the posterior parietal peritoneum)

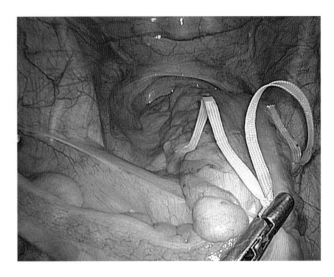

6.2.6

(**Figure 6.2.4**). The retroperitoneum is then incised medial to the left ureter, and the left hypogastric nerve identified (**Figure 6.2.7**). The presacral space is entered at a plane anterior to the left presacral hypogastric nerve, which is located around 1–2 cm lateral to the midline at the level of the sacral promontory. The lateral dissection is now completed.

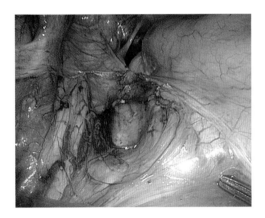

6.2.7

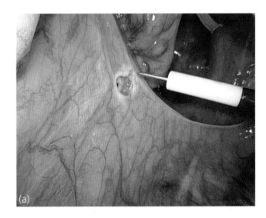

The sigmoid colon is then swung to the left side, the right ureter is outlined, and the retroperitoneum at the base of the sigmoid mesentery is incised, first at the level of the sacral promontory. Care must be taken to avoid any damage to the underlying right hypogastric nerve. If adequate lateral dissection has been previously performed, a generous retromesenteric window is easily made at the base of the mesosigmoid which should by now look paper-thin (**Figure 6.2.8a**). The left ureter is recognized once again through this retromesenteric window (**Figure 6.2.8b**). Division of the retroperitoneum can safely continue superiorly anterior to the aorta, until the inferior mesenteric artery (IMA) is encountered. The

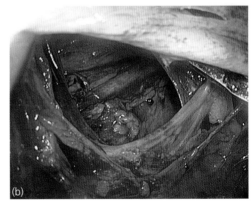

6.2.8

IMA can be controlled with either a linear endostapler or clips (**Figure 6.2.9**); alternatively, a Ligasure™ device can be used instead, although the hemostasis is sometimes suboptimal in arteries with extensive atherosclerosis. If it is intended to use the sigmoid colon for the subsequent bowel anastomosis, it is preferable to divide the IMA distal to the left colic artery take-off. The inferior mesenteric vein (IMV) lateral to the artery is likewise divided. This mesenteric division is continued for a few centimeters, until it is judged that the vascular pedicle can be subsequently delivered to the skin surface without tension. Caution needs to be exercised here to avoid inadvertent division of the marginal artery.

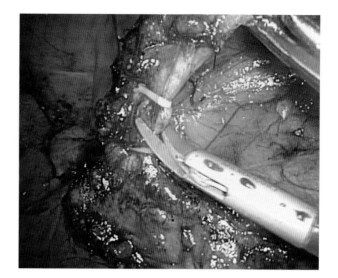

6.2.9

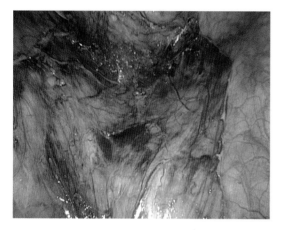

6.2.10

Pelvic dissection

Following pedicle control, attention is now turned to the pelvis. The rectum is retracted upwards and forwards, and the loose areolar plane between the mesorectum and the presacral fascia (with the hypogastric nerves lying on it) is identified. The right and left hypogastric nerves should be clearly visualized on the presacral fascia as two structures radiating downwards and diverging outwards in the pelvis (**Figure 6.2.10**). Wide opening of this presacral space is continued posteriorly, respecting the presacral fascia, up to approximately 5 cm distal to the tumor. Laterally, left and right rectal dissection is likewise performed by dividing the posterior parietal peritoneum in a direction parallel to the rectal tube. A point 5 cm

distal to the tumor (i.e. usually in the midrectum) is then chosen for subsequent rectal transection, and at this level the posterior mesorectum is slowly thinned down using ultrasonic dissectors or Ligasure™ (**Figure 6.2.11**), until the rectal tube is exposed. The assistant surgeon now pulls the rectum in a cephaloid direction. The rectum is

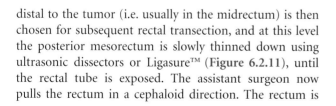

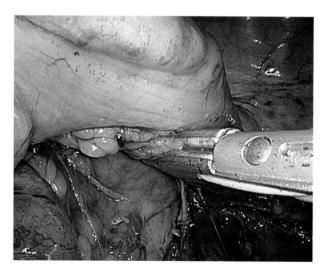

6.2.11

temporarily clamped with laparoscopic forceps below the tumor, and following cytocidal lavage through the anus, it is then transected with a linear endostapler (usually blue or gold cartridge) introduced via the 12 mm right iliac fossa port (**Figure 6.2.12**). Two to three firings are sometimes required. An angulating stapler is preferred, especially in lower resections. After this, a trial descent is performed to estimate whether enough length has been obtained for subsequent anastomosis. Provided the sigmoid is healthy without severe diverticular disease and there is good blood supply and adequate length, splenic flexure take-down is not essential. The sigmoid can be used for bowel anastomosis in most cases.

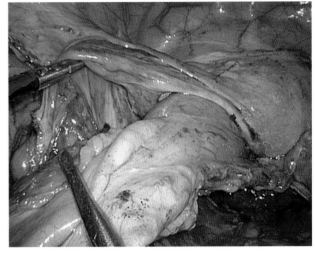

6.2.12

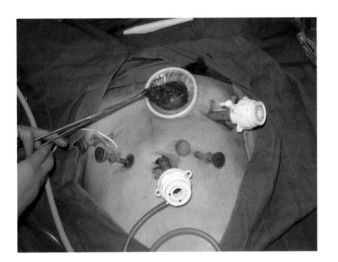

6.2.13

Specimen retrieval and intracorporeal anastomosis

This is the final stage of the entire operation. The pneumoperitoneum is abolished, and the specimen is delivered and excised via a 5–6 cm Pfannenstiel or left iliac fossa gridiron incision. In our experience, a muscle-splitting incision is less painful than a muscle-cutting incision, and results in less postoperative hernia. A sterile zip-lock bag is installed in the wound serving as protective drape during specimen extraction; alternatively Alexis® wound retractor can be used, which in our experience provides excellent wound retraction additionally (**Figure 6.2.13**). The colon is checked for the level of disease. Mesocolic division is done at the intended level of proximal colon transection, with at least a 5 cm mural margin, and marginal artery is ligated.

The length of the colon is doubly checked; if a left iliac fossa retrieval incision is made, a tension-free anastomosis requires approximately 15 cm of colon length outside the abdomen. The intended site of colonic transection is prepared, and following this the colon is transected and the specimen removed. An automatic or handsewn purse string is performed with 00 prolene suture. The colon is cleaned with iodine, and the anvil of a circular stapler (usually size 29 or above) is introduced and the purse-string tightened. The colon is replaced in the abdomen, and the retrieval wound is closed. If an Alexis® wound retractor was used, this can be temporarily closed with a sterile surgical glove; a gas-tight closure is ensured (**Figure 6.2.14**). Pneumoperitoneum is resumed and the small bowel is repositioned. After anal dilatation, the circular stapler is carefully inserted transanally. Intracorporeal anastomosis can now proceed in a similar fashion as in open surgery.

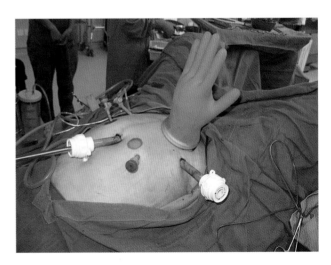

6.2.14

The tissue doughnuts are inspected, and air-leak test is performed using perioperative colonoscopy to confirm the integrity of the anastomosis. Endoscopic examination also helps to exclude staple line bleeding which might require endoscopic intervention at the same time (**Figure 6.2.15**). A drain is usually not necessary; if required, a suction drain is placed in the presacral space via a 5 mm port. Similarly, a covering stoma is usually not required. Definite indications for pelvic drainage and covering stoma include (1) incomplete proximal or distal doughnut or (2) a positive air-leak test (i.e. the anastomosis is not airtight) that persists after laparoscopic suture reinforcement.

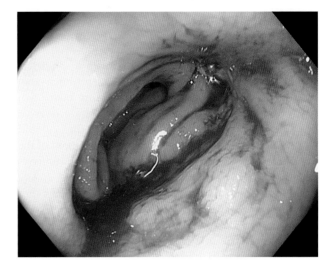

6.2.15

LAPAROSCOPIC SPHINCTER-SAVING TOTAL MESORECTAL EXCISION

Laparoscopic sphincter-saving total mesorectal excision (TME) should be performed with curative intent for most lesions in mid and low rectum where a sphincter-saving resection is considered feasible. For dubious lesion in mid rectum, the decision as to whether an ordinary anterior resection or a TME should be performed is made after full rectal mobilization – if, after full rectal mobilization, the distance between the tumor and the pelvic floor is less than 5 cm, a TME is considered mandatory. In practice, this implies almost all low anterior resections, i.e. resections that necessitate complete incision of pelvic peritoneal reflection and division of lateral ligaments, should potentially be total mesorectal excision if these resections are performed with curative intent. On the other hand, if the operation is performed with palliative intent, for instance in patients with metastatic disease, a 'total' mesorectal excision is then unnecessary; laparoscopic low anterior resection with 2 cm distal mural margin usually suffices in these circumstances.

Like laparoscopic anterior resection, contraindications of laparoscopic sphincter-saving TME include locally advanced disease with contiguous organ involvement; these patients necessitate an extensive *en bloc* resection more than that of a TME. In fact, in patients with radiological T3 or T4 disease, preoperative chemoirradiation should be considered; patients are reviewed afterwards to assess whether laparoscopic sphincter-salvage excision is still possible.

The entire operation is conveniently described in four stages.

Splenic flexure mobilization

After initial laparoscopy, splenic flexure take-down is usually required once it is decided to proceed with a sphincter-saving TME, especially when a colonic pouch–anal anastomosis is contemplated. Splenic flexure take-down is strongly recommended in patients who have received neoadjuvant chemoirradiation, in whom the sigmoid might be diseased due to radiotherapy. The positions of the operating team are shown in **Figure 6.2.16**; both surgeons and the camera assistant operate using monitor 2. The patient is put into a Trendelenburg position. The port sites are shown in **Figure 6.2.2**. Compared to laparoscopic high anterior resection, an additional 5 mm port is positioned over the epigastrium. The assistant surgeon continues to provide countertraction using the two 5 mm left iliac fossa ports. The camera assistant can use the subumbilical and the right iliac fossa 5–12 mm ports interchangeably, while the chief surgeon operates via the remaining ports. If the stomach is distended, a nasogastric tube can be placed by the anesthetist to facilitate mobilization of the transverse colon and splenic flexure.

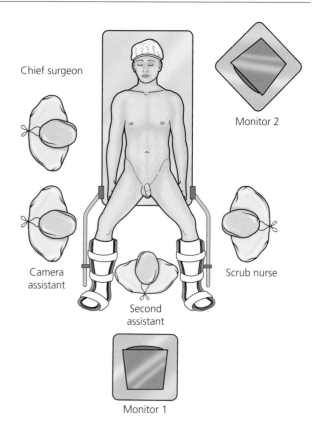

6.2.16

We favor a medial-first approach in splenic flexure take-down. The small bowel is kept in the right-side of the abdomen by tilting the operating table to the right (right-side-down position). The IMV is identified lateral to the duodenojejunal flexure, and is controlled and divided with Ligasure™ (**Figure 6.2.17**). Using the same device, blunt dissection is then carried out in the avascular plane between the mesentery of descending colon and the retroperitoneal

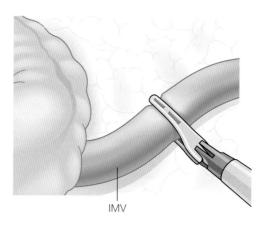

IMV

6.2.17

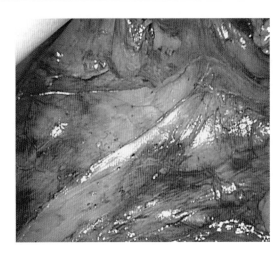

6.2.18

fascia (**Figure 6.2.18**). This dissection is continued laterally towards the splenic flexure for as far as possible, until the Gerota's fascia is exposed. The inferior border of the pancreas is identified (**Figure 6.2.19**), and caution is taken to keep the plane of dissection above the pancreas. If the above medial dissection has been adequately performed, then the subsequent lateral dissection is simple and straightforward. Starting from mid-transverse colon, the greater omentum is peeled off from the colon by incising the fascia just above the transverse colon. The posterior wall of the stomach should be clearly seen once the lesser sac is entered (**Figure 6.2.20**). By keeping close to the colon, further incision along the upper and lateral border will bring down the splenic flexure entirely. A head-up (reverse Trendelenburg) tilt helps improve exposure of the flexure during the final stage. Mobilization is considered adequate if the splenic flexure can be swung to the midline.

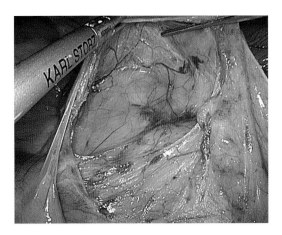

6.2.19

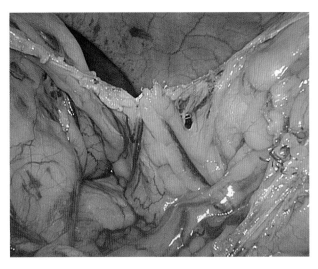

6.2.20

Sigmoid and pelvic dissection

The initial sigmoid and upper rectal mobilization are carried out as described for laparoscopic anterior resection. Medially, the mesenteric division (following IMA division) is continued proximally to join the previous window from the divided IMV (**Figure 6.2.21**). The ascending branch of the left colic artery, if not yet divided, should now be divided as proximally as possible to ensure maximal mobilization, caution being taken to avoid injury to the middle colic artery as well as the marginal artery.

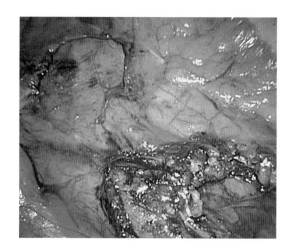

6.2.21

Different from laparoscopic high anterior resection, a much more extensive pelvic dissection should be carried out since total mesorectal excision is contemplated. Posteriorly, the presacral plane is dissected and followed as far as is comfortable. A combination of sharp and gentle blunt dissection is employed to separate or strip the mesorectum from the presacral fascia, caution being taken at all times not to breech the fascial envelope of the mesorectum (fascia propria) and the presacral fascia (**Figure 6.2.22**). The dissection next moves first to the right and then to the left of the rectum. By grasping the cotton tape and pulling the rectum to either side, the assistant surgeon can provide the necessary exposure and retraction for the chief surgeon and allow visualization of the correct plane of dissection. Distally, dissection deep down in the true pelvis is facilitated by turning the 30° laparoscope 180° upwards (**Figure 6.2.23**a and b); by so doing, a much better view can be obtained, and the sacrum and presacral fascia can be seen curving downwards and forwards.

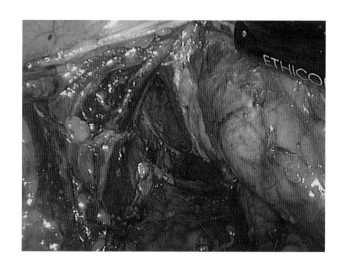

6.2.22

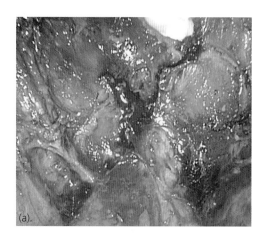

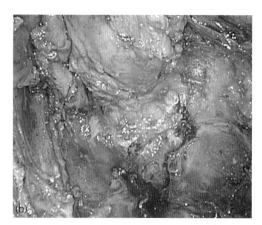

6.2.23

Attention is then turned to the anterior dissection. The rectum is pulled up (i.e. in a cephaloid direction) to expose the rectovesical or rectouterine pouch. The anterior peritoneal reflection is then incised. In male patients, the plane is developed between the rectum and the Denovilliers' fascia that covers the seminal vesicles (**Figure 6.2.24**), and in female patients between the rectum and the fascia covering the upper vagina. In female patients, a useful practice here is to have a second assistant's finger in the vagina (**Figure 6.2.25**); by retracting the vagina upwards from below, the rectovaginal plane can be easily established.

Next, the lateral ligaments on either side of the rectum are divided, and the whole rectum is mobilized down to the pelvic floor muscles. By this point, total rectal and mesorectal mobilization is completed, and the distal rectum should consist of a denuded muscle tube that is relatively free of mesorectum. The rectum is then divided with an endostapler (usually blue or gold cartridge) just above the pelvic floor after cytocidal lavage. In our experience, a smaller size stapler (30 mm) works better in the restricted space of the true pelvis. Several firings might be required. For those patients who have neoadjuvant irradiation, often the tissue is thicker and more edematous. Endostaplers of longer staple height (green cartridge) are more desirable in these cases. After rectal transection, a trial descent is performed to assess whether enough length of colon has been obtained for coloanal anastomosis.

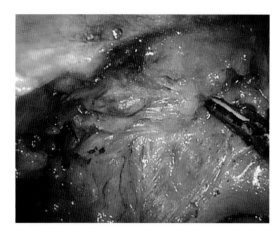

6.2.24

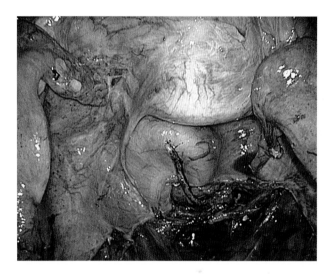

6.2.25

Exteriorization and resection of the specimen and creation of the colonic J-pouch

A 4–6 cm gridiron, musle-splitting incision is made in the left iliac fossa. Alternatively, a Pfannenstiel incision can be used. If the tumor is small, the specimen can also be extracted via the intended ileostomy site in the right iliac fossa. The wound is protected with a plastic bag or Alexis® wound retractor, and the specimen is retrieved and excised. The adequacy of the length of the colon is doubly checked. Normally, if the intended point of anastomosis in the colon can reach the symphysis pubis, then it should reach the anal verge without tension (**Figure 6.2.26**). Either a side-to-end anastomosis (L-pouch) or a colonic J-pouch can be constructed to improve subsequent bowel function. For colonic J-pouch, a 5 cm long pouch is fashioned with

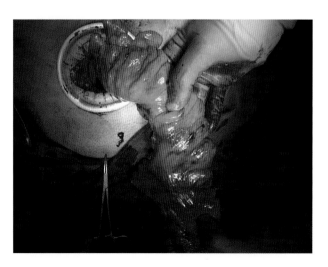

6.2.26

a 60 mm linear cutter using either the descending or the proximal sigmoid colon (**Figure 6.2.27**). The detachable anvil of a circular stapler is then inserted into the apex of the pouch and secured with a 00 prolene purse-string suture. The pouch is put back into the peritoneal cavity, and the gridiron incision is closed in layers. Alternatively, if an Alexis® wound retractor was used, this can be temporarily sealed with a sterile surgical glove.

Intracorporeal anastomosis and creation of covering ileostomy

Pneumoperitoneum is re-established. As the intracorporeal pouch-anal anastomosis is performed with the circular stapler under laparoscopic view, extreme caution must be exercised to avoid inadvertent stapling of the levator muscles or adjacent structures. In female patients, a second assistant can 'lift' the vagina upwards with a finger while closing the circular stapler. This manoeuver helps to exclude the vaginal vault from the anvil and prevents an otherwise unintentional rectovaginal fistula. In our experience, in some cases it is not possible to advance the stapler more than a few centimeters from below; under these circumstances, stapling is performed without having the stapler head fully accommodated in the distal anal stump. After construction of anastomosis, perioperative colonoscopy is carried out to exclude staple-line bleeding; air-leak test is performed simultaneously.

A covering stoma is recommended in laparoscopic sphincter-saving TME. We routinely perform loop ileostomy. A point in the terminal ileum about 20 cm from

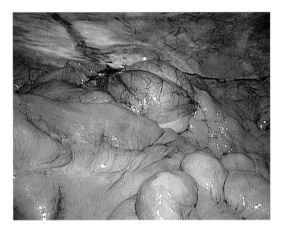

6.2.28

the ileocecal valve is then identified for the formation of a loop ileostomy. The antimesenteric border is marked lightly with bipolar cautery at two different points to differentiate the proximal and distal limbs. A cotton tape is tied around this segment via a mesenteric window, and the ileal segment is retracted by grasping the cotton tape, taking care to ensure that the ileum is not twisted during extraction. As the patient has been in a right-side down position, it is also important to make sure no small bowel loops are trapped in the 'lateral space' of the ileostomy (**Figure 6.2.28**). The presacral space is then drained via the left lower quadrant 5 mm port using a 'railroad' technique (**Figure 6.2.29**). The pneumoperitoneum is abolished,

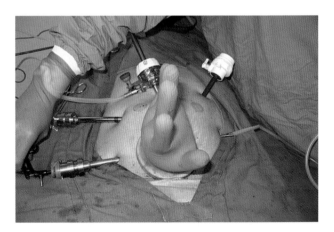

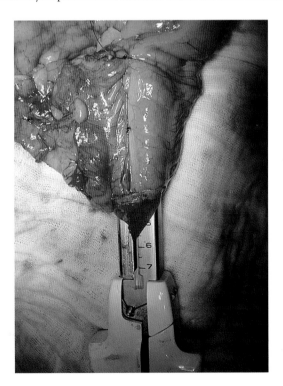

6.2.27

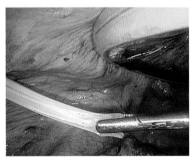

6.2.29

and a covering ileostomy is finally fashioned over the premarked stoma site. The minilaparotomy wound is closed in layers. All trocar sites above 5 mm require closure of the fascia to prevent trocar site hernia.

POSTOPERATIVE MANAGEMENT

Management of patients after laparoscopic anterior resection is essentially similar to that following traditional operations. Nasogastric tube is not usually required; if placed during surgery, it can be removed towards the end of the operation. The urinary catheter is kept for 1–2 days. Pneumatic compression stockings are removed and replaced by elastic stockings.

Patients can take liquids after the operation. Most advance to a regular diet by the second or third day. They are encouraged to ambulate on the day after the operation. The stockings are removed once the patient is walking. Drains, if any, are usually removed on the second postoperative day if the output is not excessive. Stoma care is taught to patients with covering ileostomy.

In patients with covering stoma, outpatient contrast study is arranged to ascertain the integrity of the anastomosis. Ileostomy closure can be arranged as early as 2 weeks after the initial operation.

Anterior resection – hand-assisted laparoscopic surgery

CHRISTOPHER J YOUNG

PRINCIPLES AND JUSTIFICATION

An anterior resection is usually carried out for a neoplastic growth of the sigmoid colon or rectum, or for recurrent diverticulitis, involving an anastomosis of the colon with the rectum. In the case of malignancy, it removes the primary tumor, the inferior mesenteric artery (IMA) and its accompanying lymph nodes, and joins bowel either end which has a good blood supply with no tension. Many surgeons have moved from 'pure' or straight laparoscopic colorectal surgery to routine use of the hybrid hand-assisted laparoscopic surgery (HALS). This is due to the advantages of shorter operating time, increased spatial awareness and tactile feedback, direct surgical access to the region under the handport, a reduced conversion rate, and an expanded ability to deal with the transverse colon and more advanced pathology, without loss in measured pain levels or recovery time.

Indications and contraindications

For those surgeons who selectively use HALS, indications include obese patients, cases where proximal pathology has not been able to be assessed preoperatively, and in bulky disease cases. If a handport is going to be used its advantages should be used from the start of the case.

During an anterior resection-HALS, the colon can be operated on laparoscopically and the rectum can be operated on laparoscopically or open if needed through the open handport, with minimal need or reason for conversion. Some 90 percent of rectal cancers can be treated with an anterior resection, and the HALS technique should allow all cases that can be performed and anastomosed open to be done as a HALS case.

Consent

Consent should be obtained, with discussion covering general risks of surgery and anesthesia, and specific complications of the entry wounds, risk of conversion to open procedure, and anastomotic and intra-abdominal complication risks.

PREOPERATIVE ASSESSMENT AND PREPARATION

Patients routinely have colonoscopy and computed tomography (CT) scans performed, and for rectal lesions may have magnetic resonance imaging (MRI), transrectal ultrasonography (TRUS), and/or positron emission tomography (PET) scans. A mechanical bowel preparation with sodium phosphate or polyethylene glycol-based preparations is taken by the patient. Prophylactic antibiotics are used in the perioperative period covering Gram-positive and Gram-negative organisms. Deep vein thrombosis (DVT) prophylaxis is achieved with calf compressors and 5000 units subcutaneous heparin twice daily. Abdominal marking by enterostomal therapy should occur if there is the chance or intention of a temporary or permanent stoma.

ANESTHESIA

General anesthesia is followed with endotracheal intubation and complete muscle relaxation.

OPERATION

Equipment

The equipment consists of a handport, two 12 mm and one 5 mm laparoscopic ports, two bowel grasping forceps, laparoscopic linear stapling device, energy source (harmonic scalpel, diathermy, scissors with diathermy), 10 mm laparoscopic camera with 30° lens.

If a 5 mm camera is available three 5 mm ports can be used in combination with the handport and a hemolock device for vessel ligation.

Position of patient

The patient is placed supine with a gel mat between the mattress and the patient's torso, with the legs in 'flat' lithotomy position in Allen stirrups. The arms are secured by the side with towels wrapped under the body, with an indwelling urinary catheter and nasogastric tube inserted. The monitor is placed on the left-hand side and if two monitors are available, the other monitor is placed at the head of the patient.

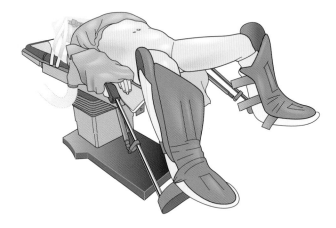

6.3.1

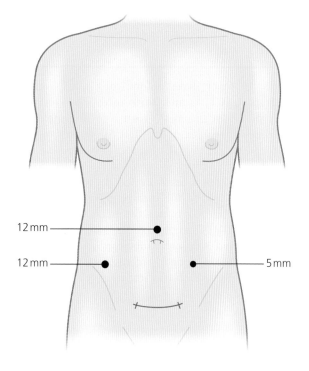

12 mm
12 mm
5 mm

6.3.2

Preparation of abdomen

The entire abdominal skin from nipples to upper thigh is prepared with a 10 percent povidone–iodine solution, with square draping of abdomen and leg drapes placed.

Incisions

A Pfannenstiel incision is made of 7–8 cm diameter, two fingers' breadth above the pubic symphysis, the width of the surgeon's hand at the level of the metacarpophalangeal joints. A 12 mm supraumbilical port, 12 mm RIF, and 5 mm LIF port site in the midclavicular line, supracristal plane are placed. Because the handport is placed first, an umbilical Hasson cannula is not required, and placing a supraumbilical port as the main camera port decreases clashing.

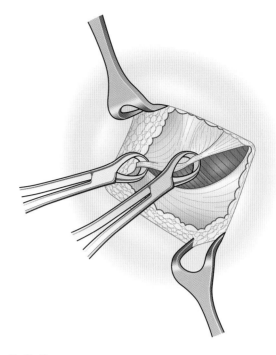

PFANNENSTIEL INCISION

The skin is incised transversely, continuing though the fat down to the anterior rectus sheath, and then through that transversely.

6.3.3

SEPARATION OF THE RECTI

The anterior rectus sheath is held up by forceps on the inferior lip of incision and the superior lip, and dissection anterior to the rectus abdominis muscle bellies, posterior to the anterior rectus sheath, is carried out down to the pubic symphysis and superior to the same height as the width of the Pfannenstiel incision. The left and right rectus abdominis muscle bellies are then held up with forceps and separated in the midline.

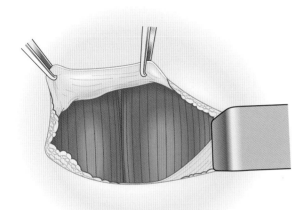

6.3.4

POSTERIOR RECTUS SHEATH

The posterior rectus sheath is then held up anteriorly either side of the midline with forceps and a vertical incision made and the peritoneum is entered. The incision is lengthened, avoiding the bladder and continuing to where mobilization is extended anterior to the recti.

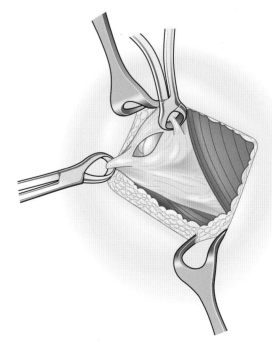

6.3.5

CHECK OF PFANNENSTIEL INCISION FOR HAND FIT

The left hand is placed through the defect to ensure the hand fits the hole. It must be kept in mind that the dominant hand is slightly larger in volume than the non-dominant hand, and therefore not to make too tight a fit when the hole fits the non-dominant hand but not the dominant hand. However, the wound retractor of the handport is usually easier to fit a hand through than the wound itself.

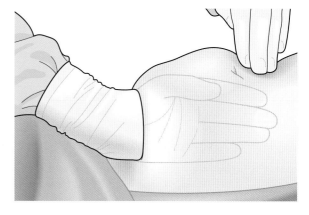

6.3.6

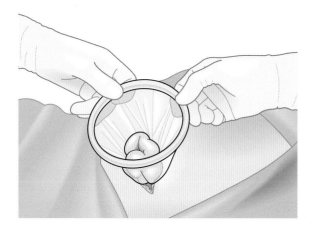

6.3.7

HANDPORT DEVICE PARTLY INSERTED

The wound retractor component of the handport is then inserted through the Pfannenstiel incision. The ring of the wound retractor should be checked to ensure it is in the peritoneal cavity and not anterior to the posterior rectus sheath. The wound retractor is then rolled to ensure a snug fit.

COMPLETE HANDPORT CONSTRUCTION

The top seal of the handport device is placed, then a 12 mm port through the handport, a pneumoperitoneum is created, and the abdominal contents are inspected. If adhesions are significant, one or two 5 mm ports can also be placed through the handport and the adhesions dissected all through the single Pfannenstiel incision and handport. A 12 mm supraumbilical port can then be placed under direct vision, angled more towards the left-hand side, and the CO_2 insufflation and laparoscope can be moved to this port, with removal of the 12 mm port from the handport.

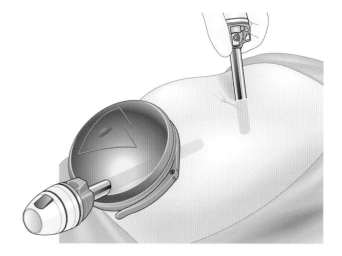

6.3.8

PLACING HAND THROUGH HANDPORT AND COMPLETING PORT INSERTIONS

The central hole in the handport is opened with the right-hand index and middle finger, then the left hand is placed through the device (and vice versa for right-hand insertion). A slurry of lubricant and water in a dish is useful, lubricating the back of the hand first before insertion. Having the inserting hand assume the position of an obstetrician's hand will aid insertion through the handport, as will running the opposite index finger under the lip of the handport device close to the inserting wrist to avoid the device telescoping into the peritoneum and pushing the wrist out of the abdomen, which can get tiresome if it is necessary to push against the device for the entire case. A longer pair of gloves will help ease movement through the handport and minimize any 'bunching' of material in the forearm which may increase forearm diameter. If longer gloves are not available, the fingers of a glove can be cut off and the remainder used as an extension of the glove on the forearm. This will be useful during the transverse colon and splenic flexure mobilization. With the hand and forearm through the handport, the LIF 5 mm and RIF 12 mm ports can be inserted using the palm and fingers of the opposite hand via the handport to control entry. A further RUQ 5 mm port may be required in some cases.

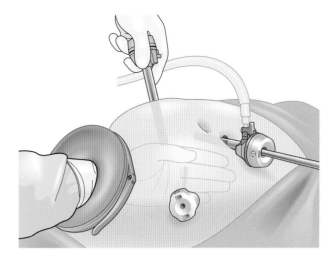

6.3.9

EXPLORATION OF THE PERITONEAL CAVITY

With all ports inserted and the left hand in the handport, a full inspection can be performed of normal anatomy and pathology. The surgeon stands between the legs with the cameraman to the patient's right side. If using a single monitor it will vary in position, at the patient's left or towards the head for the left-sided and splenic flexure mobilization, to the left if during rectal dissection the surgeon is between the legs, or at the feet if the surgeon moves to the sides of the patient.

Descending colon mobilization

With the patient placed in 15–20° left side up tilt, the left hand grasps the left colon with medial traction, not bringing the colon towards the camera or pulling inferiorly and potentially causing splenic injury. The addition of head up position usually does not aid retraction or view at this stage. Dissection commences with a harmonic scalpel on the line of Toldt. Keeping the retracting hand as flat as possible, and not obscuring the camera view, especially with the knuckles is beneficial. While the left colon is picked up first between thumb and palm in the pronated position, the hand then supinates to expose the lateral peritoneum and continues supinating more as dissection progresses. Commonly, the left hand if retracting properly will not be in the field of view. Tissue can often be splayed or retracted out between fingers as well.

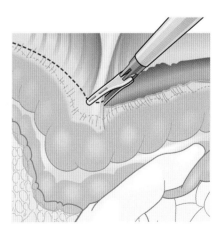

6.3.10

Slow, continual and gentle traction combined with dissection, both sharp and blunt but in small amounts, will expose the plane between the medial structures of the descending mesocolon and the contained left colic vessels, and identify and preserve the retroperitoneal structures including the left gonadal vessels, the left ureter, Gerota's fascia, the left kidney, and the tail of the pancreas.

An abdominal sponge can be placed via the handport and used to soak up blood, or can be used as a retractor, commonly of small bowel.

Splenic flexure mobilization

For splenic flexure mobilization see Chapter 5.8, Figures 5.8.2 and 5.8.3.

Dissection and ligation of inferior mesenteric vein

Whether this is done before or after the splenic flexure mobilization, the patient is placed in a 30° head up position, which in conjunction with the left side up keeps the small bowel away from the fourth part of duodenum and the paraduodenal fossa. The transverse colon is held up superiorly and anteriorly with a 5 mm grasper via the RIF 5 mm port. The left hand in a pronated position picks up the inferior mesenteric vein (IMV) between the thumb and forefinger, and retracts the IMV in a curve convex anteriorly. The ligament of Treitz and the paraduodenal fossa are dissected, incising posteriorly behind the IMV. After the fine web of fibers under the peritoneum posterior to the IMV are dissected by combination of sharp and blunt dissection, the left index finger is then placed behind and under the IMV with the hand slightly supinated, so that the window into the paraduodenal fossa can be enlarged, and the dissection onto or immediately adjacent to the index fingertip under the IMV and showing through the peritoneum in the left lateral position to IMV can be completed. The thumb and index finger should now be encircling the IMV. A linear cutting stapler with vascular staples is then inserted through the RIF 12 mm port and the left hand used to guide it around the IMV and ligate and transect the IMV. Often at this point the middle, ring, and little fingers of the left hand can be used to keep any small bowel or transverse colon away. Following vessel ligation, the left hand can be used for potential hemostasis of the IMV stump if necessary as the 5 mm grasper through the LIF 5 mm port is usually holding away the transverse colon. It is important that staplers are placed and closed without any stretch on the vessels, as the vessels will remain stretched in the staplers grasp after closure and be more likely to bleed from quick retraction following transection, even if the stretch is relaxed after the stapler is applied.

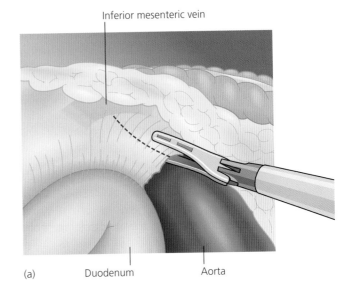

(a)   Inferior mesenteric vein

Duodenum   Aorta

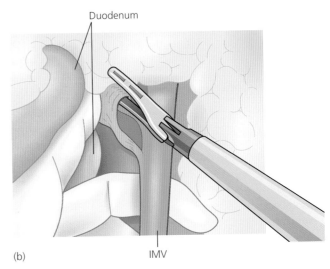

(b)   Duodenum

IMV

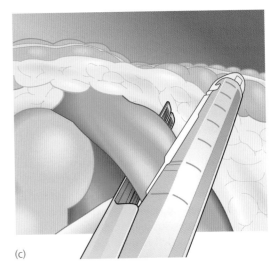

(c)

6.3.11

Sigmoid colon mobilization if not completed already

The sigmoid colon mobilization is an extension of the descending colon mobilization going inferiorly, and of the left upper rectal mobilization going superiorly; however, if standing between the legs the surgeon is presented with a reversed image on the monitor. The surgeon may want to stand on the right side, and retract with the right hand and dissect with the left hand.

The lateral peritoneal attachments of the sigmoid colon are more inconsistent than the descending colon and the right upper rectum, and staying in the correct plane can be enhanced by performing those stages first. A difficult sigmoid, or difficult adhesions, may need to be dealt with first and may be done directly through the open handport. Sigmoid mobilization progresses with identification of the sigmoid vessels, and identification and preservation of the left gonadal vessels, the left ureter, and the common and internal iliac vessels.

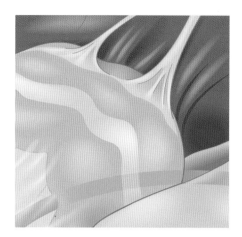

6.3.12

Right side of upper rectum mobilization

Once the descending colon, splenic flexure, and IMV are complete, the patient will be placed in steep head down, usually 30° but up to 45°, to remove the small bowel from the pelvis. Standing between the legs and with the left hand through the handport, the thumb and index finger can be used to pick up the IMA so that it curves convex anteriorly, and the peritoneum is incised with the harmonic scalpel parallel to the curve of the IMA approximately 1 cm posterior to the IMA, at the site of junction of the mesosigmoid and posterior parietal peritoneum, so that the pneumoperitoneum dissects in the avascular retrorectal fascial plane. The peritoneal incision is extended and the fine cobweb of fibers between the retrorectal fascia and the presacral tissue with the superior hypogastric nerves and nervi erigentes and its adjacent peritoneum is dissected and preserved, while preserving intact the retrorectal fascia and the mesorectum.

Much of the dissection behind the retrorectal fascia is completed from the right across to the left-hand side, so that when the left upper rectum is approached there is usually only peritoneum left intact adjacent to mesorectum. Dissection from the right upper rectum should not proceed too far left laterally though and end up behind the left ureter.

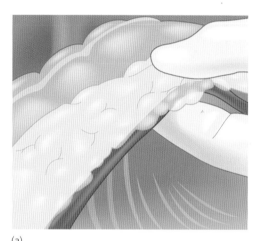

(a)

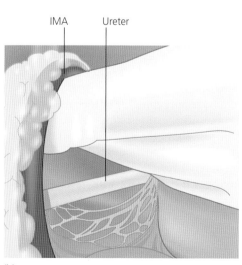

IMA   Ureter

(b)

6.3.13

Left side of upper rectum mobilization

The left hand is than supinated with the palm placed under the IMA and mesorectum and the rectum pulled to the right. The thin peritoneum with gas behind it should then be visible on the left, and the left peritoneum is incised,

joining the right-hand side dissection. Dissection continues up to the root of the IMA with the aorta posteriorly.

Along with complete left-sided colon and rectum mobilization, identification, and preservation of the left gonadal vessels, the left ureter, and the common and internal iliac vessels is ensured.

Ligation of IMA

Following dissection of the IMA and identification of the retroperitoneal structures including the left gonadal vessels and the left ureter, the IMA can be transected near the aorta with a laparoscopic stapler with vascular staples, passed through the RIF 12 mm port. The left-hand thumb and index finger present through the handport can control any potential bleeding, or DeBakey forceps via the LIF 5 mm port, or both. The left ureter's position and clear separation from the IMA and stapler is always checked one more time before firing the stapler.

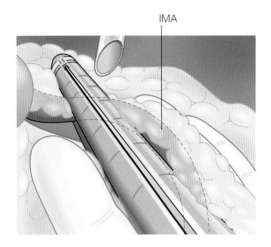

6.3.14

Distal mobilization of rectum below upper rectum for low and ultra-low anterior resection

The distal limit of resection is determined by the pathology and its site. Tumors of the sigmoid and rectosigmoid region, and diverticular disease usually require resection of the upper one-third of rectum and colorectal anastomosis, referred to as a high anterior resection. For practical reasons of circular stapler access or thickening of the upper rectal wall, or extension of inflammation, a low anterior resection through or below the mid rectum may be required for the same pathologies. All mid and low rectal tumors require complete or total mesorectal excision (TME), necessitating transection of the muscular rectal tube at or just above the anorectal junction, followed by colorectal or coloanal anastomosis, and is referred to as an ultra-low anterior resection.

A surgeon who can work with reverse image should

stand between the legs, as this aids getting the left hand out of the visual field. Otherwise, if using the handport with hand through it, the surgeon who can dissect with the hand out of the visual field should stand on the left side for right rectal mobilization. Likewise, the surgeon should stand on the right for left rectal mobilization if he can dissect with hand out of the visual field. An extra port inserted through the handport may also be used and the rectal mobilization completed laparoscopically without hand assist.

Posterior dissection continues down the avascular retrorectal plane, creating the so-called 'buttocks' of the mesorectum, continuing until the mesorectum is no longer, and the rectum is a straight tube of muscle, and the levator ani is exposed. At the point of the anorectal junction, white radial fibers between the muscularis propria as it becomes the internal anal sphincter and the levator ani and external sphincter complex will be seen, and signify the distal limit of TME dissection.

Lateral rectal dissection is an extension of the posterior dissection, and as the lower one-third of the rectal lateral dissection is approached, visualization and preservation of the nervi erigentes and the inferior hypogastric plexus should be a focus, especially at the anterolateral positions adjacent to the lateral edge of the seminal vesicles where the neurovascular bundle passes. Middle rectal vessels will occasionally be found and require ligation during the lateral dissection, more often in younger males.

Anterior dissection between the posterior vaginal wall and anterior rectum is usually performed immediately on the vaginal wall side of fascia in tumor cases, or in a male on the seminal vesicle and prostate side of Denonvilliers' fascia.

The right ureter is usually in less of a close relationship to the rectum than the left ureter, but is routinely identified and preserved, even if seen through the peritoneum.

Adjuncts to complete rectal dissection and mobilization

Females tend to have a more generous pelvis allowing full rectal mobilization laparoscopically through the handport, either using a hand or instruments through the handport.

If rectal mobilization becomes more difficult, as in a large male with a narrow pelvis, the surgeon can progress from the laparoscopic approach with a hand through the handport (**Figure 6.3.15**a); to the laparoscopic approach with instruments in the handport, a St Mark's pelvic retractor can be placed through the handport with control of the pneumoperitoneum by using a glove sealing the handport (**Figure 6.3.15**b); to the open approach with instruments through the wound retractor of the handport (**Figure 6.3.15**c); to the open approach with a non-muscle cutting extension of the Pfannenstiel incision and a circular self-retainer (Turner-Warwick with four small wound retractors) in the wound (**Figure 6.3.15**d). The Pfannenstiel incision can be enlarged after removing the handport wound retractor. It is best to then lengthen the transverse skin incision and the vertical separation of the recti and the peritoneal incision.

If the colon mobilization has been completed laparoscopically, there is almost never an advantage with pelvic access from a midline extension, converting a transverse Pfannenstiel incision into an inverted T incision (Pfannenstiel and midline incision together). In the author's experience this is a disadvantage with higher rates of pain, wound bleeding, and wound infection if there is any muscle cutting of the recti or conversion to open.

Specimen resection and anastomosis

For lesions between the mid sigmoid and rectum, the proximal bowel transection will be at the junction of the descending and sigmoid colon. After two Kocher bowel clamps are applied, a 2-0 polypropylene (prolene) 'whipstitch'-type purse-string is inserted, and the head of the circular stapling device inserted.

Distal limits depend on whether the anastomosis is to be high, mid or low rectum. About 60 percent of cases can be completed directly through the open handport wound retractor using a St Mark's retractor.

Mesorectal transection is required for high and low anterior resections, but not for ultra-low as this will be below the mesorectum and there is only the muscular tube of the rectum to deal with. It is not essential whether the muscular tube of rectum or the mesorectum is transected first, and often laparoscopically it is easier to transect the rectal tube first, after dissecting close to muscle wall and encircling the rectal wall.

The author routinely performs a double-stapling colorectal anastomosis technique. When distal bowel transection is suitable laparoscopically, a laparoscopic linear cutting stapler is introduced through the RIF 12 mm port. If distal bowel transection is required through the open handport wound retractor, the TL30 easily fits, but the TL60 usually has to be rocked gently through the Pfannenstiel wound retractor.

The pelvis is irrigated with normal saline after rectal transection and inspected for hemostasis.

A double-stapled colorectal or coloanal anastomosis with a circular end to end stapler is performed, followed by checking of donuts, and an air and water test for anastomotic patency. A drain is placed through the LIF 5 mm port site.

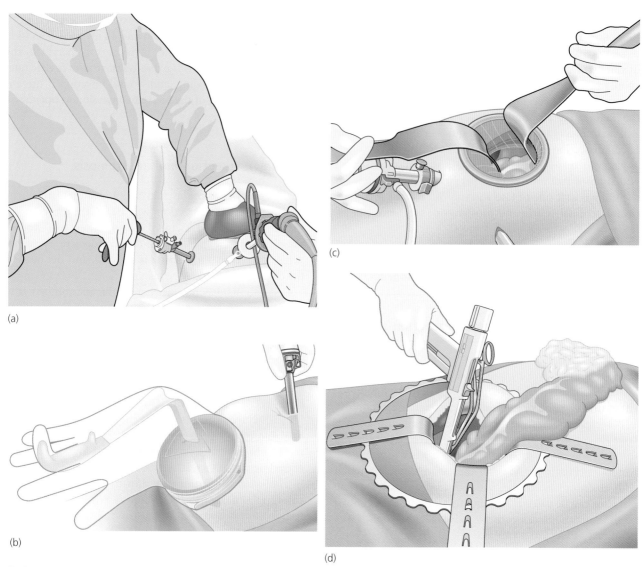

(a)

(b)

(c)

(d)

6.3.15

Wound closure

The Pfannenstiel incision is closed in layers, initially with the posterior rectus sheath and peritoneum closed with a 1 polyglactin continuous suture, and then the rectus abdominis muscle bellies are closed with interrupted 0 polyglactin, just picking up the medial body. A continuous 1 PDS suture closes the anterior rectus sheath, and the skin is closed with a 3-0 monocryl subcuticular suture. All port sites >5 mm are closed at the anterior rectus sheath level with 1 Biosyn™ on a J-shaped needle using S-shaped retractors for exposure.

If a temporary loop ileostomy is made in the RIF, ensure that the anterior rectus sheath is pulled down towards the pubis when the ileostomy site is made, or the trephine can

be made too low through the anterior rectus sheath. If that occurred, following Pfannenstiel wound closure, the small bowel at the ileostomy would be pulled and kinked towards the pubis.

POSTOPERATIVE CARE

Anesthesia will usually instill transversus abdominus plane blocks and a patient-controlled analgesia machine. DVT prophylaxis is maintained with thromboembolic deterrent stockings and subcutaneous heparin 5000 units twice daily. Nasogastric tube if used intraoperatively is removed except in cases with large bowel obstruction. Early mobilization is encouraged with fluids day 1 postoperatively as tolerated.

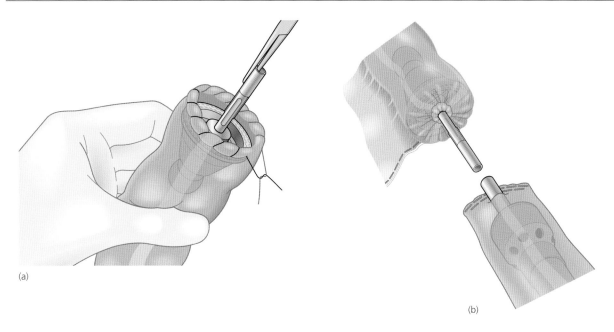

(a)

(b)

6.3.16

FURTHER READING

Lee SW, Sonoda T, Milsom JW. Expediting of laparoscopic rectal dissection using a hand-access device. *Diseases of the Colon and Rectum* 2007; **50**: 927–9.

Marcello PW, Fleshman JW, Milsom JW *et al.* Hand-assisted laparoscopic vs. laparoscopic colorectal surgery: a multicenter, prospective, randomized trial. *Diseases of the Colon and Rectum* 2008; **51**: 818–26.

Milsom JW, de Oliveira O, Trencheva KI *et al.* Long-term outcomes of patients undergoing curative laparoscopic surgery for mid and low rectal cancer. *Diseases of the Colon and Rectum* 2009; **52**: 1215–22.

Nakajima K, Lee SW, Cocilovo C *et al.* Hand-assisted laparoscopic colorectal surgery using GelPort. *Surgical Endoscopy* 2004; **18**: 102–5.

Sonoda T, Pandey S, Trencheva K *et al.* Longterm complications of hand-assisted versus laparoscopic colectomy. *Journal of the American College of Surgeons* 2009; **208**: 62–6.

Tjandra JJ, Chan MK, Yeh CH. Laparoscopic- vs. hand-assisted ultralow anterior resection: a prospective study. *Diseases of the Colon and Rectum* 2008; **51**: 26–31.

Anterior resection – robotic

ALESSIO PIGAZZI AND JULIO GARCIA-AGUILAR

PRINCIPLES AND JUSTIFICATION

Laparoscopic low anterior resection (LAR) for rectal cancer offers short-term advantages compared with the open approach. However, the procedure is technically challenging and has not gained wide acceptance among rectal cancer surgeons around the world. The major limitation of laparoscopic rectal surgery is due to the need to perform a circumferential dissection in the confined pelvic space, which renders optimal retraction and visualization difficult. The technical features of robotic technology facilitate the minimally invasive approach to rectal surgery. With three working arms, the robot provides superior retraction without having to rely heavily on a skilled assistant. The articulation of the robotic instruments allows the surgeon to follow the contour of the rectum and mesorectum with greater ease than with straight conventional laparoscopic instruments. In addition, the high-definition, three-dimensional camera gives an ideal visualization of all pelvic structures.

Our preferred approach is to perform a hybrid laparoscopic/robotic procedure, with laparoscopic mobilization of the flexure and descending colon, and subsequent robotic total mesorectal excision (RTME). The entire operation is performed with a minimally invasive approach without the use of hand assistance or open techniques. A suprapubic minilaparotomy is used in some cases only for specimen extraction; however, an entirely intracorporeal procedure with transanal extraction and no abdominal incision will also be described.

SURGEON SELECTION

While the robot facilitates pelvic dissection, the RTME technique can be technically demanding and there is undoubtedly a learning curve with this procedure.

Surgeons wishing to embrace RTME should ideally meet the following criteria:

- Be comfortable performing laparoscopic segmental colon resections without hand assistance and with reasonably low conversion rates.
- Have had robotic experience with inanimate models, animal and cadaveric sessions in order to be able to effectively utilize and troubleshoot the robotic system.
- Have a thorough understanding of the principles of total mesorectal excision (TME) and an overall rectal volume of at least ten cases per year.

PATIENT SELECTION

We use robotic LAR for any patient that presents with non-sphincter invading mid and low rectal cancer. It must be emphasized, however, that surgeons at the beginning of their learning curve should offer the procedure more selectively. Ideal cases at the beginning of one's robotic experience are female patients of normal body mass index (BMI) and with higher tumors. For a double stapled anastomosis after LAR, a distance of at least 2 cm between the lower edge of the tumor and the anorectal ring is ideal.

PREOPERATIVE

Preoperative imaging of all patients with rectal cancer should involve chest x-ray, computed tomography (CT) scan of the abdomen and pelvis, and endorectal ultrasound or pelvic magnetic resonance imaging (MRI). Neoadjuvant chemoradiation treatment should be offered to patients with locally advanced tumors according to the surgeon's preference and experience. A bowel preparation is recommended the day before surgery to render manipulation of the intestine easier.

OPERATION

Patient positioning

We routinely place a large foam mat under the patient to prevent sliding during positional changes of the operating bed. The upper chest is further secured with a velcro strap. After induction of general anesthesia, the patient is moved to a modified lithotomy position. A digital rectal examination to confirm tumor location is performed; rectal irrigation with water or iodine-based solution is done if bowel preparation is not optimal. A urinary catheter is inserted. The perineum is prepped sterile only if a transanal extraction and handsewn coloanal anastomosis are anticipated.

Hybrid laparoscopic/robotic LAR

It is our preference to perform the splenic flexure takedown and colon mobilization laparoscopically. This is due to the fact that current robotic systems do not allow the operating bed to be moved after the cart has been docked. Although we have performed and described a fully robotic procedure, in our experience a robotic flexure mobilization with the patient in a fixed position can be challenging, especially when operating on patients of high BMI. In addition, the fully robotic LAR requires a high degree of experience with robotic port placement and cart positioning in order to avoid collisions of the robotic arm.

Port placement

Pneumoperitoneum is created with the Verres needle inserted in the left subcostal region (Palmer's point). The abdomen is insufflated to 15 mmHg. A 12 mm camera port C is placed halfway between the pubis and the xiphoid and the abdomen is inspected (**Figure 6.4.1**). For the laparoscopic part we utilize a 30° telescope. A general principle is that all robotic ports need to be at least 8–10 cm apart from each other in order to avoid collisions. A 12 mm trocar (R1) is then placed in a point roughly halfway between C and right anterior superior iliac spine

(ASIS) which usually corresponds to the midclavicular line (MCL). Care needs to be taken to avoid the inferior epigastric vessels in this area. R1 will be the main stapling/clipping port for vessels, mesentery, and bowel and usually serves as the site for the protective ileostomy if one is created. It will be used by the surgeon's right hand during the laparoscopic part and will be the first robotic arm site during the RTME. The newly designed endo-wrist robotic stapler requires a special 15 mm robotic trocar. A robotic 8 mm trocar (R2) will be inserted in the same position on the left side. The third robotic port (R3) will be about 8–10 cm more lateral to R2 usually just above the left ASIS. A first 5 mm laparoscopic port (L1) is placed 8–10 cm above R1 in the MCL. A second 5 mm port (L2) will be halfway between the MCL and the midline, usually just to the right of the falciform ligament. It must be stressed that some variations in this port set-up will be necessary depending on the patient's gender, body habitus, and tumor location. For instance, in large male patients with low tumors, the position of the three robotic ports (R1–R3) will be shifted more medially in order to prevent the robotic arms from hitting the narrow pelvic sidewalls and reach the levator plane more easily.

Laparoscopic mobilization of splenic flexure and left colon

Both surgeon and assistant stand on the patient's right side. The surgeon will mainly use R1 and L1, while the assistant has the camera and L2. In order to better reach a high splenic flexure the surgeon can also easily utilize R2. A medial-to-lateral mobilization of the left and sigmoid colon is carried out. The inferior mesenteric vein (IMV) is used as the initial anatomic landmark. To expose the IMV, the ligament of Treitz and the attachments between the proximal jejunum and the descending mesocolon may need to be divided sharply so that the small bowel can be retracted towards the right upper quadrant (**Figure 6.4.2**).

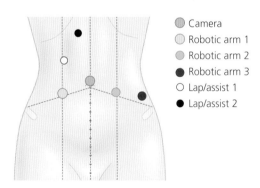

Camera
Robotic arm 1
Robotic arm 2
Robotic arm 3
Lap/assist 1
Lap/assist 2

6.4.1 Port site placement.

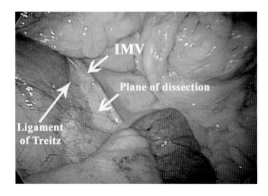

6.4.2 Exposure of the inferior mesenteric vein (IMV).

Next, the peritoneum just under the vein is incised, and the medial-to-lateral dissection is begun by separating the mesocolon from Toldt's fascia. The dissection proceeds toward the abdominal wall identifying and preserving the ureter and gonadal vessels. In order to avoid traction injuries we recommend early division of the IMV near its insertion posterior to the pancreas where the IMV is azygous, traveling without a paired artery (**Figure 6.4.3**). More distally, the IMV runs parallel to the left colic artery (LCA). Therefore the IMV/LCA pedicle should be followed inferiorly and freed from its posterior attachments to the aorta until the origin of the inferior mesenteric artery (IMA) is identified. The peritoneum over the sacral promontory just medial to the right common iliac vessels is incised entering the areolar plane posterior to the superior rectal artery. By extending this dissection plane to the left, the origin of the IMA is identified and the vascular anatomy creates a characteristic T-shaped structure (**Figure 6.4.4**).

After identifying the ureter and gonadal vessels in the retroperitoneal plane, the IMA can now be divided. We routinely divide the artery with an energy sealing device between clips at the origin to obtain a full mesocolic mobilization and ensure a tension-free low anastomosis. The medial-to-lateral dissection is taken laterally towards the abdominal wall. The colon is then retracted medially and the peritoneum along the white line of Toldt is opened freeing completely the descending and sigmoid colon. Next, the splenic flexure is taken down by opening the gastrocolic omentum just below the gastroepiploic vessels or by dividing the avascular coloepiploic attachments next to the bowel wall. The splenocolic ligament is divided (**Figure 6.4.5**). An energy-based vessel sealing device is recommended for these steps of the operation. Finally, the attachments of the body and tail of the pancreas to the colonic mesentery are carefully divided obtaining a full splenic flexure release.

The mesentery of the descending colon is then divided from the stump of the IMA towards the colon at the point

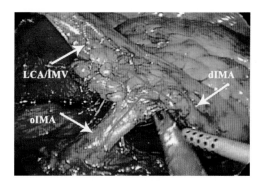

6.4.4 Identification of inferior mesenteric artery (IMA). The IMA origin (oIMA) gives off two main branches: the left colic artery (LCA) which travels with the inferior mesenteric vein (IMV) and the distal IMA which gives sigmoidal branches and becomes the superior rectal artery.

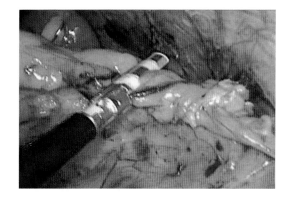

6.4.5 Division of the splenocolic ligament.

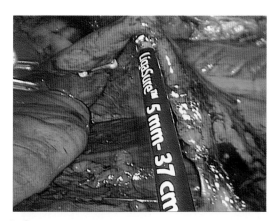

6.4.3 The clip shows the divided inferior mesenteric vein traveling with the left colic artery. The medial to lateral dissection plane can be seen beneath the vessels.

of future division of the bowel, usually at the junction of the descending and sigmoid colon. The mesentery can be divided with an energy source or with several fires of a vascular stapler. Alternatively, the mesentery can be divided with electrocautery clipping the mesenteric vessels. It is recommended to divide the marginal artery at this time, particularly if extraction of the specimen though the anus is anticipated, to avoid tearing the vessels during the extraction maneuvers.

Robotic total mesorectal excision

After completing the colonic mobilization, the robotic pelvic dissection can begin. A significant degree of Trendelenburg position is often necessary to maintain the small intestine out of the pelvis. A four-arm da Vinci® robotic system is now the system of choice. These newer surgical robots can be docked over the patient's left hip, permitting access to the anus and perineum during the entire procedure (**Figure 6.4.6**). With the first-generation standard da Vinci, this approach is not possible because the arms' reach and range of motion are limited; thus the cart must be brought into the field in between the patient's legs.

The camera arm with a 0° telescope is first docked to trocar C. Next, we attach a robotic trocar to arm one and 'piggyback' this into the 12 mm R1 port. Arms 2 and 3 will be docked to trocars R2 and R3, respectively. For robotic instruments we choose scissors for arm 1, a fenestrated bipolar grasper in 2, and a 'prograsp' grasper in 3. The assistant remains on the right side using ports L1 and L2 for suctioning and retraction of the rectum out of the pelvis.

With the assistant elevating the rectosigmoid junction the dissection begins posteriorly at the sacral promontory entering the plane between the fascia propria of the rectum and the presacral fascia (**Figure 6.4.7**). Care is taken to identify and preserve the hypogastric nerves on both sides. The dissection is carried out almost exclusively with monopolar cautery applied with the scissors in short bursts to prevent excessive smoke accumulation and injuring the nerves. The TME proceeds along the areolar plane down to the rectococcygeal ligament which is opened.

It is important to avoid grasping the mesorectum with any robotic graspers as the strength of these instruments is

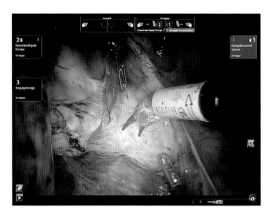

6.4.7 Development of the posterior mesorectal plane at the sacral promontory.

considerable and will result in undesirable injuries to the fascia propria and bleeding. Our preference is to use the bipolar grasper in arm 2 chiefly as a retracting device.

Anteriorly, the peritoneal reflection is incised and the dissection is continued along the rectovaginal septum in women or the rectovesical/rectoprostatic (Denonvilliers) fascia in men. Arm 3 is extremely useful to retract the bladder and other anterior structures as the dissection proceeds distally (**Figures 6.4.8** and **6.4.9**). The articulation of the robotic scissor tips allows the surgeon to carry out the dissection utilizing ideal angles of attack.

Laterally, the dissection proceeds along the sidewalls medial to both ureters. Care must be taken to avoid injuring the autonomic pelvic plexus. The middle hemorrhoidal vessels are identified and controlled with bipolar cautery in arm 2 and subsequently cut (**Figure 6.4.10**).

The dissection proceeds down to the pelvic floor separating the fatty mesorectum from the levators. Digital rectal examinations are performed regularly to ascertain the level of the tumor in preparation for rectal division.

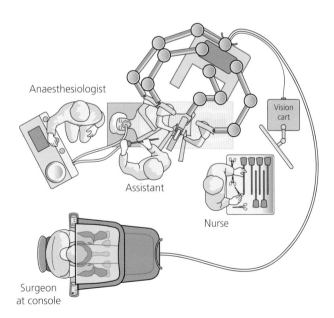

6.4.6 Position of the da Vinci robot using a left hip approach.

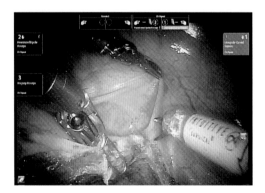

6.4.8 Incision of the peritoneal reflection. Note the position of the third working arm holding the anterior peritoneum.

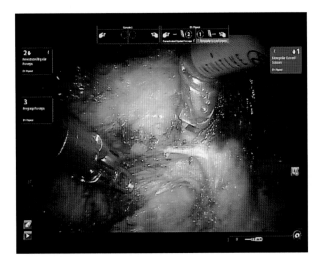

6.4.9 Development of the anterior dissection plane behind Denovilliers' fascia.

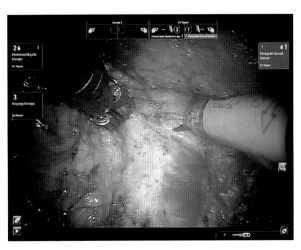

6.4.11 Exposure of the pelvic floor on the right side.

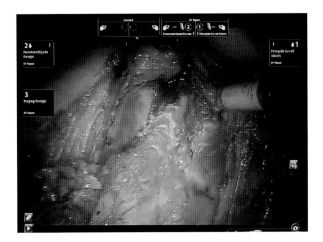

6.4.12 Completed dissection of the distal rectum to the level of the anal hiatus. Note the absence of mesorectum at this level.

6.4.10 Dissection of the right middle rectal vessels.

The rectum is lifted off the levator muscle and prepared circumferentially (**Figures 6.4.11** and **6.4.12**).

Before dividing the rectum, one member of the team performs a digital rectal examination under direct visualization to fully assess the distal margin. In selected cases, we have tied a suture around the distal rectum to close off the rectal lumen and ensure the application of the stapler below the level of the tumor. This maneuver is not technically challenging thanks to the articulation of the robotic arms (**Figure 6.4.13**).

The rectum can be divided with a standard endoscopic stapler introduced through the 12 mm laparoscopic trocar, or the endo-wrist robotic stapler introduced through the 15 mm R1 trocar. Stapler cartridge length should not exceed

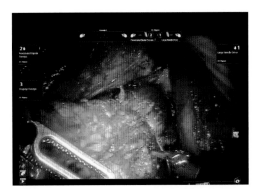

6.4.13 Closure of the rectum with an absorbable suture distal to the tumor prior to stapling.

45 mm in order to easily apply the jaws over the bowel. Usually two or three applications are necessary and it is important to maintain proper alignment in order to avoid crossing staple lines (**Figure 6.4.14**). A green cartridge is indicated given the thickness and pliability of the rectum, especially after neoadjuvant chemoradiation.

After dividing the rectum, the robotic cart can be undocked. We routinely extract the specimen through a 3–4 cm suprapubic Pfannenstiel mini-laparotomy covered with a plastic wound protector. The proximal bowel is divided and an anvil secured to the proximal colon with a handsewn purse-string suture. After closing the fascia with interrupted absorbable sutures, the anastomosis is created with a circular stapler under direct laparoscopic visualization (**Figure 6.4.15**). A diverting loop ileostomy is indicated in the case of very low anatomosis, especially after neoadjuvant chemoradiation therapy.

Transanal extraction techniques

In lieu of a LAR with a traditional double stapled anastomosis and transabdominal extraction, it is also possible to extract the specimen transanally and perform the anastomosis manually. This technique is indicated when the tumor is very close to the anorectal ring and applying the linear stapler safely can be difficult. The rectal wall is divided at the beginning of the case transanally with a clear view of the distal margin. The transanal dissection is then carried outside of the rectum and the mesorectum as far as possible. The open lumen of rectum distal to

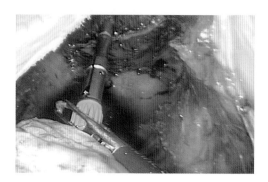

6.4.15 Completion of the coloanal anastomosis.

the tumor is closed off with interrupted sutures to avoid spillage during the pelvic dissection (**Figure 6.4.16**). The robotic dissection proceeds until the perineal dissection is met and the bowel is passed through the rectal stump, covered with a wound protector and delivered to the outside. The proximal bowel is divided outside the anus at the point where the mesentery and the marginal vessels have been previously divided and the anastomosis can then be accomplished manually with interrupted sutures (**Figure 6.4.17**).

These techniques avoid an abdominal incision and the potential for wound complications and incisional pain but require a higher degree of technical expertise thus are not recommended at the beginning of the learning curve.

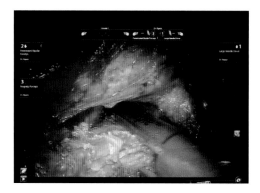

6.4.14 Division of rectum. The stapler is applied through a right lower quadrant port and the rectum is sequentially divided.

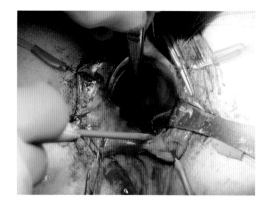

6.4.16 Transanal division of the rectal wall at the beginning of the procedure and closure of the rectum distal to the tumor.

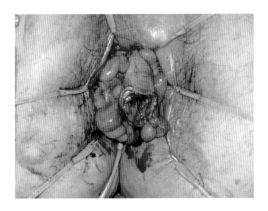

6.4.17 Divided proximal colon ready for handsewn anastomosis.

POSTOPERATIVE

Most patients will only experience mild discomfort after RTME and patient-controlled analgesia is usually not necessary. Nasogastric suctioning is not indicated after robotic LAR. Patients can be started on clear liquids on postoperative day 1 and advanced as tolerated. If a protective ileostomy is placed intravenous fluids are continued until the day of discharge and proper patient education about fluid replenishment is given to prevent dehydration when recovering at home.

Coloanal anastomosis with intersphincteric resection and colon J-pouch construction

JÉRÉMIE H LEFÈVRE AND YANN PARC

PRINCIPLES AND JUSTIFICATION

Sphincter-saving low anterior resection is now widely accepted for the treatment of cancer of the middle and lower thirds of the rectum. Long-term survival and local recurrence rates after low anterior resection are similar to those obtained by total excision of the rectum, once the distal resection margin is at least 1 cm. After rectal excision with very low colorectal and coloanal anastomosis (CAA), patients often experience a degree of urgency and increased frequency of defecation which results from loss of the rectal reservoir. In order to improve the functional results, a J-shaped colonic reservoir may be constructed[1, 2] and an anastomosis performed between the apex of the reservoir and the anal canal. For ultra-low tumor, an intersphincteric resection may be performed in selected patients to avoid an abdominoperineal resection and a permanent colostomy.[3] The authors' practice is to reserve intersphincteric resection for tumors for motivated patients with T1 or T2 tumors confined to the upper part of the anal canal such that a 1 cm distal margin is feasible.

INDICATIONS

This technique is indicated for malignant tumors of the rectum located at a distance of 1–8 cm from the dentate line, and in some benign lesions of the rectum, such as circumferential villous tumors where the lower margin of the lesion extends 0–2 cm above the dentate line.

PREOPERATIVE MANAGEMENT

A low residue diet is started 2 days before surgery. Bowel preparation is carried out using 3–5 liters of polyethylene glycol or one single dose of X-Prep® the day before surgery. Enemas are given if necessary to complete bowel cleaning. The abdomen is shaved from nipple to the pubic symphysis, as is the perineum, on the morning of surgery. Patients shower with povidone–iodine soap the day before the operation. General anesthesia with muscle relaxant is required and an epidural anesthesic may be used as a supplement. A nasogastric tube is inserted into the stomach.

OPERATIONS

LAPAROTOMY

Position of the patient

The patient is positioned in the modified lithotomy-Trendelenburg position, with the hips flexed at 30° for the abdominal phase and 100° for the perineal phase. Great care should be taken in positioning the legs to avoid deep vein thrombosis, compartment syndrome or external peroneal nerve paralysis. The legs are protected with a spongy cover and mobilized every hour during the procedure. A Foley catheter is placed into the bladder. Alternatively, a percutaneous suprapubic catheter may be placed after the abdomen has been opened.

The skin of the abdomen and the perineum is prepared with povidone–iodine and drapes are adjusted, excluding the penis and scrotum or the vulva from the operative field. When the skin is dry, the drapes are placed over the abdomen.

During the laparotomy, the surgeon stands on the left side of the patient, the first assistant on the right, the second assistant between the legs, and the assistant nurse on the right of the surgeon (**Figure 6.5.1**).

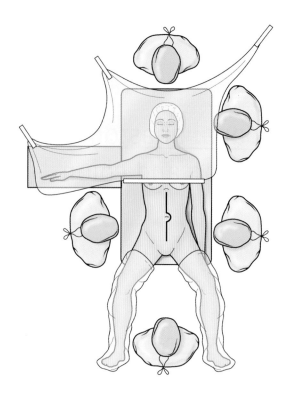

6.5.1 Position of the patient and the surgical team for open approach.

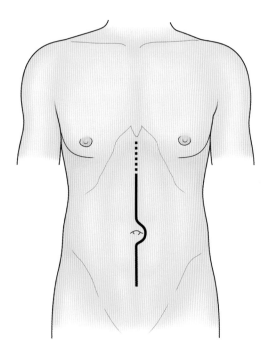

6.5.2 Midline incision.

Incision and abdominal exploration

A midline incision is made, extending from the pubic symphysis to the mid-epigastrium. The incision should reach the pubic symphysis to give good exposure into the pelvis. The upper part of the incision may reach higher than the mid-epigastrium if required for better exposure during the mobilization of the splenic flexure (**Figure 6.5.2**). A self-retaining retractor is used to retract the edges of the abdominal wall. The peritoneal cavity is explored to assess the location, size, and fixity of the lesion and to look for a synchronous colonic lesion, peritoneal spread, or hepatic metastasis. Ascitic fluid, if present, is collected for cytological examination.

Exposure, ligation, and division of the inferior mesenteric vessels

The small intestine is packed in moist pads and kept to the right of the abdominal cavity by the first assistant. The sigmoid colon is lifted up by the surgeon. The lower part of the abdominal aorta is then exposed and the peritoneum incised on its right border. The inferior mesenteric vein (IMV), which lies some 2–3 cm lateral to the aorta, is ligated and divided at this level (**Figure 6.5.3**a). An essential part of the technique is division of the inferior mesenteric artery (IMA) near its origin and the IMV at the border of the pancreas. This permits good mobilization and further descent of the left colon to the pelvis without traction. However, in elderly patients, the IMA can be ligated distal to the left ascending artery to ensure a good arterial blood supply to the descending colon (**Figure 6.5.3**b). The IMA is ligated and divided close to its origin. A distance of 1–2 cm should be maintained to avoid lesion of the hypogastric superior nerves.

Mobilization of the left colon

Once the IMA and IMV are divided, the surgeon changes position to the right of the patient for mobilization of the splenic flexure, which is an essential step that permits the colonic reservoir to reach the pelvis without tension. The splenic flexure is easier to mobilize after dissection of the left third of the transverse colon from the great omentum, which opens the lesser sac. Care should be taken not to damage the middle colic artery and its arcades. Once the left part of the transverse colon is free, the surgeon begins the dissection from the posterolateral abdominal wall. Adhesions between the spleen and the flexure should be divided gently before proceeding to fully mobilize the flexure. The mesentery on the left part of the transverse colon must be mobilized at the lower border of the tail of the pancreas. Two technical points that help to mobilize the splenic flexure are retraction of the left costal margin and tilting the table into the reverse Trendelenburg position.

The sigmoid colon is then mobilized by division of the developmental adhesions on the left side of the sigmoid colon. The first assistant holds the sigmoid colon in a forward direction, while the surgeon incises the peritoneum on its lateral side at the 'white line'. At this stage, the left ureter must be visible but not mobilized to avoid injury.

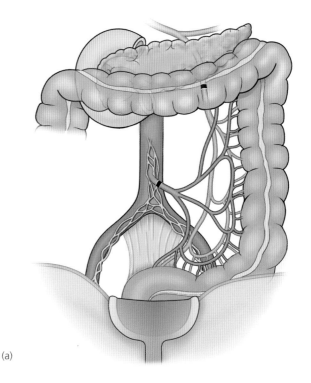

(a)

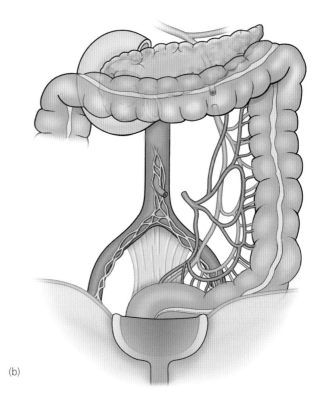

(b)

6.5.3 (a) Blood supply of the left colon; (b) ligation of both inferior mesenteric artery and vein.

Mobilization of the descending colon continues by division of the peritoneal reflection in the left paracolic gutter towards the spleen. There is a good avascular plane for this dissection, which passes between the perinephric fat and the mesocolon. The first assistant pulls the colon to the right and the surgeon, using blunt and sharp dissection, separates the mesocolon from the perinephric fat. Care should be taken not to injure the mesocolon and to keep the vascular arcades intact.

The left colon thus mobilized is attached to the posterior abdominal wall by a thin peritoneal fold of mesocolon crossing in front of the abdominal aorta. This peritoneal attachment is incised 2 mm from the aorta from the level of the transverse mesocolon downwards to the vessels of the aortic bifurcation. Bleeding from the fine vessels crossing this peritoneal fold may be controlled using electocoagulation.

Mobilization of the rectum

The self-retaining retractor is moved towards the upper part of the incision. A retractor is fixed to the self-retaining retractor and used to keep the small intestine packed with moist pads in the upper part of the abdominal cavity. The surgeon should be on the left side of the patient, the first assistant on the right. The second assistant stands between the patient's legs holding a retractor to keep the bladder (and uterus in females) forward. These arrangements give good exposure into the pelvis. At the bifurcation of the aorta, the lower end of the peritoneal incision is extended downwards to the right side of the rectum, crossing the common iliac vessels and taking care not to injure the right ureter. An important point is not to skeletonize the bifurcation of the aorta to preserve the superior hypogastric (genitourinary) plexus (**Figure 6.5.4**).

The left rectal gutter is thus opened and the 'holy plane' entered (see Chapter 6.1). The surgeon using sharp dissection follows the mesorectal fascia thus avoiding injury to the hypogastric nerves genitourinary plexus.

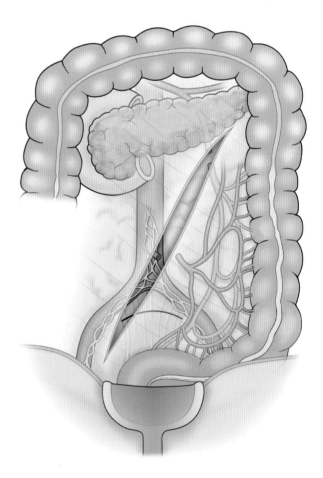

6.5.4 Posterior dissection of the mesorectum below the aortic bifurcation

It is very important to carry out the dissection laterally in the same plane to preserve the inferior hypogastric plexus nerves and to ensure total mesorectum excision (see Chapter 6.1).

The peritoneum of the pouch of Douglas is incised (**Figure 6.5.5**), and the dissection is carried downwards in the plane between the rectum and the urinary bladder, prostate, and Denonvilliers' fascia. In males, specific care should be taken to avoid injury to the neurovascular bundles (of Walsh), or between the rectum and the posterior wall of the vagina in women. Great care should be taken not to injure the vagina, particularly when using electrocoagulation. The dissection is continued as low as possible below the level of seminal vesicles in men and far along the posterior wall of the vagina in women. Dissection proceeds downward to the level of the levator ani.

Several technical points aid dissection in the lower pelvis:

1   Bimanual examination: the surgeon introduces the left finger into the rectum, holding the rectum with the right hand, thus assessing the distance remaining between the level of completed rectal dissection and the upper limit of the anal sphincter. The surgeon then changes gloves aseptically and continues to mobilize the rectum if necessary.
2   Pressure should be exerted on the perineum (by the first or second assistant) to push the whole pelvic floor upward.
3   The application of a malleable retractor behind the rectum will pull it anteriorly and to the right or the left.
4   A right-angle crushing clamp can be applied below the lower margin of the tumor and used for traction on the lower rectum. The anus is dilated and the rectum is washed with a mixture of saline, water, and povidone–iodine.

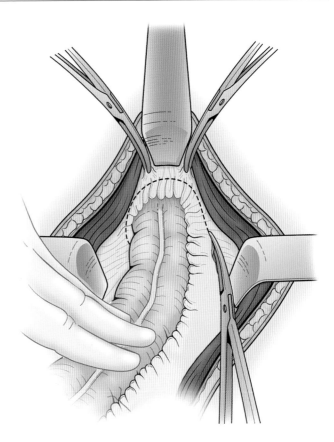

6.5.5 Incision of the pouch of Douglas.

LAPAROSCOPIC PROCEDURE

Position of the patient

The right leg should be extended by 10° to facilitate the movements of the right hand of the surgeon. The surgeon and the first assistant position themselves on the right side of the patient facing the screen placed on the left side. The second assistant stands between the patient's legs with the assistant nurse on his left (**Figure 6.5.6**).

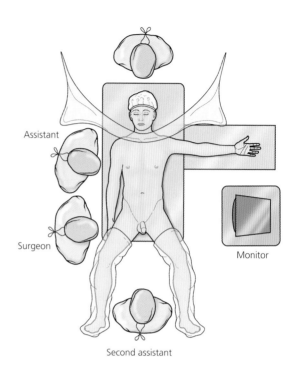

6.5.6 Position of patient and operating team for laparoscopic proctectomy.

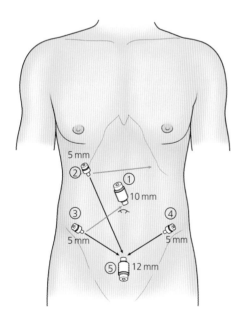

6.5.7 Trocar placement for laparoscopic proctectomy.

Port placement

Two centimeters above the umbilicus, a 10 mm port for the telescope is inserted by open technique. The peritoneal cavity is insufflated to an intraperitoneal pressure of 12 mmHg and explored. A 5 mm port is inserted at McBurney's point in the right iliac fossa, a second 3 cm below the ribs in the midclavicular line and a third symmetrically opposite to the first in the left iliac fossa. Finally, a 12 mm port is placed just above the pubis on the midline (**Figure 6.5.7**).

Inferior mesenteric vein division

The patient is placed in a Trendelenburg position and rotated with right side down. The omentum is placed in the front of the stomach as is the transverse mesentery. The duodenojejunal flexure is identified. Some adhesions may have to be freed to allow the IMV to be identified. The peritoneum below the IMV should be opened and the dissection continued between the left colon mesentery and the peritoneum covering the retroperitoneal space pushing towards the splenic flexure. The IMV can then be divided between clips (**Figure 6.5.8**).

Mobilization of the splenic flexure

The transverse mesocolon is opened above the pancreas. It is then possible to dissect the peritoneum from the lower edge of the pancreas to the splenic flexure. To complete mobilization, the omentum is dissected off the transverse colon from its mid-point to the splenic flexure. The lateral attachments of the descending colon are then easily divided.

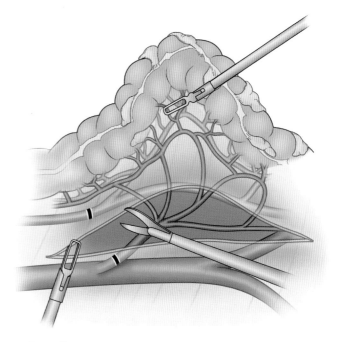

6.5.8 Laparoscopic dissection of the inferior mesenteric vein.

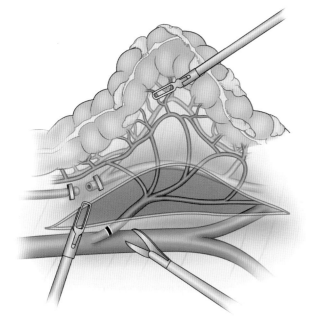

6.5.9 Laparoscopic dissection of the inferior mesenteric artery (IMA).

Inferior mesenteric artery division

The sigmoid colon is elevated by the assistant and peritoneum at the junction of the sigmoid colon and upper rectum is opened at the level of the sacral promontory. The plane between the upper part of the mesorectal fascia and the presacral and retroperitoneal fascia is identified and the dissection is extended between these layers laterally to identify the left ureter and gonadal vessels. By extending this dissection proximally, the root of the IMA is identified. The IMA is then divided between clips (Hemo-o-lock®; Teleflex Medical, Limerick, PA, USA) 2 cm from its root, thus limiting the possibility of injury to the hypogastric plexus (**Figure 6.5.9**).

Mesorectum dissection

Retraction of the upper rectum using tissue holding forceps inserted through the 5 mm ports facilitates posterior dissection of the mesorectum. Dissection on the lateral and the anterior aspects of the mesorectum is conducted as by laparotomy (**Figure 6.5.10**). Once the levator ani is reached and mobilization of the mesorectum complete, a 5 cm lower midline incision above the pubis or a Pfannenstiel incision is performed. This allows placement of a clamp below the tumor, rectal irrigation (see Mobilization of the rectum above). The rectum is then divided with a single stapling device (TA™ 30DST series; Tyco Healthcare, Norwalk, CT, USA) in the same manner as in a case performed by laparotomy. It is the authors' view that division with a single staple line reduces the risk of later anastomotic dehiscence compared to that associated with use of two or more applications of an endoscopic stapling instrument.

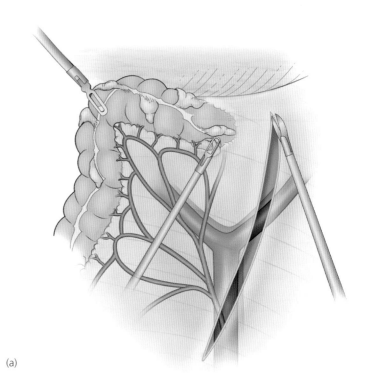

(a)

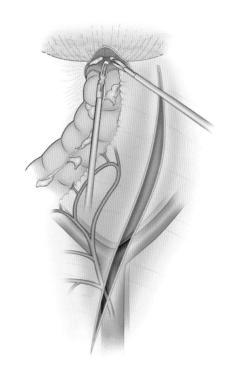

(b)

6.5.10 (a) Laparoscopic dissection of mesorectum. Dotted line (peritoneal reflexion of the Douglas pouch). (b) Laparoscopic dissection in the front of the Denonvilliers' fascia.

SELECTION OF COLORECTAL OR COLOANAL ANASTOMOSIS

Once the entire rectum and mesorectum is mobilized, a crushing clamp is applied just below the lower border of the tumor. Using a ruler, the distance between the lower border of the tumor and the upper border of the anal sphincter is measured. For tumors of the mid-third rectum, a distal resection margin of 5 cm is required. A colonic pouch is used if the distance between the level of resection and the upper border of the anal sphincter is less than 4 cm. Otherwise, a standard low anterior resection with end to end colorectal anastomosis using a circular stapling device is performed. It is the authors' view that that a coloanal pouch anastomosis provides better functional results than a direct colorectal anastomosis constructed just above the sphincter.[4] For a tumor of the lower third of the rectum, a coloanal with confection of a reservoir should be performed.

Choosing a stapled or handsewn anastomosis

If a coloanal pouch anastomosis is chosen, two anastomotic techniques are available. If a stapler can be placed below the clamp then a stapled anastomosis can be performed (see Chapter 6.1). If a stapler cannot be safely placed below the clamp, a handsewn anastomosis should be performed.

Rectal stump mucosectomy

If a handsewn coloanal anastomosis is to be performed, as it is impossible to place a crushing clamp and a stapler below the tumor, the mucosa of the rectal stump, below the level of the clamp must be removed. Once the rectal stump has been irrigated after application of a right-angle crushing retractor, a Lone Star™ retractor (Lone Star Medical Products, Houston, TX, USA) is applied. Subsequent mucosal dissection is facilitated by injection of saline containing adrenaline (1:10 000) into the submucosal plane to 'float' the mucosa away from the underlying muscle (**Figure 6.5.11**). The mucosa is removed from 5 mm above the dentate line in a circumferential manner using sharp-pointed scissor dissection and simultaneous coagulation of all bleeding points. The mucosectomy continues upwards until the upper part of the sphincter is reached, corresponding to the point reached during the abdominal dissection. This allows the specimen to be removed from the abdomen *en bloc* with the rectum before transection of the colon. Hemostasis of the anorectal muscular stump is reviewed as well as hemostasis in the lower pelvis, after irrigation with warm saline from the abdomen.

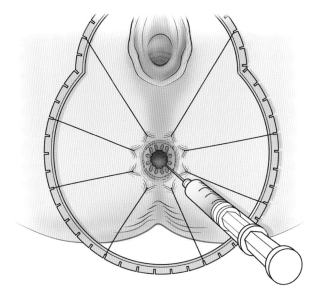

6.5.11 Lone Star™ retractor and adrenaline injection in the submucosal plane.

Intersphincteric resection

The intersphincteric plane may be dissected from the pelvic dissection or transanally. From above, the plane is entered at the anorectal junction, and if possible, the intersphincteric dissection is performed until a sufficient distal margin (at least 1 cm below the inferior extent of the tumor) is obtained.[5] If this dissection is technically difficult, a transanal approach can be used after perineal exposure with a Lone Star™ retractor. A mucosal and muscular incision is performed circumferentially at least 1 cm below the inferior extent of the tumor. If the incision is made at the level of the dentate line or 1–2 mm distally, the resection removes the upper half of the internal anal sphincter. The dissection is continued in the plane between the internal and external anal sphincters proximally to reach the abdominal dissection (**Figure 6.5.12**). If the resection is performed just above the dentate line but below the anorectal junction, the resection removes the upper third. A gauze swab with tumoricidal solution (povidone–iodine) is then inserted in the anal canal and the proximal rectum closed transanally as soon as possible to reduce the risk of tumor-cell dissemination, as in such a situation no crushing clamp can be placed below the tumor. The rectum is removed through the abdomen.

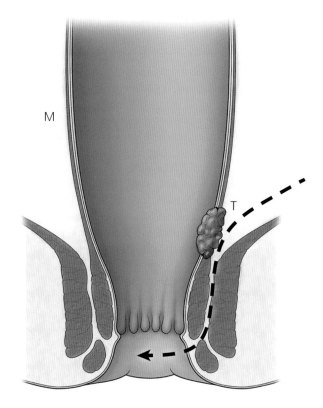

6.5.12 Evaluation of the distance between the lower border of the tumor and the external sphincter for intersphincteric resection. Dotted line: plane of dissection for intersphincteric resection allowing a 1 cm distal margin (T, tumour, M, mesorectum).

Preparation and division of the colon

A suitable site for division of the colon is chosen which ensures a good blood supply and allows construction of a pouch that will descend easily into the pelvis without tension. The pouch apex should come very easily to the level of the lower border of the pubic symphysis without traction. Usually, the site for division is in the descending colon just proximal to the sigmoid. The mesocolon is spread out to display the vessels and it is then divided obliquely from the site of the ligation of the colonic division. While doing this, great care should be taken not to jeopardize the vascularity of the colon. Before division, any arterial branch coming from the left ascending colic artery should be temporarily clamped, using a bulldog non-crushing clamp, and arterial pulsation in the arcade checked to be sure that vascularity is preserved.

The colon is then divided at the selected site after application of a transverse linear stapler on the proximal part and a crushing clamp distally. The resected specimen is removed from the operative field and opened so that the distance between the lower border of the tumor and the level of the muscular division in the anal canal can be measured to ensure that a margin of 1 cm has been achieved. Frozen-section examination should be requested at this time if dealing with a very low lesion and there is concern regarding the distal resection margin. The stapled end of the colon is under-sewn using a continuous 4-0 polyglycolic acid suture.

Construction of the colonic J-pouch

The distal 12 cm of the colon are brought together in a J-shaped manner to construct the pouch. Each limb measures 5–6 cm. The descending limb is positioned on the left, the ascending one on the right, and the mesentery behind the pouch. A pair of Allis forceps is applied to the antimesenteric border of the colon at the apex of the future pouch. Two other Allis forceps are placed equidistant from the first (5–6 cm) at the base of the pouch: one on the stapled end of the colon and one on the descending limb of the pouch. Two incisions are made by stab puncture on the antimesenteric side of each limb at equal distances from the top of the future pouch, close to the Allis forceps (**Figure 6.5.13**). The two limbs of a GIA 90™ stapler are introduced into the lumen of the colon, each through one hole, toward the apex of the pouch (**Figure 6.5.14**). The two proximal Allis forceps are applied to the edge of the holes posterior to the stapler to maintain slight traction upwards while the instrument is fired in a caudal direction. Care must be taken while firing not to include the mesentery between the two limbs; this must be checked by looking behind the stapler. The mesentery must be kept away from the stapler, usually by the index finger. The bowel is then everted to expose the remaining bridge, which is divided with a GIA 50 stapler. Hemostasis is secured at the site of anastomosis and the pouch is inverted. The Allis forceps are removed and the hole is closed by continuous 4-0 polyglycolic acid suture. The pouch is again tested to ensure that its apex can reach the lower border of the pubic symphysis. If there

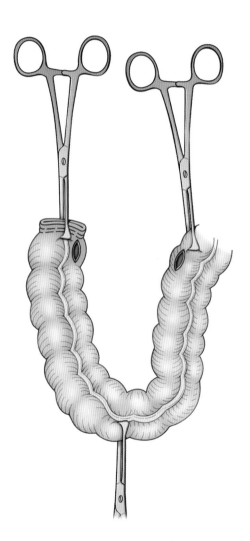

6.5.13 J-pouch confection. Openings of the colon before stapling.

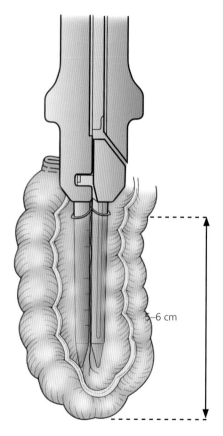

6.5.14 Confection of a J-pouch with a GIA stapler.

5–6 cm

is tension, more length can be gained by careful division of the mesocolon between the vessels. This maneuver provides both length and laxity. If a stapled anastomosis is proposed, the anvil of the circular stapling device is placed at the apex of the J-pouch.

Coloanal anastomosis

To perform a handsewn anastomosis, the pouch is directed towards the lower pelvis, with great care taken not to twist the mesentery. From the perineum, a Babcock forceps is introduced through the anus to grasp the apex of the pouch, and is guided through the anal stump aided by gentle squeezing from above. The pouch is then fixed to the anal sphincter by three interrupted sutures of 4-0 polyglycolic acid, each at one cardinal point just above the mucosal section. The apex of the pouch is opened and the anastomosis is performed between the mucosa of the anal canal and the full thickness of the colonic pouch, using interrupted sutures of 4-0. Four stitches are initially placed at 3, 6, 9, and 12 o'clock and then four further stitches are added to each of the quadrants thus formed (**Figure 6.5.15**).

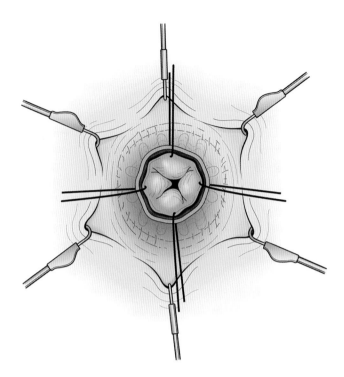

6.5.15 Handsewn coloanal anastomosis using a Lone Star™ retractor.

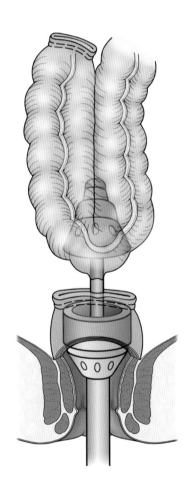

To perform a stapled anastomosis, the head of the circular stapler is inserted through the anus and fired to create the anastomosis with the pouch (**Figure 6.5.16**). Caution is again required to avoid a twist of the mesocolon.

The Lone Star™ retractor is then removed, and a Penrose drain is inserted into the pouch reservoir through the anastomosis. Care should be taken to ensure that the mobilized colon does not compress the duodeojejunal junction. If this occurs, the latter should be mobilized by division of the ligament of Treitz to avoid postoperative obstruction. It is the authors' practice to suture the free border of the mobilized colonic mesentery to the posterior peritoneal wall using absorbable sutures to reduce the possibility of internal herniation causing postoperative small bowel obstruction.

6.5.16 Double-stapled coloanal J-pouch anastomosis.

DRAINAGE, TEMPORARY ILEOSTOMY, CLOSURE

Two suction drains are placed in the pelvis anterior and posterior to the colonic pouch and brought out through lateral abdominal stab wounds, or the 5 mm port sites, in the case of a laparoscopic-assisted procedure. A loop ileostomy is then created in the right iliac fossa at the marked site (see Chapter 3.2). The abdominal wall is closed in one layer on the aponeurosis with continuous suture of 1. The skin is closed, and at the end of the procedure, the ileostomy is opened with interrupted stitches of 4-0 (**Figure 6.5.17**).

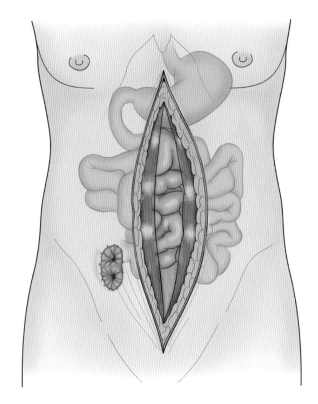

6.5.17 Ileostomy placement.

POSTOPERATIVE CARE

Postoperative care is similar to low anterior resection. The nasogastric tube can be removed on day 1 and liquid intakes are then given. The suprapubic catheter can be removed on day 5 after testing voiding in men; in women the Foley catheter can be removed on day 2. The normal hospital stay after an uncomplicated course is 7–11 days in the authors' institution. The loop ileostomy is usually performed 6 weeks after the initial surgery once a contrast enema study has confirmed normal healing of the pouch and the anastomosis.

OUTCOMES

The functional outcome after a colon pouch–anal anastomosis has been shown to be superior to that of a straight CAA or an ultralow CAA. Earliest reports[6, 7] were confirmed in initial randomized trials.[1] A meta-analysis has compared the functional results of 2240 patients from the collected series.[2] A reduction in bowel frequency and a decreased incidence of urgency has been observed in all studies. The functional results of colon pouch–anal anastomosis are comparable to those obtained with a low colorectal anastomosis.[4] The functional superiority of the colonic J-pouch is greatest within the first year after surgery[8] but is still sustained over the long term.[4]

The major drawback of the pouch is fecal retention secondary to poor evacuation. In the authors' series,[7, 9] this was observed in 20 percent of patients; these patients required enemas or suppositories to defecate. The combination of smaller J-pouches (5 cm rather than 10 cm long) constructed from the descending rather than the sigmoid colon may help overcome these problems.[10]

REFERENCES

1. Wille-Jorgensen P. Meta-analysis of colonic reservoirs versus straight coloanal anastomosis after anterior resection (*Br J Surg* 2006; 93: 19–32). *British Journal of Surgery* 2006; **93**: 639; author reply, 639.

2. Heriot AG, Tekkis PP, Constantinides V *et al.* Meta-analysis of colonic reservoirs versus straight coloanal anastomosis after anterior resection. *British Journal of Surgery* 2006; **93**: 19–32.

3. Schiessel R, Karner-Hanusch J, Herbst F *et al.* Intersphincteric resection for low rectal tumours. *British Journal of Surgery* 1994; **81**: 1376–8.

4. Dehni N, Tiret E, Singland JD *et al.* Long-term functional outcome after low anterior resection: comparison of low colorectal anastomosis and colonic J-pouch–anal anastomosis. *Diseases of the Colon and Rectum* 1998; **41**: 817–22; discussion 822–3.

5. Chamlou R, Parc Y, Simon T *et al.* Long-term results of intersphincteric resection for low rectal cancer. *Annals of Surgery* 2007; **246**: 916–21; discussion 921–2.

6. Parc R, Tiret E, Frileux P *et al.* Resection and colo-anal anastomosis with colonic reservoir for rectal carcinoma. *British Journal of Surgery* 1986; **73**: 139–41.

7. Lazorthes F, Fages P, Chiotasso P *et al.* Resection of the rectum with construction of a colonic reservoir and colo-anal anastomosis for carcinoma of the rectum. *British Journal of Surgery* 1986; **73**: 136–8.

8. Joo JS, Latulippe JF, Alabaz O *et al.* Long-term functional evaluation of straight coloanal anastomosis and colonic J-pouch: is the functional superiority of colonic J-pouch sustained? *Diseases of the Colon and Rectum* 1998; **41**: 740–6.

9. Berger A, Tiret E, Parc R *et al.* Excision of the rectum with colonic J pouch–anal anastomosis for adenocarcinoma of the low and mid rectum. *World Journal of Surgery* 1992; **16**: 470–7.

10. Lazorthes F, Gamagami R, Chiotasso P *et al.* Prospective, randomized study comparing clinical results between small and large colonic J-pouch following coloanal anastomosis. *Diseases of the Colon and Rectum* 1997; **40**: 1409–13.

Proctocolectomy for inflammatory bowel disease – open

W DONALD BUIE AND ANTHONY R MACLEAN

INTRODUCTION

Total proctocolectomy with end ileostomy was for many years the procedure of choice for inflammatory bowel disease (IBD) patients who required surgery. However, additional options have evolved over the past 40 years, including colectomy with ileorectal anastomosis (which should generally only be used in patients with rectal sparing), restorative proctocolectomy with continent ileostomy, or reconstruction with an ileal pouch-anal anastomosis (IPAA). The latter has become the most frequently performed procedure for patients with ulcerative colitis (UC) who require surgery. Total proctocolectomy was initially conceived as a four-stage procedure (ileostomy, right hemicolectomy, left hemicolectomy, and abdominoperineal resection) eventually becoming a two-stage procedure (total abdominal colectomy and proctectomy) and, finally, the modern one-stage procedure due to advances in anesthesia, antibiotics, and surgical technique.

INDICATIONS

The most common indication for proctocolectomy in patients with inflammatory bowel disease is failure of medical management. Although this term may represent several scenarios, in general it indicates that patient symptoms are inadequately managed by maximal medical therapy. Other indications for proctocolectomy include complications of medical therapy, complications of disease (including stricture and fistula formation in Crohn's disease), neoplastic transformation, and occasionally severe extraintestinal manifestations of IBD.

While a restorative procedure is a desired option for most of these situations, in others total proctocolectomy with end ileostomy should be considered the preferred procedure. These situations include patients with Crohn's disease and rectal involvement, those with poor continence, and some with rectal neoplasia, particularly those with distal rectal involvement and those requiring chemoradiation, although the latter is only a relative contraindication for IPAA.

CONTRAINDICATIONS

Total proctocolectomy is contraindicated in patients presenting with fulminant colitis or toxic megacolon. In these patients, a subtotal colectomy with end ileostomy should be considered the procedure of choice. The rectosigmoid is handled as a closed Hartmann stump, or a closed or open mucous fistula. Total proctocolectomy is also contraindicated in patients who desire an IPAA. Relative contraindications also include patients who wish to avoid any risk of surgery-induced sexual dysfunction and females who wish to avoid increasing their risk of infertility. Patients with active perianal infections should generally not undergo proctectomy until the infection is under control as the risk of perineal wound infection and subsequent delayed perineal wound healing is increased.

PREOPERATIVE ASSESSMENT AND PREPARATION

Prior to surgery, the surgeon should assess each patient for comorbidities, such as cardiopulmonary problems, diabetes and hypertension that may affect postoperative recovery and surgical outcomes. Routine blood work should be checked. Appropriate consultation should be requested to help optimize or correct any reversible medical condition.

All patients undergoing a total proctocolectomy with permanent ileostomy should have a preoperative consultation with an enterostomal therapist, if available. The purpose of this consultation is to provide preoperative stomal education, marking the ideal ileostomy position, and possibly arranging for peer group meetings. When an enterostomal therapist is not available, these roles should be undertaken by the surgeon, particularly the preoperative marking of the stoma site. The site is generally in the right lower quadrant overlying the rectus abdominus muscle, but depends on factors such as body habitus, presence of pannus, or skin folds, typical height of belt line, occupation, and pre-existing scars.

Patients undergoing a proctocolectomy do not generally require a mechanical bowel preparation. They should, however, receive preoperative intravenous antibiotics administered within 60 minutes of the skin incision. A variety of antibiotics have been investigated and there is no dominant strategy. The choice of antibiotics should be largely determined by the local patterns of antibiotic resistance. We typically utilize cefazolin 1 g and metronidazole 500 mg i.v. There is no benefit to continuing antibiotics postoperatively.

Patients with IBD who will be undergoing a proctocolectomy should be considered at high risk for thromboembolic complications, and should receive thromboprophylaxis. We generally employ pneumatic compression stockings and daily prophylactic doses of low molecular weight heparin started preoperatively.

When patients have active disease, their IBD medications should in general be continued up to the time of surgery. While some of these medications, particularly corticosteroids, have been shown to increase perioperative complications, it is important to keep the disease under good control if possible. Perioperative stress-dose steroids should be provided for patients who may have adrenal suppression due to long-term treatment.

There is no indication for routine placement of ureteric stents or nasogastric tubes. A closed suction drain is generally placed into the pelvis either transabdominally (which we prefer) or transperineally. A urinary catheter is placed at the time of surgery to monitor fluid balance and to prevent retention in the early postoperative period, especially in males. Patients should be crossmatched for blood.

Sexual dysfunction following pelvic surgery occurs in both men and women. In young patients with benign disease, this rate should be very low. An increased rate of infertility has also been recognized in women who undergo pelvic surgery, and should be discussed preoperatively.

ANESTHESIA

The operation is performed under general anesthetic. Placement of an epidural catheter may be considered for postoperative pain control, although patient-controlled analgesia (PCA) or bolus narcotics are also acceptable. This may be augmented by a transversus abdominis plane (TAP) block placed while under anesthesia.

OPERATION

Positioning

The operation can be performed in one of two approaches. The combined lithotomy position is preferred when two operating surgeons are available such that mobilization and resection of the colon and rectum can proceed simultaneously. The patient is positioned in lithotomy with the buttocks slightly over the edge of the operating table. When placing the legs in stirrups, care is required to ensure there is no pressure on the peroneal nerve where it passes lateral to the knee over the head of the fibula, as this can lead to neuropraxia and resultant foot drop.

The second approach requires two separate positions. The abdominal colectomy and end ileostomy are performed in lithotomy. Following complete mobilization of the colon and rectum, the rectosigmoid junction is divided with a transverse linear cutting stapler. The abdomen is closed and the ileostomy constructed. The patient is repositioned in prone jack-knife position and reprepped and draped for the perineal dissection to complete the proctectomy. The major advantage for this second position is improved visibility for the perineal surgeon and his first assistant.

Incision

A midline incision is used from the pubic symphysis skirting the umbilicus to the left. The upper limit must allow easy access to both flexures. An abdominal exploration is performed to assess any unsuspected pathology.

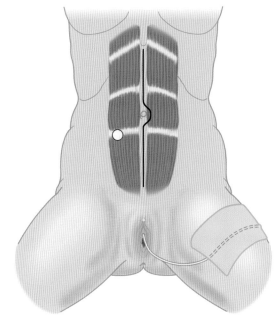

6.6.1

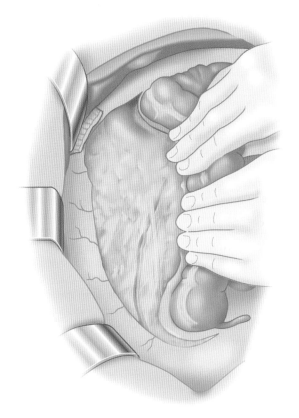

Mobilization of the colon

Mobilization of the colon should proceed in a sequential manner. The authors prefer to start at the cecum. The right colon is lifted up and retracted medially placing the lateral peritoneum under tension. The peritoneum in the left paracolic gutter is incised inferolateral to the cecum continuing cephalad just medial to the reflected line of the retroperitoneal fascia. Using cautery, the right colon and its accompanying mesentery is separated from the investing retroperitoneal fascia. The dissection should be relatively bloodless and excessive bleeding means that the surgeon has broken through the fascia into the retroperitoneum or alternatively that the dissection is too shallow and is within the mesentery of the right colon. The gonadal vessels and the right ureter are located below the investing fascia of the retroperitoneum and must be identified and preserved. The ureter is best identified where it crosses the bifurcation of the common iliac vessels. The peritoneal incision is extended up and around the hepatic flexure.

6.6.2

Using gentle traction, the hepatic flexure is reflected inferomedially, while cautery is used to mobilize it off the retroperitoneal fascia. The lateral edge of the duodenum is identified and the dissection proceeds medially leaving the duodenum in the retroperitoneum. The mobilization is continued until the right colon is supported on its mesentery near the midline. As the anterior surface of the second portion of the duodenum comes into view along with the pancreas, care must be taken not to tear the anterosuperior and anteroinferior pancreatic duodenal veins through excessive traction. These veins enter the lateral aspect of the superior mesenteric vein just proximal to the confluence of the ileocolic vein at the head of the pancreas. If torn, they should initially be packed and pressure applied followed by careful suture ligation if they are still bleeding.

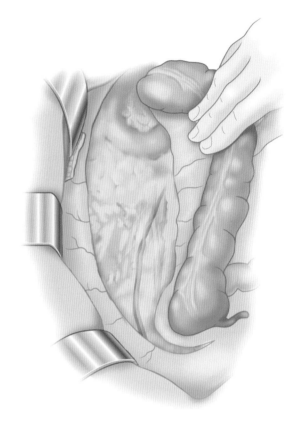

6.6.3

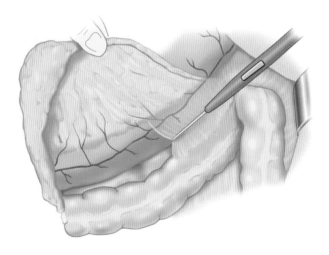

6.6.4

At this point, a decision must be made to either preserve or excise the omentum. When possible, the authors prefer to preserve it. Although the dissection may be started at the right transverse colon, the dissection plane is often more easily identified near the mid-transverse colon. The omentum is lifted superiorly while the transverse colon is distracted inferiorly. Using traction and counter-traction, the plane between the omentum and the transverse mesocolon is identified. Using cautery, the omentum is lifted off the transverse colon. Entry into the lesser sac facilitates the dissection which proceeds across the entire transverse colon towards each flexure until the omentum is completely separated, exposing the root of the transverse mesocolon. This should be relatively bloodless if the correct plane is identified. In obese patients, the surgeon must differentiate the large epiploicae of the colon from the omentum.

In some cases, the omentum cannot be separated from the transverse colon due to acute and chronic transmural inflammation secondary to Crohn's disease and must be excised with the colon. In this situation, the omentum is opened over the lesser sac superior to the transverse colon, divided between clamps and tied preserving the gastroepiploic arcade along the greater curve of the stomach. Again, entrance into the lesser sac facilitates the dissection which proceeds laterally separating the remaining omentum from the transverse colon out to and including the hepatic and splenic flexure.

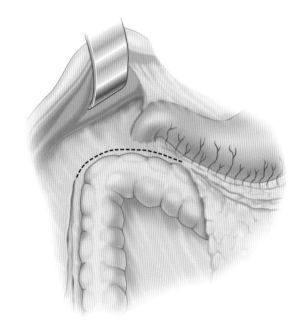

6.6.5

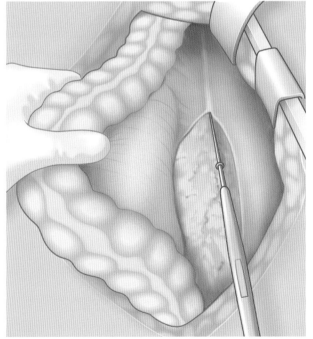

6.6.6

Attention is now turned to the left colon. It is retracted medially and the peritoneum is incised just medial to the line of Toldt (the reflected edge of the retroperitoneal fascia) at the level of the sigmoid colon. Sharp dissection with cautery is used to lift the left colon and its accompanying mesentery which is rotated medially away from the retroperitoneum progressing upwards towards the splenic flexure mobilizing towards the midline. Again the dissection should be relatively bloodless and the retroperitoneal investing fascia should be left intact identifying and preserving the left gonadal vessels and the left ureter beneath it. The latter is identified at the bifurcation of the common iliac artery. If the ureter is not identified, look on the underside of the sigmoid mesorectum as the dissection plane may have been too deep. As on the right side, excessive bleeding implies an incorrect dissection plane.

Prior to mobilizing the splenic flexure, any attachments between the spleen and the colon are divided to prevent tearing of the splenic capsule. Avoid pulling down on the splenic flexure as this may cause bleeding. When mobilizing the flexure, it is often easiest for the surgeon to perform this maneuver while standing between the legs of the patient. The peritoneal incision is extended superiorly towards the splenic flexure approximately 1–2 cm lateral to the edge of the colon medial to the reflected edge of the retroperitoneal fascia and inferomedial to the spleen.

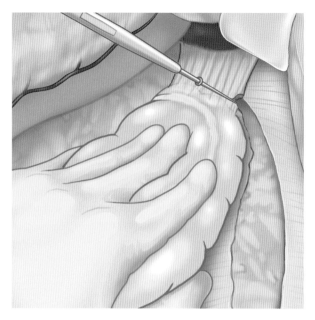

6.6.7

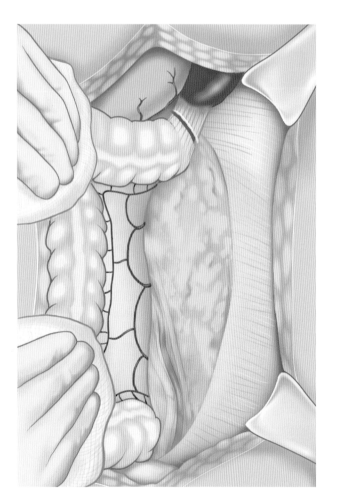

6.6.8

The flexure is lifted medially to expose the retroperitoneal fascia, along with the renocolic ligaments and the splenocolic ligaments which are divided sharply with cautery to release the splenic flexure from Gerota's fascia. The mobilization is continued medially until the left colon is suspended on its mesentery at the midline.

In the case of an unsuspected local perforation with omental or peritoneal seal in the transverse colon or splenic flexure region, the area should be left intact until all other areas are mobilized. In the case of omental involvement, the omentum should be resected with the colon. When mobilizing the involved colon take steps to minimize local contamination with gentle dissection, packs, and suction.

When the entire colon is mobilized and suspended on its mesentery, it is devascularized starting with the ileocolic vessels which are skeletonized near their origin and taken between clamps. All major vessels are doubly ligated with absorbable suture for security. The ileal mesentery is divided to the left of the ileocolic tie, radially out towards the terminal ileum between clamps and tied with absorbable suture. A suitable resection site 5 cm proximal to the ileocecal valve at the intestinal site is cleared of fat for a distance of 2 cm and a transverse linear cutting stapler is applied across the terminal ileum and fired to separate the small intestine from the colon. The colon is devascularized dividing the mesentery of the colon in a logical fashion. Often it is easiest to transilluminate the mesentery to identify the vessels to facilitate the dissection. At this point we find it easier to lift the colon out of the abdomen placing the devascularized section in a towel on the chest. The left colic is taken along with the sigmoid branches between clamps and tied with absorbable suture. We do not take the inferior mesenteric at its origin but instead carry our dissection through the mesosigmoid preserving the superior rectal vessels to the level of the sacral promontory.

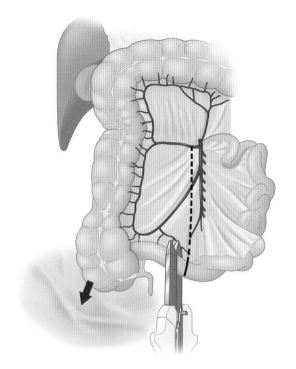

6.6.9

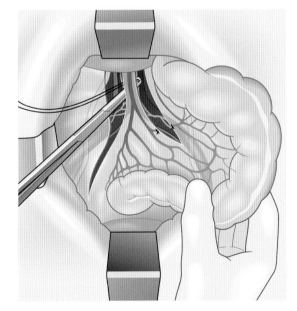

6.6.10

Mobilization of the rectum

The superior rectal vessels are skeletonized and divided at the level of the sacral promontory. The mesorectal plane is identified posterior to the vessels by placing upward traction on the mesorectum revealing the areolar tissue between the mesorectal fascia and the presacral fascia. The ureter should be identified prior to starting the pelvic dissection. Dissection proceeds in the midline from the sacral promontory downwards using cautery to separate these two layers. Care is taken to identify the hypogastric nerves, separating them from the mesorectum leaving them in the retroperitoneum. This should be done sharply to avoid thermal injury from cautery. The nerves are most vulnerable at the entrance to the pelvis on the posterolateral aspect of the mesorectum where they can be very intimate as they give off branches to the rectum.

The peritoneum is incised bilaterally in the lateral sulcus at the base of the rectal mesentery. The two peritoneal incisions are extended lateral to the mesorectum down into the deep pelvis where they arc around the rectum anteriorly to connect with each other in the cul de sac.

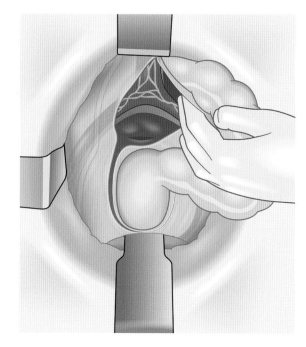

6.6.11

The dissection is continued posteriorly and laterally staying on the mesorectal fascia down to the pelvic floor to the bare area of the rectum below the mesorectum. The rectosacral fascia must be incised sharply to ensure the dissection can proceed to the pelvic floor. The authors continue this dissection through the levator hiatus preserving the fascia over the levators and dividing the median raphe at the level of the anococcygeal ligament to expose the tip of the coccyx.

Anteriorly the dissection is carried through Denonvilliers' fascia onto the rectum to protect the nervi erigentes or parasympathetic pelvic nerves which in the male run between Denonvilliers' fascia and the posterior aspect of the seminal vesicles and prostate. In the female, dissection in this plane protects the back wall of the vagina. The dissection is continued down anteriorly through the levator hiatus. Extending the abdominal dissection through the hiatus as far as possible on all sides of the rectum makes the perineal dissection much easier.

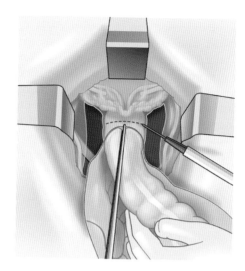

6.6.12

When the perineal dissection is to be completed in the prone jack-knife position, the colon is separated from the rectum at this point with a transverse linear stapler and handed off. The abdominal portion of the operation is completed as outlined below prior to repositioning the patient. When the perineal dissection is to be completed in the lithotomy position, the perineal surgeon begins the dissection as the abdominal surgeon is starting the rectal mobilization, so that the abdominal and perineal surgeons meet below the levators. This allows the abdominal and perineal closures to occur simultaneously.

To complete the abdominal portion, a disk of skin is removed at the previously marked ileostomy site. The underlying rectus sheath and rectus muscle are divided longitudinally taking care to avoid injury to the inferior epigastric vessels, and the stapled end of the ileum is brought through the abdominal wall. The defect in the abdominal wall is made just large enough to comfortably bring the intestine through. We do not recommend a cruciate incision nor do we use the 'two-finger rule'. We ensure that at minimum a 2 cm band of anterior and posterior fascia is left intact between the ileostomy and the midline wound to reduce herniation. A closed suction drain is placed in the pelvis through a separate stab wound and sutured in place. If the patient is to be repositioned in

the prone jack-knife, the end of the drain is sutured to the top of the rectum. The abdomen is irrigated with copious amounts of saline and suctioned dry. Complete hemostasis is obtained with cautery and suture ligation. The abdomen is closed with a heavy slowly absorbable suture in a single layer. The skin is closed with suture or staples and covered with a suitable dressing. Finally, the ileostomy is matured in a Brooke fashion with interrupted absorbable sutures. The stoma should be everted 1–2 cm above the level of the skin to facilitate pouching.

In the case of an associated colonic malignancy, all resection margins should follow general oncologic principles with wide peritoneal dissection around the tumor and proximal division of the attendant blood supply near its origin to ensure adequate nodal sampling. All extraintestinal involvement is excised *en bloc* to ensure an R0 resection. If a rectosigmoid or rectal cancer is present, the inferior mesenteric artery is taken 1–2 cm distal to its origin. The inferior mesenteric vein is taken just inferior to the margin of the pancreas as described in Chapter 5.6. If an abdominoperineal resection is required, the pelvic dissection should proceed only to the level of the levators and not down to or through the levator hiatus, so that a cylindrical resection can be performed (see Chapter 6.10).

Perineal dissection

The perineal dissection can be performed in lithotomy or prone jack-knife position and is meant to remove only the anorectal tissue. The former is quicker as two surgeons can work simultaneously. The authors do not recommend suturing the anus closed prior to dissection as this distorts the normal anatomy. After identification of the intersphincteric groove, cautery is used to incise the overlying skin in a circumferential fashion starting posterolateral where the intersphincteric groove is most pronounced. The intersphincteric groove is most often identified with palpation. When the groove is indistinct, placing the anal canal on stretch with the Pratt bivalve may facilitate dissection. Once the intersphincteric plane has been clearly established, the anal margin is oversewn or grasped with clamps to prevent leakage of stool during manipulation.

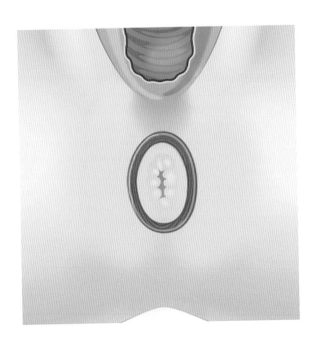

6.6.13

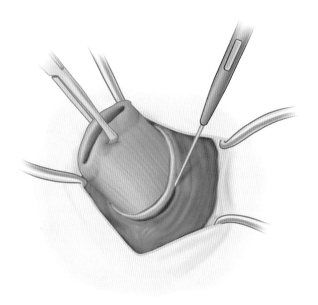

Two self-retaining retractors (Gelpi or similar) are placed and the anus is grasped with an Allis or a Kocher clamp. The dissection is continued cephalad between the internal and external sphincters. Typically, there is very little bleeding. In cases of pre-existing perianal Crohn's disease, this plane can be difficult to identify.

6.6.14

Anatomically, the external sphincter becomes the levator ani muscle and the internal sphincter becomes the inner circular muscle of the rectum. If the abdominal dissection has been carried through the levator hiatus, the perineal dissection is much easier and moves quite quickly. Continuity between the abdominal and perineal dissection is established posteriorly. It is helpful in lithotomy for the abdominal surgeon to place his hand posteriorly down to the coccyx pulling the rectum anteriorly to guide the perineal surgeon into the pelvis. Once the pelvis is entered, the dissection is extended circumferentially around the anorectum.

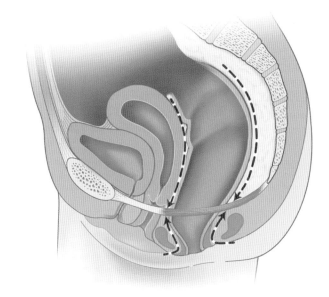

6.6.15

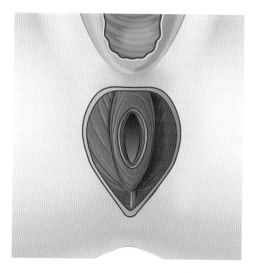

The anterior dissection can be difficult as the external sphincter muscle decussates and becomes attached to the rectourethralis. In men, some of the external sphincter muscle must be divided to expose the posterior surface of the prostate.

6.6.16

In women, the vagina is dissected anteriorly off the anal canal and the lower rectum. Once the anorectum is separated from the levators and the surrounding pelvic tissue, the entire specimen is brought out through the anus. If the patient is in the prone jack-knife position, the suction drain is drawn down when the specimen is removed and the suture is cut.

The pelvis is irrigated with copious amounts of saline and suctioned dry. Complete hemostasis is obtained. The closed suction drain is positioned in a dependent position down into the pelvis. The levators and external sphincter are closed with an absorbable monofilament suture. The authors close the skin with an absorbable 3-0 or 4-0 subcuticular suture.

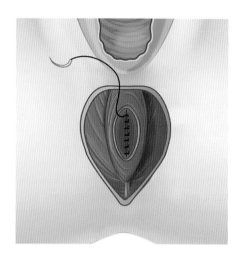

6.6.17

In patients with extensive perineal Crohn's disease, every attempt should be made to settle any acute infectious process prior to proctectomy. This may require incision and drainage of abscesses, use of draining setons, and partial or complete unroofing of sinuses and fistula tracts where appropriate, in addition to maximizing medical therapy and the use of adjunctive antibiotics. If the disease is extensive, consideration may be given to an abdominal colectomy and ileostomy to defunction the area with delayed proctectomy. At the time of proctectomy, short fistula tracts may be excised *en bloc*. Long and complex fistula tracts should be unroofed or curetted out. Extensive excision and debridement should be avoided.

In the case of a low rectal cancer that requires an abdominoperineal resection, the perineal dissection is started outside the sphincter complex. It proceeds laterally to include the entire levator complex to avoid taking a narrow waist in close proximity to the tumor (see Chapter 6.10).

POSTOPERATIVE CARE

Patients should be allowed to progress their diet as they tolerate it early in the postoperative period. There is no need for nasogastric tube drainage unless a mechanical obstruction was present preoperatively. Physiologic intravenous fluids are administered until the patient is tolerating adequate oral intake and the ileostomy is functioning well with outputs of less than 800–1000 mL/day.

There is no need for routine postoperative antibiotic prophylaxis. The urinary catheter can generally be removed on the third or fourth postoperative day. The pelvic drain can generally be removed when the drainage is serous and

less than 50 mL/day. Skin staples are removed and replaced with steristrips as the patient is leaving the hospital which is typically around 6–8 days.

LONGER-TERM OUTCOMES

Patients with ulcerative colitis who undergo a total proctocolectomy and end ileostomy are cured of their disease and typically do very well. Patients who have a permanent ileostomy have similar quality of life to those who undergo a restorative procedure with an ileal pouch-anal anastomosis. However, it should be recognized that up to 10 percent of patients thought to have UC will subsequently be found to have Crohn's disease, and thus the procedure in those patients will not have been curative.

In patients with Crohn's disease, the rate of recurrent disease following total proctocolectomy and end ileostomy is the lowest of any operative procedure used. The rate of reoperation for symptomatic recurrence is generally felt to be 20–30 percent at ten years, and may be even lower now with the advent of improved medical therapy.

Despite appropriate wound care measures, the perineal wound may take several months to heal, especially in situations of extensive perianal Crohn's disease or postoperative perineal infection. Small wound sinus tracts are usually relatively asymptomatic and can be left alone. In situations where the perineal wound has failed to heal leaving a cavity or a static granulating wound, consideration should be given to wide debridement and vascularized musculocutaneous flap reconstruction with the rectus abdominus, gracilis, or gluteus maximus depending on wound size, the need for skin coverage and muscle availability.

Proctocolectomy for inflammatory bowel disease – laparoscopic

TONIA M YOUNG-FADOK

HISTORY

Proctocolectomy (PC) for inflammatory bowel disease (IBD) is most commonly performed for ulcerative colitis (UC) and infrequently for Crohn's disease (CD) with associated pancolitis. This chapter will focus primarily on PC for UC, with additional comments pertaining to CD.

Currently, in centers that perform high volumes of laparoscopic colorectal surgery, a laparoscopic procedure is the approach of choice for patients requiring PC, either with Brooke ileostomy in UC or CD, or with the more common ileal J-pouch anal anastomosis (IPAA) reconstruction in UC.

This is a major development from early recommendations. Initial descriptions of laparoscopic PC and IPAA indicated feasibility, but were not terribly encouraging about the wisdom of continuing to proceed along this path. One must review these early studies in the context of early experience and rudimentary instruments. For example, Wexner *et al.* reported a comparative study of five open versus five laparoscopic IPAAs, and found that duration of ileus and length of stay were actually longer in the laparoscopic group, which was counter to the perceived benefits of the approach. Careful review of the technical details in the manuscript, however, reveals that the mobilized colon was extracted via a Pfannenstiel incision and that the authors speculated whether traction on the mesentery may have contributed to postoperative ileus. Soon thereafter it was realized that the mobilized colon and rectum may be extracted via a periumbilical incision, avoiding such traction, and subsequent to that, vessel-sealing devices became more sophisticated, dividing vessels up to 7 mm in diameter, allowing for safe intracorporeal division of the major mesenteric vessels, including the inferior mesenteric artery and the middle colic vessels.

DEFINITIONS

Proctocolectomy involves resection of the entire colon and rectum, with or without excision of the sphincter complex. The word 'total' as used by some authors in 'total proctocolectomy' is redundant. PC is performed most commonly for UC. In about 10 percent of such procedures, the indication is familial adenomatous polyposis (FAP), and in a lesser percentage, the diagnosis is CD. In the vast majority of cases of UC, a reconstructive procedure is performed with an IPAA. In the case of pancolonic CD, a reconstructive procedure is contraindicated secondary to the high risk of subsequent complications, and a proctocolectomy is performed with Brooke ileostomy and either excision of the sphincter complex, or (according to the author's preference) preservation of the sphincter in the event that subsequent pharmacologic advances permit the construction of an ileal pouch without the risk of devastating side effects from the development of pouch fistulas.

Following PC, the terminal ileum may be matured as a Brooke ileostomy (in CD and selected cases of UC), or, in most cases of UC, used to reconstruct a 'neo-rectum' to re-establish bowel continuity. This is most commonly in the form of an ileal J-pouch which is anastomosed to the anal canal. PC and construction of an ileal pouch is referred to as either restorative proctocolectomy (favored in the UK and by the Cleveland Clinic) and proctocolectomy and IPAA, the term used by the Mayo Clinic. The author's preference is the latter as it describes the means of restoration of bowel continuity. An alternative form of reconstruction using the terminal ileum is a continent ileostomy, although this is used infrequently and is generally not recommended because of the high complication and reoperative rate, and it is contraindicated in CD.

With specific reference to laparoscopic PC with or without IPAA, a laparoscopic-assisted procedure would utilize a 3–5 cm periumbilical incision to extract the specimen and construct the ileal pouch through this incision. A completely laparoscopic PC ± IPAA is used to describe complete laparoscopic mobilization of the colon and rectum, transection of the rectum and mesentery intracorporeally, followed by extraction of the specimen via the planned ileostomy site. Thus, no additional incision is employed for specimen extraction. The pouch is also constructed extracorporeally via the ileostomy site.

Single-incision laparoscopic PC can use a periumbilical incision for placement of the multiport device and subsequent specimen extraction, but would then need a separate ileostomy site. True single-incision PC deploys the port device via the planned ileostomy site.

INDICATIONS AND CONTRAINDICATIONS

Proctocolectomy may be indicated in both UC and CD manifesting as pancolitis. Reconstruction of intestinal continuity with an ileal pouch is used for most individuals with UC and contraindicated in CD.

In both UC and CD, reasons for recommending PC include: medically refractory disease; the presence of colonic dysplasia or neoplasia; side effects of medications, e.g. diabetes resulting from the use of steroids, or anaphylaxis with biological agents; inability to wean steroids despite successful response; growth retardation in pediatric patients; and patient desire in individuals who prefer to avoid long-term immunosuppression.

Contraindications to PC and to laparoscopic PC are dependent upon the timing of the procedure (emergent versus elective), patient factors, and disease process (UC or CD). In UC in the emergent setting, with perforation, toxic megacolon, and hemorrhage, PC is contraindicated. Total colectomy with Brooke ileostomy (TCB) (open or laparoscopic at the discretion of the surgeon) is the procedure of choice. The symptoms will resolve postoperatively and the tissue planes in the pelvis are not disturbed, allowing a subsequent completion proctectomy, with or without IPAA. Patient factors indicating potential need for an initial total colectomy include malnutrition, recent use of biologic agents, and obesity. Malnutrition (low serum albumin, low serum pre-albumin, World Health Organization definition of >10 percent weight loss) should dictate TCB rather than PC. Recent data suggest that surgical intervention within the treatment duration of a biologic agent/anti-tumor necrosis factor (TNF) agent results in increased risk of pouch complications. Thus, a three-stage procedure should be considered in patients within 8 weeks of receiving infliximab or 2 weeks of adalimumab. One additional contraindication is obesity. Although UC is considered a wasting disease, that is not always the case in the United States. In the morbidly obese patient, the pouch may not reach or even fit into the pelvis. In such patients, a total colectomy with Brooke ileostomy may be performed. Being given a goal body mass index (BMI) before completion proctectomy and pouch are performed is highly motivational for appropriate weight loss!

PREOPERATIVE PLANNING

All outside data are obtained, specifically previous colonoscopy reports, pictures, and the original pathologic slides for review by our pathologists. When indicated, the patient is seen in consultation by one of our gastroenterology colleagues with an interest in IBD, if there is concern that medical management options have not been fully explored. Colonoscopy with biopsy is repeated if indicated. All patients undergoing an elective operation have a formal preoperative assessment which includes: evaluation in our preoperative clinic to clear the patient for anesthesia; blood tests which include electrolytes, complete blood count, and albumin and prealbumin when indicated by history; chest x-ray and electrocardiogram (EKG) when appropriate; type and screen within 72 hours of operation; and pregnancy test when applicable. Consultation with an ostomy nurse provides information for the patient and marking of the most appropriate site for an ileostomy. Regarding bowel preparation, some data suggest that this is not necessary, but the data are from open cases. Laparoscopic handling of the bowel is facilitated by a bowel preparation, and exteriorization via a small incision demands it. A 4-liter polyethylene glycol (PEG) solution appears to be the most effective. This author does not use oral antibiotics (metronidazole and erythromycin) as part of the bowel preparation, because the nausea induced by these medications results in less effective intake of the PEG solution.

Immediately preoperatively, patients who are taking steroids, typically prednisone, receive an intravenous dose of methylprednisone 10–20 mg greater than their current dose of prednisone. This is then tapered over the next 3 days back to the preoperative dose. Patients who have been treated with steroids within the preceding 6–12 months, but are currently not taking them, receive methylprednisone 20 mg intravenously and then a rapid taper over 3 days.

Guidelines of the National Surgical Quality Improvement Program (NSQIP) are followed. Ertapenem 1 g i.v. is administered within 60 minutes prior to the incision in patients without a penicillin allergy. No postoperative doses are required secondary to the 24-hour duration of action. Metronidazole 1 g i.v. and ciprofloxacin 500 mg i.v. are used in combination in the patient allergic to penicillin. A warming blanket is used preoperatively and during the induction of anesthesia for the maintenance of normothermia.

OPERATION

Positioning

Safe and secure positioning is essential for the success of the operation. Three factors have to be addressed: (1) the patient must be safely secured to the table without concern for slipping with the steep position changes required during laparoscopic procedures; (2) access to the perineum is required for construction of the anastomosis, whether stapled or sutured; and (3) it must be possible to deploy laparoscopic instruments in all four quadrants of the abdomen. Modified combined synchronous position (modified lithotomy) is used. Medical grade pink egg-crate foam taped to the operating room (OR) table ensures the patient does not slip. The foam is taped to the bed over a drawer sheet which is used for securing the arms. The legs are placed in stirrups and positioned with the thighs parallel to the abdominal wall to avoid interference with laparoscopic instruments during mobilization of the hepatic and splenic flexures. Hands are padded with foam and the drawer sheet is used to tuck the arms alongside the torso. A warming blanket device is placed over the chest, covered by a regular blanket, and the chest is secured to the table with linen tape wrapped entirely around the patient's chest and the table. Before draping, a 'tilt test' is performed by moving the OR table into extreme Trendelenburg, reverse Trendelenburg, and right and left tilt, to ensure the patient is secure in these positions.

A Foley catheter is placed in the bladder. An orogastric rather than a nasogastric tube provides gastric decompression and is removed at the end of the operation.

SURGICAL TECHNIQUE

Rationale

Both lateral-to-medial and medial-to-lateral approaches may be used for mobilization of the colon. The author prefers the lateral-to-medial approach for multiple reasons. First, open procedures in most teaching institutions are performed lateral-to-medial and thus trainees are more familiar with the tissue planes. Second, a medial-to-lateral approach for mobilization of the right colon

requires division of the ileocolic pedicle. In order to obtain adequate pouch 'reach' (the ability of the pouch to reach the planned level of anastomosis without tension), either the ileocolic pedicle or the adjacent arcade may be the length-limiting structure and require division. This cannot be determined accurately until the pouch is created; hence the author prefers to preserve the ileocolic pedicle during mobilization of the colon. Third, a medial-to-lateral approach devascularizes the colon; a lateral-to-medial approach avoids ischemic colon sitting in the abdomen while the rectal mobilization is performed. Finally, the mesentery may be divided wherever it is most convenient, avoiding the large proximal vascular pedicles if desired, in patients with tissues friable from steroid use. In thin patients, the mesentery need not be divided at all, as the colon and rectum, once mobilized, can be exteriorized via a periumbilical incision, and the mesentery divided extracorporeally.

Breaking the procedure down as simply as possible, there are three steps to the initial laparoscopic part of the procedure: mobilization of the left colon, the right colon, and the rectum. A rationale exists for this order too: as mobilization of the right colon is less technically demanding than the left colon, this provides a break before the challenges of the pelvic dissection.

Laparoscopic approach

A diamond-shaped configuration is used for port placement. A supraumbilical cutdown is employed for insertion of a 12 mm blunt port and a pneumoperitoneum is achieved to 13 mmHg. A Veress needle technique is never used. After exploration of the abdominal cavity, two 5 mm ports are placed, one in the suprapubic midline and one in the left lower quadrant. At the planned ileostomy site in the right lower quadrant, a disk of skin and subcutaneous fat are excised and a 12 mm port is placed through this site. Additional 5 mm ports may be placed as required.

For a single incision procedure, the ileostomy site is prepared by excising a disk of skin and subcutaneous fat. The anterior rectus fascia is divided, the rectus muscle fibers separated, and a 3 cm incision is made in the posterior fascia to allow for placement of the multiport device.

LEFT COLON MOBILIZATION

Mobilization of the left colon commences at the left pelvic brim. The OR table is placed in Trendelenburg with the left side inclined up. The left lateral peritoneal reflection alongside the sigmoid colon is opened by incising immediately medial to the white line of Toldt with cautery scissors (**Figure 6.7.1**). The peritoneal reflection itself is 'left with the patient' as the dissection proceeds in the plane between the posterior aspect of the left colon mesentery and the retroperitoneal structures. Remaining

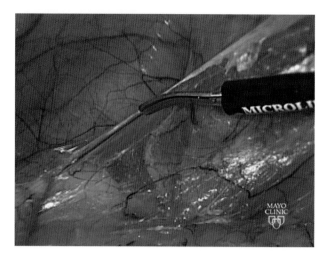

6.7.1 Lateral-to-medial mobilization of the sigmoid colon. Photo courtesy of Mayo Clinic.

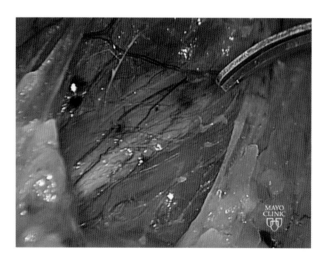

6.7.2 Identification of the left ureter. Photo courtesy of Mayo Clinic.

in the correct plane of dissection brings one to the left ureter which is carefully swept laterally and protected (**Figure 6.7.2**). Once the sigmoid colon is fully mobilized from the retroperitoneum, the left lateral peritoneal reflection alongside the descending colon is incised and the descending colon is mobilized medially, taking care to identify the correct plane anterior to Gerota's fascia and avoid undermining of the left kidney.

The OR table is moved to reverse Trendelenburg, still with the left side inclined up. There are several options for mobilization of the splenic flexure, related to direction of dissection and treatment of the omentum. The direction of dissection can be retrograde (from descending colon to transverse colon), antegrade (transverse colon to descending colon), or a combination of the two. The omentum can be retained with the patient, or taken with the colon. Any approach may be used in the patient with normal BMI. In the obese patient, it is usually easier to use the combination approach and to take the omentum with the colon.

In the retrograde approach, the proximal descending colon is dissected off Gerota's fascia and as the plane of dissection turns medially and superior to the splenic flexure, the lesser sac is entered at its lateral aspect, and the gastrocolic ligament is divided in a retrograde fashion. A vessel-sealing device is helpful around the splenic flexure, as the planes are different from the bloodless retroperitoneal plane. In the antegrade approach, the lesser sac is entered superior to the distal transverse colon, either by elevating the omentum and entering the lesser sac between the transverse colon and the omentum, or by dropping the omentum into the pelvis and incising the gastrocolic ligament to gain entry into the lesser sac (**Figure 6.7.3**). The dissection is then continued distally along the transverse colon and around the splenic flexure. In the combination approach, which is helpful in the heavier patient, the lateral dissection alongside the proximal descending colon is carried as far around the splenic flexure as possible. Attention is then turned to the mid-transverse colon, where the lesser sac is identified and entered above the mid-transverse colon and the dissection is continued towards the splenic flexure to join the lateral dissection. It is usually easier to take the omentum with the colon in the obese patient as the plane between the transverse colon and the omentum is often not clearly visualized having been obliterated by fat deposition.

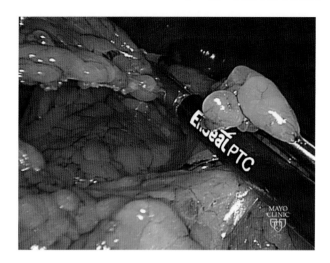

6.7.3 Entry into the lesser sac for mobilization of the splenic flexure. Photo courtesy of Mayo Clinic.

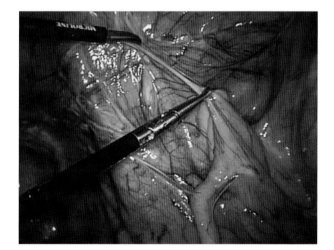

6.7.4 Initial mobilization of the right colon commencing at the appendiceal attachments.

RIGHT COLON MOBILIZATION

The OR table is placed in Trendelenburg with the right side inclined up. Commencing at the right pelvic brim, the peritoneum is scored around the medial aspect of the base of the terminal ileal mesentery and around the cecum with the cautery scissors, and the correct retroperitoneal plane is entered (**Figure 6.7.4**). In patients with normal BMI, the ureter can often be visualized through the peritoneum, whereas in heavier patients this is easier after opening the retroperitoneal plane. The white line of Toldt alongside the ascending colon is incised with cautery scissors and the ascending colon is mobilized medially to the midline, again taking care to remain in the correct retroperitoneal plane anterior to Gerota's fascia to avoid undermining the kidney. Along the medial aspect of the terminal ileal mesentery, the peritoneum is scored up to the level of the duodenum. Throughout the dissection, care is taken to identify and protect the right ureter, inferior vena cava, and the duodenum.

With the patient in reverse Trendelenburg, and right side still inclined up, a vessel-sealing device is used to divide the hepatocolic attachments, again identifying and protecting the duodenum. Management of the omentum should mirror the treatment of the omentum at the splenic flexure, either taking the omentum with the colon or leaving it with the patient.

DISSECTION OF THE RECTUM

With the OR table in Trendelenburg, the left side is inclined upwards slightly. The left side of the rectosigmoid mesentery is grasped and elevated towards the anterior abdominal wall and the left side of the pelvis. The left ureter is again identified and protected. Careful inspection of the left side of the rectum identifies a subtle differentiation between 'white tissue' laterally and 'yellow tissue' medially that indicates fatty tissue within the mesorectal fascial envelope. The line between the two parallels the course of the rectum and marks the point of entry into the presacral plane. The prior line of dissection along the distal sigmoid colon is continued over the sacral promontory, scoring the left pararectal peritoneum along this subtle line.

The presacral space is thus entered and developed with cautery scissors medially and distally as far as visualization permits. The left hypogastric nerve should be identified and protected. It is possible to enter the presacral space too close to the promontory in a plane that is actually posterior to the nerve, so it is important to enter the plane immediately posterior to the mesorectum, and anterior to the nerve.

After the left side of the presacral space is developed as far as visualization permits, the right side of the presacral space is entered by scoring the right pararectal peritoneum after identifying the right ureter. The dissection is joined with that already performed from the left side and the right hypogastric nerve is identified and swept posteriorly.

Attention is turned to the anterior dissection of the rectum. This is often the most technically demanding aspect of the rectal mobilization and is facilitated by the mobilization of the posterior and lateral aspects of the rectum which allow tension to be placed on the anterior attachments by appropriate retraction of the rectum out of the pelvis. In male patients, the seminal vesicles and prostate are identified and protected. In female patients in whom the uterus is obscuring the view of the pelvis, several options are available. A uterine retractor may be placed, but requires dilation of the cervix. The most simple and effective option is to place a transabdominal suture through the fundus of the uterus to retract it superiorly and anteriorly. Also, a sponge stick placed in the vagina to retract it anteriorly facilitates dissection in the rectovaginal septum. As each quadrant of dissection of the rectum proceeds, this allows for more effective retraction of another quadrant and thus dissection proceeds circumferentially. Thus, the rectum is completely dissected circumferentially down to the level of the pelvic floor which is confirmed by digital examination (**Figure 6.7.5**). It is actually possible to dissect into the intersphincteric space, especially in slim patients, and thus digital examination to confirm the level of dissection is important.

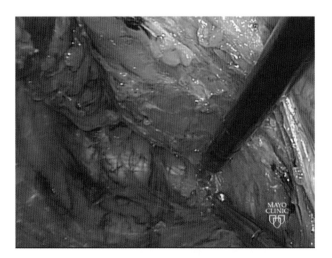

6.7.5 Completing the posterior dissection of the rectum to the level of the pelvic floor. Photo courtesy of Mayo Clinic.

In UC patients, it is possible to transect the rectum and perform either stapled anastomosis, or mucosectomy and handsewn anastomosis. The author's preference is for stapled anastomosis at the top of the anal canal, with preservation of the anal transition zone as evidence suggests better function in such cases. Mucosectomy is reserved for ulcerative colitis with rectal dysplasia or rectal cancer, a relatively uncommon indication. In CD patients, the rectum may be transected at the top of the anal canal, thus not burning any bridges for later reconstruction, versus performing either intersphincteric dissection or abdominoperineal resection.

To transect the rectum at the level of the pelvic floor, an articulated laparoscopic stapler is deployed via the right lower quadrant 12 mm port creating a transverse staple line. Some surgeons prefer to use a suprapubic port (this should influence initial port placement). The choice of staple cartridge is determined by the confines of the pelvis and thus by the gender of the patient. In female patients, it may be possible to deploy a 45 or even a 60 mm cartridge, whereas male patients with a narrow pelvis may require several firings of a 30 mm cartridge.

TRANSECTION OF THE MESENTERY

In the patient with a normal BMI, the following is the simplest approach. After transection of the rectum at the pelvic floor, the mobilized colon and rectum become a midline structure centered beneath the umbilicus. The entire colon and rectum can actually be exteriorized through a 3–5 cm periumbilical incision. The supraumbilical port-site incision is extended around the left side of the umbilicus (to avoid interference with an appliance for the ileostomy) and the mesentery is transected extracorporeally.

In the obese patient, or for a 'completely laparoscopic' approach, the mesentery is divided intracorporeally. In the infrequent cases of cancer or dysplasia, the vascular pedicles should be divided at their bases. In most patients, the mesentery may be divided where convenient. Commencing at the top of the presacral dissection, at the sacral promontory, a vessel-sealing device is used to transect the mesentery sequentially from the rectosigmoid to the right colon, preserving the ileocolic pedicle. The transected end of the rectum is grasped with a laparoscopic instrument and inspection is performed to ensure small bowel does not lie over the colon.

EXTERIORIZATION AND POUCH CREATION

Several options exist at this point:

- In the slim patient, without cancer or dysplasia, and in whom the mesentery has not been divided (the simplest and least technically demanding approach), a 3–5 cm periumbilical incision is made by extending the supraumbilical port site incision around the left side of the umbilicus. The colon is exteriorized and the mesentery is divided extracorporeally.

- In the obese patient in whom the mesentery has been divided intracorporeally, it is better to extract the specimen via a periumbilical incision rather than try to extract it via the ileostomy site, as the diameter of the colon will enlarge the ileostomy site. It is also difficult to gauge the reach of the pouch in an obese patient in whom the specimen has been extracted via the ileostomy site.

- In slim patients, with intracorporeal division of the mesentery, the specimen may be extracted via the ileostomy site for a 'completely laparoscopic' approach (**Figure 6.7.6**). This also applies to the single incision approach. The 12 mm port in the planned ileostomy site is removed, the anterior rectus fascia is incised in a cruciate fashion, the rectus muscle fibers are separated, and the posterior fascia is elevated and incised in a cruciate fashion. The rectum is passed up through this ileostomy incision and the entire specimen is exteriorized.

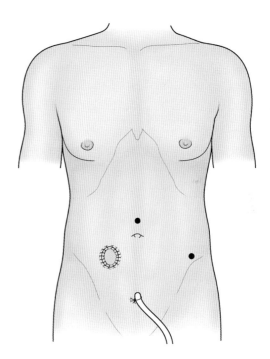

6.7.6 Final result after 'completely laparoscopic' approach, with exteriorization of the colon via the ileostomy site.

- In single-incision PC, the transected end of the rectum is held with a grasper, the port device removed, with the grasper still deployed through it and the entire specimen is exteriorized via the ileostomy site.

In each instance, the remaining mesentery is divided, preserving the ileocolic pedicle. The terminal ileum is transected with a linear stapler (a reload of the laparoscopic stapler may be more cost-effective than using a separate linear stapler). The distal ileum, approximately 15 cm from the transected end, is examined to determine whether it reaches to the pubis. In a slim patient, exteriorization of the ileum via a non-midline incision (the ileostomy site) does not affect this test. In a patient with a thicker abdominal wall, experience should determine whether pouch-lengthening techniques are necessary. A 15 cm J-pouch is constructed with two firings of either an 80 or a 100 mm linear stapler via an enterotomy at the apex of the pouch. The anvil of a circular stapler is secured within the enterotomy at the apex with a monofilament suture. The blind (efferent) limb of the pouch is tacked to the adjacent afferent limb, burying the staple line.

The pouch is returned to the abdominal cavity, which is irrigated and aspirated. The fascia of the extraction site (periumbilical incision or ileostomy site) is closed with sutures, and the 12 mm port is secured within the incision again, between two of the sutures, allowing the pneumoperitoneum to be re-established. In single incision cases, the port is replaced in the ileostomy site.

CREATION OF THE ILEAL J-POUCH ANAL ANASTOMOSIS

The anus is dilated and the stapler inserted. The spike is brought out adjacent to the staple line rather than through it. The cut edge of the pouch mesentery is traced to the duodenum to ensure there is no twisting of the pouch. The anvil is docked onto the handle and the stapler is reapproximated. In female patients, digital examination confirms that the posterior wall of the vagina has not been trapped in the staple line. The stapler is then fired and removed. Both tissue rings are examined and the distal ring is sent to pathology.

A 15-Fr round Jackson-Pratt drain is placed in the pelvis via the suprapubic port. Distal ileum, approximately 10–12 inches proximal to the pouch, is brought up through the ileostomy site. The remaining ports are removed and inspected for hemostasis. The fascia of the supraumbilical extraction site or 12 mm port site is closed. Skin incisions are approximated with subcuticular monofilament 3-0 suture, and the ileostomy is matured in loop fashion with 3-0 monofilament suture. In single-incision cases, there are no incisions to close, only an ileostomy to mature! A 20–24-Fr red rubber catheter is placed transanally into the pouch for decompression.

POSTOPERATIVE MANAGEMENT

The orogastric tube is removed at the end of the operation. Scheduled i.v. ketorolac and oral acetaminophen are used if not contraindicated, and patient-controlled analgesia (PCA) with morphine, fentanyl, or hydromorphone, is used for breakthrough pain. If ertapenem is infused preoperatively, no further antibiotic coverage is required. If ciprofloxacin and metronidazole were used preoperatively,

two additional doses are given, ensuring discontinuation of antibiotics by 24 hours postoperatively. On the first postoperative day (POD 1) the patient may have limited oral clear liquids (500 mL) and unrestricted clear liquids on the morning of POD 2. Diet is advanced as tolerated, to an ileostomy diet (low residue diet with thickening snacks) later on POD 2 or the morning of POD 3. The PCA is stopped when solid food is tolerated and the Foley is removed after the PCA is discontinued. Ostomy teaching starts on POD 1, and home health services are requested to assist with post-discharge ostomy management. Discharge is appropriate when the patient is tolerating 2000 mL oral intake, and output from the ileostomy is less than 1000 mL. Patients are instructed to take loperamide 2–4 mg 30 minutes prior to meals and at bedtime to prevent dehydration.

Complications

Potential intraoperative complications include bleeding, ureteral injury, and injury to the hypogastric nerves, although these risks are low. There is the possibility of conversion to an open operation, but patients are counseled that this is an intraoperative decision not a 'complication'. The potential postoperative complications are similar to the standard open approach, although some complications may be less frequent compared with an open operation. The most common immediate complications are postoperative ileus, high ileostomy output, small bowel obstruction, wound infection, urinary tract infection, and pouch leak. Evidence suggests that the wound infection rate may be reduced in laparoscopic cases. Long-term complications, such as pouch dysfunction and pouchitis, are similar to open PC and IPAA. One exception may be small bowel obstruction, because fewer adhesions form after a laparoscopic approach, and this may eventually manifest as a reduced risk of small bowel obstruction, and also maintenance of fecundity in women of child-bearing age.

Results

Postoperative length of stay is reduced compared with the open approach, with the vast majority of patients being discharged between POD 3 and 5. From the patients' perspective, following closure of the ileostomy, the vast majority have acceptable bowel frequency, especially when compared to the frequency, pain, and urgency experienced during active colitis. The surgical literature suggests a range of four to six bowel movements during the day and none to two at night. Many younger patients, particularly teenagers and patients in their twenties, will attain a daily frequency of between two and four bowel movements, dependent on dietary intake.

SUMMARY

A laparoscopic approach is feasible for proctocolectomy with or without IPAA. This chapter has concentrated on laparoscopy-assisted, completely laparoscopic, and single incision laparoscopic approaches. A lateral-to-medial approach duplicates the open approach, allows a choice regarding the level of mesenteric vessel transection, and avoids ischemic bowel remaining in the abdominal cavity while the pelvic dissection is performed. The cosmetic results are favorable, length of stay is shorter, and functional outcomes are similar to open procedures.

FURTHER READING

Ahmed Ali U, Keus F, Heikens JT *et al*. Open versus laparoscopic (assisted) ileo pouch anal anastomosis for ulcerative colitis and familial adenomatous polyposis. *Cochrane Database of Systematic Reviews* 2009; (1): CD006267.

Bemelman WA. Laparoscopic ileoanal pouch surgery. *British Journal of Surgery* 2010; 97: 2–3.

Chung TP, Fleshman JW, Birnbaum EH *et al*. Laparoscopic vs open total abdominal colectomy for severe colitis: impact on recovery and subsequent completion restorative proctectomy. *Diseases of the Colon and Rectum* 2009; 52: 4–10.

Indar AA, Efron JE, Young-Fadok TM. Laparoscopic ileal pouch-anal anastomosis reduces abdominal and pelvic adhesions. *Surgical Endoscopy* 2009; 23: 174–7.

Lawes DA, Young-Fadok TM. Minimally invasive proctocolectomy and ileal pouch-anal anastomosis. In: Frantzides CT, Carlson MA (eds). *Atlas of minimally invasive surgery*. Philadelphia: Saunders Elsevier, 2009: 139–46.

Polle SW, Dunker MS, Slors JF *et al*. Body image, cosmesis, quality of life, and functional outcome of hand-assisted laparoscopic versus open restorative proctocolectomy: long-term results of a randomized trial. *Surgical Endoscopy* 2007; 21: 1301–7.

Vivas D, Khaikin M, Wexner SD. Laparoscopic proctocolectomy and Brooke ileostomy. In: Asbun HJ, Young-Fadok TM (eds). *American College of Surgeons Multimedia atlas of surgery*. Colorectal surgery volume. Chicago: American College of Surgeons, 2008: 111–16.

Wexner SD, Johansen OB, Nogueras JJ, Jagelman DG. Laparoscopic total abdominal colectomy. A prospective trial. *Diseases of the Colon and Rectum* 1992; 35: 651–5.

Young-Fadok TM, Nunoo-Mensah JW. Laparoscopic proctocolectomy and ileal pouch-anal anastomosis (IPAA). In: Asbun HJ, Young-Fadok TM (eds). *American College of Surgeons Multimedia atlas of surgery*. Colorectal surgery volume. Chicago: American College of Surgeons, 2008: 117–29.

Continent ileostomy (Kock reservoir ileostomy)

R JOHN NICHOLLS AND PARIS P TEKKIS

HISTORY

The operation was developed in the 1960s by Nils Kock of Gothenburg, Sweden, with the original intention to create an artificial urinary bladder from small intestine. The resulting construction was subsequently applied to patients who required a proctocolectomy for ulcerative colitis (and selected patients with Crohn's disease). Its aim was to improve quality of life, by creating a continent ileostomy which did not require the use of a stoma appliance. This was achieved by the formation of a reservoir combined with an inverted nipple valve fashioned from the terminal segment of the small bowel.

Until the description and general use of restorative proctocolectomy in the late 1970s, the continent ileostomy was often used, particularly in Scandinavia, for patients who required a permanent ileostomy after proctocolectomy. In the last 20 years, its application has declined considerably, but it still has a place in selected patients.

PRINCIPLES AND JUSTIFICATION

Continent ileostomy is applicable to patients who require or already have had a permanent ileostomy after proctocolectomy with removal of the anal sphincter. Its only purpose is to improve quality of life by allowing the patient to be free of a stoma appliance at least during the day. It can be carried out at the same time as the proctocolectomy or it can be performed as a procedure secondary to a previous proctocolectomy. In both circumstances, open abdominal access is required. It is therefore a major undertaking. In addition, slippage of the nipple valve and fistulation can occur. The operation should therefore be carried out in selected patients, who have a strong desire to have the benefits while being aware of the risks. Today the number of surgeons capable of performing the operation is small. The procedure should therefore be carried out in a specialist unit.

Indications are as follows:

- Patients with a permanent ileostomy who do not have an anal sphincter mechanism.
- Selected patients with Crohn's disease. These include patients with large bowel involvement with a normal small bowel.
- Selected patients with a restorative proctocolectomy who have failed and require removal of the ileoanal reservoir. Great thought should be given to this decision. The patient has already experienced the suffering leading to failure. A second operation with potential morbidity and the further possibility of failure could prolong the patient's suffering and subsequent removal, if necessary, would increase the chance of short bowel syndrome. There is no place for carrying out such a procedure outside a specialist unit.

Contraindications are as follows:

- Most patients with Crohn's disease.
- Patients who have had a small bowel resection. Since the continent reservoir requires a length of 45 cm of small intestine, there is a risk of short bowel syndrome if the operation fails and resection of the reservoir is necessary.
- Patients who require urgent surgery for acute severe colitis. These should be treated by a colectomy with ileostomy to allow them to recover their health. If, several months later, a total proctectomy (rather than a restorative proctectomy) is decided upon, the patient could have a continent ileostomy constructed at the same time.
- Patients with low intelligence or psychological instability, or children too young to be able to manage the stoma. In the last instance, the patient can be considered for a continent ileostomy when considered to be sufficiently mature.

PREOPERATIVE ASSESSMENT AND PREPARATION

The preoperative preparation is identical to any major intestinal open operation including antibiotic cover and thromboembolic prophylaxis (see Chapter 6.9).

The site of the stoma is marked. This should be done by the surgeon, unless the stomatherapist is familiar with the operation. The position is lower and more medial than for a conventional ileostomy. It should be medial to the linea semilunaris of the rectus abdominis muscle and lie about 5 cm above the inguinal ligament just below the bikini line.

ANESTHESIA

This is identical to that used for any major intestinal open operation.

OPERATION

Position of patient

The patient is placed in the reversed Trendelenburg position with the legs raised (Lloyd-Davies) as described in Chapter 6.5, p. 498.

Incision

If the operation is part of a conventional proctocolectomy, a midline incision is used. If it is carried out secondary to a previous proctocolectomy, the ileostomy is circumcised and dissected from the subcutaneous fat and rectus sheath and its end is closed with a suture or stapling device with minimum loss of terminal ileum. The abdomen is then opened through the previous midline incision (**Figure 6.8.1**).

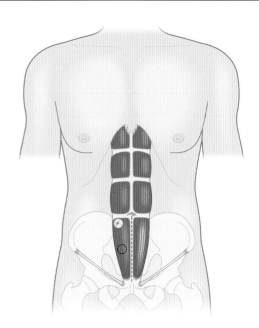

6.8.1

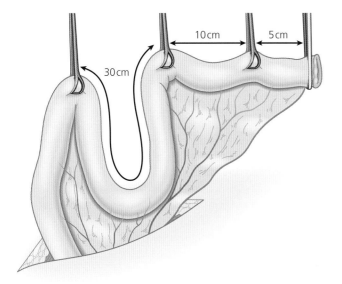

6.8.2

Formation of the ileal reservoir

Having removed the colon and rectum, the terminal 45 cm of small intestine are measured (**Figure 6.8.2**). The following illustrations show the operating field with the surgeon standing on the patient's right.

The terminal ileum is brought out through the abdominal incision to face the head of the patient. Three 15 cm segments are measured. The most distal is divided into a 10 cm proximal length for construction of the nipple valve and a 5 cm distal length which will pass through the anterior abdominal wall. In an obese patient, the terminal segment will need to be more than 5 cm long. A suitable length is estimated leaving the other measurements as stated above.

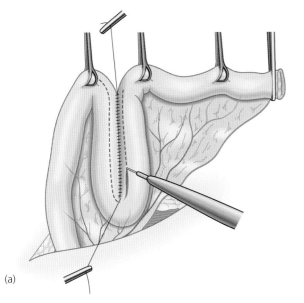

(a)

6.8.3

(b)

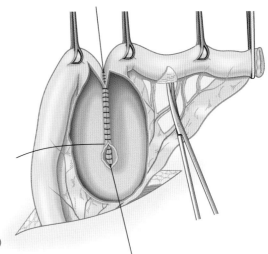

The antimesenteric border of the two proximal 15 cm segments is approximated by an absorbable seromuscular (2-0 polyglactin, 20 PDS) suture. The loops are then opened using the cutting diathermy extending this for a further 3 cm (**Figure 6.8.3**a, b).

The posterior layer is then sutured using a full-thickness continuous suture.

Using sharp dissection, the peritoneum is removed from the mesentery which will be invaginated during formation of the nipple valve. Care must be taken to avoid damage to the mesenteric vessels.

Formation of the nipple valve

A light tissue forceps (e.g. Babcock's pattern) is applied to the mucosa of the segment planned to form the nipple valve. On gentle traction, the intestine is invaginated to produce a spout about 5 cm long (**Figure 6.8.4**).

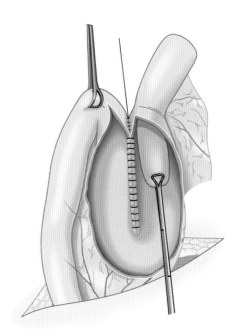

6.8.4

The nipple is then fixed in position by the application of four lines of staples using the bladeless 55 mm linear stapler (S-GIA™; Covidien, Dublin, Ireland) (**Figure 6.8.5**).

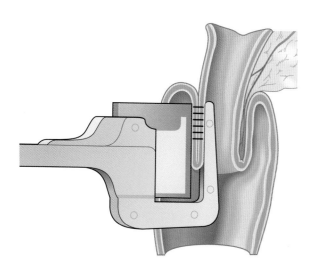

6.8.5

Two firings are made on each side of the mesentery and the other two on the antimesenteric side of the intestine about the same distance apart (**Figure 6.8.6**). The nipple may become cyanosed, but it will remain viable.

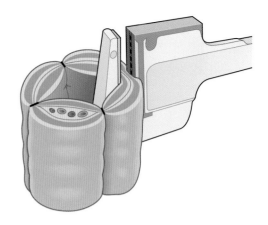

6.8.6

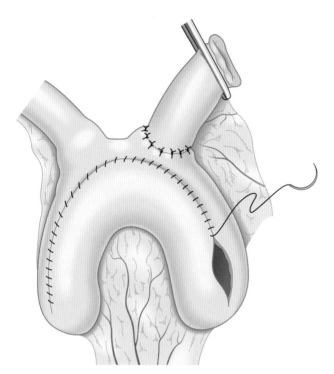

6.8.7

Completion of the reservoir

The ileal reservoir is folded and closed with a continuous absorbable suture starting at the apex and continuing towards the corners on each side (**Figure 6.8.7**). A series of interrupted non-absorbable seromuscular sutures is placed around the circumference of the external point of invagination of the valve.

Orientation of the reservoir

The reservoir is turned through the leaves of the mesentery by gentle pressure on its corners, reversing its position enabling it to lie comfortably in the right iliac fossa. (**Figure 6.8.8**). The integrity of the suture lines is tested by distending the reservoir with saline solution to identify any point of leakage.

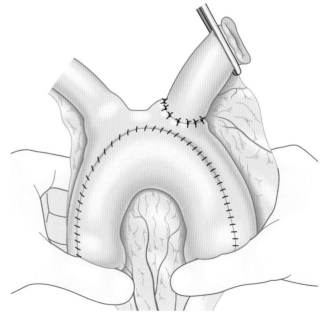

6.8.8

The ileostomy trephine and fixation of the reservoir to the anterior abdominal wall

A disk of skin of about 15 mm diameter is excised at the site marked for the ileostomy. The incision is deepened through the anterior rectus sheath and the rectus muscle splitting its fibers to the peritoneum. The opening should take no more than one and a half fingers.

The reservoir is positioned in the right iliac fossa supported by the iliac bone with its overlying muscles. Four or five interrupted non-absorbable sutures are then placed between the lateral aspect of the ileostomy trephine and the reservoir along the external line of invagination of the nipple valve. These are tied and the distal ileal segment is then drawn through the ileostomy trephine (**Figure 6.8.9**). Further interrupted non-absorbable sutures are placed to form a complete ring (**Figure 6.8.10**). Care must be taken not to damage the mesentery. This step is important since it attaches the reservoir to the anterior abdominal wall taking the strain off the terminal ileal segment which would result in dislocation of the nipple valve.

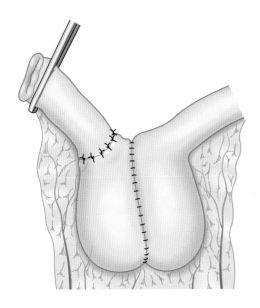

6.8.9

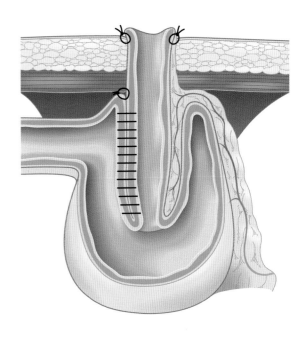

6.8.10

The stoma is fashioned flush with the skin by the insertion of interrupted mucocutaneous sutures.

Before the abdomen is closed, a Medina (28 Fr) catheter is passed through the ileostomy into the reservoir. This has a blunt tip with two large side holes through which the contents of the reservoir will drain (**Figure 6.8.11**). The competence of the nipple valve is tested by instilling 100 mL of saline down the catheter into the reservoir and after its removal the stoma is inspected for any leakage. If satisfactory the catheter is then reinserted and is anchored in place by two loose sutures placed through the edge of the ileostomy.

A protective ileostomy is sometimes used according to the judgment of the surgeon. The abdomen is closed and the catheter connected to tubing leading to a drainage bag.

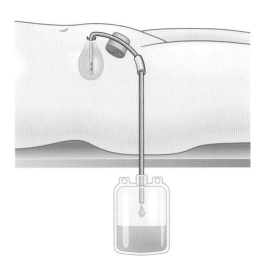

6.8.11

POSTOPERATIVE CARE

Other than management of the catheter, the postoperative care is identical to that for any other intestinal operation. This varies in detail from one unit to another. In the authors' practice, the catheter remains *in situ* for 4 weeks. During the immediate postoperative period, satisfactory continuous drainage should be confirmed by observation. Irrigation may be necessary if there is a blockage. On discharge from hospital between days 7 and 10, the patient should be given instructions on irrigation and should be in easy contact with the unit. He or she is provided with a catheter and a 60 mL bladder syringe and pads to cover the ileostomy.

At an outpatient visit 2–3 weeks after discharge (one month from the procedure), the catheter is removed and the patient is taught to reinsert it. On returning home, the patient catheterizes the stoma every 4 hours and leaves it on free drainage at night. The interval between emptying is gradually extended until catheterization is performed three to four times per day and not at night. Many patients use an ileostomy appliance at night for security.

COMPLICATIONS AND OUTCOME

Early

Early complications include breakdown of the suture line with peritonitis, enterocutaneous fistula and ischemia of the stoma. Peritonitis requires laparotomy with peritoneal irrigation and creation of a proximal loop ileostomy. Fistulation and ischemia can usually be managed conservatively. It may be necessary to carry out a revisional operation a few months later.

Late

The most important late complication is sliding (subluxation) of the nipple valve. This occurs in less than 10 percent to over 30 percent of cases. It is suggested by difficulty in intubation and incontinence of the stoma. The complication is usually associated with detachment of the reservoir from the anterior abdominal wall. Surgical revision of the nipple valve is required.

Fistulation from the base of the valve occurs in less than 5 percent of cases. It will have presented in the early postoperative period. It requires surgical closure at an interval of several months to allow local inflammatory changes to have settled.

Stoma complications include stenosis, herniation, and prolapse. Stenosis may result in patients who develop ischemia. It can usually be treated conservatively by dilatation, but if this is not successful, a revision operation is required. This is rare. Herniation is uncommon and may occur if the diameter of the ileostomy trephine was too wide. Management is difficult. A local mesh insertion may be successful. Prolapse can consist of the entire nipple valve. Reduction should be performed. Surgical revision may be necessary.

Pouchitis was described in continent ileostomy before it was after restorative proctocolectomy. After formation of any ileal reservoir, there is a million-fold increase in the fecal bacterial concentration. This overgrowth may contribute to mucosal inflammation in the reservoir with a cumulative incidence of 40 percent over five years. Clinically significant pouchitis is present in only a minority (5 percent) of patients. Pouchitis is an uncommon reason for removal of the reservoir and establishment of a conventional stoma.

REVISIONAL SURGERY

Revisional surgery is required for patients with subluxation of the nipple valve, fistulation, and a few with stenosis. These operations should only be carried out in a unit familiar with continent ileostomy.

Valve subluxation (slippage)

This involves an abdominal procedure in which adhesions are divided and the reservoir is opened. The nipple valve is then restored and fixed by further stapling either as described above or by incorporation of the nipple with the wall of the reservoir. The postoperative management is similar to that described above under the heading Postoperative care. Sometimes a complete revision of the valve is necessary as described for fistulation at the base of the valve (see below).

Fistulation and stenosis

An abdominal revision is necessary. Adhesions are divided and the reservoir is identified. Fistulation from the body of the reservoir is closed. A temporary loop ileostomy may be considered necessary. Where the fistula is located at the base of the valve, simple closure is not possible. In this circumstance, the valve should be excised. The reservoir is then rotated through 180°. A new nipple valve is made by invagination of what was until this moment the afferent ileal loop. Intestinal continuity is then restored by an anastomosis between the reservoir at the site of the previous valve and the divided proximal small bowel.

FURTHER READING

Dozois RR, Kelly KA, Beart RW, Beahrs O. Improved results with continent ileostomy. *Annals of Surgery* 1980; **192**: 319–24.

Kock NG. Intra-abdominal 'reservoir' in patients with permanent ileostomy. *Archives of Surgery* 1969; **99**: 223–31.

Kock NG Myrvold HE, Nilsson LO, Philipson BM. Continent ileostomy: an account of 314 patients. *Acta Chirurgica Scandinavica* 1981; **147**: 67–72.

Myrvold HE. The continent ileostomy. *World Journal of Surgery* 1987; **11**: 720–6.

Restorative proctocolectomy with ileal reservoir

R JOHN NICHOLLS AND PARIS P TEKKIS

HISTORY

Restorative proctocolectomy, also known as ileal pouch-anal anastomosis (IPAA), is suitable for diffuse mucosal diseases of the large bowel, such as ulcerative colitis and familial adenomatous polyposis. The mortality of the former was 50 percent up to the introduction of colectomy with ileostomy in the late 1930s and 1940s, when it fell precipitously to under 5 percent. The resulting stoma was usually well accepted by patients in exchange for the recovery of health. Attempts to avoid a permanent stoma were, however, made from the early 1940s. Colectomy with ileorectal anastomosis left the rectum, which in many colitic patients led to continued poor function and also the risk of malignant transformation. This operation has largely been replaced by restorative proctocolectomy, originally described by Nissen in 1934 and subsequently developed by Ravitch, Bacon, Kock, and Parks. The present form of the operation resembles that described by Parks (1978) with subsequent modifications of the type of ileal reservoir used and the method of performing the ileoanal anastomosis. Restorative proctocolectomy is now the most frequently used operation when surgery is indicated in ulcerative colitis.

In familial adenomatous polyposis, colectomy with ileorectal anastomosis and restorative proctocolectomy are used depending on the perceived risk of rectal cancer which is dependent on age, genetic disposition, family history, the number and extent of adenomas in the rectum, and considerations of female fertility.

PRINCIPLES AND JUSTIFICATION

The only reason for restorative proctocolectomy (IPAA) is to avoid a permanent ileostomy. A conventional proctocolectomy gives excellent results except for this. Where there is no medical objection, the choice lies between a restorative or conventional proctocolectomy and is almost entirely the patient's to make. This is possible only if the disadvantages are fully discussed. These include failure and complication rates, total treatment time, the possibility of pouchitis occurring, and the likely functional outcome. The operation is a specialist procedure and should be carried out in a unit experienced in performing it.

The principle of the operation is to remove all diseased tissue and to restore intestinal continuity to avoid a permanent stoma. This is achieved by a proctocolectomy identical to that described in Chapter 6.6 until the pelvic floor is reached by the dissection. The rectum is then divided at the level of the anorectal junction to preserve the anal sphincter. An anastomosis is performed between the terminal ileum and the anal stump after construction of a reservoir of terminal ileum to act as a neorectum to optimize function. The ileoanal anastomosis can be carried out using a manual or stapled technique. Most surgeons add a protective ileostomy which is closed after 8 weeks if all suture lines are satisfactorily healed.

PREOPERATIVE ASSESSMENT AND PREPARATION

Antibiotic cover should be by single dose perioperative injection, but if the duration of operation exceeds 3 hours, a second dose of antibiotic is advisable, particularly if the antibiotic has a short half-life. In immunosuppressed patients receiving drugs such as cyclosporin or biologicals sulfonamides may still have a role in protecting against *Pneumocystis carinii* pneumonia.

Thromboembolic prophylaxis using subcutaneous heparin, pneumatic leg gaiters, and thromboembolic deterrent stockings should be employed.

Blood (usually 4 units) should be cross-matched and available if necessary.

A fast track management program should be offered.

ANESTHESIA

The operation is carried out under general anesthesia with full relaxation. If a central venous line is needed for total parenteral nutrition, this should be inserted at the end of the operation. If an open technique is used, the abdominal wound will be an important cause of pain and an epidural anesthetic should be given. The bladder is routinely catheterized.

OPERATION

Position of the patient

The patient is placed in the reversed Trendelenburg position with the legs raised (Lloyd-Davies) as described in Chapter 1.2. Whether an open or laparoscopic technique is used, this gives excellent access to the abdomen and perineum and allows the suitable deployment of surgeon and assistants around the patient.

Drainage of the rectum

It is helpful to insert a proctoscope before starting, to drain the rectum of any excessive liquid feces and flatus.

Incision

For an open operation a midline incision is made. This should be long enough to allow safe access to the pelvis and should be taken down to the pubis. In ulcerative colitis, the splenic flexure may be drawn down by longitudinal contraction of the colon by chronic fibrosis when it may be possible to mobilize it using an incision taken above the umbilicus by only 2–3 cm.

On entering the peritoneal cavity, abdominal exploration is performed, the wound margins are protected and a Balfour retractor with a central blade is inserted.

The incision for a laparoscopic operation is described in Chapter 6.7.

In patients who have had a previous colectomy with ileostomy, and a rectosigmoid mucous fistula, these are circumcised and mobilized as far as possible down to the fascia. Each is then closed by a running suture. The abdomen is recleaned with skin preparation and opened through the previous skin incision. (**Figure 6.9.1**)

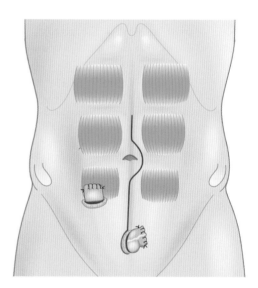

6.9.1

Mobilization of the colon

This has been described in detail in Chapter 6.6. It is helpful to follow a routine.

The dissection starts with the right colon. The surgeon stands on the patient's left side. The right colon is mobilized and the ileocolic vessels are divided. The terminal ileum is divided at the ileocecal junction. This frees the right colon and allows the surgeon to divide the right colic vessels and the vessels supplying the transverse colon as far towards the splenic flexure as is convenient.

The surgeon then changes to the patient's right side and mobilizes the sigmoid and descending colon. In ulcerative colitis the splenic flexure is often drawn down owing to shortening by chronic fibrosis. Mobilization may be easy as a consequence. After full mobilization of the entire colon, the middle and left colic vessels are divided.

Mobilization of the rectum

Two techniques are available. The first is the classic anatomical dissection in the presacral plane (total mesorectal excision), for example, see chapter 6.1, the second is close rectal dissection along the rectal wall. With the former there is a small (2–3 percent) risk of damage to the pelvic nerves which in theory is avoided in the latter.

DISSECTION IN THE PRESACRAL PLANE (TOTAL MESORECTAL EXCISION)

In ulcerative colitis, it is obligatory to use this method in the presence of cancer or dysplasia anywhere in the large bowel. With dysplasia, invasion unrecognized before operation can sometimes be found on histological examination of the operative specimen.

It should also be used in familial adenomatous polyposis except in patients with only a few small rectal adenomas.

Dissection of the rectum in the presence of malignancy or dysplasia is identical to that used for anterior resection.

CLOSE RECTAL DISSECTION

The dissection is carried out close to the rectal wall within the arcade of the superior rectal vessels.

The sigmoid mesocolon is dissected from the retroperitoneal structures and the left gonadal vessels and ureter are identified and safeguarded.

The sigmoid branches of the inferior mesenteric vessels are divided close to the mesenteric border of the colon. The first few branches of the superior rectal vessels are divided at the upper rectal level bringing the dissection to within their arcade.

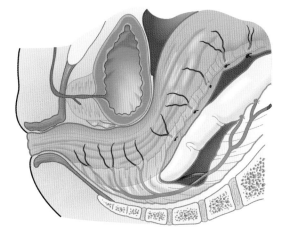

6.9.2

The superior rectal artery bifurcates giving rise to two leaves of the mesorectum. These can be separated by inserting a finger in the midline immediately posterior to the rectum and by blunt dissection an avascular plane between the two leaves of the mesorectum is developed down to the level of the pelvic floor. (**Figure 6.9.2**)

THE ANTERIOR RECTAL DISSECTION

In the male, the peritoneum is divided anteriorly on the base of the bladder anterior to the rectoprostatic sulcus (**Figure 6.9.3**a). A long-lipped retractor (St Mark's pattern) is then placed in the peritoneal incision and gently angled to elevate the anterior layer of the divided peritoneum. By blunt dissection using a Lahey peanut dissector, the seminal vesicles are identified and gently pushed anteriorly. (**Figure 6.9.3**b) The rectoprostatic septum is thus entered to show Denonvilliers' fascia on the anterior surface of the rectum. This is divided transversely. The anterior dissection is continued distally behind the fascia to the level of the apex of the prostate (**Figure 6.9.3**c).

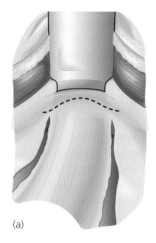

(a)

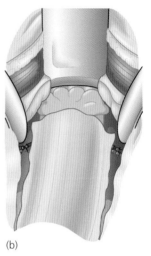

(b)

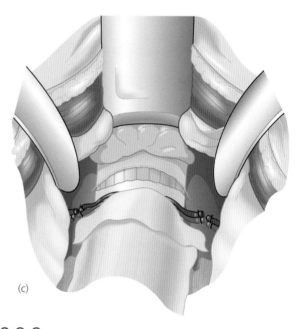

(c)

6.9.3

In the female, the peritoneum is divided transversely at the point of its inflection in the rectovaginal sulcus to avoid damage to the posterior vaginal venous plexuses (**Figure 6.9.4**). The peritoneum is mobilized by a combination of sharp and blunt dissection towards the vagina to identify the post-vaginal veins. Denonvilliers' fascia is less apparent than in the male and may not be seen. The dissection is continued distally in the rectovaginal septum

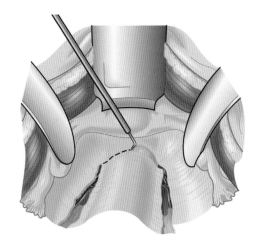

6.9.4

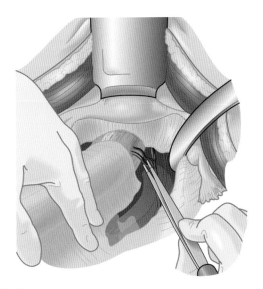

In both sexes at this level, the blood vessels entering the rectal wall laterally on each side and any left posteriorly are identified and coagulated close to the rectal wall by diathermy or the LigaSure device. (**Figure 6.9.5**).

6.9.5

The level of the mobilization is determined by inserting a gloved finger into the anus allowing an assessment per abdomen of the level of division (**Figure 6.9.6**).

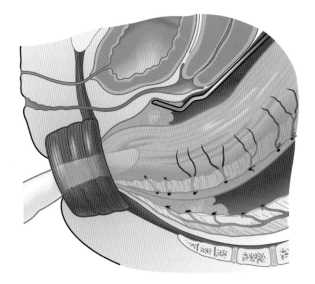

6.9.6

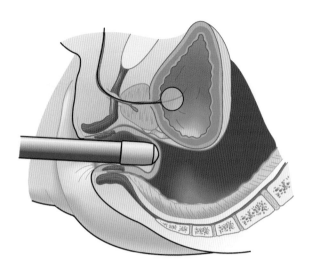

6.9.7

FINDING THE RECTUM AFTER PREVIOUS COLECTOMY

When the rectum or rectosigmoid stump is evident on opening the abdomen, mobilization will proceed as described above. In some cases, however, part of the rectum will have been removed previously along with the colon. In this circumstance, the rectum may lie below the pelvic peritoneum and may not therefore be visible. This is a difficult situation especially if the rectal stump is short.

Dissection should be determined by the need to avoid damaging the vagina, the urogenital system in the male, or the lateral pelvic wall veins.

A rectoscope with its obturator left in place will help to identify the position of the rectal stump (**Figure 6.9.7**).

In the female, insertion of a finger into the vagina will allow it to be elevated anteriorly facilitating identification of the rectovaginal septum and the subsequent anterior dissection (**Figure 6.9.8**).

Once the rectal stump is found, dissection proceeds as described above.

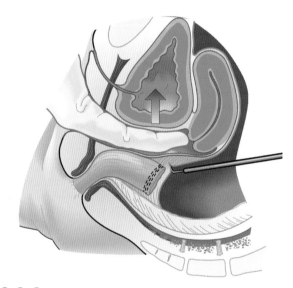

6.9.8

Division of the rectum

The technique for division of the rectum depends on whether a manual or a stapled ileoanal anastomosis is to be performed. It is generally agreed that the gut tube should be divided at the level of the anorectal junction.

MANUAL ANASTOMOSIS

When fully mobilized, the rectum is clamped above the pelvic floor (**Figure 6.9.9**). The anorectal stump in then cleaned with povidone-soaked swabs introduced by an assistant *per anum*.

The anorectal junction is at about 2 cm above the dentate line. A perineal surgeon inserts an anal retractor (e.g. Eisenhammer pattern) or a finger and identifies the dentate line anteriorly.

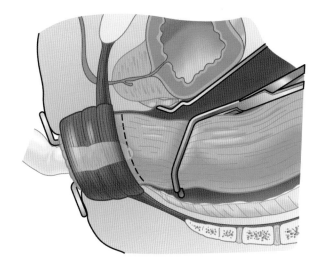

6.9.9

The abdominal operator then pushes the angled point of a diathermy needle through the anterior rectal wall as directed by the perineal operator. The bowel is then divided via the abdomen at this level using cutting diathermy or scissors (**Figure 6.9.10**).

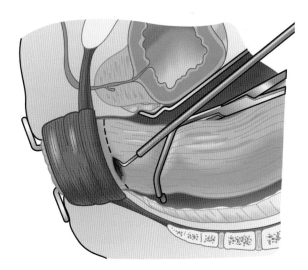

6.9.10

On dividing the bowel, the surgical specimen is removed. Bleeding from the perimuscular and submucosal vessels in the opened anorectal stump can be brisk and should be secured by diathermy coagulation.

A pack is left in the pelvis, firmly applied to the divided stump.

STAPLED ANASTOMOSIS

In this circumstance, the rectum is divided by a transverse stapling instrument (**Figure 6.9.11**a and b).

Care should be taken to ensure that the level of division is at the anorectal junction. There should be no retained rectal stump.

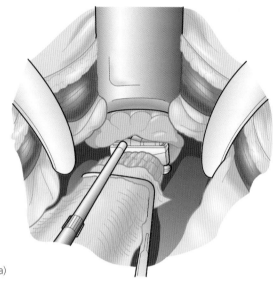

(a)

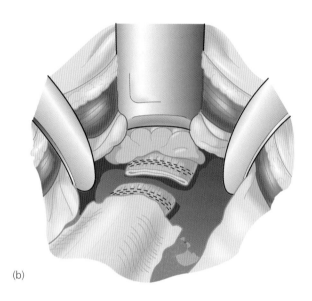

(b)

6.9.11

Mobilization of the terminal ileum

The operation depends on adequate mobility of the ileal reservoir to descend to the level of the anal canal. It is essential to achieve adequate mobility before constructing the reservoir.

DIVISION OF ADHESIONS

In the case of a previous colectomy, all small bowel adhesions should be divided. This includes all adhesions intrinsic to the mesentery.

MANEUVERS TO INCREASE MOBILITY

The mesentery can be made more mobile if necessary by various maneuvers (**Figure 6.9.12**).

The free edge of the mesentery can be divided. The peritoneum on each surface of the mesentery can be incised by a series of short transverse cuts. The duodenum can be mobilized by Kocher maneuver.

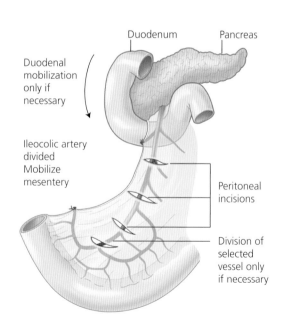

6.9.12

Occasionally, it may be necessary to divide a branch of the superior mesenteric artery showing tension. This should be done with great care. The end of the terminal ileum should be carefully inspected for any change in color when the vessel is temporarily occluded by a bulldog clamp. If there is no evidence of ischemia, the vessel can be divided.

Having obtained adequate mobilization, a pack is placed in the pelvis to discourage minor bleeding.

TESTING MOBILITY (TRIAL DESCENT)

The free edge of the mesentery is followed to the duodenum where adhesions at this level are divided. The most dependent part of the terminal ileum is identified. This is usually about 15–18 cm proximal to the ileocecal junction. This point is gently held over the pubis to test the mobility of the mesentery.

It can also be taken down into the pelvis by a suture which is grasped by an artery forceps inserted into the anus by a perineal surgeon (**Figure 6.9.13**a). Gentle traction on the suture will draw the loop of small bowel into the anal canal. If the apex of the loop reaches the dentate, it will do so after the reservoir is formed (**Figure 6.9.13**b).

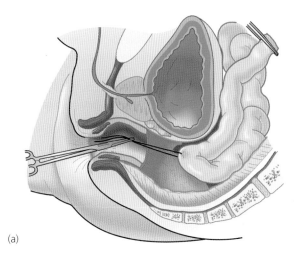

(a)

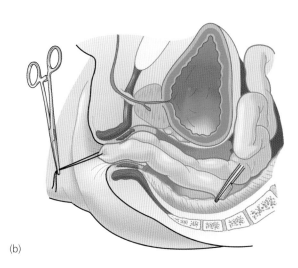

(b)

6.9.13

Ileal reservoir

PRINCIPLES OF RESERVOIR FORMATION

There are three main principles in construction of the reservoir. First, there should be minimal tension in the mesentery when it is brought down to the anal level. Second, it should be of adequate capacitance. Third, it should be anastomosed directly onto the anal canal without any distal ileal segment or retained rectum.

CHOICE OF RESERVOIR

There are no particular indications other than surgeon preference which type of reservoir should be used except for the S-reservoir, use of which has almost died out as the distal ileal segment often caused evacuation difficulty.

In practice today, therefore, the J-pouch predominates, with a much smaller proportion of patients having a W-pouch. The latter is used in some units and in recent years it may have increased in popularity following some evidence that long-term function is better. The length of small intestine used for each is similar (40 cm) and the mobility of the mesentery which determines whether or not there will be some tension on the anastomosis, is also similar for both J- and W-reservoirs.

As long as an ileoanal anastomosis is possible, there is no particular preoperative planning required for the reservoir. The choice of configuration is unaffected by general factors such as the patient's condition or medication requirements. There are no local anatomical or pathological factors which would lead to one or other type being preferred. Thus the width of the pelvis, mobility of the mesentery, the state of the anal sphincter, and the extensiveness of any adhesions do not influence the choice of reservoir.

J-reservoir

STAPLED CONSTRUCTION

The distal end of the terminal ileum will have already been closed by a linear stapling device.

The last 40 cm of terminal ileum are folded into two loops. These are held together by three lightly applied atraumatic tissue forceps (**Figure 6.9.14**).

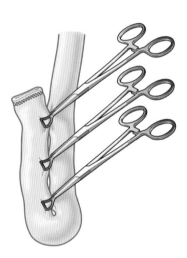

6.9.14

The apex, which will form the ileal component of the ileoanal anastomosis, is opened by a transverse incision about 2 cm long (**Figure 6.9.15**).

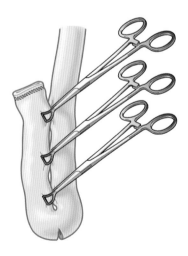

6.9.15

A linear stapler with a shaft length of 80 cm is introduced into the small intestine through the opening created. This is usually easier if the instrument is dismantled first and each shaft is introduced separately. The shafts are then brought together (**Figure 6.9.16**a and b).

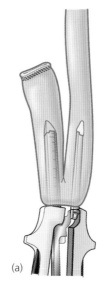

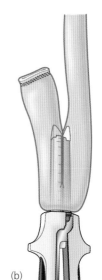

(a)

6.9.16

(b)

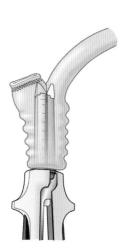

6.9.17

The small intestine of each limb is gently fed over the length of the shafts of the stapler (**Figure 6.9.17**).

The stapler is closed, ensuring by placing a finger or blunt instrument between its two leaves, that the mesentery is not included in the closed shafts (**Figure 6.9.18**).

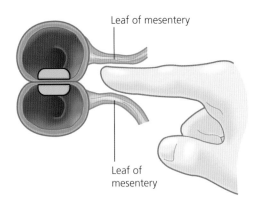

Leaf of mesentery

Leaf of mesentery

6.9.18

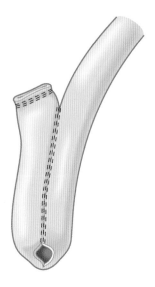

6.9.19

The stapler is fired and removed for recharging the cartridge. This procedure is repeated two more times to create a suture line of about 17–18 cm (**Figure 6.9.19**).

The suture line should be carefully inspected for any defect, especially next to the distal opening where there may be a deficiency of staples (**Figure 6.9.20**).

There will be a short free segment of bowel, 'dog ear', just proximal to the closed terminal ileum. This is fixed with seromuscular sutures to the afferent small intestine above the reservoir, to prevent torsion.

MANUAL CONSTRUCTION

The last 40 cm of terminal ileum are folded into two loops and are approximated by light tissue forceps. The bowel is opened. A full thickness suture is placed to create the posterior layer of the pouch. This is continued to allow the terminal ileum to be incorporated end-to-side into the reservoir. This maneuver avoids the 'dog ear' described for a stapled reservoir. The suture is then continued along the anterior wall of the reservoir.

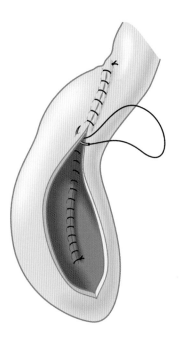

6.9.20

The continuous suture is continued onto the anterior layer of the reservoir (**Figure 6.9.21**).

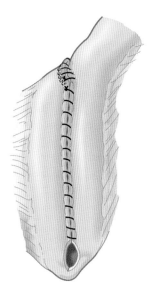

6.9.21

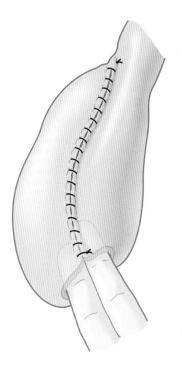

6.9.22

Manual ileoanal anastomosis

When a manual ileoanal anastomosis is to be made, the continuous suture is taken to the distal end of the reservoir to leave an opening that comfortably takes two fingers (**Figure 6.9.22**).

Two 2-0 polyglactin sutures mounted on a heavy duty 25 mm taper-cut needle are placed at the open end (**Figure 6.9.23**). One suture incorporates each edge of the anterior suture line. The other is inserted diametrically opposite. These will be subsequently passed through the pelvis and anal canal to the perineal operator.

The anterior layer is completed by a seromuscular suture.

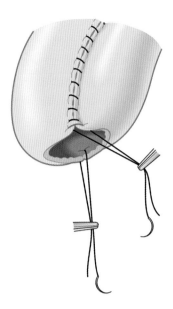

6.9.23

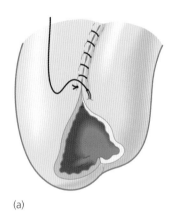

(a)

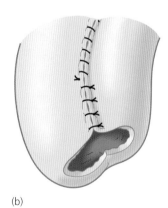

(b)

6.9.24

Stapled ileoanal anastomosis

For a stapled ileoanal anastomosis, a modification of the anterior layer is necessary. The continuous suture of the anterior layer should be terminated about 2 cm shorter than for a manual anastomosis and the remaining part of the reservoir completed with interrupted sutures (**Figure 6.9.24**).

The opening at the distal end of the reservoir should be wide enough to take the anvil of a circular stapling instrument.

The anterior layer is completed by a seromuscular suture.

Ileoanal anastomosis

The ileoanal anastomosis can be stapled or hand-sutured. The former is technically easier and is therefore used more frequently. A manual anastomosis with mucosectomy is more distal and has the advantages that the sutures are accurately placed under direct vision and that removal of the mucosa of the upper anal canal avoids leaving any retained rectal mucosa. The disadvantage is increased tension in a few cases and the possibility of a greater incidence of minor continence disturbance, although the studies in which the stapled and manual techniques have been prospectively compared have not shown any significant difference. In performing a stapled anastomosis, there is the danger of making it too proximal leaving a small area of diseased mucosa. This may not matter in most cases, but in some patients there is severe inflammation and ulceration of the distal mucosa. Function after closure of the ileostomy may be poor with anal burning, urgency, and blood due to the presence of the inflamed mucosa itself and the frequent passage of small volume stool due to incomplete evacuation. A stapled ileoanal anastomosis must therefore be sufficiently distal to avoid this complication. Direct inspection of the anal canal at operation is advisable, and if the inflammation is severe with ulceration, a manual anastomosis should be performed.

STAPLED ILEOANAL ANASTOMOSIS

Double stapled anastomosis

The distal anorectum will have already have been closed with a transverse stapling instrument (see above).

A purse-string suture of 0 gauge Prolene is placed through the open end of the reservoir. The anvil of a 28 or 29 mm circular stapling device is detached and inserted into the reservoir. The purse-string suture is tied (**Figure 6.9.25**).

The head of the instrument is advanced through the anal sphincter taking care not to rupture the transverse staple line on the anorectal stump. The trocar is advanced through the stump and the anvil is engaged. The instrument is closed and fired (**Figure 6.9.26**). The 'donuts' are removed and inspected for completeness.

Single stapled anastomosis

As described above, a purse-string suture of 0 gauge Prolene is placed through the open end of the reservoir. The anvil of a 28 or 29 mm circular stapling device is detached and inserted into the reservoir. The purse-string suture is tied.

A purse-string suture of 0 gauge Prolene is placed in the anorectal stump in a manner identical to that used in anterior resection. In cases where the stump is inaccessible through the abdomen, the suture can be inserted endoanally.

The head of the instrument is inserted through the anal canal. The shaft is unscrewed and the distal purse-string suture is tied. The anvil is advanced into the reservoir and the proximal purse-string suture is tied. The instrument is closed and fired. The 'donuts' are inspected for completeness.

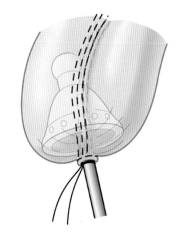

6.9.25

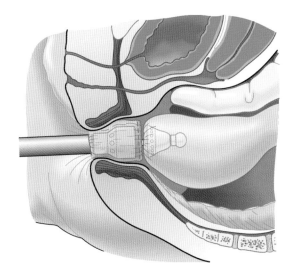

6.9.26

MANUAL ILEOANAL ANASTOMOSIS WITH MUCOSECTOMY

Positioning and visual access (Figure 6.9.27)

The patient's perineum should project a short distance (5 cm) beyond the edge of the table. The buttocks are strapped laterally. The perineal operator takes up a seated position facing the perineum. The scrub nurse is deployed on the surgeon's left side and an assistant on the right.

A Mayo table is brought up to the end of the operating table and the skin drape is attached to the leg covers with towel clips. The surgeon adopts a relaxed upright sitting position with the spine extended and the operating table is raised to bring the anus to the level of the surgeon's eyes. A 30° angle of head down tilt allows the surgeon to see directly along the axis of the anal canal. A high intensity headlight should be used. Cleaning blood from the operating field is best done by the surgeon using swabs rather than by suction. Median length instruments (10–15 cm) should be used.

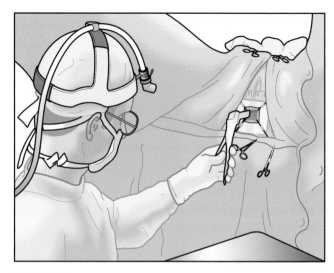

6.9.27

Mucosectomy

An anal retractor or a Lone Star™ retractor is inserted (**Figure 6.9.28**). The latter gives excellent exposure for the mucosectomy but should not be used for the anastomosis itself since it will increase tension on the small bowel mesentery owing to the distal displacement of the anal canal, which it causes.

The Eisenhammer pattern is also a suitable anal retractor. Anal retraction should be gentle and used only when access is needed. The anal retractor is inserted and the anorectal stump is inspected and any obvious bleeding vessels from its divided end are coagulated. The abdominal surgeon simultaneously secures hemostasis in the pelvis.

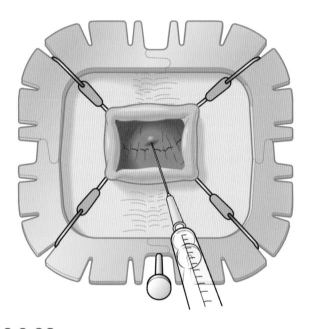

6.9.28

An anastomosis just above (5 mm) the tips of the papillae of the dentate line should be planned (**Figure 6.9.29**). The submucosal plane is infiltrated in the midline posteriorly with a solution of saline containing adrenaline (1:300 000) using a long spinal needle (22 gauge) mounted on a syringe.

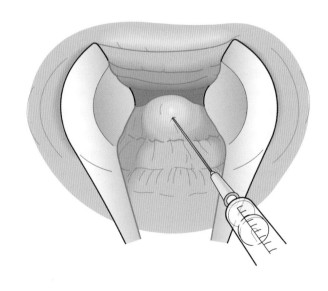

6.9.29

An incision in the form of an inverted T is made in the posterior midine and its vertical limb is continued to the top of the short anorectal stump (**Figure 6.9.30**).

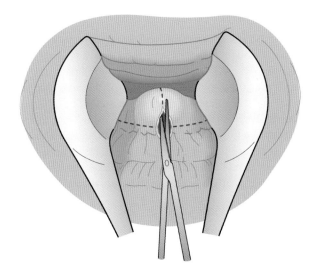

6.9.30

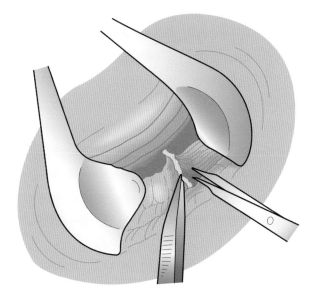

6.9.31

The retractor is removed and reinserted to expose the right posterior aspect of the anal canal. Further submucosal injection is made and the mucosa is separated from the underlying internal sphincter by sharp scissor dissection (**Figure 6.9.31**). Miltex scissors (American fistula pattern), which have serrated blades, are ideal. With repeated insertion of the retractor and submucosal injection the anal canal is exposed throughout 360° and the mucosa excised to yield a complete strip of tissue which is sent for histological examination. The mucosectomy is now complete.

When a Lone Star™ retractor is used, the entire anal canal is exposed and there is no need to remove and replace the instrument (**Figure 6.9.32**). Otherwise the technique is identical. On completing the mucosectomy, the Lone Star™ retractor is removed.

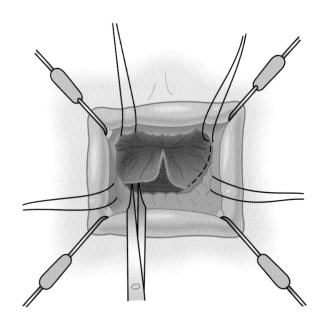

6.9.32

The ileoanal anastomosis

Figure 6.9.33: Two pairs of long artery forceps are then inserted through the anus and their tips advanced into the upper pelvis. The abdominal operator holds out the sutures previously placed in the end of the reservoir and checks that the mesentery is not twisted. The reservoir is constructed in such a way that the suture placed into the seam lies to the left (3 o'clock) and the diametrically opposite suture lies on the right (9 o'clock). The sutures are then grasped by the artery forceps and are drawn down through the anal canal to the exterior, maintaining the orientation of the reservoir.

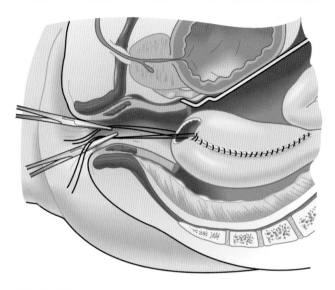

6.9.33

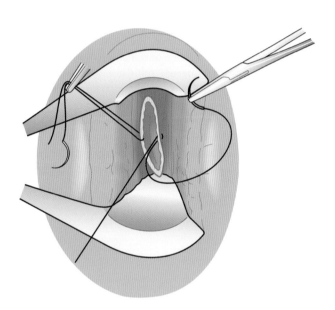

6.9.34

The perineal operator takes the 3 o'clock suture in a needle holder. The anal retractor is inserted to expose the lateral aspect of the anal canal and the edge of the mucosectomy is identified. The suture is placed through the anal epithelium taking an ample bite of subepithelial tissue and internal sphincter (**Figure 6.9.34**).

The retractor is withdrawn and the suture is tightened to bring the edge of the reservoir to the edge of the anal canal epithelium (**Figure 6.9.35**). Apposition is judged to be satisfactory when there is no longer any palpable gap between them. The suture is then tied with four throws.

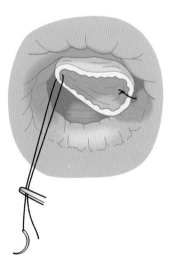

6.9.35

The suture at 9 o'clock (on the right side of the anus) is then placed in the anal canal in an identical manner and tied after removing the anal retractor (**Figure 6.9.36**).

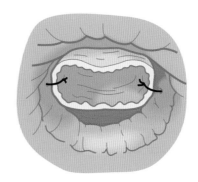

6.9.36

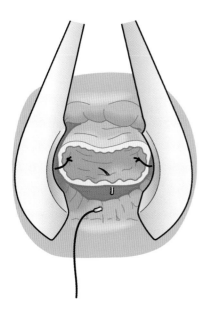

6.9.37

The anal retractor is reinserted and any blood obscuring vision is swabbed away. The anterior or posterior edge of the reservoir, or both, should come into view. The surgeon places a suture of 2-0 polyglactin mounted on a 25 mm taper-cut needle (Johnson & Johnson W9350; Ascot, Berkshire, UK) through the edge of the anal epithelium at 12 or 6 o'clock depending which is more accessible. The needle is then passed through the full thickness of the edge of the reservoir in the same sector (**Figure 6.9.37**).

With sutures placed at three cardinal points, it is easy to insert the retractor directly into the reservoir (**Figure 6.9.38**). This will expose the remaining cardinal point which is then sutured.

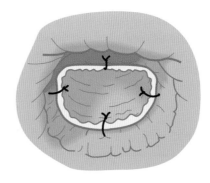

6.9.38

The intervening sectors between the four sutures are then closed in turn placing two sutures into each gap (**Figure 6.9.39**). At the end anastomosis will have been formed by 12 sutures, one for each hour of the clock. The anastomosis is checked for completeness and hemostasis. Further sutures should be inserted if necessary.

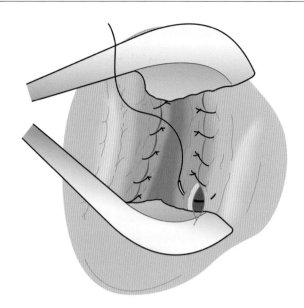

6.9.39

Closure of the abdomen

When a defunctioning ileostomy is to be used, the exteriorized ileum should be the most adequately mobile loop nearest to the reservoir. If there is too much tension in the mesentery on attempted exteriorization, the ileostomy should not be performed.

Use of a drain is optional.

The abdomen is closed using a mass suture technique.

POSTOPERATIVE CARE

The postoperative management is similar to that for any major abdominal surgery. The vital signs, urine and ileostomy output, and losses from any drain should be monitored.

Early mobilization and oral alimentation are encouraged. Early stomatherapy support encourages the patient to take part in their care and may reduce the inpatient stay.

Antibiotics should only be continued if clinically indicated. Thromboembolic prophylaxis is maintained until discharge from hospital and the patient is asked to wear the stockings for a further 2 weeks.

Complications

EARLY

These include complications resulting from any intestinal operation. Complications more specific to the operation include pelvic sepsis, leakage from the reservoir, and ileostomy complications such as high output.

Pelvic sepsis

This occurs in 5–15 percent of patients. It is the most frequent cause for failure (50 percent of failures).

Early warning of septic complications should prompt rapid assessment, diagnosis, and treatment. A fever in the early postoperative period is very likely indeed to be due to a pelvic collection with or without a degree of breakdown of the ileoanal anastomosis. The passage of bright (not altered) blood *per anum* is indicative of this. A digital examination is essential and this should be followed by a computed tomography scan. A collection should be drained endoluminally at a site depending on whether the collection is separate from the anastomosis or associated with it.

Leakage from the reservoir

Intra-abdominal sepsis can arise occasionally from leakage of the 'dog ear' of a stapled reservoir. If peritonitis is present, laparotomy is indicated. If peritonitis is not present, but there is no temporary ileostomy, then an ileostomy should be carried out. In all cases adequate drainage should be secured.

High ileostomy output

High ileostomy losses of water and electrolyte should be replaced. Occasionally the 24 hour output may be several liters. This will gradually settle but can take weeks to do so in some cases.

LATE

Most late complications are the same as those which occur after any abdominal intestinal operation. Complications specific to restorative proctocolectomy include pouchitis, late sepsis, stenosis of the ileoanal anastomosis, and retained anorectal stump. The last of these is the result of too high an anastomosis between the reservoir and the distal bowel and may cause distal outlet obstruction.

OUTCOME

Most patients regain their health with quality of life assessments showing levels similar to the normal population and, in ulcerative colitis, better than that of unoperated patients in whom the disease is not adequately controlled. Median frequency of defecation over 20 years is stable at about six to seven evacuations/24 hours. Urgency in colitic patients is abolished by the operation in over 90 percent. There is a gradual increase in minor continence disturbance from under 10 percent to more than 20 percent at 5–20 years. Episodes of inflammation of the reservoir (pouchitis) occur cumulatively in 50 percent of patients over five years but the prevalence of clinically significant chronic pouchitis requiring regular or long-term antibiotics is less than 10 percent.

Failure (defined as the need for a definitive or indefinite stoma) is progressive being around 10 percent at ten years and 10–20 percent at 20 years. Failure is due to sepsis in half the cases, poor function in a third, and pouchitis in 10 percent. In patients having restorative proctocolectomy for ulcerative colitis, the long-term incidence of neoplastic transformation in the reservoir is rare, and is largely confined to patients who had dysplasia or an established malignancy at the time of the original surgery. In patients with polyposis, adenoma formation occurs in the reservoir in up to 50 percent of patients over a five- to ten-year period. These are usually not troublesome.

FURTHER READING

Dozois RR, Kelly KA, Welling DR *et al.* Ileal pouch-anal anastomosis: comparison of results in familial adenomatous polyposis and chronic ulcerative colitis. *Annals of Surgery* 1989; **210**: 268–71.

Fazio VW, Ziv Y, Church JM *et al.* Ileal pouch-anal anastomoses complications and function in 1005 patients. *Annals of Surgery* 1995; **222**: 120–7.

Hahnloser D, Pemberton JH, Wolff BG *et al.* Results at up to 20 years after ileal pouch-anal anastomosis for chronic ulcerative colitis. *British Journal of Surgery* 2007; **94**: 333–40.

Heuschen UA, Allemeyer EH, Hinz UH *et al.* Outcome after septic complications in J pouch procedures. *British Journal of Surgery* 2002; **89**: 194–200.

Parks AG, Nicholls RJ. Proctocolectomy without ileostomy for ulcerative colitis. *British Medical Journal* 1978; **2**: 85–8.

Tekkis PP, Lovegrove RE, Tilney HS *et al.* Long-term failure and function after restorative proctocolectomy – a multi-centre study of patients from the UK national ileal pouch registry. *Colorectal Disease* 2010; **12**: 433–41.

Tulchinsky H, Hawley PR, Nicholls J. Long-term failure after restorative proctocolectomy for ulcerative colitis. *Annals of Surgery* 2003; **238**: 229–34.

Abdominoperineal excision of the rectum and anus

PAUL J FINAN

HISTORY

Abdominoperineal excision of the rectum and anus (APER) was popularized by Ernest Miles at the beginning of the last century. This procedure, that of combining the abdominal and perineal phases of the operation, was a natural extension of the staged procedure of a loop colostomy followed, several weeks later, by a perineal proctectomy performed with the patient in the left lateral position. Despite the inability to extend the excision much above the sacral promontory, this latter operation was the generally accepted procedure for rectal carcinoma, particularly in the pretransfusion era. Miles' operation of combined abdominoperineal excision of the rectum and anus was developed in order to take account of the lymphatic spread of cancer in a cephalad direction and to obtain a wider clearance of the lymphovascular structures together with the tissues immediately adjacent to the tumor. A greater understanding of the mode of spread of rectal cancer, advances in stapling techniques, and the desire to avoid a permanent stoma has led to the procedure being performed less often; yet population-based audits[1,2] have indicated its continued use in approximately 25 percent of patients with rectal cancer. There has been a resurgence of interest in APER in recent years following the publication of several studies which demonstrated that inadequate 'clear surgical margins' were associated with poor local cancer control. Recent technical advances in the performance of APER include sequential rather than combined abdominal and perineal phases to the operation, the use of the prone position for the perineal phase and adaptation of the planes of dissection to obtain a more cylindrical specimen with a wider circumferential clearance in the vicinity of the primary tumor.

PRINCIPLES AND JUSTIFICATION

The selection of patients with rectal cancer for APER should be made preoperatively. An exception can be made in patients who have received preoperative chemoradiotherapy and, although the primary tumor appears 'fixed', a trial dissection can be undertaken as the fixity may be attributable to fibrosis rather than tumor. APER is reserved for primary tumors of the distal portion of the lower third of the rectum, where the levator ani muscle or external anal sphincter musculature is involved, where there is involvement of the fat within the ischiorectal fossa, or for recurrent or residual tumors of the anal canal. It may also be necessary for selected cases of recurrent rectal cancer. In principle, if one can obtain adequate clearance below the tumor, an APER should not be necessary as distal spread within the bowel wall is uncommon and the mesorectum is removed in its entirety. Although a restorative resection may be ill-advised because of concerns over the functional outcome, the low rectum can be cross-stapled below the tumor: the 'ultra-low' Hartmann's procedure. There is some concern that such a procedure might be associated with an increased rate of postoperative pelvic sepsis, but this might be preferable to the unhealed perineal wound which can complicate an APER. Preoperative radiotherapy is likely to increase the incidence of this complication and postoperative difficulty with the perineal wound is something that needs to be specifically mentioned to the patient.

With the exception of the specific problems relating to the perineal wound, there are few problems specific to this procedure. Urethral injuries during the perineal phase are not common, but equally are not unknown. Damage to the pelvic autonomic nerves is a complication of any pelvic surgical procedure, but specifically during rectal mobilization lateral to the prostate gland. Pelvic collections are not uncommon and are a cause of postoperative morbidity.

Absolute contraindications to APER are rare, however small, relatively asymptomatic tumors in patients associated with metastatic disease are probably better managed without an APER. Locally advanced lesions with fixity to the low sacrum may still be resected if only for local control, but widespread disease within the pelvis is a relative contraindication for fear of recurrent disease in the perineal wound.

PREOPERATIVE ASSESSMENT AND PREPARATION

All patients with a suspected carcinoma of the rectum require histological confirmation. The height of the lower border of the tumor from the anal verge should be measured using a rigid sigmoidoscope. Complete imaging of the remaining colon and rectum can be achieved with colonoscopy or computed tomography (CT) colonography. It is now routine to image biopsy-proven carcinomas of the rectum with both CT scanning of the thorax, abdomen, and pelvis with additional magnetic resonance imaging (MRI) of the pelvis. Transrectal ultrasonography is used in many units and specifically gives additional information on the depth of penetration of the tumor through the rectal wall and of involvement of the anal sphincter musculature. MRI has been shown to be of use in defining those tumors that encroach on the mesorectal fascia and the proposed circumferential margin of excision. There are increasing difficulties with adequate assessment of tumors at the anorectal junction by means of MRI as the mesorectal tissues become attenuated. In addition to rectal imaging, there may also be the need for an examination under anesthetic. All cases should be discussed at a multidisciplinary meeting where a decision can be made on preoperative adjuvant therapy.

Patients should be seen in the preoperative period by a colorectal nurse specialist and, in addition to receiving further advice on the procedure, have the site for the colostomy marked on the abdominal wall. The colostomy site should avoid skin folds, previous incisions, and underlying bony landmarks. Particular attention is necessary with the proposed site if it is planned to make use of a rectus abdominis flap for perineal reconstruction.

There remains some debate over the value of preoperative bowel preparation within colorectal surgery, but there is no need, nor indeed value, in undertaking this prior to an APER. Systemic antibiotic prophylaxis at the time of surgery is appropriate, but there is a trend towards shorter duration of administration and avoidance of oral antibiotics. Prophylactic measures for the avoidance of deep vein phlebothrombosis are mandatory and may include compression stockings, as well as subcutaneous heparin or substitute.

ANESTHESIA

Full general anesthesia with appropriate venous access is required for an APER. Although blood loss is often manageable, there is the potential for rapid and large volume blood loss from the pelvis during the procedure. Additionally, an epidural catheter can be inserted for appropriate analgesia in the postoperative period. Full monitoring is employed with an increasing number of anesthetists using intraoperative, transesophageal, Doppler recording of cardiac output for appropriate fluid replacement. The anesthetist needs to be informed if it is proposed to place the patient in the prone position for the perineal phase of the operation.

OPERATION

Preparation of the patient

The patient is initially placed supine in the lithotomy-Trendelenburg position with Lloyd-Davies leg supports and initially minimal flexion of the hips (**Figure 6.10.1**).

Depending on whether the perineal part of the procedure is to be performed with the patient in the supine or prone position (the personal preference of the author), it is useful to place a support under the sacrum to lift the anus from the operating table and so allow access. A urethral catheter is introduced (unless a suprapubic catheter is to be employed) and the scrotum strapped out of the operating field. Most surgeons prefer a urethral catheter for an APER, at least during the procedure, as this can be easily felt during the perineal dissection. It is useful at this stage to perform a digital rectal examination, while the patient is under anesthetic to confirm the site of the tumor and relationship

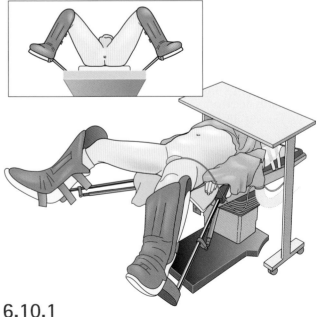

6.10.1

to the external anal sphincter. This is useful particularly in patients who have received preoperative neoadjuvant therapy. Finally, before the abdominal incision is made, the anus is occluded with two strong purse-string sutures. It is preferable to have the instrument table over the head of the patient, away from the pelvic and perineal areas.

ABDOMINAL INCISION

A lower midline incision is made extending cephalad from the symphysis pubis to the region of the umbilicus (**Figure 6.10.2**). It is unusual for there to be an extensive mobilization of the left colon or mobilization of the splenic flexure and hence a limited abdominal incision will often suffice.

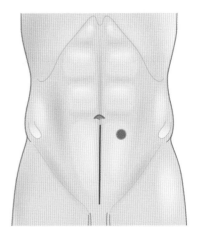

6.10.2

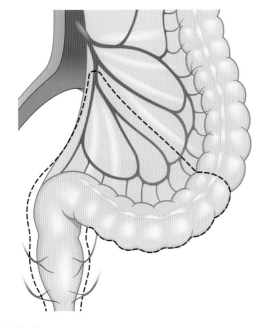

6.10.3

TECHNIQUE

On gaining entry into the abdominal cavity, a full laparotomy is performed. The primary tumor is usually impalpable, although bulky tumors extending up into the middle third of the rectum should be assessed for fixity. The liver is carefully palpated and, although it is unusual to find previously undiagnosed metastases, small lesions on the surface of the liver or the peritoneal surface may be identified. The colon should be palpated to exclude synchronous pathology. A plastic wound protector not only protects the wound, but provides useful retraction of the wound edges. The extent of colonic and rectal dissection is shown in **Figure 6.10.3**. Although a retractor can be placed in the abdomen at this stage and the small bowel packed away into the upper abdomen, an alternative is to bring the small bowel out of the abdominal cavity, wrapped carefully in a damp pack, so that the right side of the sigmoid mesentery is readily accessible. The sigmoid colon is retracted to the right side and the adhesions of the mesentery to the pelvic side wall (the white line) are dissected free (**Figure 6.10.4**). Full mobilization of the mesentery will identify the plane between the inferior

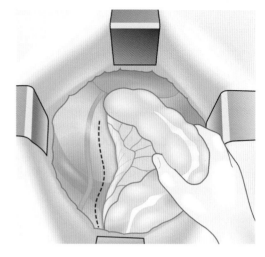

6.10.4

mesenteric vessels and the retroperitoneal structures, in particular the left ureter, gonadal vessels, and autonomic nerves. At this stage, the peritoneal incision goes no further than the pelvic brim (**Figure 6.10.5**).

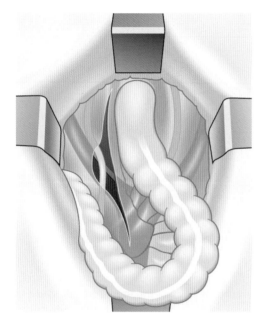

6.10.5

The sigmoid colon is now retracted to the left of the patient and a similar incision is made in the peritoneum on the right side of the colon. The right ureter may be seen at this stage, but is not usually at risk (**Figure 6.10.6**). On full mobilization of the sigmoid colon, the inferior mesenteric vessels are ligated. The proximal end is ligated twice and the tie on the distal end left long as a marker for the pathologist. Unlike a restorative resection, where well-vascularized colon has to be taken down to the pelvis, the ligation of the pedicle may be low and below branches of the left colic artery.

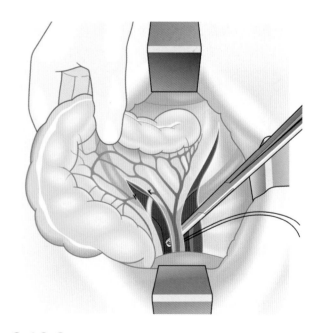

6.10.6

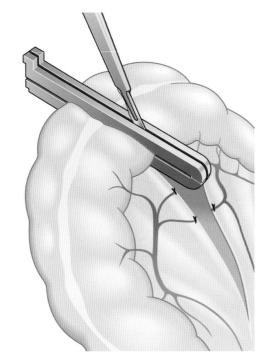

6.10.7

At this stage, it is advantageous to divide the mesentery of the sigmoid colon as far as the proposed line of division of the colon, often at the junction of the descending colon and sigmoid or, in the presence of a long sigmoid loop, in the proximal sigmoid. Division of the bowel at this stage facilitates the pelvic dissection with complete mobility of the distal end of the bowel. The bowel is transacted either with a linear stapler or a Zachary Cope clamp (**Figure 6.10.7**). The proximal end of the bowel is covered with a cetrimide-soaked swab. A self-retaining retractor is placed in the abdomen, the patient is put in the 'head-down position' and the small bowel and proximally divided colon packed away for the remainder of the abdominal phase of the procedure.

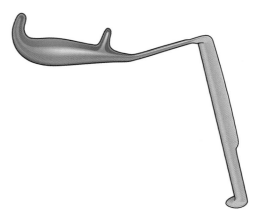

6.10.8

The surgeon now turns his attention to the pelvic dissection. A St Mark's lipped retractor (**Figure 6.10.8**) is placed in the midline by an assistant standing between the patient's legs. A second retractor is placed on one side and then the other as the peritoneal incisions are extended down on each side of the rectum and curve forward just above the reflection onto the back of the seminal vesicles or posterior fornix of the vagina (**Figure 6.10.9**).

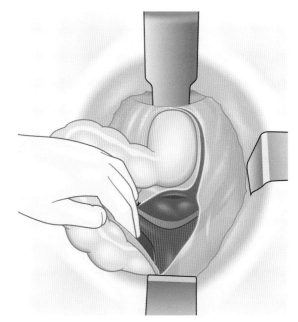

6.10.9

Moving from side to side, and with retractors providing traction and counter-traction, and having identified the hypogastric nerves on either side of the pelvic brim, the rectum and surrounding mesorectal package are dissected from the side wall of the pelvis and from the sacral hollow taking care to stay anterior to the presacral fascia. The dissection posteriorly is in loose areolar tissue, but is performed under direct vision with scissors or a bladed diathermy (**Figure 6.10.10**). At this stage, the St Mark's retractor may be used to retract the mobilized rectum away from the pelvic side wall structures.

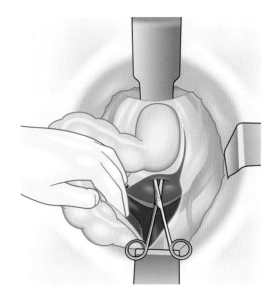

6.10.10

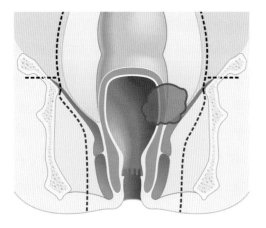

6.10.11

Unlike the dissection for a low restorative resection, there is a need to stop the lateral dissection as one approaches the superior aspect of the levator musculature. Any further dissection inevitably guides the dissection towards the primary tumor and contributes to 'waisting' of the specimen. The lateral ligaments may be formally divided, but are often taken piecemeal with the diathermy (**Figure 6.10.11**).

The peritoneal dissection is completed anteriorly and further dissection reveals the seminal vesicles or posterior fornix of the vagina.

In the narrow male pelvis, a narrow bladed St Mark's retractor is very often of use as the anterior dissection continues (**Figure 6.10.12**). If the tumor in a female is anteriorly placed and possibly involving the posterior vaginal wall, then the abdominal dissection stops at this point. In the male patient, the plane of dissection can continue anterior to the fascia of Denonvillier if the tumor is anteriorly placed or the fascia can be incised transversely to enter the space leading down to the apex of the prostate

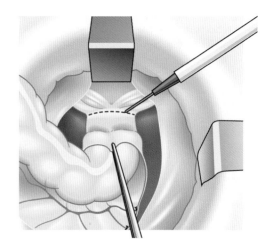

6.10.12

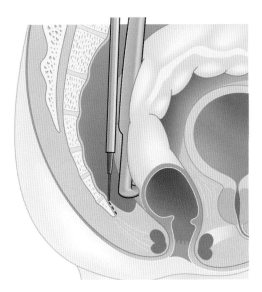

6.10.13

gland. Once identified, this dissection is better performed during the perineal phase of the procedure if the prone position is used. Posteriorly, the dissection continues down until the coccyx is palpable (**Figure 6.10.13**).

The abdominal phase of the rectal dissection is now complete and further dissection is performed from the perineum. If the perineal phase is performed with the patient in the prone position, then a swab is placed posterior to the mobilized rectum, and a couple of suction drains are placed into the sacral hollow, leaving enough length to reach to the perineal wound. It is not necessary to reperitonealize the pelvis. If a rectus abdominis flap has been raised, this can be rotated into the pelvis and attached to the proximal, transected, end of the mobilized rectum for delivery into the perineal wound as the specimen is removed (see Chapter 7.1). In the absence of a pedicled flap, the omentum can be mobilized from the greater curvature of the stomach, based on the left gastroepiploic vessels and placed into the pelvic cavity. A left iliac fossa colostomy (as described below) is fashioned and the wound closed with a mass suture of monofilament absorbable suture and skin closure with staples or a continuous subcuticular stitch (**Figure 6.10.14**).

As previously mentioned, the perineal phase may be performed with the patient in the prone or supine position. The advantage of the former is ease of access, good illumination, better access for an assistant, and ease of dissection of the rectum from the urogenital structures. Continuing the perineal dissection with the patient in the supine position reduces the time for the procedure and allows assistance from the abdominal operator during the dissection.

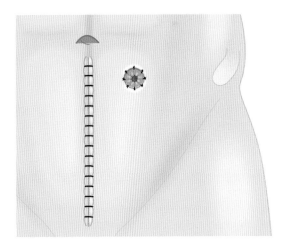

6.10.14

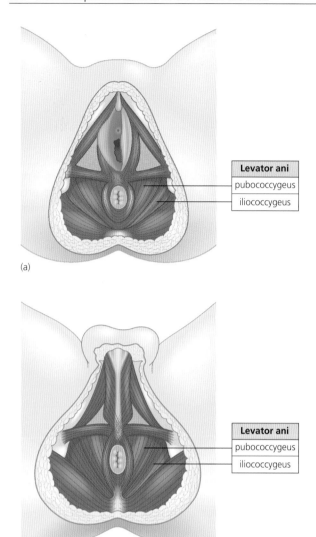

(a)

(b)

6.10.15

Perineal dissection in the supine position

Although a synchronous procedure was performed in the past, the competitive phases of the operation led to the term of 'combined asynchronous avulsion of the rectum and anus'. It is usual to perform the abdominal phase as previously described and for the abdominal operator to merely be present to offer guidance as the perineal dissection is performed. The posterior dissection is the same in both males and females, but there are major differences in the anterior dissection. A schematic diagram of the muscles of the pelvic floor in the male and female are shown in **Figure 6.10.15** (parts a and b respectively).

An elliptical incision is made around the anus and extends posteriorly towards the coccyx. If the posterior wall of the vagina is to be removed, the incision stops at the posterolateral aspect of the labia. Otherwise, the incision is completed and dissection proceeds into the ischiorectal fossa on both sides (**Figure 6.10.16**).

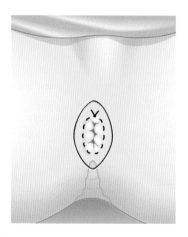

6.10.16

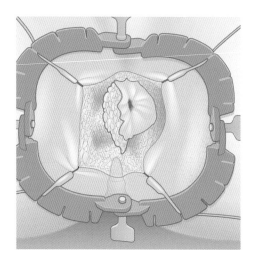

Unless the tumor is perforating the levator muscles or is locally advanced and extending into the anal canal, the dissection remains just outside the external sphincter muscle. Initially, a ring retractor with hook attachments or Lone Star™ retractor is of use for the initial stage of the perineal dissection (**Figure 6.10.17**).

6.10.17

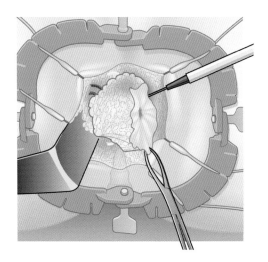

6.10.18

A self-retaining retractor is placed into the wound and lateral dissection proceeds in a cephalad direction. Branches of the pudendal artery and the nerves to the external sphincter are usually dealt with by diathermy or suture ligation (**Figure 6.10.18**).

On encountering the inferior surface of the levator ani muscles, the dissection continues to the insertion of the levator ani muscle on the lateral side wall of the pelvis, on the fascia overlying obturator internus.

Posteriorly, the coccyx is palpated and the anococcygeal ligament is divided. An alternative is to flex the tip of the coccyx and remove it with the specimen. With guidance from the abdominal operator, Waldeyer's fascia is incised and the abdominal and perineal dissections meet (**Figure 6.10.19**).

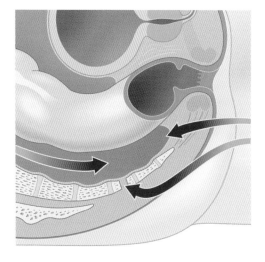

6.10.19

The rectum and anus are now free in the midline posteriorly. The levators (iliococcygeus) on either side of the midline can now be divided as far lateral as possible ensuring a good clearance of tissue surrounding the tumor (**Figure 6.10.20**).

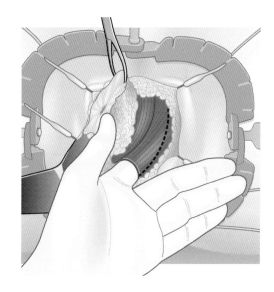

6.10.20

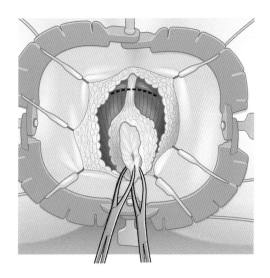

6.10.21

Attention is now turned to the anterior dissection. The rectum is retracted posteriorly and both the superficial and deep transverse perineal muscles identified (**Figure 6.10.21**).

The plane of dissection is posterior to both these muscles and inadvertent dissection anteriorly may lead to urethral injury. Anterolaterally, the pubococcygeal portion of the levator complex is divided under direct vision (**Figure 6.10.22**) and can also be facilitated by inserting the index finger over the superior aspect to guide the dissection.

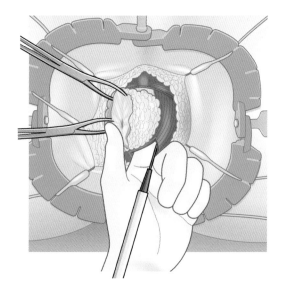

6.10.22

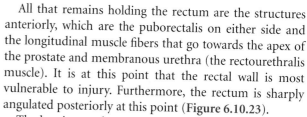

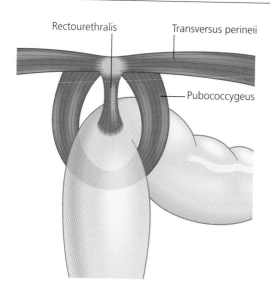

6.10.23

All that remains holding the rectum are the structures anteriorly, which are the puborectalis on either side and the longitudinal muscle fibers that go towards the apex of the prostate and membranous urethra (the rectourethralis muscle). It is at this point that the rectal wall is most vulnerable to injury. Furthermore, the rectum is sharply angulated posteriorly at this point (**Figure 6.10.23**).

The barrier can be separated into two bundles with an artery forceps and again the correct plane can be found,

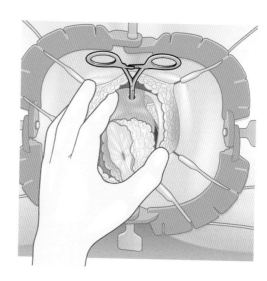

6.10.24

lying parallel to the posterior aspect of the prostate, with the aid of the abdominal operator (**Figure 6.10.24**).

Alternatively, this can be done by a single operator with the left index finger in the perineal wound guiding an artery forceps introduced from the abdomen in the previously dissected plane between the seminal vesicles and the anterior surface of the rectum. Any remaining attachments laterally are now divided and the specimen is removed through the perineal wound.

If a pedicled flap is not being used, the perineal wound is closed in layers, although the wide excision of the levators

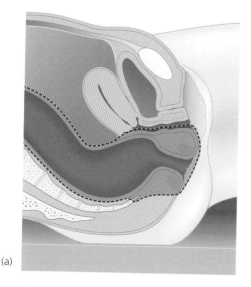

(a)

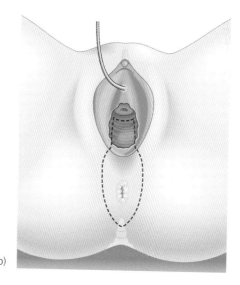

(b)

6.10.25

from the lateral side wall makes approximation of any muscle impossible. The previously mobilized omentum can be placed in the perineal defect and the wound closed with suction drains inserted per abdomen.

The perineal dissection in the female is the same in both the posterior and lateral planes. For anything other than small posterior tumors, the posterior wall of the vagina is included in the excision (**Figure 6.10.25a,b**).

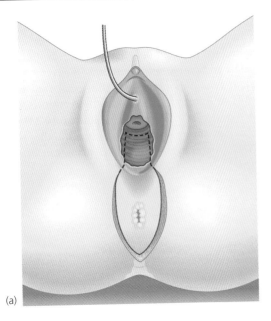

(a)

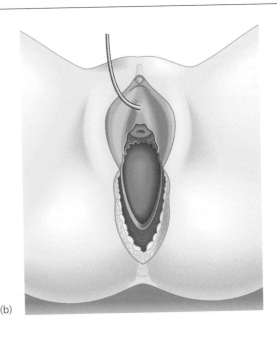

(b)

6.10.26

After the levators have been divided, the skin incision on either side extends through the full thickness of the vaginal wall (**Figure 6.10.26**a,b). A full thickness transverse incision at the level of the posterior fornix completes the dissection. Troublesome bleeding from the cut edge of the vagina is controlled with a continuous absorbable suture or by employing modern sealing devices e.g. the harmonic scalpel. Most surgeons do not attempt reconstruction of the vagina and the remaining part of the perineal wound is closed as in the male (**Figure 6.10.27**).

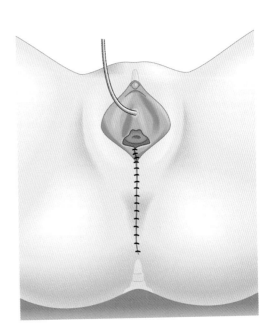

6.10.27

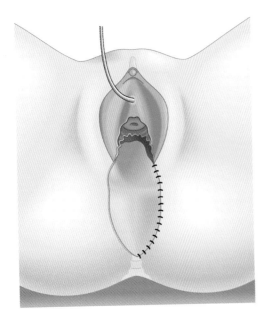

6.10.28

In the sexually active female, and particularly when the pelvic reconstruction includes a pedicled rectus abdominis flap, then vaginal reconstruction is possible. Once the flap is delivered to the perineal wound, the skin of the flap can be folded into the vaginal defect and direct suturing of the vaginal remnant to the flap can be achieved. Any excess skin on the flap is de-epithelialized prior to reconstruction (**Figure 6.10.28**).

A colostomy is fashioned, at the previously marked site, in the left iliac fossa. A disk of skin is removed with sharp dissection down to the underlying fascia. It is not usually necessary to remove any subcutaneous fat.

A cruciate incision is all that is necessary in the anterior rectus sheath and the underlying muscle is split using scissors (**Figure 6.10.29**). On reaching the pre-peritoneal space, a short tunnel can be made before entry into the abdominal cavity. A Babcock forceps is introduced

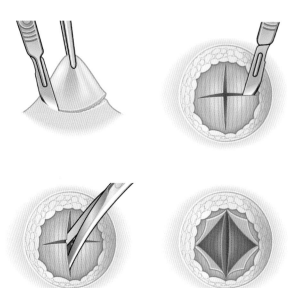

6.10.29

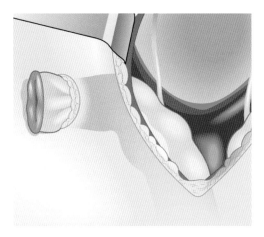

6.10.30

through the wound and the divided proximal end of colon delivered, without tension, to the abdominal surface (**Figure 6.10.30**). Although the author has no personal experience, some surgeons employ a mesh at this stage to encircle the colon as a means of prevention of parastomal herniation.

The cut edge of the colon is sutured to the subcuticular part of the abdominal wall once the main abdominal wound has been closed and covered with a dressing (see Chapter 3.2).

Perineal dissection in the prone position

For the reasons previously mentioned, the prone position for the perineal phase of the procedure is gaining in popularity. Prior to closure of the abdomen a swab is left in the depths of the pelvis posterior to the mobilized rectum. If an omentopexy is to be employed, this is placed in the pelvis prior to closure.

The patient is placed in the prone jack-knife position. If the operating table allows, the legs may be abducted to allow the operator to stand between the legs, although this is not essential (**Figure 6.10.31**).

The dissection actually mirrors that performed with the patient in the supine position. A circumanal incision with an upward extension over the coccyx is made. The plane immediately lateral to the external sphincter is identified and dissection proceeds cephalad with ligation of the pudendal vessels. The transverse perineal muscles are identified, but no further dissection is needed in this area.

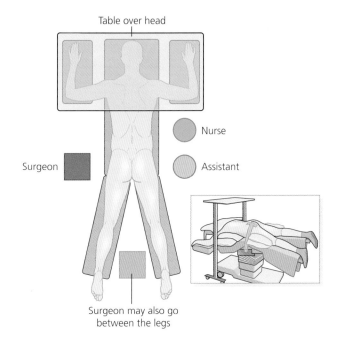

6.10.31

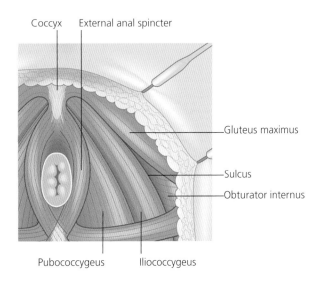

6.10.32

The plane of dissection, retracting the ischiorectal fat laterally, leads to the inferior surface of the levator ani and this is followed out to the insertion of the levators on the lateral side wall of the pelvis. It is usual to see the obturator internus, covered by its fascia, laterally and the lower border of gluteus maximus superiorly. Care should be taken not to extend the dissection too far anterolaterally in the sulcus between the levators and the obturator internus (**Figure 6.10.32**).

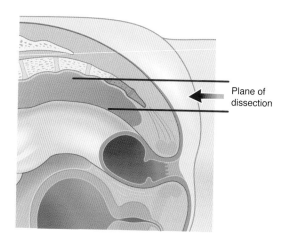

Plane of dissection

The tip of the coccyx may be removed to gain access to the true pelvis, but if this is not performed then the ano-coccygeal raphe is divided under direct vision. The coccyx can be elevated with a bone hook at this stage. It is important to direct the dissection immediately behind the coccyx, parallel to the plane of the operating table. Any dissection away from this plane risks damage to the posterior wall of the rectum (**Figure 6.10.33**).

Continued dissection in this plane divides Waldayer's fascia and the swab, left during the abdominal phase, is encountered and removed.

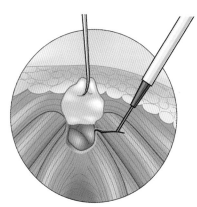

6.10.33

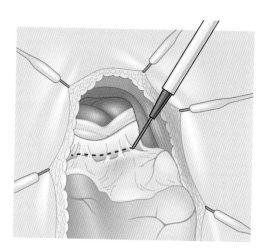

6.10.34

Having gained access to the pelvis and the superior aspect of the levators, the iliococcygeal muscle on either side is divided as far laterally as possible. It is important not to deliver the mobilized rectum out of the perineal wound too soon. Such a maneuver leads to an acute angulation of the rectum with the attachments to the prostate. Any division of the lower part of the lateral ligaments, not divided during the abdominal phase, are dealt with at this point.

After mobilization on both sides, the rectum can be delivered and the plane of dissection immediately behind the seminal vesicles (or posterior fornix of the vagina) is identified and extended (**Figure 6.10.34**).

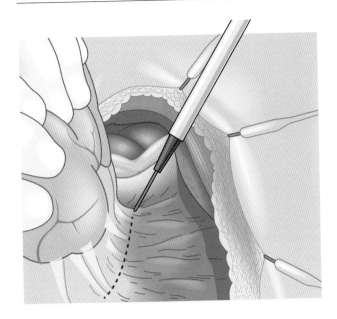

6.10.35

Once the rectum and anus are removed, any bleeding from the back of the prostate is easily dealt with under direct vision (**Figure 6.10.36**). As with the perineal dissection in the supine position, the wound is closed in layers, accepting that the levators cannot be approximated. Mobilized omentum, a pedicled flap (See **Figure 6.10.28**), or prosthetic mesh may be used during the closure (**Figure 6.10.37**).

It has to be appreciated that there are several components to the perineal wound with a wide defect at the outlet, and a large dead space. There is also the need to obtain primary skin healing. With the tendency to use preoperative chemoradiation, flaps of one variety or another are being increasingly utilized. They have the advantage of filling the dead space and bringing well-vascularized, non-irradiated skin to the perineum (see Chapter 7.1).

The urogenital structures are easily identified in the wound and the autonomic nerves lateral to the prostate identified and preserved. Gentle traction of the rectum inferiorly, with continued reflection allows the attachments to the prostate to be divided under direct vision and, following division of the pubococcygeal portion of the levator complex, the specimen is removed (**Figure 6.10.35**).

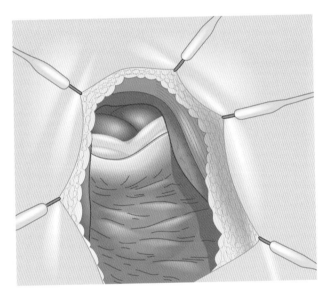

6.10.36

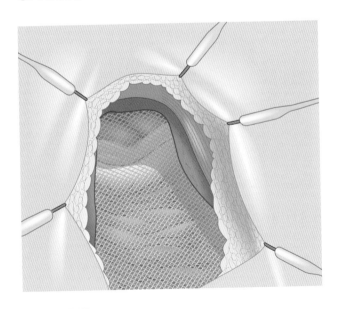

6.10.37

POSTOPERATIVE CARE

Like other major colorectal procedures, patients should be enrolled into an enhanced recovery program. This has seen the early introduction of fluids and food without the time-honored delay waiting for flatus from the colostomy. Urinary retention is not uncommon, but there is no reason to continue catheter drainage of urine once the patient is mobilizing. If an epidural catheter has been placed, this is discontinued on about the second postoperative day and non-opioid oral analgesics commenced. A common problem and one that can contribute to the morbidity of this operation is the occurrence of a pelvic collection. The suction drains, exiting per abdomen but lying in the pelvis, are left *in situ* for up to a week. The perineal sutures can comfortably be left for 12–14 days, although it is reasonable to assume that perineal wound healing, or lack thereof, is likely to be related to many other factors. Despite preoperative visits from the stoma care nurses, it is often stoma management which delays the discharge of the patient.

OUTCOME

There is good evidence in the literature that the operation of APER for low rectal cancer compares unfavorably with anterior resection of the rectum.[3] Local recurrence rates are higher, circumferential margins are more frequently involved with tumor, and five-year survival rates are lower. Comparisons between the two procedures are invidious when one accepts that the two procedures are performed for tumors at different levels in the rectum. What one can observe is that the operation of APER, a difficult procedure particularly within the male patient, is less likely to achieve surgical clearance of the tumor. While non-surgical therapies are employed with increasing frequency, there is also good recent evidence that concentration on clearance, adoption of the principle of cylindrical excision, and perhaps performance of the perineal phase of the operation in the prone position will reduce intraoperative perforations of the rectum, lower the margin positivity rates, and increase the volume of tissue removed from around the tumor.[4, 5] Whether this translates into reduced local recurrence rates and contributes to an increase in overall five-year survival remains to be seen with more prolonged follow-up.

REFERENCES

1. Harling H, Bulow S, Kronborg O *et al.* Survival of rectal cancer patients in Denmark during 1994–99. *Colorectal Disease* 2004; **6**: 153–7.
2. Tekkis PP, Heriot AG, Smith J *et al.* Comparison of circumferential margin involvement between restorative and nonrestorative resections for rectal cancer. *Colorectal Disease* 2005; **7**: 369–4.
3. Marr R, Birbeck K, Garvican J *et al.* The modern abdominoperineal excision: the next challenge after total mesorectal excision. *Annals of Surgery* 2005; **242**: 74–82.
4. West NP, Finan PJ, Anderin C *et al.* Evidence for the oncological superiority of cylindrical abdominoperineal excision for low rectal cancer. *Journal of Clinical Oncology* 2008; **26**: 3517–22.
5. West NP, Anderin C, Smith KJE *et al.* Multicentre experience with extralevator abdominoperineal excision for low rectal cancer. *British Journal of Surgery* 2010; **97**: 588–99.

Operative technique for pelvic exenteration

KIRK KS AUSTIN AND MICHAEL J SOLOMON

INTRODUCTION

Despite its first description in 1948, pelvic exenteration (PE) still remains a surgical challenge associated previously with a high mortality and significant morbidity.[1, 2, 3] Such extensive radical surgery aims to completely resect all malignant disease to achieve an R0 resection (i.e. a clear resection margin). In order to accomplish this, complete or partial removal of all the pelvic viscera, vessels, muscles, ligaments, and part of the pelvic bone (ileum, ischium, pubic rami, sacrum, or coccyx) may be required. While the role of PE still remains somewhat controversial, without resection patients have a poor prognosis with less than 4 percent surviving four years.[4] Non-surgical treatments, such as radiotherapy and chemotherapy, provide only temporary relief of symptoms in most cases, with continual disease progression resulting in pain, bleeding, intestinal and urinary fistulae and obstruction prior to death.

PRINCIPLES AND JUSTIFICATION

The evolution of PE surgery over the past decade has shown that this procedure can be done safely with acceptable morbidity and mortality, but requires careful planning and a multidisciplinary approach.[5, 6, 7] Consistent with other published studies, our review of 160 patients who underwent PE over the past decade for recurrent rectal cancer demonstrated a 36–46 percent five-year survival, with the ability to achieve a clear resection margin (R0 resection) predictive of survival.[8, 9] Radical excision for lateral extension into the iliac vasculature with *en bloc* vascular resection is also possible with R0 resection rates of 53 percent.[9]

Radical colorectal pelvic exenterations are done for recurrent rectal cancer, advanced T4 primary rectal cancers, and a variety of soft tissue tumors and other recurrent genitourinary tumors. Rarely exenteration can be done for palliation and includes uncontrollable malignant masses with small and large bowel to vesical, vaginal, and/or cutaneous fistulae, unmanageable malignant cutaneous and vaginal wounds, as well as intractable sciatic nerve or pelvic soft tissue pain. Indications for curative PE surgery include a relatively fit patient (e.g. American Society of Anesthesiologists score of 3 or less) and localized disease to the pelvis (i.e. the absence of unresectable distant metastatic disease). All decisions regarding the management of patients considered for PE surgery should be made in a multidisciplinary setting with all involved relevant medical and surgical specialties. All patients should have localized pelvic disease confirmed by computed tomography (CT scan), magnetic resonance imaging (MRI), and positron emission tomography (PET) prior to consideration of proceeding to surgery. While CT scan and PET imaging give vital information regarding metastatic disease, MRI imaging is most useful in determining resectability and meticulous planning of the surgical approach. The multidisciplinary team meetings should optimally not only involve the various surgical, perioperative anesthesiology, and oncological specialties but allied health including stomal therapy, rehabilitation, nutrition, as well as psycho-oncology support and expertise are necessary. The malignant indications for radical exenteration can guide the decision to proceed but the anatomical limitations of the pelvis as well as quality of life implications and patient choice are all important for informed consent. The traditional anatomical limits of resecting with a clear margin, such as involvement of any bone other than S2 down, major vasculature and lumbosacral, sciatic, or femoral nerve involvement remain the contentious issues of this century rather than the issues of any resection at all debated in the preceding decades. An understanding of outcomes both with and without exenteration including long-term survival data, operative morbidity and mortality, length of hospital stay and time for rehabilitation, as well as quality of life all need to be discussed in detail. Hospital stays average close to 3 weeks with recovery taking three to six months before a stable quality of life is achieved.

ANATOMICAL CONSIDERATIONS

Patients who present with localized advanced primary or recurrent pelvic cancer are a heterogeneous group of patients in terms of the involved pelvic structures and, as such, the definition of extent of resection is debatable. As a result, there is no standard defined surgical procedure that is performed, instead the type of operation is dependent on the site of tumor, size of tumor, and number of organs involved. This means that a number of different pelvic organs, vasculature, muscles, ligaments, nerves, and pelvic bone components are excised.

In order to help understand the operative approaches the pelvis can be divided into four main compartments (**Figure 6.11.1**):

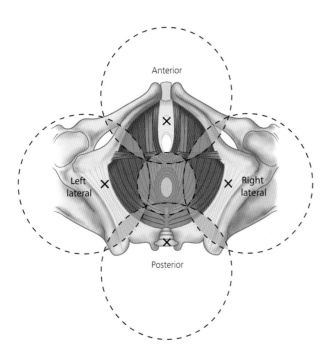

6.11.1

1 Anterior compartment: consists of the bladder, prostate, seminal vesicles, vas deferens, urethra, urogenital diaphragm, dorsal vein complex, obturator internus and externis muscle, anterior pelvic floor muscle (pubococcygeus and puborectalis part of the levator ani), and pelvic bone (symphysis pubis, superior and inferior pubic rami).

2 Axial compartment: consists of the vagina, uterus, ovaries, Fallopian tubes, broad ligament, round ligament of uterus, rectum, and pelvic floor muscle (iliococcygeus part of levator ani).

3 Posterior compartment: consists of the rectum, pelvic floor (coccygeus muscle), branches of the internal iliac vessels and tributaries, piriformis muscle, sacral nerves S1–S4, pelvic bone (sacrum and coccyx), anterior sacrococcygeal ligament, medial sacrotuberous and sacrospinous ligaments.

4 Lateral compartment: consists of the pelvic sidewall structures, ureter, internal iliac vessels, external iliac vessels, piriformis and obturator internus muscle around the ischial spine, coccygeus muscle, lateral sacrotuberous and sacrospinous ligaments attached to ischium, ischium including tuberosity and spine, lumbosacral trunk and sciatic nerve distal to ischial spine, obturator nerves and vessels.

In broad surgical anatomy, the four compartments can be best understood by their central points with some degree of overlap of their peripheries. The anterior is the urethra, axial the tip of the coccyx, posterior is the third sacral vertebra, and lateral the ischial spine. In view of this heterogeneity, the type of resection can also be broadly defined as either a partial or complete PE. A complete PE is defined as removal of the primary or recurrent tumor (with or without attached bone) with all remaining pelvic viscera, that is, involving aspects of all four anatomical components of the pelvis. Partial PE is defined as removal of the primary or recurrent tumor (with or without attached bone) with *en bloc* resection of up to three anatomical components of the pelvis.

Pelvic exenteration always involves an abdominal approach, usually with a perineal completion phase that can be done in lithotomy or prone (see Chapter 6.12). The anterior, axial, and lateral compartments are best done through an abdominal combined with a perineal lithotomy approach. Posteriorly, resection of the sacrum from S4 down and the sacrospinous ligaments allows radical excision of posterior pelvic floor that is approached from the abdominal side and is often better visualized than prone. Involvement of S3 and above by nature of the sacroiliac joint attachment requires a prone approach unless only the anterior cortex of the midline bones of L5 and upper sacrum are necessary, which can be done abdominally. Lateral higher sacrum and full vertebral excision of S2 and S3 requires the posterior prone approach.

This chapter aims to describe a schematic approach via the abdominal phase to the various compartments of the pelvis in order to achieve a clear resection margin without disruption of the tumor during exenteration. The lithotomy perineal approach and finally the prone approach to higher sacrectomy are described in Chapter 6.12. The approaches of total mesorectal excision and abdominoperineal resection for primary rectal cancer are described in other chapters. Surgical approaches to radical resection of the four compartments will be described in detail and an overview of restoration after resection will be discussed in less detail (e.g. conduit techniques, perineal closure utilizing myocutaneous flaps).

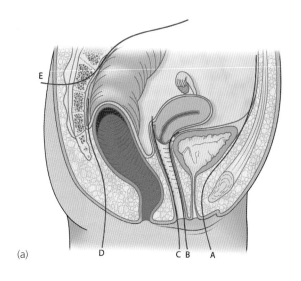

(a)

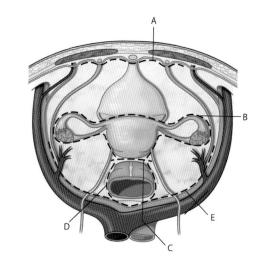

(a)

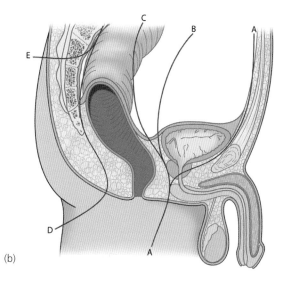

(b)

6.11.2

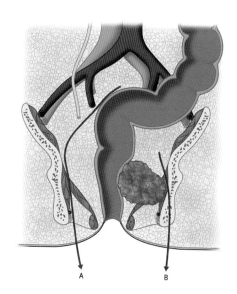

(b)

6.11.3

CLASSIFICATIONS AND PLANES OF DISSECTION

Figure **6.11.2**a and **6.11.2**b illustrate the sagittal planes of dissection for females and males, respectively:

- **A:** Anterior plane for total pelvic exenteration
- **B:** Anterior plane for axial pelvic exenteration with subtotal vaginectomy
- **C:** Anterior plane for axial pelvic exenteration with posterior vaginectomy
- **D:** Posterior plane for total pelvic exenteration or axial pelvic exenteration
- **E:** Posterior plane for abdominosacral exenteration

Figure **6.11.3**a illustrates in sagittal view the planes of dissection previously demonstrated in **Figure 6.11.2**a.

Figure **6.11.3**b illustrates the planes of dissection for lateral pelvic involvement.

- **A:** Lateral plane of dissection for lateral pelvic tumour extension not involving the muscle or bone, or any exenteration requiring sacrectomy.
- **B:** Lateral plane of dissection for bone involvement requiring excision of ischium.

OPERATION

ABDOMINAL PHASE

Perioperative preparations

Stoma sites are marked. If necessary, the elliptical cutaneous incision for the vertical rectus myocutaneous flap is marked with a surgical skin marker. If the patient already has a colostomy, this is covered with a swab and impervious plastic dressing so that it is not removed during the lengthy procedure. Bowel preparation is usually advisable. Preparation can be avoided only in patients with pre-existing stomas but is important if a colostomy is to be converted into a colonic conduit.

Positioning

The patient is placed directly on a gel mattress to secure their position and prevent unexpected slippage during steep Trendelenburg positioning. The abdominal phase of pelvic exenteration is performed in the modified Lloyd-Davies position with both arms secured at the patient's side. The perineal phase can also be performed in the modified Lloyd-Davies or in the prone position. Sacrectomy above S3 is performed in the prone position. However, partial anterior sacrectomy or a distal sacrectomy below S3 can be performed from a transabdominal approach. The anus if present is sutured, preventing soiling during the operation. The vagina is also included in the skin preparation. When draping the patient, exposure should include the groin and thigh if vein harvest is necessary for an interposition graft or patch.

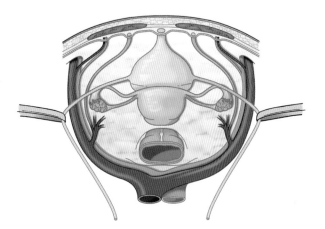

6.11.4

Laparotomy

Despite resectability being determined preoperatively by CT, MRI, and PET in a multidisciplinary setting, the initial role of surgery is to exclude metastatic peritoneal disease that may have been missed by preoperative testing. A thorough laparotomy and adhesiolysis is performed meticulously and 'cautiously' to prevent enterotomies to radiotherapy-damaged small bowel. If negative for missed small volume peritoneal metastatic disease then the planned exenteration surgery begins. Of note, lateral pelvic sidewall involvement and bone fixity are not contraindications for pelvic exenteration surgery and are best assessed by MRI preoperatively rather than by palpation at laparotomy.

Preparing the pelvis

Adhesiolysis is necessary for relaparotomies. The small bowel is mobilized out of the pelvis; however, it is often adherent to the tumor in recurrent disease. The involved segment(s) of small bowel is disconnected from the rest of the small bowel with a linear gastrointestinal stapling and cutting device to resect the involved segment(s) *en bloc*. Of note, the appendix is usually removed in view of the perceived potential difficulty with access after exenteration with stomas and conduits, abdominal wall mesh reconstruction, and surgery often involving myocutaneous flaps with the threat of injury to the inferior epigastric vascular pedicle in the future.

URETEROLYSIS

The ureters are identified at the pelvic brim as they cross the bifurcation of the common iliac artery and sacroiliac joint. They are mobilized proximally and distally, ensuring that the surrounding ureteric connective tissue with its blood supply is preserved. The dissection can be performed via sharp dissection or with diathermy using a right-angle forceps to keep the heat source clear of the ureter and its blood supply. Vessel loops are placed around the mobilized ureters and used to retract them laterally (**Figure 6.11.4**). Distal mobilization is continued distally for as far as feasibly possible. If radical cystectomy or partial cystectomy with ureterectomy is necessary, transection of the ureter(s) is usually delayed for as long as possible. However, if early ureteric transection is necessary, infant-feeding tubes can be secured to the proximal cut ureter(s) and into a urinary catheter to measure urine output and prevent long hours of complete obstruction.

GONADAL VESSELS

The gonadal vessels are ligated in complete or anterior compartment exenterations. They are usually preserved in males and posterior compartment exenterations. Often, in females, they are ligated when radical hysterectomy is necessary. Of note, we preserve the abdominal portion of the gonadal vessels as it gives crucial arterial supply to the ureter, important for healing of ureteric anastomoses (**Figure 6.11.5**).

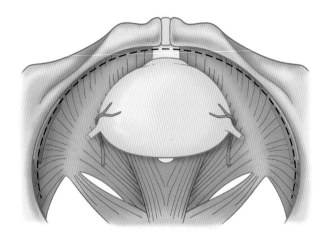

6.11.6

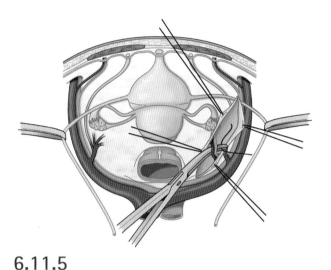

6.11.5

A: ANTERIOR PLANE FOR TOTAL PELVIC EXENTERATION

Radical cystectomy

The bladder is mobilized in the standard fashion. Anteriorly, the prevesical space of Retzius is opened and continued laterally to the endopelvic fascia and levator muscles (**Figure 6.11.6**).

The endopelvic fascia must be opened in order to elevate the prostate and gain access to the dorsal venous complex (**Figure 6.11.7**).

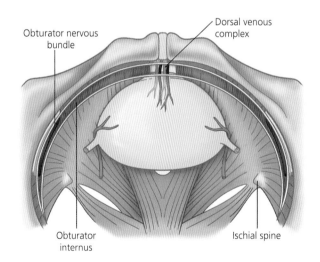

6.11.7

The vas deferens, superior vesical, and inferior vesical vascular pedicles may have already been ligated during the lateral pelvic wall dissection. If not ligated before they should be done in the same order as above. Laterally, the obturator neurovascular bundle will be seen as it runs along the superior border of the obturator internus muscle. Bilateral obturator lymphadenectomy is performed with the preservation of the neurovascular bundle (**Figure 6.11.8**).

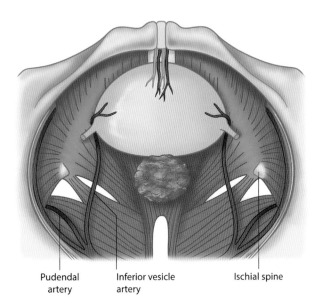

Pudendal   Inferior vesicle   Ischial spine
artery   artery

6.11.8

Anterior tumors invading the pubic bone will be excised *en bloc* with the pubic bones (see Chapter 6.12). Furthermore, anterior recurrent tumors require *en bloc* excision of levators and obturator internus muscles back to ischial spine with or without preservation of the obturator neurovascular bundle.

MALE

After incising the endopelvic fascia the dorsal venous complex is exposed and is ligated. This then allows mobilization of the prostate inferiorly to the urethra (**Figure 6.11.9**).

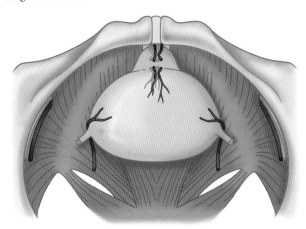

6.11.9

Of note, the urethra (as it exits the prostate and traverses the urogenital diaphragm) can be identified by palpating the urinary catheter. A urethrotomy is then performed, the catheter divided, and the distal portion removed from the penis. The distal cut portion of the urethra is sutured closed with a braided absorbable suture (**Figure 6.11.10**).

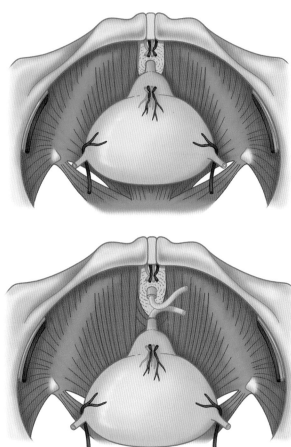

6.11.10

For anterior tumors involving the urethra, urethral resection may be done in continuity from the perineum with transection of the urethra at the base of the penis. This allows *en bloc* excision of the membranous urethra. If the rectum is *in situ* then the dissection is continued to rectovesical fascia of Denonvilliers. If bowel continuity is a possibility then an ultra-low anterior resection is performed. If bowel continuity is not an option then perineal dissection proceeds as per an abdominoperineal excision. Occasionally, the ligation of the urethra occurs at the distal prostatic urethra through the apex of the prostate and therefore a minute amount of the apex of the prostate will be left *in situ*. The prostate is suture ligated to minimize bleeding.

FEMALE

Mobilization continues inferiorly after the ligation of the venous plexus. Palpating the urinary catheter identifies the urethra. The rest is the same procedure as in the male. The plane of resection for anterior-based recurrent cancers in the female is adjacent to the inferior pubic rami and symphysis with *en bloc* excision of obturator internus, levators muscle, bladder, and vagina. This complete excision bounded only by the anterior bones is often less vascular than preserving the anterior structures. This anterior excision is usually performed in combination with a perineal lithotomy approach and can include *en bloc* removal of the pubic rami and posterior symphysis.

B: ANTERIOR PLANE FOR AXIAL PELVIC EXENTERATION WITH SUBTOTAL VAGINECTOMY (PRESERVATION OF URETHRA AND BLADDER)

This plane of dissection requires radical hysterectomy and bilateral salpingoophrectomy *en bloc* with the malignant mass and other involved structures. To begin, Kocker's clamps can be placed on either side of the uterus at the junction between the uterus and the Fallopian tubes (**Figure 6.11.11**).

This helps to suspend and retract the uterus in all planes of dissection. The gonadal vessels are then ligated just beyond the pelvic brim. The round ligaments are ligated at the deep ring where they exit the peritoneal cavity to enter the inguinal canal. This frees the superior lateral attachment of the uterus. Next, the visceral peritoneum is divided over the periuterine and perivesical spaces. This allows for the lateral dissection plane to be entered and the Fallopian tubes and uterus to be freed from the lateral pelvic sidewall by transecting the transverse cervical (cardinal) ligaments.

Following this, bilateral ureterolysis is continued to identify the ureters as they pass below the uterine vessels to enter the bladder (**Figure 6.11.12**).

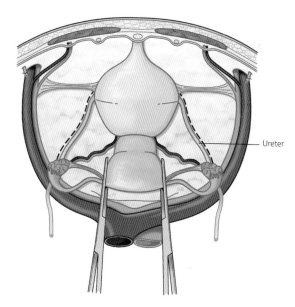

Ureter

6.11.12

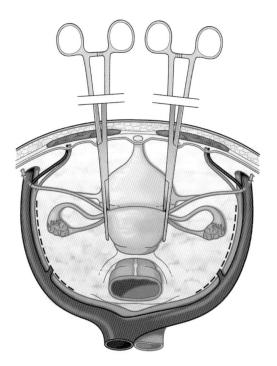

6.11.11

The ureters are retracted laterally and anteriorly and the uterine vessels along with their vaginal branches transected and suture ligated (**Figure 6.11.13**).

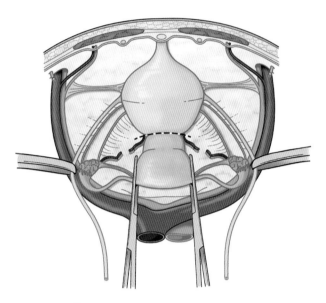

6.11.13

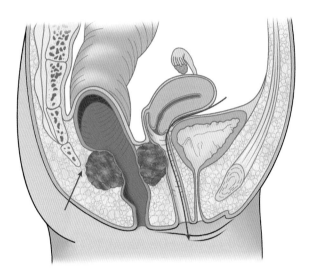

6.11.14

A St Mark's lipped pelvic retractor is inserted to retract the bladder anteriorly. With diathermy or scissors the anterior plane between the bladder and vagina is dissected with a combination of sharp and blunt dissection and the pubocervical ligaments transected. Dissection is continued through the levator ani muscle to the urogenital diaphragm. Placing a 'swab on a stick' or narrow deep retractor into the vagina and palpating the balloon of the urinary catheter can help in finding the plane between the vagina and bladder, which can be difficult to identify in irradiated tissue. At the level of the urogenital diaphragm, the vagina is entered anteriorly (**Figure 6.11.14**).

At this stage, in combination with the perineal dissection, two 1-inch long vaginal gauzes can be placed from the abdominal incision through the anterior colpotomy incision and tied bilaterally to the abdominal retractor. This elevates the anterior vagina, trigone of the bladder, and distal ureters and allows safer and more lateral radical vaginectomy that is continued down the vaginal wall to a wide perineal and vulvae skin incision. This now completely frees the uterus, tubes, and anterior vagina leaving the anterior wall of the vagina supporting the urethra. Of note, the attached posterior vaginal wall and the rectovaginal septum is not entered and resection is completed by the perineal phase of the operation that also incorporates the posterior labia majora and minora but leaves the urethra and clitoris. The perineal and vaginal defect is then reconstructed by the anterior aspect of the rectus myocutaneous flap to reconstruct the posterior and lateral walls of the vagina.

C: ANTERIOR PLANE FOR AXIAL PELVIC EXENTERATION WITH POSTERIOR VAGINECTOMY OR ANTERIOR PLANE FOR POSTERIOR EXENTERATION IN THE FEMALE

The approach is similar to (B) except that vaginectomy only includes the posterior vaginal wall. Total abdominal hysterectomy and bilateral salpingoophrectomy is not usually required. However, if they are involved in the malignant process they need to be resected as above. This has the advantage of using the uterus to help 'fill' the defect created by resection. The anterior vagina and distal ureters need not be dissected extensively if the uterus is to be preserved. Once the uterus has been mobilized the posterior fornix or wall of the vagina is entered at the level of the cervical os. This is identified by placing a narrow deep retractor or 'swab on a stick' into the vagina and guiding it into the posterior fornix. Using diathermy, the vagina is entered by cutting onto the retractor or swab. Once the vagina has been entered, the dissection is then continued down to the posterolateral vaginal wall. At this point, the vagina is incised down towards the pelvic floor on either side (**Figure 6.11.15**).

D: POSTERIOR PLANE FOR TOTAL OR AXIAL PELVIC EXENTERATION

Rectal mobilization

This is usually performed in the standard fashion; however, if a 'neorectum' is present dissection in the mesorectal plane is more difficult due to previous surgery and radiotherapy (**Figure 6.11.16**).

The exenteration plane for recurrence is bounded by the bony pelvis. Tumors abutting or invading these bones require *en bloc* or composite bone excision (see Chapter 6.12). Posteriorly, the plane of dissection is on the presacral fascia or ligaments of the sacrum and an ultrasonic or diathermy hemostatic device is often employed to minimize presacral bleeding.

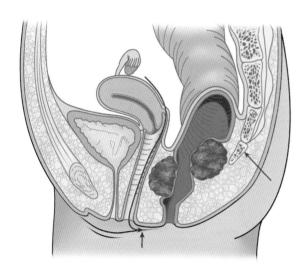

6.11.15

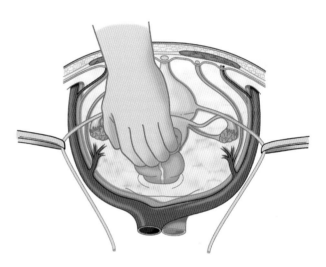

6.11.16

This then leaves the uterus and tubes 'only' attached to the anterior vaginal wall with the anterior and lateral walls of the vagina free. As described above, the final resection occurs in the perineal phase of the operation. Once the tumor has been removed, the vagina can usually be closed in the multiparous female or a rectus myocutaneous flap used to reconstruct a posterior wall of the vagina.

The posterior dissection stops approximately 1–2 cm proximal to the level of the primary or recurrent tumor (**Figure 6.11.17**). If sacrum is involved above S3 a metal sacral pin (11 × 15 mm, Smith & Nephew™ fixation staple; London, UK) is inserted into the sacral bone 1 cm proximal to the primary or recurrent tumor.

This aids in localization of the level of sacral transection when the patient is placed in the prone position. The level of the sacral pin is found using fluoroscopic imaging.

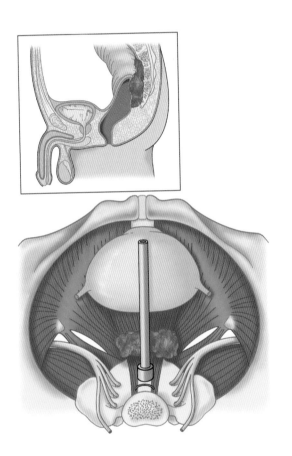

6.11.17

E: POSTERIOR PLANE FOR ABDOMINOSACRAL EXENTERATION

The dissection in the posterior plane is the same as above, but the dissection stops above the proximal margin of the recurrent tumor which is adherent to the sacrum. Abdominosacral exenteration requires lateral pelvic dissection which includes the ligation and transection of the internal pelvic vasculature and the exposure of the pelvic nerves and bones. Abdominosacral exenteration is discussed in Chapter 6.12.

URINARY DIVERSION: ILEAL AND COLONIC CONDUITS

It is vital to preserve the blood supply to the ureters. Sharp dissection is preferred in order to avoid thermal injury with diathermy. The 'abdominal' ureter is preferred for the anastomosis rather than the pelvic ureter. The pelvic ureter is more susceptible to injury, preoperatively by radiation and perioperatively during pelvic dissection (**Figure 6.11.18**).

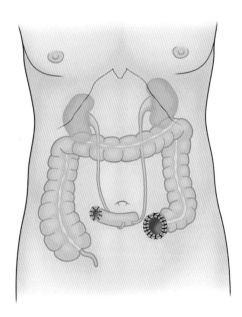

6.11.18

The distal ileum is most often used as the conduit internationally. The conduit is prepared by disconnecting it from the rest of the ileum with a gastrointestinal stapling and cutting device. The small bowel is reconstituted. It is necessary to make sure the small bowel anastomosis is at least 15–20 cm proximal to the ileocecal valve. This diminishes the backpressure exerted by the ileocecal valve on the anastomosis, reducing the risk of a leak. The ureters are implanted and sutured into the conduit where they lie comfortably under no tension. The options include bilateral (Wallace) and single (Bricker) implantation. The latter involves spatulation and uretero-ureteric anastomosis. This single ureteric end is anastomosed to the conduit. Bilateral ureteric stents are always inserted to protect the anastomoses. The distal end is used to mature the stoma and often fashioning the Brooke stoma utilizing the antimesenteric side 2–3 cm proximal to the distal staple line particularly in radiated, shortened, or fat mesenteries.

The left colon can be used as a conduit and is the preferred conduit when there is chronically radiated small bowel and an already established left colostomy, thus avoiding an extra anastomosis (entero-enterostomy) in radiated small bowel. The rationale is that this part of the bowel has not been exposed to radiation therefore healing is better. If there is a pre-existing colostomy, transection of the descending colon is performed approximately 20–25 cm from the stoma after ensuring full mobilization of the splenic flexure, with vascularity reliant on the marginal branches of middle colic. The proximal right colon becomes the end colostomy, which will be fashioned and matured on the right side based on the right colic and ileocolic arteries. The ureters are implanted into the proximal end of the colonic reservoir (the transected part of the 'old' colostomy). Wet colostomies have been reported in the literature. This type avoids double stomas but has higher urinary tract sepsis rates (**Figure 6.11.19**).

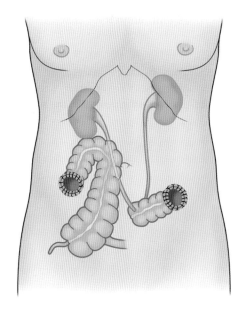

6.11.19

PERINEAL RECONSTRUCTION

Perioperative assessment occurs by a plastic surgeon when a myocutaneous flap is necessary to fill the perineal or perineal sacral defect created by resection. The vertical rectus abdominis myocutaneous flap (VRAM) is best as it provides good tissue bulk for the perineal defects and is easier to swing into the perineal space compared to other flaps. Elsewhere (see Chapter 7.1) the VRAM flap with an oblique paddle of skin and subcutaneous fat has been described. In this chapter, a VRAM flap with a vertical paddle of skin is briefly described as the authors prefer this technique when there is a need for two stomas. Gracilis myocutaneous flaps are less robust and usually too small for exenteration wounds. Gluteus myocutaneous flaps can be utilized for prone completions; however, if lateral internal iliac vasculature excision or ligation are performed then they are devascularized and relying on collaterals and should be avoided. Rectus flaps are easier when the anterior compartment is excised but can still be used if the bladder is preserved but requires medialization of one side of the bladder to pass the flap through the anterior pubovesical space.

VRAM is done with the patient in the modified Lloyd-Davies position. The skin incision for the VRAM flap as well as the marked stoma site (sited by the stomal therapist) and the expected stoma site after the rectus flap is harvested, are marked prior to making the midline incision. As a guide, the stoma is below and lateral to the umbilicus 5 cm from the midline planned incision. A line is then drawn from the midline incision line through the stoma site and then a further 5 cm laterally. The expected stoma site is then marked 5 cm laterally to the old marked site and a 5 cm wide VRAM (i.e. approximately 10 cm from the midline incision). If the patient requires two stomas, the stoma site on the contralateral side from the VRAM flap is also marked prior to laparotomy. During the abdominal phase of surgery, care is taken to ensure that the rectus muscle is only gently retracted so that minimal pressure is exerted on the inferior epigastric vessels. Of note, during mobilization of the external iliac artery to the inguinal ligament precaution is taken not to injure the origin of the inferior epigastric artery.

After the specimen has been removed and pelvic hemostasis achieved, the VRAM flap is harvested.

The skin is incised with a knife along the marked line in an elliptical fashion (**Figure 6.11.20**).

The subcutaneous tissue is dissected to the anterior sheath with diathermy. The anterior sheath is then separated from the posterior sheath at the midline (linea

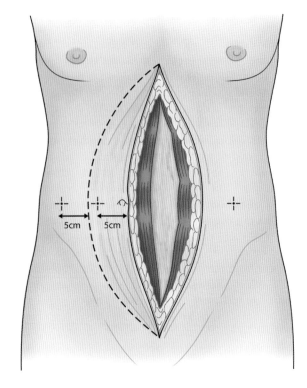

6.11.20

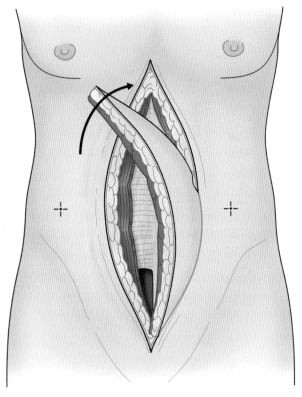

6.11.21

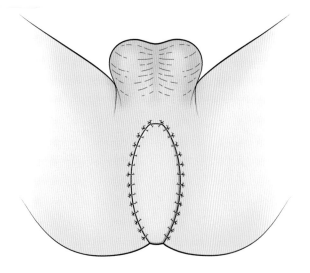

6.11.22

alba) and this begins the mobilization of the medial border of the VRAM flap. Alice clamps are placed on the posterior sheath at the midline and retracted towards the centre of the wound by the assistant. Superiorly, the anterior sheath and rectus muscle are transected at the level of the eighth costochondral junction. The superior epigastric vessels are ligated and tied. This allows for the rectus muscle to be lifted off the posterior sheath by a combination of sharp and blunt dissection. Rectus muscle mobilization should be done in a superior to inferior fashion to minimize injury to the inferior epigastric vessels. All perforator vessels are diathermied when encountered during mobilization. The lateral border of the flap is also mobilized from superiorly to inferiorly by incising the anterior rectus sheath at the linear semilunaris as mobilization occurs. Extreme caution is taken during mobilization of the lower third of the VRAM flap as the inferior epigastric vessels can be easily injured here. Inferiorly, the anterior sheath and rectus muscle are transected 2 cm above the pubic symphysis taking care not to damage the inferior epigastric pedicle.

This then allows for complete mobilization of the VRAM flap and rotation of the inferior epigastric pedicle when the flap is passed through the pelvis and into the perineal wound. Position, tension, and viability are checked once the flap is positioned. The flap can then be trimmed if necessary and is then sutured in place (**Figures 6.11.21** and **6.11.22**).

Reconstruction of the posterior vaginal wall with a VRAM flap is shown in **Figure 6.11.23**. Depending on the planned perineal phase of the exenteration (see Chapter 6.12), the mobilized VRAM is rotated down and secured with the caudal end of the flap now the anterior and the cephalad end is posteriorly placed in the perineal wound. If the bladder and anterior compartment is preserved then the bladder is mobilized free of the inferior pubic rami on the ipsilateral side and the VRAM brought down anteriorly to prevent angulation and stretching of the inferior epigastric pedicle. The VRAM is secured with dermal sutures and skin clips combined with non-absorbable interrupted 3-0 nylon. If the perineal exenteration is to be completed prone then the mobilized VRAM is placed at the pelvic inlet above the planned resected specimen then secured in the prone position after resection.

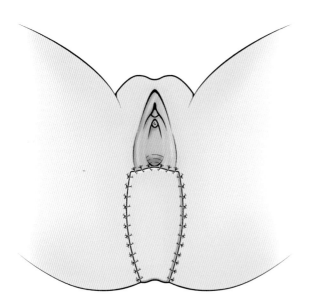

6.11.23

ABDOMINAL WALL RECONSTRUCTION

The skin and subcutaneous fat is mobilized bilaterally free of muscle to close the defect under less tension. The stoma on the donor VRAM flap site is brought through the external oblique muscle and the contralateral stoma fashioned (**Figure 6.11.24**).

The posterior sheath is then sutured to the linea alba. This provides some strength but mainly provides a tissue layer of cover between mesh and the intra-abdominal contents (see **Figure 6.11.24**).

It is the authors' preference to lay polypropylene mesh onto the posterior sheath and cut to fit the flap defect in the abdominal wall. It is then sutured laterally to the linear semilunaris and medially to the linea alba with continuous 2-0 prolene. Inferiorly, it is sutured to pubic symphysis well over and clear of the inferior epigastric pedicle and to

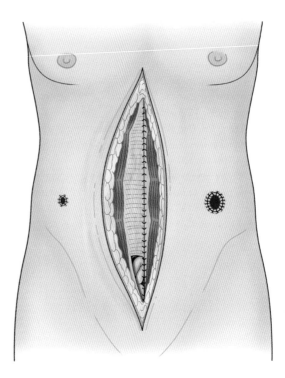

6.11.24

the 2 cm remnant of the rectus muscle and anterior sheath (**Figure 6.11.25**).

The wound is washed with chlorhexidine and a 7 Fr Jackson Pratt drain is then inserted and laid on top of the mesh. The skin is then closed with a combination of skin clips and interrupted vertical non-absorbable sutures.

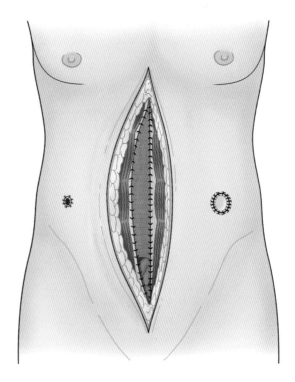

6.11.25

REFERENCES

1. Rodriguwz-Bigas MA, Petrelli NJ. Pelvic exenteration and its modifications. *American Journal of Surgery* 1996; **171**: 293–8.
2. Lopez MJ, Standiford SB, Skibba JL. Total pelvic exenteration. A 50-year experience at the Ellis Fischel Cancer Center. *Archives of Surgery* 1994; **129**: 390–6.
3. Yu HH, Leong CH, Ong GB. Pelvic exenteration for advanced pelvic malignancies. *Australian and New Zealand Journal of Surgery* 1976; **46**: 197–201.
4. Dobrowshy W, Schmid AP. Radiotherapy of presacral recurrence following radical surgery for rectal carcinoma. *Diseases of the Colon and Rectum* 1985; **28**: 917–19.
5. Moore HG, Shoup M, Reidel E *et al.* Colorectal cancer pelvic recurrences: determination of resectability. *Diseases of the Colon and Rectum* 2004; **47**: 1599–606.
6. Hahnloser D, Nelson H, Gunderson LL. Curative potential of multimodality therapy for locally recurrent rectal cancer. *Annals of Surgery* 2003; **237**: 502–8.
7. Yamada K, Ishizawa T, Niwa K *et al.* Patterns of pelvic invasion are prognostic in the treatment of locally recurrent rectal cancer. *British Journal of Surgery* 2001; **88**: 988–93.
8. Heriot AG, Byrne CM, Lee P *et al.* Extended radical resection: the choice for locally recurrent rectal cancer. *Diseases of the Colon and Rectum* 2008; **51**: 284–91.
9. Austin KKS, Solomon MJ. Pelvic exenteration with en-bloc iliac vessel resection for lateral pelvic wall involvement. *Diseases of the Colon and Rectum* 2009; **52**: 1223–33.

Pelvic exenteration: radical perineal approaches and sacrectomies

PETER J LEE AND MICHAEL J SOLOMON

PERIOPERATIVE PREPARATION AND PLANNING

The surgical approach is planned using magnetic resonance imaging. The abdominal approach is performed prior to the perineal approach. Stomas, conduits, and the myocutaneous flap are performed prior to or during the perineal approach. The location of the primary or recurrent tumor determines the operative approach for a perineal or prone dissection. Tumors involving the posterior compartment and the sacrum above the junction of the S3–S4 disc space require a prone abdominosacral excision in most cases (always for lateral combined with posterior compartments). If the tumor is centrally placed on the sacrum, dissection of the upper sacral nerves first (to free them laterally) can allow an anterior central sacral vertebral body excision between the sacral foramina without lateral or prone excision. The anterior compartment excision and planes are best performed radically in modified Lloyd-Davies and can be performed prior to prone positioning for the posterior and lateral completions. This also allows access into the pelvis from the prone position to guide excision of the sacrum radically with identification and preservation of the sciatic nerves. This maneuver of disconnecting the anterior compartment, anterolateral muscles, and ligaments during the abdominal and perineal resections means when prone disconnection of the sacrum is performed, access can be more readily achieved into the pelvis by rotating the transected sacrum caudal to expose the anterior pelvis free of muscular and ligamentous anterior attachments and direct visualization of the preserved lumbosacral trunks.

POSITIONING

The transabdominal component is performed in the modified Lloyd-Davies position. The perineal dissection can be performed in either the modified Lloyd-Davies (two surgeon technique) or prone position but is better performed in the former, if the anterior compartment is to be removed as well. The sacrectomy is usually performed in the prone position, especially if the recurrence is above S4. A partial anterior sacrectomy (L5–S3 or a distal sacrectomy at S3 or S4 and distally) can be performed transabdominally. The patient lies directly on a gel mattress to secure their position. Steep Trendelenburg positioning will not result in any unexpected slippage of the patient. The anus if present is sutured, preventing soiling during the operation and the vagina is included in the skin preparation.

LATERAL PELVIC DISSECTION (FOR EXCISION OF LATERAL TUMORS OR IN COMBINATION WITH PROXIMAL SACRECTOMY)

Lateral pelvic dissection with vascular ligation is essential for lateral tumors, recurrences that require proximal sacrectomy (S1–S3) and the extended lateral excision of the pelvic bone, the ischium. This is necessary for exposure, identification of pelvic nerves (especially lumbosacral and S1 nerves), and vascular control. Catastrophic hemorrhage is a potential risk if these vessels are not ligated. However, in the partial anterior sacrectomy or distal sacrectomy (S4–S5) vascular ligation may be avoided.

This dissection usually commences after ureterolysis and 'floatation' of the common iliac vasculature (see Chapter 6.11). Lateral pelvic dissection begins with ligation of the internal iliac vasculature. This provides exposure of the lumbosacral nerves, sacral nerve roots, and obturator nerves. Ligation of the internal vessels inherently involves the dissection and *en bloc* resection of the lateral pelvic lymph nodes. This extensive dissection and ligation is essential for an *en bloc* resection of the pelvic tumor. Lateral pelvic dissection is necessary for laterally located tumors and in preparation for a proximal sacrectomy (S1/2, S2/3). The aim in this latter group is to avoid massive pelvic bleeding during the sacrectomy. In the former group, this lateral plane gives wider access to the neurovascular and muscular structures that exit from the sciatic foramen and hence, increase the probability of achieving a clear resection margin for lateral tumors.

Pelvic devascularization

Pelvic devascularization is achieved by division and suture ligation of the IIA and IIV on the recurrent side or often on both sides if sacrectomy is necessary. The iliac system is mobilized from the retroperitoneal structures. Dissection commences with the common iliac vessels proximally and the external iliac vessels distally with each completely freed and vessels loops placed for gentle retraction (**Figure 6.12.1**).

Lateral exposure is often easier in previously undissected and less radiated planes. Dissection of the external and common iliac veins can be done at this stage and vessel loops placed. However, the planes may not be clearly dissected until the internal iliac artery is ligated and transected, floating the common iliac artery and external iliac artery free, with now complete exposure of the iliac venous system.

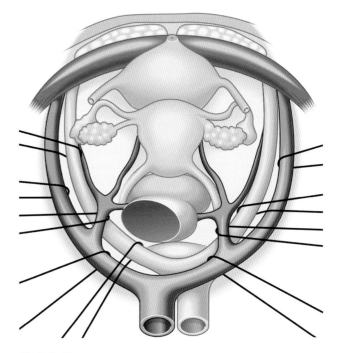

6.12.1

Ligation of the internal iliac artery

Total pelvic exenteration with proximal sacrectomy requires bilateral proximal ligation of the internal iliac vessels. Lateral recurrences may only require ipsilateral and 'selective' distal ligation of the branches of the internal iliac vessels. Proximal ligation of the internal iliac artery for a total exenteration with sacrectomy is performed just distal to the bifurcation of the common iliac artery. It is necessary to make sure there is a sufficient cuff. Transection will 'float the arterial system' exposing the venous system, aiding venous dissection (**Figure 6.12.2**).

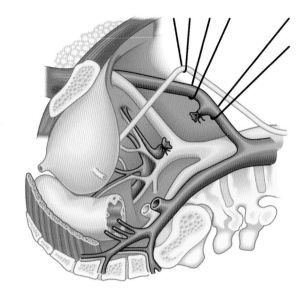

6.12.2

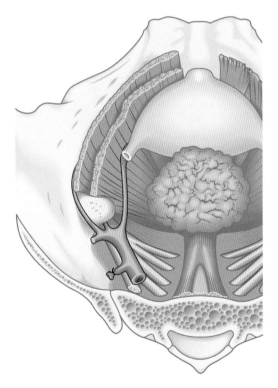

6.12.3

Distal ligations occur at:

- The branches of the **posterior** division of the internal iliac artery (**Figure 6.12.3**): the superior gluteal artery just proximal to where it bisects the lumbosacral nerve and the S1 nerve root as it exits the greater sciatic foramen; the iliolumbar and lateral sacral arteries. The iliolumbar vessels are variably located close to the bifurcation of the common iliac and may be preserved if high but usually transected.
- The branches of the **anterior** division of the internal iliac artery: the superior and inferior vesical, uterine and vaginal, middle rectal, inferior gluteal, and internal pudendal arteries. These are usually dissected and resected *en bloc* and distally ligated. This is important for exposure of the venous system, which lies just deep to these arteries. The internal pudendal arteries are not approached until the internal iliac veins are ligated and the lumbosacral nerve dissected to the ischial spine. Ligation of the internal pudendal vessels at the ischial spine exposes the junction of the distal piriformis and the proximal obturator internus muscles. This is the central aspect of the lateral compartment exposure.

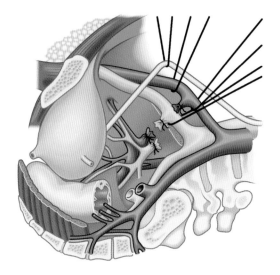

6.12.4

Ligation of the internal iliac vein

The venous system is variable. The internal iliac vein may be single or multiple. When it is multiple, the major tributaries will drain into one to three veins that drain directly into the common iliac vein. The distal dissection and ligations are similar to the arterial system, but it is necessary to be aware of the anatomical variations. Meticulous dissection of the posterior and sacral foramina branches with suture ligation rather than clips is recommended, as these tend to interfere with further ligation and dissection and are often displaced in close dissection of the sacrum.

Double ligation of the internal iliac vein is recommended, especially if a significant vascular cuff is not possible. The second ligation is often best with a 4-0 non-absorbable stitch tie (**Figure 6.12.4**).

The ligation of the venous system exposes the pelvic nerves (**Figure 6.12.5**).

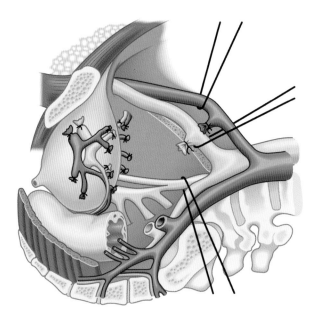

6.12.5

Exposure of the pelvic nerves

Ligation of the internal iliac vasculature will expose the pelvic nerves. The most important nerves in terms of preservation of lower limb motor function include the lumbosacral nerves, S1 (±S2) nerve roots, and the final sciatic nerve as these exit the pelvis through the greater sciatic notch. Vessel loops are placed around the confluence of the lumbosacral and S1 nerve root, which helps in locating them during the sacrectomy in the prone position. If tumor extends to the level of the sciatic nerve, that portion of the nerve is taken *en bloc* with the specimen. Under direct vision, the dissection is continued through this plane and into the piriformis muscle, coccygeus portion of pelvic floor muscle to free them off the lateral pelvic bone.

This allows access into a 'fresh' plane and helps achieve a clear macroscopic resection margin in the lateral dissection particularly if the posterior lateral recurrence is in the internal iliac nodal system (**Figure 6.12.6**).

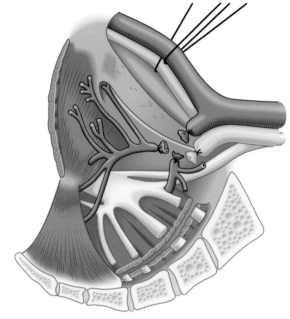

6.12.6

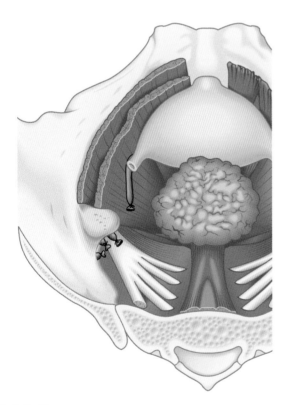

6.12.7

Ligation of the internal pudendal vessels will expose the confluence of the sacral nerves (the 'sacral plexus') as they enter the greater sciatic foramen, deep to the obturator internus muscle and lateral to the ischial spine, as the sciatic nerve (**Figure 6.12.7**).

Transecting the ischial spine with a Gigli saw will allow a wider margin of clearance and greater exposure of the sciatic nerve (see below under Abdominoperineal excision of ischium). This is performed by pulling the Gigli saw around the ischial spine with a curved angle forceps. A metal spatula is then placed between the saw and sciatic nerve to protect the nerve during transection of the ischial spine (**Figures 6.12.8, 6.12.9** and **6.12.10**).

In addition, it helps 'free' the lateral aspect of the sacrum by releasing the coccygeus muscle with the sacrospinous ligament attachment to the ischial bone, thus assisting sacrectomy. This also exposes the sacrotuberous ligament and this can be transected and resected abdominally if needed.

Excision of the ischial tuberosity as well as the ischium up to the acetabulum can be achieved in combination with a perineal lithotomy approach if necessary. This approach, when complete, can expose the sciatic nerve well into the thigh from the original lumbar and sacral foramina via exposure of the lumbosacral and sacral nerves. The gateway to exposure of these nerves and bony excision is by *en bloc* excision of the internal iliac vasculature.

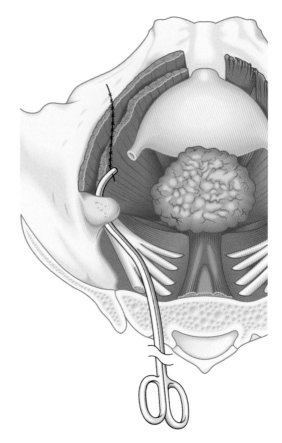

6.12.8

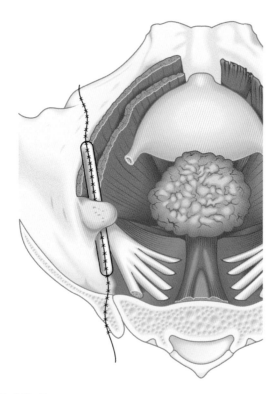

6.12.9

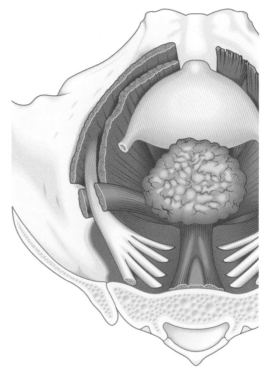

6.12.10

ABDOMINOPERINEAL RESECTION FOR EXENTERATIONS

For the general principles of abdominoperineal resection for rectal cancer and the infralevator planes of dissection, see Chapter 6.11. The anterior plane of dissection for abdominoperineal resection during pelvic exenteration has been described in detail in the abdominal phase of exenteration in Chapter 6.11 and, in particular, the approaches to partial and complete vaginectomy in females.

The fundamental principle of perineal pelvic exenteration surgery is the peripheral plane of resection at the pelvic floor. The TME plane should be completely ignored by the exenteration surgeon. The plane for recurrent rectal cancer surgery for the involved compartment is, at a minimum, the soft tissue attachments to the bones of the pelvis, and when the tumor involves or abuts the bone, the excision plane is partial or complete bone removal (see below). Planned close margins are to be completely avoided as: R0 margins are the major predictor of survival; recurrent tumors are usually in previous surgical planes and in more depth than expected with no tumor 'capsule'; recurrent tumors can be multifocal at the margin with satellite tumor deposits (NB recurrent anal squamous cell carcinoma after radiotherapy); the planes of soft tissue and bone are often less vascular with less blood loss than the previous surgical planes.

The anterior APE plane for exenteration without bone involvement depends on whether the bladder is being preserved but even if this is the case the bladder often needs to be mobilized medially on the tumor side to expose the pelvic floor and obturator internus muscle. For complete pelvic exenteration, the urethra has been transected during the bladder mobilization, however if the tumor extends to the urethra then the urethra needs to be excised completely in females or transected distally in the penis during this perineal approach. This allows the pubis to be exposed completely.

Extending anterolaterally for an anterolateral tumor, the plane from the perineal approach is the attachment of the levator muscle to the inferior pubic ramus moving posteriorly to the ischium and excision of the obturator internus muscle laterally to the level of the obturator canal, or including the canal and neurovascular bundle for tumors involving the lateral compartment more extensively. These lateral compartment tumors will already have the internal iliac vasculature excised *en bloc* and the lumbosacral trunk dissected free down to the ischial spine. Once the obturator internus and anterior levators are freed from the inferior pubic ramus, this exposes bone back to the ischial spine and the sacrospinous ligament. The posterior level of anterior radical excision is excision of all muscle anterior and deep down to the level of the sacrospinous ligament.

True lateral compartment tumors require excision of the sacrospinous ligament and sometimes deep to this the sacrotuberous ligament which can be excised with a heat source free off the ischium. This is all possible and best performed abdominally after excision of the internal iliac vasculature and exposure of the lumbosacral and sacral nerves as they lie on the posterior muscle, the piriformis. In general, the posterolateral (piriformis, lumbar and sacral nerves, sacrospinous ligaments and obturator internus) are best performed abdominally with levator, sacrotuberous ligament and anterolateral bones through the perineum. The tumor is removed then with a synchronous combined perineal and abdominal approach and the closure is dependent on the need for vertical myocutaneous flaps.

ABDOMINOPERINEAL SACRECTOMY S4–S5

Central (axial) and low posterior tumors require wide excision of the entire posterior levator floor from the level of the ischial spine laterally to the junction of the S3–S4 vertebra medially (defined by the sacrospinous ligament more deeply). These tumors may require excision of the lower piriformis muscle and sacral nerves laterally if the mass extends to the lateral compartment.

Once these structures have been disconnected laterally, the junction of S3 and S4 is exposed using diathermy, at a high coagulation setting, to transect the longitudinal ligaments and midline muscles.

The sacrum is then transected transabdominally, using a 20 mm extended length osteotome and hammer, from medial to lateral along the sacrospinous ligament to the ischial spine. The lumbosacral trunk and upper sacral nerve trunks on the piriformis are preserved if they are not abutting or involved with the tumor. The perineal surgeon has dissected posterior to the coccyx and sacrum up to the level of S3 prior to bone transection. The anterior perineal plane is then connected to this posterolateral plane by combined abdominal and perineal dissection. The specimen is removed through the perineal wound (**Figure 6.12.11**).

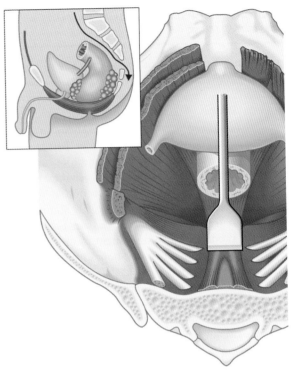

6.12.11

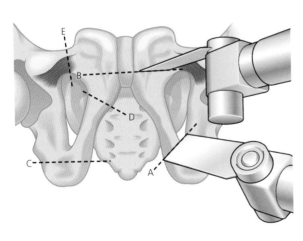

6.12.12

ABDOMINOPERINEAL EXCISION OF PUBIS

For anterior compartment tumors abutting or infiltrating the pubic bone, a more radical margin than in Chapter 6.11 becomes necessary for the excision of the anterior compartment. Wide exposure, but not incision, of anterior levator muscles are performed out to the inferior ramus of the pubic bone and extended back to the ischial tuberosity. The adductor and gracilis muscles are separated from their attachments to the lateral border of the inferior pubic rami with diathermy and extended through the obturator fascia into the exposed pelvis. The inferior pubic ramus is transected free from the ischial bone (**Figure 6.12.12, Line A**) and anteriorly from the pubis (**Figure 6.12.12, Line D**) with an oscillating saw or, alternatively, a Gigli saw can be used. If the pubis and symphysis needs excising this can be done partially for the inferior half (**Figure 6.12.12, Line B**) or the whole central pubis can be excised (**Figure 6.12.12, Line E combined with Line A**). Excision of the ischial tuberosity (**Figure 6.12.12, Line C**) can be performed from the perineal lithotomy approach with preservation of the whole pubic bone.

The superior half of the pubis and symphysis combined with the superior pubic rami maintains stability of the pelvis if preserved, however excision of the whole pubis requires no metallic prostheses and is structurally repaired by a polypropylene mesh joining the cut ends of all four pubic rami and covering this with a myocutaneous and/or rotation flap.

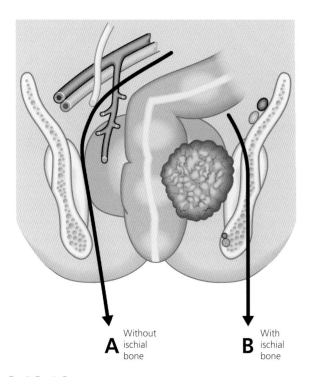

A Without ischial bone   **B** With ischial bone

6.12.13

ABDOMINOPERINEAL EXCISION OF ISCHIUM

Excision of the ischium can be performed as transection of the ischial spine through an abdominal approach only to give wider access to the lumbosacral trunk where it becomes the sciatic nerve as it exits the greater sciatic foramen to enter the thigh. This also exposes for the lateral resection of obturator internus and piriformis outside the pelvis with exposure of the gluteus muscle lateral to the bony pelvic margin. This procedure follows excision of internal iliac vasculature and dissection of the lumbosacral trunk free of the lateral bone of the ischial spine. This dissection is only possible after ligation of the internal pudendal vessels at the sciatic notch. Once this has been performed a large curved right angle (SEMBS modified 26 cm ligature carrier is good for this) is placed from greater to lesser sciatic notches and a Gigli saw brought back. A metal malleable spatula is placed between the Gigli saw and the nerve deep to the ischial spine prior to transaction for protection of the nerve.

For wider excision of the medial wall of the ischial bone a 20 or 10 mm osteotome can be used either abdominally vertically or horizontally through the perineal exposure (**Figure 6.12.13**, Line B). Excision of the whole ischial tuberosity from below the acetabulum posteriorly to the inferior pubic ramus can be performed by a combination of perineal and abdominal exposure (**Figure 6.12.12**, Line C). First, the abdominal dissection of the sciatic nerve free of the ischium (often requiring initial transection of the ischial spine for lateral exposure) is performed as previously described (see **Figures 6.12.8, 6.12.9** and **6.12.10**). The perineal surgeon then exposes the lateral ischial tuberosity by releasing the attachments of the posterior adductor magnus, semimembranosus and quadratus femoris. The ischium can now be transected with the oscillating saw through the perineum always with protection of the sciatic nerve. Alternatively, a Gigli saw can be placed with one end abdominally and the other from the perineal wound. The ischial tuberosity can be excised individually (**Figure

6.12.12, Line C) or *en bloc* with the inferior pubic ramus (**Figure 6.12.14**).

Ligation of the internal pudendal vessels will expose confluence of the sacral nerves (the 'sacral plexus') as

they exit through the greater sciatic foramen, deep to the obturator internus muscle and lateral to the ischial spine, as the sciatic nerve, and is integral to the exposure of this central portion of the lateral compartment.

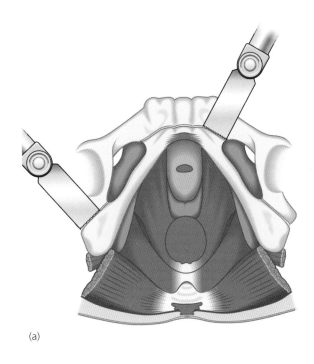

(a)

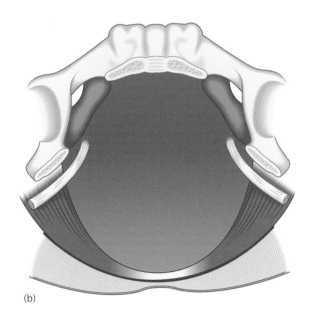

(b)

6.12.14 (a) Axial view of the lateral planes for anterior and lateral recurrences or any exenteration requiring pubic and ischial bone resections in combination with sacrectomies; (b) post-excision of the pubic bone and ischial tuberosities bilaterally.

ABDOMINOPRONE SACRECTOMY S1–S3

Prone position

The patient is placed in the prone jack-knife position for the sacrectomy after the abdominal component is completed. Completion of the transabdominopelvic component includes mobilization of the rectus abdominis myocutaneous flap (which is placed in the pelvis above the mass), vessel loops tied around the lumbosacral and S1 nerve roots and secured with metal clips, the placement of a sterile pack in the pelvis above the plane of sacral resection to protect small bowel loops as the saw enters the pelvis, insertion of a pelvic drain, closure of the abdominal wound, and maturation of the colostomy and conduit. A polypropylene mesh is used to reinforce the fascial defect secondary to the rectus abdominis flap as per Chapter 6.11. The level of sacral planned transection is marked abdominally prior to closure utilizing a sacral

pin (11 × 15 mm Smith & Nephew fixation staple, **Figure 6.11.16** in Chapter 6.11). This allows lateral radiological confirmation of the level of transection of the sacrum prior to commencing transection of the sacrum.

Completing the anterior dissection through the perineum in the modified Lloyd-Davies position with temporary closure of this wound using a continuous stitch for transfer into the prone position can greatly enhance the prone dissection. Alternatively, the perineal incision becomes the extension of the midline sacral incision ('racquet' incision) with the patient in the prone position. Complete transection of S1 disrupts the support of the pelvis and, as yet, cannot be performed and restored successfully despite attempts with fixation devices. The anterior body of the S1 can be mobilized horizontally (cephalad to caudad) with an osteotome abdominally prior to prone transection vertically (posteriorly to anteriorly) through the S1–S2 disc space allowing the stability of the pelvis to be maintained through the posterior S1 vertebral body.

Incision

A midline sacral incision is made. It is extended distally to encompass the perianal skin 'racquet' incision (**Figure 6.12.15**).

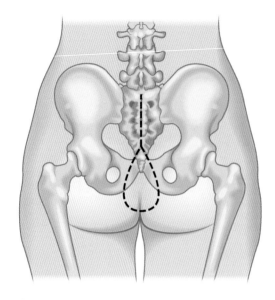

6.12.15

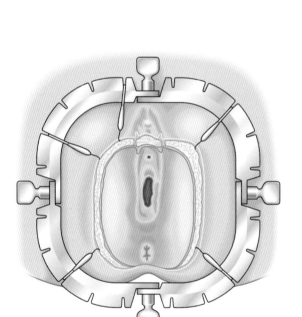

6.12.16

Alternatively, the sacral incision can be joined with previous perineal incision, which was performed by the 'perineal' surgeon with the patient in the lithotomy position. This becomes the perineal dissection of an abdominoperineal resection, which is incorporated with the sacrectomy. The cephalad extent of the incision depends on the level of sacrectomy (**Figure 6.12.16**).

Useful surface anatomy includes:
- the posterior superior iliac spine = superior border of the sacrum;
- the posterior inferior iliac spine = the level of the third segment of the sacrum (S3).

Exposure of the sacrum

Diathermy dissection is performed onto the median crest of the sacrum (**Figure 6.12.17**).

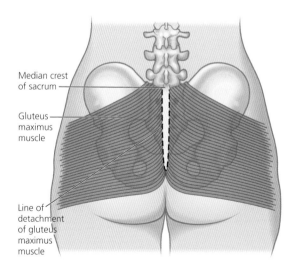

Median crest of sacrum

Gluteus maximus muscle

Line of detachment of gluteus maximus muscle

6.12.17

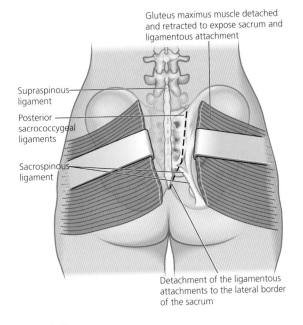

Gluteus maximus muscle detached and retracted to expose sacrum and ligamentous attachment

Supraspinous ligament

Posterior sacrococcygeal ligaments

Sacrospinous ligament

Detachment of the ligamentous attachments to the lateral border of the sacrum

6.12.18

The gluteus maximus muscles are detached from the sacrum bilaterally and mobilized laterally. This exposes the posterior and lateral sacrococcygeal ligaments inferiorly, and the posterior sacroiliac and sacrotuberous ligaments laterally. The sacrospinous lies deep to the sacrotuberous ligaments (**Figure 6.12.18**).

All ligaments are divided to free the lateral borders of the sacrum. When the sacrospinous ligament is divided the piriformis muscle will be exposed. The sacral nerve roots and the sciatic nerves lie deep to the piriformis muscle. It is important to stay close to the bony lateral borders of the sacrum if possible to avoid injury to the sciatic nerves. The operator's finger is placed deep to the piriformis muscle and superficial to the sacral nerve roots to protect these nerves from injury. Usually for S2 resection prone, the inferior nerve roots (S3, S4, S5) will be sacrificed due to the nature of the pathology (**Figure 6.12.19**).

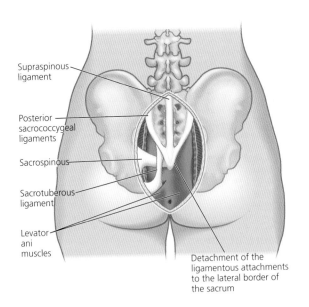

Supraspinous ligament

Posterior sacrococcygeal ligaments

Sacrospinous

Sacrotuberous ligament

Levator ani muscles

Detachment of the ligamentous attachments to the lateral border of the sacrum

6.12.19

SACRECTOMY

The level of the sacrectomy is estimated by the placement of an artery forceps on the median sacral crest. A mobile lateral x-ray is taken to correlate with the sacral pin (inserted during the transabdominal dissection; **Figure 6.11.16** in **Chapter 6.11**). The aim is to resect the sacrum with the pin *in situ* in the specimen to ensure a clear sacral margin.

After the level of sacrectomy has been determined, the median crest is resected to expose the dura mater after gradual transection of posterior ligaments. This level can also be confirmed by digital palpation through the previous anterior lithotomy incision, which is now opened and included in the prone exposure. The cauda equina and occasionally the lower canal is identified and ligated with a heavy tie and transected distally (**Figure 6.12.20**).

The sacrectomy is completed with an oscillating saw. The sacrum is retracted to expose the pelvic cavity. This retraction caudad is made more easily by previous lateral and anterior lithotomy dissection. The sterile pack will first become evident and then the rectus abdominis flap will become evident. The vessel loops around the lumbosacral and S1 nerve roots should be intact.

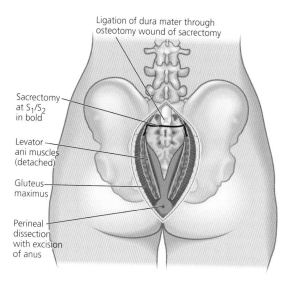

Ligation of dura mater through osteotomy wound of sacrectomy

Sacrectomy at S_1/S_2 in bold

Levator ani muscles (detached)

Gluteus maximus

Perineal dissection with excision of anus

6.12.20

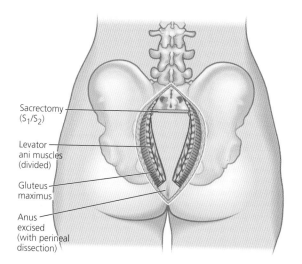

Sacrectomy (S_1/S_2)

Levator ani muscles (divided)

Gluteus maximus

Anus excised (with perineal dissection)

6.12.21

PERINEAL DISSECTION

The lateral pelvic excision is continued until the pelvic floor is identified and connected to the previous anterior compartment resection performed in lithotomy. If this was not performed, the anterior plane of dissection is done through the prone approach, which can be confusing (reversed) unless the surgeon is familiar with this approach. The increased utilization of the prone approach to abdominoperineal resection for primary tumors may facilitate this dissection (see **Chapter 6.10**).

The inferior and lateral borders of the resection are determined by the extent of the tumor into the lateral compartment. The vessel loops around the lumbosacral and S1 nerve roots can be used as a good lateral resection guide while completing the division of the piriformis, lower sacral nerve roots, lateral aspect of the obturator internus, and lateral pelvic floor. This is performed bilaterally, and continued to the anterior lateral border of the levator excision. During the total cystectomy, this part of the levator can be divided transabdominally, thus helping with the anterior part of the perineal dissection.

The specimen is delivered *en bloc* with the sacrum after the levator muscles have been transected circumferentially (**Figure 6.12.21**).

Hemostasis is secured. The abdominal drain is placed to the level of the previous pelvic floor and the vessel loops removed. The rectus flap is placed in the pelvic, perineal, and sacral defect and sutured ensuring there is no twist or tension (**Figure 6.12.22**).

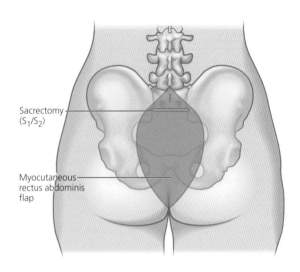

Sacrectomy (S_1/S_2)

Myocutaneous rectus abdominis flap

6.12.22

Lateral pelvic lymph node dissection in low rectal cancer

HIDEAKI YANO

HISTORY

In contrast to western countries, lateral pelvic lymphadenectomy (LPLD) has been continuously promoted, performed, and refined in Japan. Key refinements have been a more selective approach and nerve preserving surgery.[1]

PRINCIPLES AND JUSTIFICATION

A recent, large retrospective multicenter review from Japan reported lateral node involvement in 20.1 percent of patients with T3/4 low rectal cancer.[2]

Controversy exists as to whether involved lateral pelvic nodes represent systemic disease or localized disease amenable to curative resection. This bears an analogy with liver metastasis. Undoubtedly, a proportion have localized disease as demonstrated by favorable five-year survival in patients with involved lateral pelvic nodes who had LPLD.[1]

The latest Japanese guidelines suggest LPLD for T3/4 cancer with its lower edge lying at, or below, the peritoneal reflection.[3]

PREOPERATIVE ASSESSMENT AND PREPARATION

Advances in pelvic imaging, particularly computed tomography (CT) and magnetic resonance imaging (MRI), with the ability to visualize lymph nodes, has renewed interest in pelvic sidewall nodal disease not only in Japan but in western countries. The author reported a high diagnostic accuracy in predicting lateral pelvic nodal status in low rectal cancer using CT scans.[4]

An informed consent should be obtained, in particular regarding the risk of urinary and sexual impairment.

OPERATION

LPLD is usually performed following completion of rectal resection using the principles of total mesorectal excision (TME) or sphincter resection in those who require abdominoperineal excision. In restorative procedures, LPLD is performed before the anastomosis.

If there are worries about the margins of the suspicious node(s), the internal iliac artery and/or vein should be excised *en bloc*.

The following steps outline the main aspects of LPLD on the right pelvic sidewall.

The hypogastric nerve is secured using a vessel loop or tape. Caudally, the inferior hypogastric plexus and the pelvic splanchnic nerves (nervi erigentes) are dissected off the parietal endopelvic fascia and preserved. The ureter is then secured using a vessel loop or tape to reduce risks of inadvertent damage (**Figure 6.13.1**).

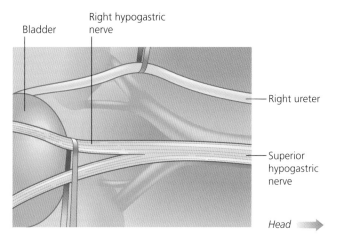

6.13.1

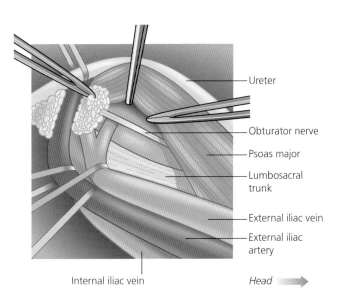

6.13.2

The external iliac artery is exposed and secured using a vessel loop or tape. By exposing the medial aspect of the psoas major muscle, the fat tissue between the external iliac artery and the psoas major is dissected and the obturator nerve is identified. Care should be taken not to damage the fifth lumbar vein that drains into either the inferior vena cava or the external iliac vein (**Figure 6.13.2**).

Prior to the dissection of the obturator region, the anterior aspect of the internal iliac artery is exposed and the fat tissue surrounding the external iliac vein is dissected from the cranial to the caudal direction. There is no need to follow the external iliac vessels to their distal ends unless necessary as it may increase the risk of lymphedema of the leg (**Figure 6.13.3**).

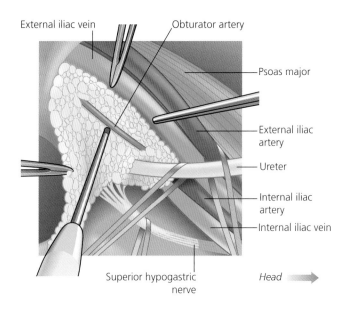

6.13.3

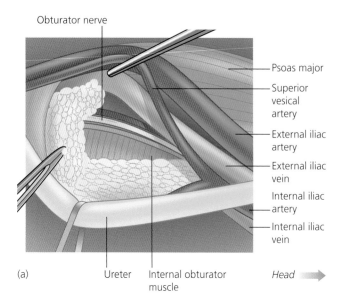

(a)   Ureter   Internal obturator
                          muscle   *Head* ➡

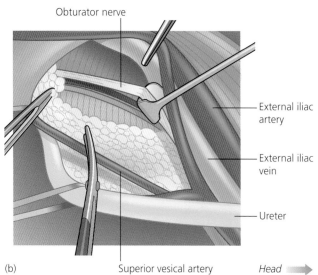

(b)   Superior vesical artery   *Head* ➡

6.13.4

By retracting the ureter and the external iliac vessels laterally, the optimal surgical field will be obtained. The dissection of the obturator region is commenced from where the internal and external iliac arteries branch off the common iliac artery. The superior vesical artery and the obturator vessels are then identified, both of which can be excised if necessary. Retracting the superior vesical artery medially, dissection is continued by exposing the obturator nerve and the internal obturator muscle as far as the point where the nerve enters the obturator canal. When using diathermy dissection, local perineural injection of lidocaine is very helpful to prevent stimulation of the adductor muscles. Alternatively, ultrasonic coagulating shears may prove useful (**Figure 6.13.4**).

On the craniomedial aspect, the lymphatic tissue is dissected off the internal iliac vessels that are situated on the lumbosacral trunk and the sacral nerve plexus. Care should be taken, particularly if excising the internal iliac vessels, not to damage the small branches of the vein, which would cause considerable bleeding (**Figure 6.13.5**).

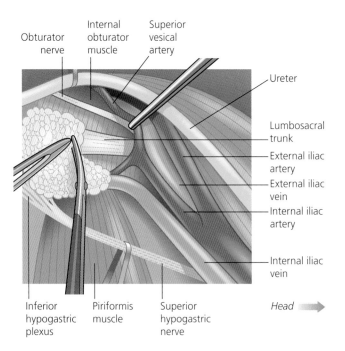

6.13.5

The caudal part of the obturator area is dissected by pulling medially the superior vesical artery and the ureter. The levator ani muscle is exposed just caudal to the internal obturator muscle (**Figure 6.13.6**).

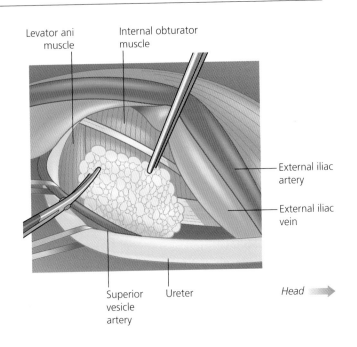

6.13.6

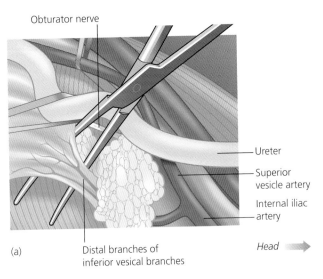

(a)

More medially, the identification of the inferior vesical vessels that are situated just lateral to the inferior hypogastric plexus is important. This is followed by division of the distal branches of the inferior vesical artery and vein at the point just proximal to the bladder. LPLD is completed by dividing the inferior vesical vessels from the internal iliac vessels (**Figure 6.13.7a–c**).

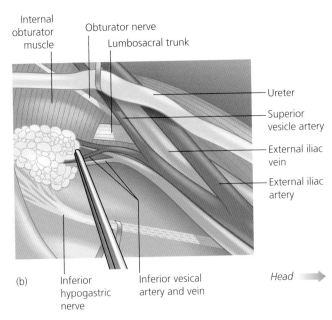

(b)

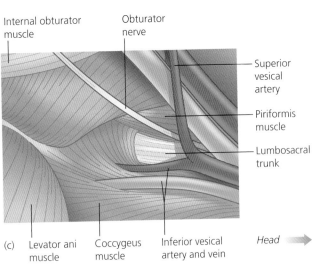

(c)

6.13.7

POSTOPERATIVE CARE

LPLD is associated with functional impairment, particularly impotence and bladder dysfunction, although recent modifications using nerve-sparing techniques have greatly reduced morbidity. A suprapubic catheter is particularly useful in male patients. Patients should be kept on anticoagulation as LPLD may increase a risk of venous thromboembolism although the evidence regarding this is unclear.

OUTCOME

In Japan, the reported five-year survival rates of patients with lateral pelvic node involvement range from 25 to 80 percent.[1] In a recent multicenter review, the five-year survival rate of patients with positive lateral nodes was 45.8 percent compared to 71.2 percent in patients with stage III disease with negative lateral nodes.[2]

REFERENCES

1. Yano H, Moran BJ. The incidence of lateral pelvic side-wall nodal involvement in low rectal cancer may be similar in Japan and the West. *British Journal of Surgery* 2008; **95**: 33–49.
2. Sugihara K, Kobayashi H, Kato T *et al.* Indication and benefit of pelvic sidewall dissection for rectal cancer. *Diseases of the Colon and Rectum* 2006; **49**: 1663–72.
3. Japanese Society for Cancer of the Colon and Rectum. *Japanese classification of colorectal carcinoma*, 2nd English edn. Tokyo: Kanehara, 2009.
4. Yano H, Saito Y, Takeshita E *et al.* Prediction of lateral pelvic node involvement in low rectal cancer by conventional computed tomography. *British Journal of Surgery* 2007; **94**: 1014–19.

Transanal resection for rectal lesions

SCOTT R STEELE

HISTORY

While total mesorectal excision (TME) and abdominal-perineal resection provide standard of care procedures for major oncologic resection of rectal cancer, the transanal approach to rectal lesions offers solutions to complex problems with the added benefits of other minimally invasive procedures. By utilizing the perianal approach, surgeons can minimize surgical stress and optimize function without compromising oncologic outcome. The potential morbidity associated with radical surgery (including major medical complications, impaired sexual and urinary function, reduced fecal continence, and the need for a permanent stoma) is in large part avoided altogether. Parks described the first transanal submucosal excision of a rectal lesion in 1966,[1] and transanal local excision (TLE) continues to serve as an option for cure in select patients who present with early tumors and favorable characteristics. In addition, it remains a palliative procedure for more advanced disease in high-risk patients. With proper selection of appropriate candidates, TLE stands as a useful and valuable tool in the surgeon's armamentarium for rectal lesions.

PRINCIPLES AND JUSTIFICATION

Benign and premalignant masses of the rectum such as sessile adenomas involve the mucosal layer of the rectal wall only, and may be removed via a submucosal excision. While other forms of local therapy such as fulguration with electrocautery, laser, or radiation are described, they do not provide a specimen for pathological examination, and are more appropriately used in a palliative or adjunctive capacity. Indications for resection include symptomatic control (e.g. bleeding, mucus seepage), as well as eliminating the inherent potential for malignant degeneration. By employing a resection in the submucosal plane, the lesion may be adequately removed while minimizing the risk

of complications. However, this approach depends upon accurate preoperative staging to avoid inadequate resection of more advanced lesions. Endorectal ultrasound has reported rates of up to 90 percent accuracy for determining tumor depth of penetration, along with sensitivity rates of 60–70 percent and specificity rates of 70–80 percent for nodal metastases. Similarly, magnetic resonance imaging (MRI) is associated with accuracy rates of up to 85 percent for primary rectal wall involvement, and nodal sensitivity rates of 60–70 percent and specificity rates of 70–80 percent.[2] For malignant or indeterminate lesions, local excision involves a full thickness resection of the mass along with 1–2 cm margins (**Figure 6.14.1**). This provides an intact specimen with its surrounding tissue,

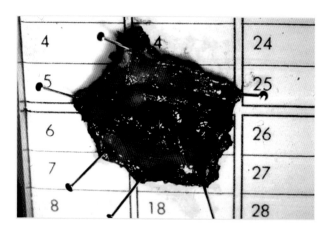

6.14.1 Full thickness excision of a rectal lesion with surrounding margin. Courtesy of Ann C. Lowry, MD.

and allows adequate primary tumor (T) staging. Radical resection offers lower recurrence rates when compared to local excision.[3] This is especially true for T2 tumors, where local recurrence has been cited to be as high as 47 percent. Early T1 tumors and specific patient populations such as elderly, high-risk patients, and young, healthy patients with low tumors who do not wish to undergo permanent diversion remain excellent candidates for TLE. In addition, very low lesions closer to the anal verge are technically more feasible for a traditional local excision than transanal endoscopic microsurgery (TEM). Depending on the nature of the specimen and depth of invasion, lymph node metastases may still be present in 6–12 percent of patients following TLE in T1 lesions. Invasion into the deeper third of the submucosal layer (Sm_3) has been reported to have even higher rates of lymph node metastases (up to 25 percent)[4] and consideration should be given to a traditional resection if the patient's risk profile tolerates it. Additionally, lesions T2 or deeper should normally not be operated with TLE, as nodal rates have been reported as high as 25–30 percent for pT2 and 30–35 percent in pT3 lesions. Similarly, those lesions possessing poor prognostic risk factors, such as lymphovascular invasion (LVI), poor differentiation, tumor budding, and mucinous or signet cell adenocarcinoma should avoid TLE.[5]

PREOPERATIVE ASSESSMENT AND PREPARATION

Sessile adenoma

Patients should undergo an initial examination to determine whether they are medically fit to tolerate an operation. Colonoscopy should be used to address or exclude synchronous lesions. In addition to a general physical examination, digital rectal examination can assess sphincter tone and palpate the lesions in many cases. Sessile adenomas are typically soft and mobile on examination. Characteristics, such as ulceration, fixation, or firmness of the lesion, are concerning for invasion and warrant further investigation to exclude malignancy. Biopsy is commonly performed for histological diagnosis, though excision of the mass is still required. Preoperative staging is again crucial to stratify which patients may safely undergo a local procedure versus those that require a more extensive resection, as well as to determine the need for full thickness versus submucosal excision.

To perform a proper TLE, the lesion must be accessible from the anal verge, which depends, in part, on patient body habitus. In general, distance from the verge limits this approach to those located in the distal half of the rectum (below 8 cm). Techniques, such as intussusception of the rectal wall using atraumatic bowel graspers or traction sutures, can aid in allowing access to more proximal lesions in the mid- to upper rectum and even

sigmoid colon that are not otherwise reachable (**Figures 6.14.2** and **6.14.3**).

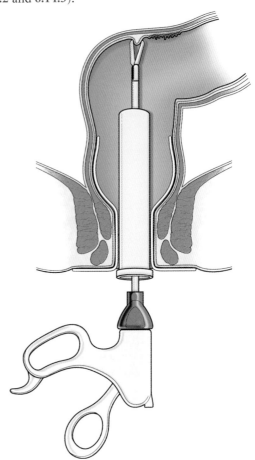

6.14.2 Atraumatic graspers allow access to higher lesions.

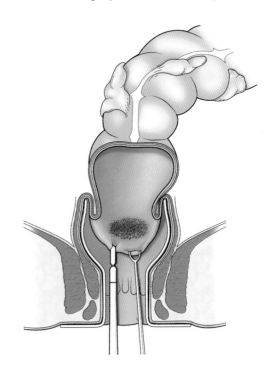

6.14.3 See legend above.

Initial preparations for a transanal local excision consist in most cases of a full mechanical bowel preparation, although some surgeons prefer the use of enemas alone. Preoperative intravenous antibiotics are routinely given. In addition, deep venous thrombosis prophylaxis including sequential compression devices and chemical prophylaxis (i.e. heparin or low molecular weight heparin) may be considered.

Rectal carcinoma

As with benign lesions, colonoscopy is used to assess for other synchronous masses. In addition to staging with endorectal ultrasound (ERUS) or MRI, a computed tomography (CT) scan of the chest, abdomen, and pelvis is commonly used to evaluate for distant spread. Standard laboratory evaluation normally involves a complete blood count, liver function tests, and carcinoembryonic antigen (CEA). In theory, a proper full thickness transanal excision of the mass that includes a surrounding 1 cm margin of normal tissue is a useful operation for T1 or T2 lesions with no lymph node or distant metastatic spread. Therefore, emphasis is placed on accurately determining the depth of invasion and lymph node status. The risk for leaving behind unrecognized lymph node disease increases in more advanced T stages, and errors in preoperative T staging can therefore affect the outcome of TLE. Pathological nodes are frequently defined on ERUS as hypoechoic lesions greater than 5 or 10 mm with similar echogenicity as the primary tumor. With MRI, a spiculated or heterogeneous appearance, and those with irregular borders are concerning for positive nodes. However, up to 20 percent of positive lymph nodes can be as small as 2 mm and over 50 percent may be less than 5 mm in diameter.[6] Apart from T and N stage, the size of primary lesion itself is another consideration when deciding on whether or not to pursue TLE, although larger (>3–4 cm) and even circumferential lesions have been reported to be successfully resected with proper experience and expertise. Indications may be modified in otherwise compromised patients who may not tolerate more standard abdominal approaches.

Use of a bowel preparation, intravenous antibiotics, and thromboembolic prophylaxis follow that of benign lesions.

ANESTHESIA

While provider preference plays a large role in anesthesia selection, a regional or general anesthetic is used for most transanal resections. The combination of conscious sedation and a perianal block with local anesthetics (i.e. lidocaine, marcaine) can be successfully used for low-lying and small lesions. Injection of a local agent with the addition of adrenaline in the rectal wall surrounding the mass can also provide improved hemostasis. Postoperatively, most patients have effective pain relief by utilizing short-term oral narcotics and/or non-steroidal medications.

OPERATIONS

As in all surgery, adequate exposure remains of paramount importance to helping achieve optimal outcomes. Taping the buttocks laterally improves perianal exposure. In addition, a Lone Star Retractor System™ (Cooper Surgical Inc., Turnbull, CT, USA) or other self-retaining retractors facilitate visualization while freeing the assistant's hands. Both the surgeon and assistant should wear headlights in order to aid in visualization.

Positioning of the patient

Patient positioning depends primarily on the location of the lesion. For posterior lesions, the lithotomy position provides excellent exposure. The prone position provides superior visualization for anterior and lateral lesions, while allowing improved access for an assistant surgeon (**Figure 6.14.4**). All bony prominences are well padded and consideration should be given for a pad under the sacrum when in lithotomy. According to physician preference, both arms may be tucked at the patient's side or extended for monitoring access.

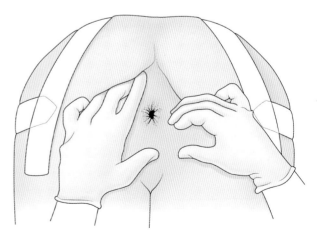

6.14.4 Prone position for anterior and lateral lesions.

Submucosal resection

For a transanal approach, a Pratt bivalve, Fansler, Parks or
Hill-Ferguson anoscope provides excellent exposure for
low-lying lesions. A Lone Star™ Retractor System (Cooper
Surgical, Turnbull, CT) may be used to facilitate exposure
for higher lesions (**Figure 6.14.5**). With the Lone Star™
Retractor System in place, its accompanying hooks are
positioned at the four corners to evert the anal verse and
provide enhanced exposure to the lesion. Additional stay
sutures may be placed at least 2 cm from the lesion and
hooked onto the retractor to further aid in this process.
Gelpi retractors are also useful in the absence of a Lone
Star™ or in difficult cases, while Deaver or Wylie renal vein
retractors are useful for more proximal lesions (**Figure
6.14.6**). Electrocautery or advanced energy devices are
commonly used for marking out the circumferential
incision as well as for the resection.

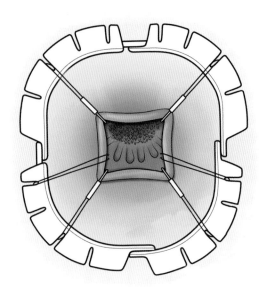

6.14.5 Stay suture on surrounding mucosa to pull the
lesion into operative field.

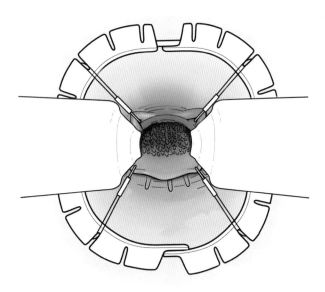

6.14.6 Retractors are useful to access more proximal
lesions.

To aid in dissection and hemostasis, the submucosal plane surrounding the lesion is infiltrated with a mixture of local anesthetic or saline with 1:100 000–1:200 000 adrenaline. For benign lesions, this will separate the mucosal–submucosal layers from the underlying muscle, helping to delineate the plane of dissection. Injection should begin distal to the tumor and extend several centimeters beyond the intended borders (**Figure 6.14.7**).

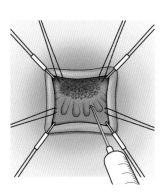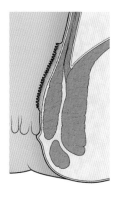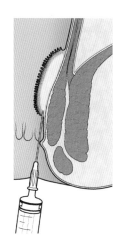

6.14.7 Injection of adrenaline solution around the lesion.

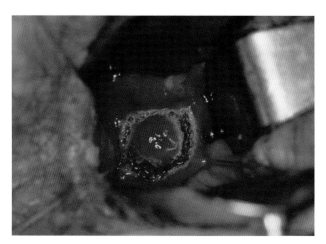

6.14.8 Photo courtesy of W Brian Sweeney, MD.

Electrocautery with either a standard or needle tip is used to demarcate 1 cm margins in the normal mucosa surrounding the lesion (**Figure 6.14.8**).

The submucosal plane is entered sharply with electrocautery, scissors, or an energy device. Dissection continues by elevating the lesion off the underlying muscle, and progressing more proximally (**Figure 6.14.9**). Downward traction aids in bringing the upper extent into view, though care must be taken to avoid fragmenting the mass. Proper specimen orientation must be maintained, and additional adrenaline can be injected as necessary to help with hemostasis. Partial thickness resections do not require closure, though this may be done at the discretion of the surgeon.

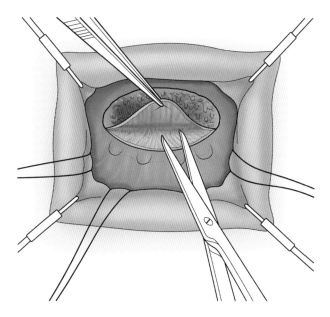

6.14.9

More diffuse and circumferential lesions can be adequately removed via the peranal route using a sleeve resection. Infiltration of the wall with an adrenaline mixture improves visualization of the extent of the adenoma, as well as aiding in separation of the layers of the rectal wall. Dissection should begin 1 cm distal to the lower edge of the lesion and continue in the submucosal plane, removing an entire cylinder of the rectal wall containing the adenomatous lesion (**Figure 6.14.10**).

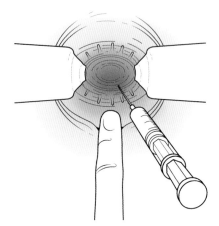
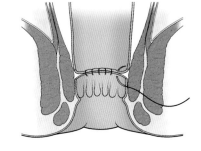

6.14.10

Care must be taken to avoid stricture formation with the large resultant defect. Similar to a Delorme resection, muscular plication is performed using absorbable sutures in each of the four quadrants to help ease tension, and approximate the mucosal edges. Additional sutures are placed as necessary with attention likewise focused on compressing the exposed muscle (**Figure 6.14.11**).

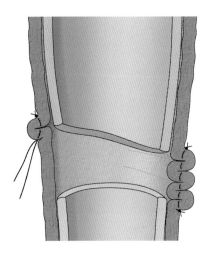

6.14.11

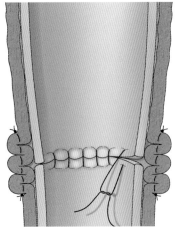

6.14.12

Following plication, the mucosal edges are closed using interrupted absorbable sutures in a separate layer. Conversely, the plication and closure of the mucosa can be performed in the same stitch. Mobilization of the proximal mucosa is often required to advance the upper rectal wall to the more distal rectum to provide a tension-free anastomosis (**Figure 6.14.12**).

Once complete, rigid proctoscopy should always be performed to ensure patency of the rectal lumen, evaluate for adequate hemostasis, and confirm complete resection of the lesion. With extensive dissection, inadvertent closure of the rectum is an unintended, yet avoidable outcome. Adequate exposure during this step allows for visualization of each suture placement and minimizes this occurrence.

The lesion is then pinned out on a corkboard or electrocautery scratch pad and labeled to properly orient the pathologist for histological assessment (**Figure 6.14.13**). In this manner, improved focus for any subsequent treatment is possible; such as in the case of positive margins, invasive malignancy, or other unexpected findings.

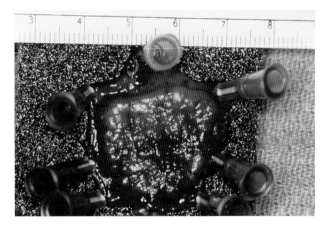

6.14.13 Photo courtesy of W Brian Sweeney, MD.

MALIGNANCY IN VILLOUS ADENOMAS

Polyps may also contain foci of invasive cancer. Depending on the depth of invasion, location of the lesion, and type of adenomatous polyp (i.e. sessile, flat, pedunculated), local excision may provide a curative option through endoscopic or traditional transanal methods. In general, full thickness resection is warranted. Deeper invasion, concerning histological characteristics (i.e. poor differentiation, lymphovascular invasion), or inability to achieve adequate margins are all indications for additional therapy such as low anterior or abdominal-perineal resection. **Figure 6.14.14** shows a pedunculated polyp with tumor invasion of the base of the stalk.

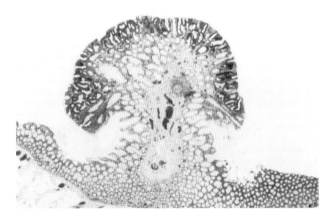

6.14.14

CARCINOIDS

Carcinoid tumors are most commonly identified as incidental submucosal masses encountered during endoscopy (**Figure 6.14.15**). Endorectal ultrasound or MRI can be used to locally stage these lesions. Additionally, full colonoscopy should be performed to exclude a synchronous malignancy. CT of the chest, abdomen, and pelvis and/or an octreotide nuclear medicine scan is normally performed to evaluate for metastatic disease. These lesions should undergo a full-thickness excision to evaluate for depth of invasion. Large tumors (>2 cm) or invasion of the muscularis propria are indications to undergo more extensive surgery.

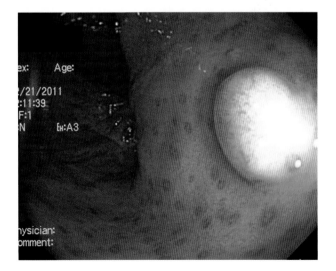

6.14.15

Full thickness excision

Unlike benign lesions, in which a submucosal excision is acceptable, invasion of the bowel wall by a rectal cancer requires full thickness excision. Visualization of the perirectal fat should be accomplished to ensure adequate resection depth (**Figure 6.14.16**). The initial steps of the operation from patient positioning, achieving exposure, and use of adrenaline solution mirror those for non-malignant lesions.

The author prefers using infiltration of adrenaline solution around the lesion in the rectal wall, not to raise the lesion as in benign lesions, but to improve hemostasis and visualization. Stay sutures and a Lone Star™ retractor once again provide optimal exposure. Electrocautery can be used to mark 1 cm boundaries around the lesion (see **Figure 6.14.8**).

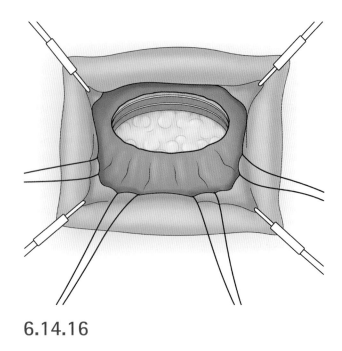

6.14.16

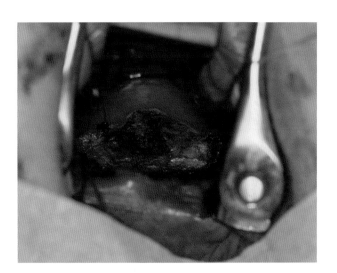

6.14.17 Photo courtesy of W Brian Sweeney, MD.

Following infiltration of an adrenaline solution, full thickness dissection of the rectal wall progresses in a distal to proximal fashion down to the level of the perirectal fat. Care should be taken to avoid tearing the lesion, as well as maintaining proper orientation.

Following excision, sterile water or another tumoricidal solution may be placed in the resulting defect to help minimize the risk of seeding the tumor bed with residual tumor cells. For extraperitoneal lesions, the resulting defect may be left open with little consequence (**Figure 6.14.17**).

In most cases, the rectal wall is closed, in a single or double layer using interrupted absorbable sutures following complete removal. Intraperitoneal defects mandate closure of the rectal wall, typically with an absorbable suture in one or two layers. This is often facilitated by full-thickness closure as the dissection progresses (**Figure 6.14.18**).

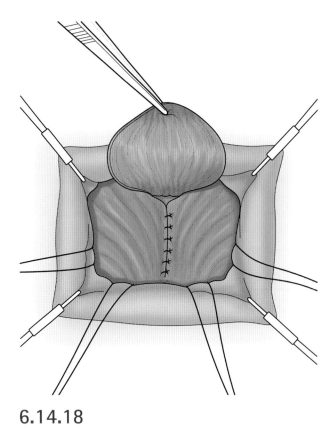

6.14.18

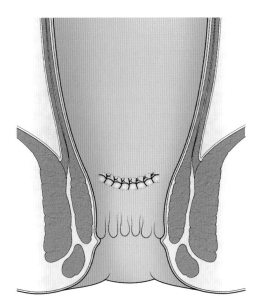

6.14.19

Downward traction is placed on the distal suture line to keep the upper extent of the resection in view and prevent recoiling of the lesion site more proximally until completely closed (**Figure 6.14.19**). When finished, rigid proctoscopy should be performed to ensure patency of the rectal lumen.

POSTOPERATIVE CARE

Typical postoperative management includes early ambulation and initiation of enteral feeding as tolerated. Nasogastric tubes are not required. The bladder catheter is removed on the day of surgery or first postoperative day, pending surgeon preference. Mild discomfort is normally controlled with oral pain medication, and aided by periodic warm sitz baths. Standard perioperative antibiotic dosing (<24 hours) is all that is necessary. Patients are usually discharged within 1–2 days with a scheduled follow-up in clinic in 1–2 weeks. Perioperative bleeding, infection, and stricture are uncommon complications, occurring in <10 percent of cases, and rarely warrant reintervention.[7]

OUTCOMES

Following TLE, the local recurrence rate for villous lesions is variable at 2–40 percent, with some large series reporting <5 percent. T1 and T2 tumors similarly have wide ranges, at 10–20 percent and 25–50 percent, respectively.[3] Factors such as size, dysplasia, margin status, and histological predictors (i.e. LVI, differentiation) play a role in this spectrum. Ten-year survival is also inconsistent, although reported rates are approximately 70–80 percent for T1 lesions and 65–75 percent for T2 lesions. In addition to the intrinsic tumor factors, the variability results from other factors, such as use of adjuvant chemo- or radiotherapy.

Villous lesions should be followed with digital rectal examination and proctoscopy every three months for one year, every six months for the following two years, and annually thereafter pending the findings at each visit. Recurrent lesions should be appropriately staged and treated with fulguration or repeat local excision if benign. Unexpected findings of malignancy on final pathology may warrant a more traditional anterior resection.

Patients with rectal carcinoma undergoing TLE should be followed with examination and proctoscopy every three months for the first two years. Some authors advocate endorectal ultrasound to aid in detecting recurrence early. Standard postoperative surveillance guidelines for malignant lesions should be followed with CT scans and laboratory evaluation (liver function tests, CEA) every six months for the first few years following surgery, and complete colonoscopy at one year.

The addition of radiation, with or without chemotherapy, in an adjuvant or neoadjuvant setting has demonstrated promise in select lesions for lowering recurrence rates. Long-term survival data in large numbers are still lacking. Theoretical advantages include sterilization of microscopic disease both within the wall as well as lymph node basins. Elderly, high-risk patients may elect to undergo observation alone following initial transanal excision.

ACKNOWLEDGMENTS

This chapter was originally written by the late Sir Alan Parks MCh, FRCS, FRCP, Consultant Surgeon, The Royal London Hospital and St Mark's Hospital for Diseases of the Rectum and Colon, London, UK, and most recently by Ann C Lowry, MD, Clinical Professor of Surgery, University of Minnesota, Minneapolis, MN, USA.

REFERENCES

1. Parks AG. Benign tumours of the rectum. In: Rob C, Smith R, Morgan C (eds). *Abdomen and rectum and anus.* Operative surgery, vol. 10. London: Butterworth, 1966: 541–8.
2. Bipat S, Glas AS, Slors FJ *et al.* Rectal cancer: local staging and assessment of lymph node involvement with endoluminal US, CT, and MR imaging – a meta-analysis. *Radiology* 2004; **232**: 773–83.
3. Paty PB, Nash GM, Baron P *et al.* Long-term results of local excision for rectal cancer. *Annals of Surgery* 2002; **236**: 522–9.
4. Nascimbeni R, Nivatvongs S, Larson DR, Burgart LJ. Long-term survival after local excision for T1 carcinoma of the rectum. *Diseases of the Colon and Rectum* 2004; **47**: 1773–9.
5. Bretagnol F, Rullier E, George B *et al.* Local therapy for rectal cancer: still controversial? *Diseases of the Colon and Rectum* 2007; **50**: 523–33.
6. Zheng YC, Zhou ZG, Li L *et al.* Distribution and patterns of lymph nodes metastases and micrometastases in the mesorectum of rectal cancer. *Journal of Surgical Oncology* 2007; **96**: 213–19.
7. Ptok H, Marusch F, Meyer F *et al.* Oncological outcome of local vs radical resection of low-risk pT1 rectal cancer. *Archives of Surgery* 2007; **142**: 649–55.

FURTHER READING

Friel CM, Cromwell JW, Marra C *et al.* Salvage radical surgery after failed local excision for early rectal cancer. *Diseases of the Colon and Rectum* 2002; **45**: 875–9.
Garcia-Aguilar J, Mellgren A, Sirivongs P *et al.* Local excision of rectal cancer without adjuvant therapy: a word of caution. *Annals of Surgery* 2000; **23**: 1345–51.
You YN, Baxter NN, Stewart A, Nelson H. Is the increasing rate of local excision for stage I rectal cancer in the United States justified?: A nationwide cohort study from the National Cancer Database. *Annals of Surgery* 2007; **245**: 726–33.

Transanal endoscopic microsurgery

NEIL MORTENSEN AND ROEL HOMPES

PRINCIPLES AND JUSTIFICATION

Transanal endoscopic microsurgery (TEM), introduced by Buess et al.[1] in 1983, was initially designed to improve the results for local resection of rectal adenomas. The most common conventional technique of local resection of rectal tumors is the Parks' per anal resection (PAR). This technique is safe and straightforward; however, the restricted view and limited range (lower rectum) are major drawbacks. The recurrence rates range from 4 to 57 percent.[2] The high recurrence rates after PAR are thought to be due to the limited view, leading to less precise excisions with a higher rate of specimen fragmentation and positive resection margins. Alternative local techniques for the resection of larger and/or tumors of the mid or upper rectum are the Kraske (suprasphincteric/transsacral) or Mason (transsphincteric) procedures. These are, however, technically demanding and associated with high postoperative morbidity rates of 24–41 percent and 11–70 percent, respectively.

In contrast, TEM offers access to the entire rectum and distal sigmoid with an unequaled view of the operative field, and low postoperative morbidity and mortality rates. With TEM, it is feasible and safe to resect tumors situated up to 20 cm posteriorly, 15 cm laterally, and 12 cm anteriorly from the anal verge. A systematic review revealed a morbidity rate for TEM of 10.3 percent (versus 17 percent for PAR).[3] Reported recurrence rates are lower than for PAR being 3–16 percent.[2]

TEM has been proven to be safe and effective for the treatment of rectal adenoma, but there is growing consensus that TEM is also a good indication for the treatment of early rectal cancers with favorable histopathological features (pT1 Sm1 lesions, well differentiated, without lymphovascular invasion, and up to 3 cm in diameter). In these carefully selected patients, survival and local recurrence rates are similar to those of more involved, traditional operations but with limited morbidity and mortality. Available data on TEM after neoadjuvant treatment for advanced rectal tumors are encouraging, but need confirmation by larger and randomized trials.

Diagnostic excision of polyps or other lesions with unclear pathology, and palliation in some advanced cancers can also be achieved with this technique.

PREOPERATIVE ASSESSMENT AND PREPARATION

Staging

A routine preoperative work up is essential to select patients appropriate for TEM. A thorough clinical examination with digital rectal examination (DRE) is important to assess tumor location, size and depth of rectal wall penetration. Preoperative colonoscopy should be performed, especially if the tumor is too proximal to assess by DRE. The lesion is accurately localized by quadrant, and distance from the anal verge and circumferential extent noted. At the same time synchronous lesions are excluded and large villous lesions can be debulked to allow better access to the base of the lesion during TEM.

For malignant lesions of the rectum, computed tomography (CT) scan of the chest, abdomen, and pelvis is necessary to exclude distant metastatic disease, but for locoregional staging endorectal ultrasound (ERUS) and magnetic resonance imaging (MRI) are better modalities. At present, ERUS has the highest accuracy for staging early rectal cancer. The sensitivity and specificity are reported to be 87.8 and 98.3 percent for T1, and 80.5 and 95.6 percent for T2 tumors, respectively.

While MRI is of limited value in assessing early T-stage, it is useful however for the locally advanced tumors, and assessment of mesorectal nodes and the relationship of the tumor to the mesorectal fascia. For lesions located anteriorly, MRI also provides the surgeon with information on the depth of fat anterior to rectum.

The role of PET for local and regional staging of rectal

cancer is limited, and should be reserved for evaluation of local recurrence or doubtful mesorectal nodes.

Patient preparation

Prior to admission, the patient is given a diet of clear fluids for 24 hours. The patient is admitted on the day of the operation and is given an enema 1 hour in advance. Consent should be obtained for the procedure and for an explorative laparoscopy or laparotomy in the case of unforeseen operative or technical events.

ANESTHESIA

The procedure can be performed under general or regional anesthesia. General anesthesia is preferable if the patient has to be positioned in the prone jack-knife position and when the surgeon is on a learning curve. Some medical comorbidities of the patient may mandate regional anesthesia.

The preference in the authors' department is for general anesthetic in all patients, if feasible, because this tends to facilitate a more stable pneumorectum.

OPERATION

Equipment

The TEM rectoscope is 40 mm in diameter and comes in two different lengths, 12 and 20 cm. The rectoscope is sealed with an airtight, removable face piece that has four entry ports: three working ports with capped rubber seals, and one port for the magnifying stereoscopic optic. There is an accessory endoscope that can be connected to a monitor to display the surgical field for the surgeon and the rest of the operating team. The lens is equipped with a separate irrigation channel for cleaning, activated by a foot pedal. The intrarectal pressure is autoregulated at a preset pressure of 12–15 mmHg by constant-flow carbon dioxide insufflation, thus maintaining a stable pneumorectum which provides excellent visibility and a steady workspace. The stereoscopic optic provides the surgeons with an unequaled three-dimensional view with a perceptible depth of field, resolution, and six-fold magnification (**Figure 6.15.1**).

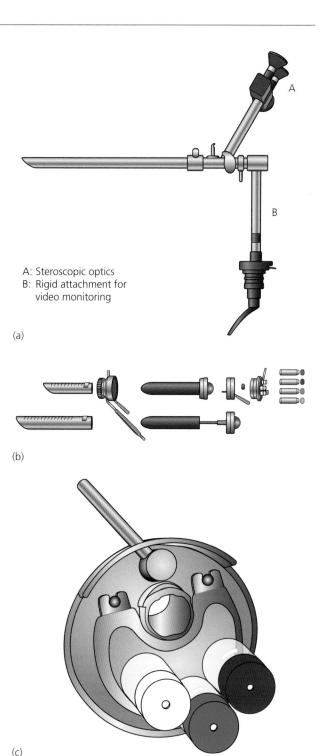

A: Steroscopic optics
B: Rigid attachment for video monitoring

(a)

(b)

(c)

6.15.1

A variety of instruments are available (forceps, high-frequency knife, scissors, suction coagulator, clip applicator, and needle holders), angled to either the right or left to compensate for the narrow working channel and bent downwards to negotiate easily the sacral cavity (**Figure 6.15.2**).

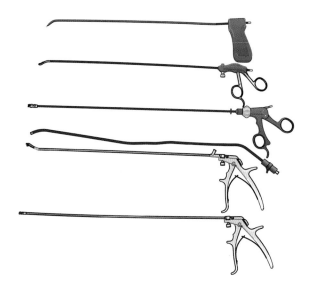

6.15.2

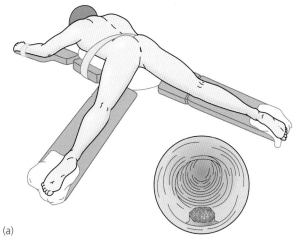

(a)

Patient installation and set-up

The bevel of the rectoscope must face downward so positioning of the patient depends on the location of the lesion. At all times the bulk of the lesion should be kept at six o'clock in the operation field; posteriorly located lesions are operated on in a lithotomy position, lateral lesions in a side position and for anterior lesions the patient is placed in extreme jack-knife position with the legs spread to allow space for the surgeon. For this reason, the authors make a final check of the position of the lesion in the anesthetic room (**Figure 6.15.3**).

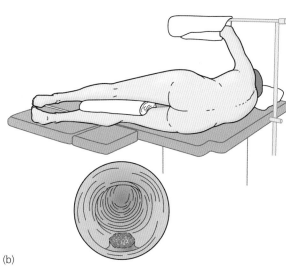

(b)

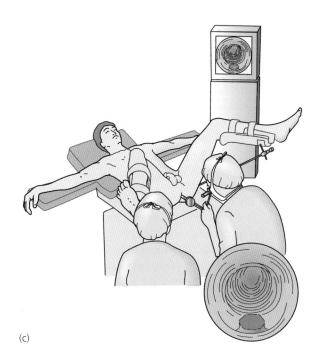

(c)

6.15.3

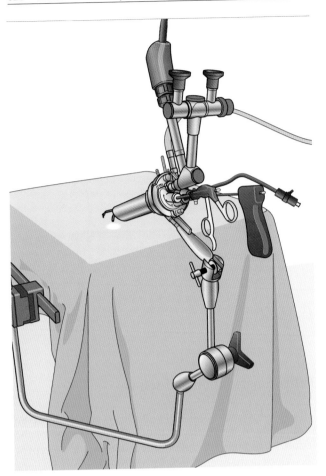

6.15.4

After a dilating DRE, the well-lubricated rectoscope is gently inserted into the rectum. An anal block (20 cc marcaine 0.5 percent) can further relax the sphincter muscle and offers additional analgesia up to 12 hours postoperatively. The obturator is replaced by a glass window, and with the rectum manually insufflated, the lesion can be identified and the rectoscope advanced under direct vision to the desired position.

Locked into position, the rectoscope is fixed to the table by the Martin arm, a supporting device, making sure that the double-ball joints and arms are in one vertical plane. Correct positioning of the rectoscope and the supporting arm are important for subsequent successful excision and suturing. As a final step, the gas insufflation (turquoise), irrigation (blue), suction (red), and pressure (green) monitoring tubes are attached and the pump/insufflator unit is turned on (**Figure 6.15.4**).

Technique of resection

RESECTION MARGIN

Before any dissection is done, the margin of clearance should be clearly defined with coagulation dots all around the tumour. All lesions should be excised with at least a 1 cm margin of normal mucosa, although a 5 mm margin is acceptable for benign lesions (**Figure 6.15.5**).

MUCOSECTOMY OR FULL-THICKNESS?

A full-thickness resection with adequate margins of clearance is preferably used in the extraperitoneal part of the rectum, thus lesions up to 20 cm from the dentate line posteriorly, 15 cm laterally, and 10–12 cm anteriorly.

Partial-thickness excisions can be performed in the case of lesions suspected to be benign, or if the procedure is done with the intent of compromise/palliation. However, partial-thickness excisions are associated with a six-fold increase in the odds of a positive margin.[4] Therefore, the authors believe that a full-thickness excision of any lesion distal to the peritoneal reflection should be considered standard, even for lesions thought to be benign.

Mixed partial- and full-thickness excisions are undertaken either to preserve the internal anal sphincter, where a lesion encroaches on the upper anal canal, or to prevent perforation into the peritoneal cavity for more proximal lesions and not increase the risk of an R1 resection.[4]

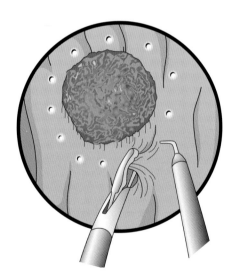

6.15.5

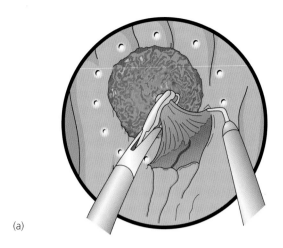

(a)

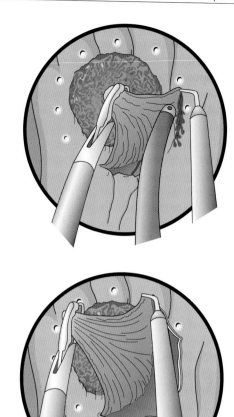

(b)

(c)

6.15.6

RESECTION

The dissection is usually started aborally in the midline by incising the rectal wall layer by layer, until reaching the perirectal fat (**Figure 6.15.6**). In the case of a lesion just above the dentate line, the initial plane of dissection is submucosally, by incising the rectal wall onto the internal sphincter muscle. These extremely distal lesions can be difficult to excise by TEM, because of frequent loss of

pneumorectum and bleeding from hemorrhoidal vessels. Once the dissection margin is marked out and the surgical plane identified, the dissection is continued orally and from left to right, dissecting tissue behind the lesion onto the proximal resection margin. Anteriorly, one should always stay close to the rectal wall to avoid damaging the vaginal wall, urethra, or accidental entry into the abdominal cavity. For posterior located lesions, part of the mesorectal fat can be resected for lymph node sampling, although this can lead to troublesome bleeding and spoil planes for any subsequent TEM (**Figure 6.15.7**).

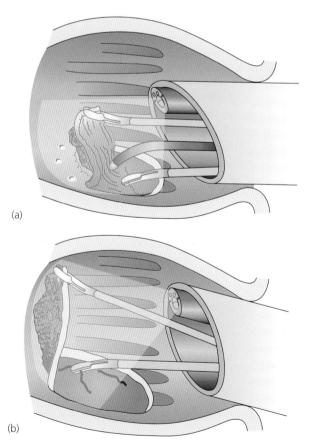

(a)

(b)

6.15.7

If during the dissection bleeding occurs, the bleeding point is best controlled by compression with the tip of an instrument and then coagulated with the tip of the suction device or grasped with a forceps and coagulated. Bleeding most often occurs when dissection extends too deep into the perirectal fat or mesorectum where larger vessels are encountered. Hemostatic devices like the harmonic scalpel may not only reduce the blood loss but also shorten operating time. The authors do not however use them regularly.

If during dissection the peritoneum is accidently opened, the defect should be immediately closed if it causes difficulty due to loss of the pneumorectum (**Figure 6.15.8**). Otherwise, it is sufficient to close the rectal wall defect after resection of the lesion. If it is thought that there has been fecal soiling in the peritoneal cavity it is prudent to consider a laparoscopic lavage of the pelvis after finishing the TEM procedure. At the same time, the closure site can be inspected and tested with a leak test.

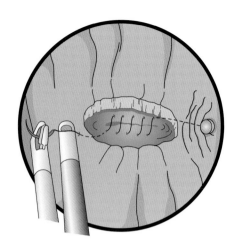

6.15.8

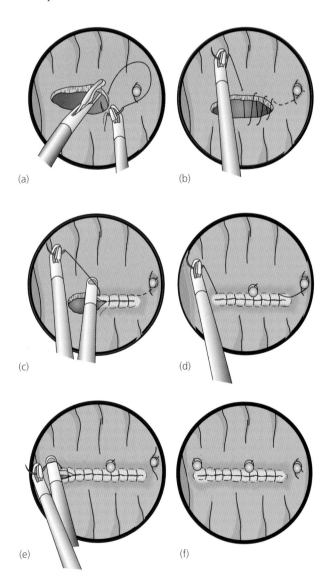

(a)

(b)

(c)

(d)

(e)

(f)

6.15.9

WOUND CLOSURE

The parietal defect created should be rinsed with a copious amount of disinfectant fluid to prevent abscess formation and the theoretical possibility of tumor implantation. The wound can be closed by a transverse continuous absorbable monofilament 2-0 suture. However, about 20 percent of sutured defects break down and for that reason the authors tend not to suture the lower lesions (**Figure 6.15.9**).

For closure of the defect, the endoluminal pressure is reduced to 10–12 mmHg to allow better tissue approximation. Instead of a knot, a silver clip is pressed onto the thread to lock the suture. Closure of the defect is easier when sewing from right to left, and aborally to orally. Only for closure of the left corner, changing the direction of suturing (orally to aborally) may help to get better access for placing the suture.

In the case of a large defect, stay sutures can be placed for orientation and correct alignment of wound edges. To keep tension on the suture within the field of vision, the sutures should be kept at 8 cm or less (length of the package of suture) (**Figure 6.15.10**).

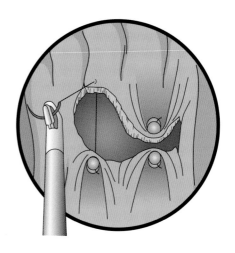

6.15.10

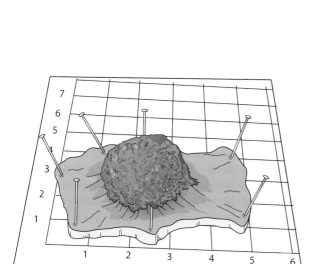

6.15.11

SPECIMEN

The specimen should be handled with care and sent fresh to the pathologist, and pinned out on a piece of cork to preserve the relationship between the normal margin and tumor (**Figure 6.15.11**).

POSTOPERATIVE CARE

Postoperative instructions

After extraction of the rectoscope, a large Foley catheter (32 Ch) is inserted to drain residual rinsing fluid, and is removed 24 hours after the procedure. Once back on the surgical ward, the patient is started on a liquid diet if tolerated. The first day after the operation, the patient is given a regular diet and discharged if no complications occur. In the case of a mucosectomy, patients can go home the same day if they are comfortable, tolerate oral fluids, and do not live alone.

Complications

Postoperative morbidity after TEM is generally low, approximately 5–10 percent. These are mainly minor complications: pain, rectal bleeding, fever, and urinary retention. Other less frequent complications that have been reported are intra- or transmural abscess formation, fistulae to perineum or vagina, and rectal strictures.

Dysuria or urinary retention usually resolve spontaneously in the first 24 hours after surgery. In the case of urinary retention, catheterization might be necessary for a short period. Wound breakdown can lead to pelvic sepsis and usually warrants an examination under anesthesia to drain the abscess. If sepsis persists, a diversion colostomy or ileostomy may be necessary. In the case of severe rectal bleeding, an emergency rectoscopy is required to deal with the focus of bleeding, which is usually at the suture line or a mucosal tear. Clinically significant bleeding has been found to occur more often if the defect has not been sutured, and in lesions located further than 8 cm from the anal verge, especially if arising from the lateral wall.

Transient fecal incontinence is present in nearly all patients undergoing TEM, and is found to correlate with the duration of the procedure. Although this has resulted in some concerns about the functional outcomes after

TEM, anal canal pressures have been shown to return to normal levels after six months, and quality of life and even continence may be improved after tumor removal.

Follow-up

After resection of an adenoma, the patient should have a flexible sigmoidoscopy after three months, with further endoscopic evaluations yearly thereafter if there are no signs of recurrence. Adenoma with high grade dysplasia warrants closer follow-up. Any recurrent adenoma can be treated by further endoscopic resection or re-TEM.

Follow-up for TEM in the case of rectal cancer is performed according to our departmental protocol: clinical examination and flexible endoscopy at three-monthly intervals for the first year, thereafter six-monthly for up to five years. Pelvic MRI is performed at three, nine, and 18 months postoperatively, and CT scan of abdomen and pelvis annually for the first three years for patients at high risk for recurrence. PET-CT is not routinely recommended. Although not part of the authors' protocol, carcinoembryonic antigen levels can be determined every three to six months for two years, then every six months for a total of five years in patients who are potential candidates for resection of isolated metastasis.

OUTCOME

TEM procedures have been performed in the Department of Colorectal Surgery, Oxford since 1993, as part of the surgical strategy for the excision of benign and selected malignant rectal lesions. Over a 12-year period, TEM was performed for excision of rectal adenoma or carcinoma in 148 and 52 patients, respectively.[5] The planes of dissection were full thickness in 170 patients (85 percent), and partial thickness in 15 patients or mucosectomy in 15 patients. The defect in the rectal wall was not routinely closed, only lesions in the upper or anterior rectum ($n = 56$, 28 percent) were closed with a running absorbable suture. In 24 patients intraoperative technical problems were encountered; breach of the peritoneal cavity ($n = 7$), bleeding ($n = 6$), difficulties with resection due to bulky lesion ($n = 5$), gas leak ($n = 3$), instrumentation failure ($n = 2$), and limited view due to poor prep ($n = 1$). In all seven patients in whom the peritoneum was opened, the resection could be carried out after closure of the defect with sutures.

The postoperative complication rate was 14 percent, and the 30-day postoperative mortality rate 0.5 percent. Hospital readmission was necessary for ten patients because of bleeding, but all settled conservatively and transfusion was necessary in only one patient. Pelvic sepsis occurred in four patients, which required a laparotomy for drainage in two patients, a defunctioning colostomy in one patient, and could be managed conservatively with antibiotics in the fourth patient. Stenosis at the resection site required dilatation in three patients, with satisfactory result in two patients. Other complications included urinary tract infection ($n = 4$), pulmonary infection ($n = 3$), urinary retention ($n = 2$), anal fissure ($n = 1$), and small bowel obstruction ($n = 1$).

Local recurrence rate after resection of rectal adenomas was 7.6 percent, with a median time to recurrence of 23 months (range 6.5–123). In two patients the local recurrence could not be controlled with a conventional transanal resection or colonoscopy and necessitated radical surgery. Radical surgery was avoided in 77 of 79 (97 percent) patients with a tumor too proximal for a conventional transanal approach.

Postoperative staging of carcinomas revealed pathological tumor (pT) stage 1 in 31 patients, pT2 in 17, and pT3 in four. Completion surgery was offered to patients when adverse histopathological features were present, including pT1 tumors with invasion into the deeper layers of submucosa (sm2 and sm3, 14 and 13 patients, respectively). Fifteen patients had salvage therapy, either radical surgery ($n = 7$) or adjuvant radiotherapy ($n = 8$), while the remaining 17 patients with adverse features declined further treatment or were deemed unfit on account of age or comorbidities. At a median follow-up of 34 (range 1–102) months, eight patients (15 percent) with carcinomas had developed local recurrence. The overall and disease-free five-year survival rates for patients with carcinomas were 76 and 65 percent, respectively.

REFERENCES

1. Buess G, Theiss R, Gunther M et al. Endoscopic operative procedure for the removal of rectal polyps. *Coloproctology* 1984; 1/84: 254–61.
2. De Graaf EJ, Burger JW, van Ijsseldijk AL et al. Transanal endoscopic microsurgery is superior to transanal excision of rectal adenomas. *Colorectal Disease* 2011 Jul; 13(7); 762–7.
3. Middleton PF, Sutherland LM, Maddern GJ. Transanal endoscopic microsurgery: a systematic review. *Diseases of the Colon and Rectum* 2005; 48: 270–84.
4. Bach SP, Hill J, Monson JR et al. A predictive model for local recurrence after transanal endoscopic microsurgery for rectal cancer. *British Journal of Surgery* 2009; 96: 280–90.
5. Bretagnol F, Merrie A, George B et al. Local excision of rectal tumours by transanal endoscopic microsurgery. *British Journal of Surgery* 2007; 94: 627–33.

Presacral resections – Kraske

RUUD SCHOUTEN

HISTORY

In 1874, Theodor Kocher (1841–1917) was the first to recommend excision of the coccyx to facilitate a posterior approach to the mid-rectum for excision of lesions located below the peritoneal reflection. According to Paul Kraske (1851–1930), removal of the coccyx alone did not provide sufficient exposure to the upper part of the mid-rectum. At the 14th meeting of the German Association of Surgeons in 1885, he reported that better exposure could be obtained by dividing the lower margin of the gluteus maximus muscle and the sacrospinous as well as the sacrotuberous ligaments. In addition, he also removed the lowermost part of the left wing of the sacrum. This posterior approach rapidly became a popular surgical option in the treatment of cancer, located in the middle and lower third of the rectum. Unfortunately, Kraske's operation was complicated by a 90 percent local recurrence rate and a 70 percent incidence of rectocutaneous fistula formation. Because of this high complication rate and the adequate local control of rectal cancer, the procedure never gained wide acceptance outside Europe. The abdominoperineal resection, introduced by Ernest Miles in 1908 and the low anterior resection, described by Claude Dixon in 1939 gradually gained popularity over Kraske's operation. However, over many decades, a modified posterior approach, without resection of the lowermost part of the left wing of the sacrum, has been used for the local excision of benign rectal neoplasm, such as villous adenoma. This modified Kraske's operation remained popular until the introduction of transanal endoscopic microsurgery in 1983. This challenging technique enables the excision of large lesions, even in the upper third of the rectum (see Chapter 6.14). Local excision of these lesions by a posterior approach is rarely now indicated. At present, there are two principal remaining indications for the modified Kraske's approach: the management of presacral tumors and the rectal sleeve procedure.

PRINCIPLES AND JUSTIFICATION

Presacral tumors

Tumors occurring in the space between mesorectum and sacrum are rare. Even large referral centers will see fewer than five or six patients in a year.

The presacral space is bounded anteriorly by the rectum, posteriorly by the sacrum, superiorly by the peritoneal reflection and inferiorly by the pelvic floor. This space is the area of embryologic fusion between hindgut and proctodeum, neural elements, and bone, and contains remnants from various embryologic tissues. Approximately two-thirds of presacral tumors are congenital, arising from these embryologic remnants. The congenital lesions include cystic and solid lesions. Purely cystic lesions can be classified as dermoid or epidermoid cysts, tailgut cysts, and rectal duplication cysts.

Dermoid cysts arise from the ectoderm and are lined with squamous epithelium combined with various cutaneous appendages. These cysts are unilocular and filled with dense muddy or fatty material. Epidermoid cysts also arise from the ectoderm and are lined with squamous epithelium alone. These cysts are unilocular and filled with clear fluid. Dermoid and epidermoid cysts may communicate with the skin, creating a postanal dimple, and have a high infection rate. Tailgut cysts, also called 'cystic hamartomas', are less common. They are caused by incomplete regression of the embryonic tailgut. Most tailgut cysts are multilocular. They are lined with columnar epithelium and other epithelia, surrounded by muscle layers without enteric nerves. Tailgut cysts are not in continuity with the rectum and are filled with mucoid material.

Rectal duplication cysts are very rare, representing only 5 percent of congenital cystic lesions. They are in continuation with the rectum and have a mucosal lining similar to rectal mucosa, surrounded by a smooth-muscle coat in two layers with enteric nerves. Although most cystic lesions are benign, malignant transformation has been reported.

Chordomas are the main solid congenital lesions. These tumors arise from the notochord and are malignant. Teratomas contain tissue from each germ-cell layer and usually present with mixed solid and cystic components. The germ-cell elements are capable of malignant degeneration.

Congenital presacral tumors, especially the cystic ones, are most common in females. The Currarino syndrome is an inherited autosomal dominant condition in which partial sacral agenesis is associated with a presacral teratoma or anterior meningocele and anorectal malformation. It is caused by a mutation in the *HLXB9* homeobox gene.

Approximately one of every three presacral tumors is acquired. The acquired tumors can be classified as inflammatory, neurogenic, osseous or miscellaneous lesions, both benign and malignant.

CLINICAL SIGNS

Most benign presacral lesions are asymptomatic and are often discovered incidentally on rectal or pelvic examination. In symptomatic patients, pain in the perineum or low back is the most common complaint. Larger benign lesions may be associated with constipation and voiding disturbances by compression of the rectum and the bladder. Malignant presacral tumors are more often symptomatic, with pain as the most common sign.

DIAGNOSIS

Digital examination

Almost all patients with a presacral tumor have a palpable mass on digital examination, which is a very effective means of identifying the tumor. Congenital cystic lesions are usually situated in the midline. They are soft, compressible, and non-tender. Chordomas and other malignant lesions are solid tumors, frequently fixed to the sacrum. Rectal examination can also reveal the proximal extension of the lesion, which is important in determining the surgical approach. Tumors with a proximal extent are palpable, do not extend above the level of the third sacral body, and are amenable to a modified Kraske's approach.

Imaging

Magnetic resonance (MR) imaging is emerging as the most sensitive and specific technique for the imaging and characterization of presacral lesions. MR imaging enables the delineation of soft-tissue planes and provides a useful tool for the evaluation of bony invasion and nerve involvement. It enables the differentiation between cystic and solid lesions. Cystic lesions are hypointense on T_1-weighted images and hyperintense on T_2-weighted images. High signal intensity in T_1-weighted images is secondary to mucoid content (tailgut cysts) or fatty content (dermoid cysts). Focal irregular wall thickening with intermediate signal intensity on both T_1- and T_2-weighted images and with enhancement after injection of contrast material is suggestive of malignant degeneration.

BIOPSY

There is no indication to biopsy a purely cystic presacral lesion. In patients with a solid or heterogeneously cystic tumor, a biopsy is mandatory if the lesion appears to be unresectable and a tissue diagnosis is required to guide adjuvant therapy. Biopsies should never be performed transrectally or transvaginally. In case of a cystic lesion, such an approach is likely to result in infection. Once infection occurs, the postoperative recurrence rate is about 30 percent, since complete excision of infected cysts is far more difficult. An inadvertent transrectal biopsy of a meningocele may result in meningitis. Since biopsy of malignant lesions may result in tumor spread, the needle track needs to be excised *en bloc* with the specimen. Therefore, a transperineal or parasacral approach is advocated if a biopsy is considered in case of a suspected lesion.

MANAGEMENT

Most presacral tumors are congenital. Although benign in the majority of patients, these lesions should be resected since they possess the potential for malignant transformation. In addition, the congenital cysts carry the risk of secondary infection. Once infected, these cysts become adherent to adjacent tissues, which increases the morbidity after later attempts at resection. Furthermore, infected cysts have been shown to be associated with a significantly higher recurrence rate.

Surgical resection is the only possible curative treatment for malignant lesions in the presacral space, which are known to be chemoradioresistant.

Based on these considerations, it is obvious that all presacral lesions, including the asymptomatic ones, should be treated surgically. The surgical approach depends on the nature of the lesion and on its location. High lesions, located in front of the sacrum between promontory and the third sacral segment require a transabdominal (anterior) approach. Low lesions, situated between the coccyx and the third sacral segment, can be resected using the modified Kraske's approach. For larger tumors or those in an intermediate position, a combined anterior and posterior approach may be necessary.

OPERATION

Position of the patient

For a modified Kraske's approach, the patient is placed in prone jackknife position with rolls under the shoulders and pelvis (**Figure 6.16.1**). The buttocks are retracted with tape prior to prepping.

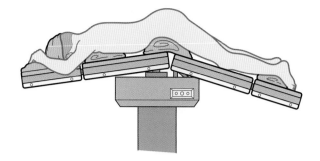

6.16.1

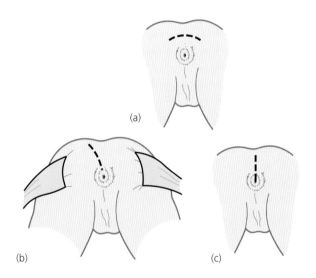

(a)

(b)   (c)

6.16.2

Incision and exploration

A curvilinear (**Figure 6.16.2a**), paracoccygeal, parasacral (**Figure 6.16.2b**), or a simple midline incision (**Figure 6.16.2c**) can be used to gain access to the presacral space. The parasacral incision (**Figure 6.16.2b**) is most often used because of the possibility of extending it upwards to incise the lower part of the gluteus major muscle to obtain wider exposure. The transverse incision, advocated by Localio, provided more direct access to the lower third of the rectum and upper anal canal. The midline incision proposed by Bevan is now seldom used.

The first layer encountered beneath the subcutaneous fat is the lumbosacral fascia. After division of this fascia, the dissection is taken down to the sacrum, the coccyx, and the anococcygeal ligament. A self-retaining retractor is utilized to facilitate exposure (**Figure 6.16.3**).

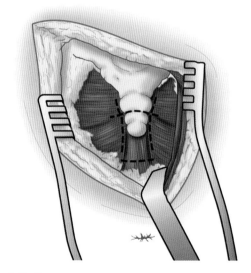

6.16.3

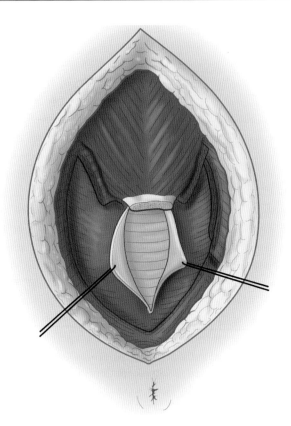

The anococcygeal ligament is divided and the coccyx is disarticulated from the fifth sacral body with electrocautery. Next, the exposed fascia of Waldeyer is divided in the midline from the end of the sacrum as far forward as the anorectal junction (**Figure 6.16.4**).

At this point, one should decide whether or not to transect the fifth and, if necessary, a portion of the fourth sacral body. This decision depends on the size of the tumor, its relationship to the sacrum, and the exposure required. If transection of these sacral segments is necessary, the gluteus maximus muscle can be detached from each side.

6.16.4

The rectum in its fascial capsule may now be separated from the hollow of the sacrum by division of some areolar tissue. If more access is required, the fascia of Waldeyer is freed from the anterior surface of the lower sacrum (**Figure 6.16.5**).

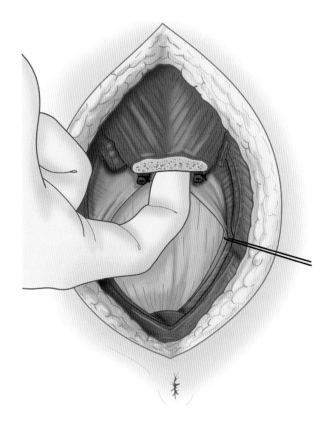

6.16.5

The fifth sacral segment is excised and, if necessary, the body of the fourth sacral vertebra medial to the fourth sacral foramina is nibbled with a rongeur forceps. Bone wax can be helpful in obtaining hemostasis. The levator ani muscle is incised in the midline and tagged with sutures. Care should be taken to avoid damage to the puborectalis muscle and the external anal sphincter (**Figure 6.16.6**).

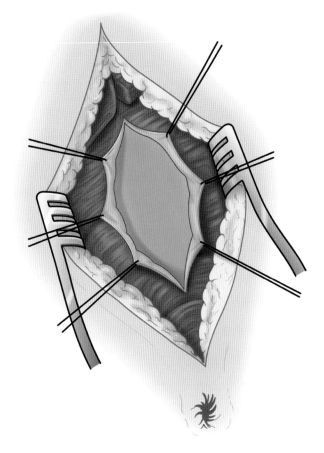

6.16.6

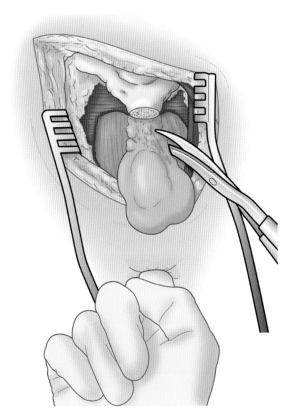

6.16.7

Next, the presacral tumor is mobilized by sharp and blunt dissection. The lesion should be dissected from the rectal wall in a plane between the retrorectal fat and the tumor mass itself. Frequently, the rectum is densely adherent to the tumor. Furthermore, it is often difficult to differentiate the fibers of the levator ani muscle from the rectal wall. With the index finger of the left hand in the lower part of the rectum, the lesion can be pushed outward to facilitate dissection without injury to the rectal wall (**Figure 6.16.7**).

The large potential space, remaining after excision of the tumor, should be drained with a suction tube.

The wound is closed in layers, including the levator ani muscle (**Figure 6.16.8**).

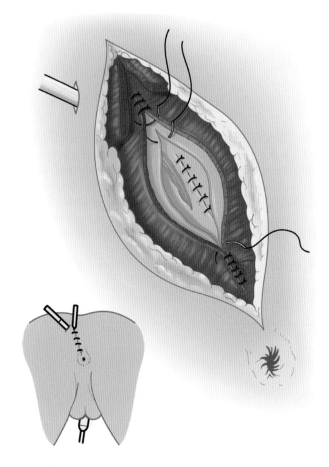

6.16.8

Rectal sleeve advancement

The modified Kraske's approach can also be used for rectal sleeve advancement in women with an obstetric rectovaginal fistula in whom the fistula persists despite previous local attempts at repair or in men with a rectourethral fistula usually following radiotherapy for prostate cancer.

After incision of the levator ani muscle, the rectum is circumferentially mobilized by freeing it from the posterior wall of the vagina. The rectum is encircled with soft rubber drains and mobilized into the wound (**Figure 6.16.9**).

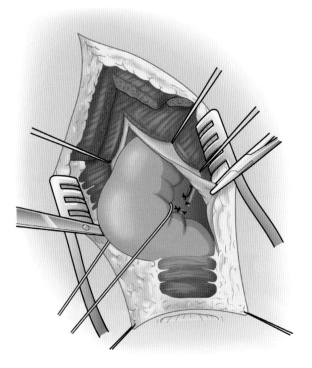

6.16.9

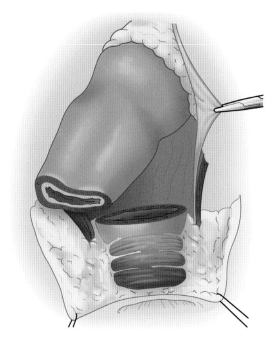

Next, the rectum is mobilized distally, until the pelvic floor is reached. At this point, the posterior wall of the rectum can be opened and the fistula tract excised and the defect repaired in two layers.

Alternatively, just above the pelvic floor, the rectum is transected (**Figure 6.16.10**).

6.16.10

Then, a Scott or Lone Star™ retractor is used, in order to gain access to the anal canal. A circumferential mucosectomy is performed from the dentate line up to the level of the pelvic floor (**Figure 6.16.11**).

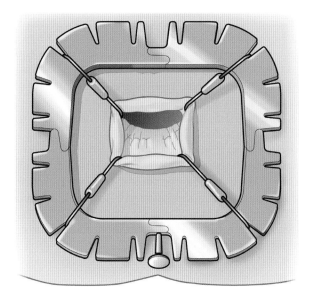

6.16.11

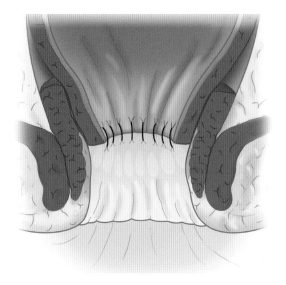

6.16.12

The opening of the rectovaginal or rectourethral fistula is enlarged by removing all fibrotic tissue, located at the edge of the opening. The enlarged opening is closed with interrupted sutures. The transected rectum is passed through the anal canal. Next, an end-to-end anastomosis is created to the dentate line with interrupted sutures (**Figure 6.16.12**).

The original anal opening of the fistula is now covered by a well-vascularized layer of full-thickness rectal wall. The fistulous opening at the vaginal side remains open.

SEGMENTAL RESECTION OF THE LOWER RECTUM

Because of technical advances with transanal resection techniques (see Chapter 6.14) and TEMS (see Chapter 6.15), it is now rarely necessary to perform a segmental resection of the lower rectum. However, the approach may be useful on occasions, particularly for circumferential villous adenoma of the lower third of rectum.

As the first step, circumferential isolation of the lower rectum is carried out as already described. Instead of incising the fascia and the rectal wall vertically, however, a horizontal incision is made at a level a little distal to the lower border of the tumor. The location of the tumor should be accurately assessed by digital examination through the intact anus.

Before completing the circular incision, at least four stay sutures should be placed through the whole thickness of the distal cut edge of the rectum, at the anterior, posterior, and both lateral sites.

At the estimated proximal incision line, the endopelvic fascia is incised, and fat tissues under it are peeled from the rectal wall. The muscle coat and mucosa are incised in the same way as the distal incision. More than four stay sutures will be required to indentify the proximal cut edge of the intestine (**Figure 6.16.13**).

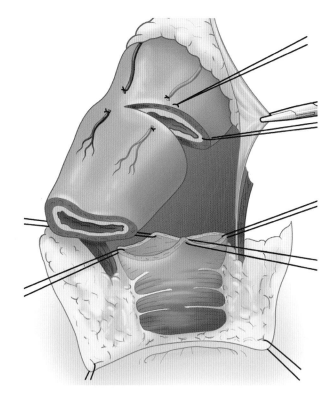

6.16.13

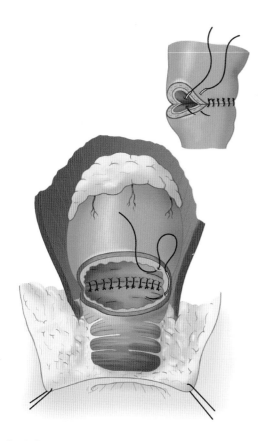

The intestinal wall is approximated at both lateral corners. By pulling up the sutures on one side, the anterior aspect of the cut edges of the intestinal wall come into direct vision and are sutured. After the muscle layer has been sutured anteriorly, the inner layers (mucosa and submucosa) are approximated from the inside. This process continues on the posterior aspect until the inner layer of sutures is completed using interrupted absorbable material. Finally, the outer layer of the posterior aspect is sutured (**Figure 6.16.14**).

6.16.14

Wound closure and drainage

After the rectal wall has been sutured or the anastomosis has been completed (being careful not to spill intestinal contents), the whole area is washed with warm normal saline. The wound is closed in layers, making certain that the layers are approximated very accurately, guided by the stay sutures previously placed. A thin, soft drainage tube is inserted through a separate stab wound near the incision line, down in the perirectal space or to the level of the levator ani muscle. The drainage tube will be removed within 4–5 days. In stout and obese patients, a thin Penrose drain is inserted into the ischiorectal space through the incision and removed once serosanguineous drainage ceases at about 48 hours.

OUTCOMES

The Kraske approach is generally well tolerated. Difficulties with wound healing are uncommon, however, if an infected presacral lesion is removed there is increased risk of wound breakdown. Patients should be warned that for some months following operation sitting on a hard surface may be uncomfortable. If a rectal anastomosis has been performed, rectocutaneous fistula is an uncommon but serious complication which may require diverting colostomy to assist in closure.

Surgery for Hirschsprung's disease

RJ RINTALA AND MP PAKARINEN

HISTORY

Hirschsprung's disease (HD) is characterized by an absence of ganglion cells in the nerve plexuses of the distal large bowel. The lack of ganglion cells produces a functional obstruction and leads to dilatation of the bowel that is proximal to the aganglionic zone. The commonly quoted incidence of HD is 1 in 5000. The classic description of HD was presented by Danish pediatrician, Harald Hirschsprung, in 1886. The absence of ganglion cells in the distal large bowel was first reported in the early 1900s but the crucial role of this finding as the primary pathology was not appreciated until the late 1940s. In 1948, the first successful operation for HD was performed by Orvar Swenson and Alexander Bill.

PRINCIPLES AND JUSTIFICATION

The functional obstruction caused by lack of enteric ganglion cells in the distal bowel results in delayed passage of meconium, severe constipation, and failure to thrive, and may be fatal because of enterocolitis. The exact embryological mechanism of the development of HD is controversial but the most favored theory is defective neuronal migration. Although defects in several genes (RET, GDNF, EDN3, ETRB) have been shown to cause HD, single gene defects explain only a minority of HD cases, and in the majority, the etiology is multifactorial and multigenic.

In its classic form, HD is restricted to the rectosigmoid segment of large bowel and this form comprises 75–80 percent of all patients. Long colon segment HD and total colonic aganglionosis (TCA) HD with a variable length of ileal involvement each occurs in 5–15 percent of patients. More extensive proximal aganglionosis is exceedingly rare.

The severity of the clinical picture of HD is variable and not necessarily related to the length of the aganglionic segment. Almost all patients have symptoms immediately after birth but symptoms may be initially alleviated and the patients present later in infancy. The variation in clinical presentation of HD is poorly understood.

There are four major types of procedures that are in common use for the repair of HD (**Figure 6.17.1**). Each procedure has unique features in terms of the need for intrapelvic dissection and preservation of anal canal length. Each of the techniques can be used as a primary operation or as part of a multistage procedure. Each is also suitable for a laparoscopic or laparoscopic-assisted approach.

Swenson's rectosigmoidectomy

Swenson's operation was the first consistently successful operative method for HD. The original concept of elimination of the functional obstruction by mobilizing ganglionic bowel to reach at or near the anus is the basis of all later surgical modifications. The sigmoid bowel and rectum are mobilized and resected transabdominally down to the anal canal. The anal canal is everted and an anastomosis between the pulled through ganglionic colon and anal canal is performed outside the anus. The level of anastomosis is 1–2 cm above the dentate line.

Duhamel's retrorectal pull-through

The Duhamel procedure, described by Bernard Duhamel in 1956, requires much less pelvic dissection than the Swenson procedure. The dissection is retrorectal and preserves the extrinsic innervation of the pelvic organs. Ganglionic bowel is brought down to the level of the anal canal behind the aganglionic rectum and anastomosed side-to-side to the rectum. The lower level of the anastomosis is about 1 cm above the dentate line.

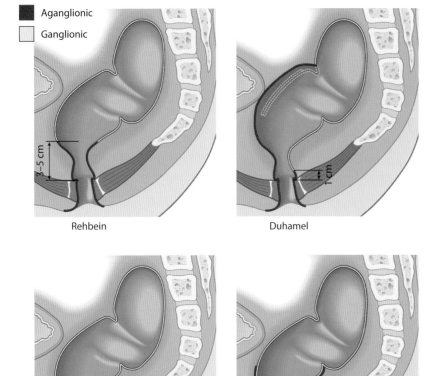

Aganglionic

Ganglionic

Rehbein

Duhamel

Swenson

Soave (ERPT)

6.17.1 Commonly performed operations for Hirschsprung's disease. The distances in the text show the level of the anastomosis in relation to the dentate line.

Soave's endorectal pull-through

The Soave endorectal pull-through operation was described in 1964. The principle of the Soave procedure is to protect pelvic innervation and organs by keeping the rectal dissection in the submucosal plane within the bowel wall. The submucosal dissection is extended down to the anal canal. Ganglionic bowel is pulled through the muscular sleeve of rectum and anastomosed to the mucosa of the anal canal about 1 cm above the dentate line. More recently, the Soave operation has been modified by performing the complete endorectal dissection transanally. Recent developments include laparoscopic-assisted transanal endorectal pull-through and totally transanal endorectal pull-through.

Rehbein's anterior resection

The Rehbein anterior resection for HD was first described by Fritz Rehbein in 1959. The operation comprises low anterior rectosigmoid resection and end-to-end anastomosis between rectum and proximal ganglionic

bowel 5–7 cm above the dentate line. There is no dissection in the lower pelvis which leaves the extrinsic innervation intact. The remaining aganglionic rectum is potentially obstructive, therefore, long-term anorectal dilatations are required in many patients who have undergone the procedure.

PREOPERATIVE ASSESSMENT AND PREPARATION

The diagnosis of HD is based on the absence of ganglion cells and increased acetylcholinesterase staining of hypertrophied nerve fibers in rectal biopsies. Rectal biopsies are usually obtained with a special suction device. Common pitfalls include an inadequate superficial biopsy sample without submucosa, especially in older children, too distal biopsy site in the very distal rectum just proximal to the dentate line with physiological aganglionosis, and weak acetylcholinesterase staining occasionally associated with long segment disease. In unclear cases, repeated rectal suction or open biopsy and/or anorectal manometry with an absent rectoanal inhibitory reflex will ultimately reveal the diagnosis. Patients should also undergo routine preoperative assessment for associated chromosomal, cardiac, and genitourinary anomalies.

The transitional zone between ganglionic and aganglionic bowel is visible in contrast enema in about 80 percent of patients. If there is any doubt of location of the transitional zone after contrast enema, frozen section mapping biopsies of the colon should be obtained either laparoscopically or by means of an umbilical minilaparotomy. Totally transanal mobilization of the colon is not possible when aganglionosis extends proximal to the rectosigmoid junction. A more proximal location of the transitional zone requires additional colonic mobilization which is performed first either laparoscopically or by means of an umbilical minilaparotomy, if a transanal approach to the rectosigmoid is to be used. If aganglionosis extends close to the cecum or to the distal small bowel, total proctocolectomy and ileoanal anastomosis is performed. The standard repairs for classic HD are all suitable to treat TCA; the most commonly used are the Duhamel operation and endorectal pull-through. The authors use endorectal pull-through with J-pouch ileoanal anastomosis.

The operation is usually performed in one stage without a diverting stoma some weeks after the birth as soon as the diagnosis is confirmed. Prior to the operation the functional obstruction is treated with daily rectal washouts with warm saline. Some pediatric surgeons prefer staged repair of HD and perform primarily a defunctioning leveling colostomy in which the most distal part of the colon with normal ganglion cells is brought out as a loop colostomy. This needs to be carefully sutured to the abdominal wall to minimize the risk of stoma prolapse.

Children with significant additional anomalies require an individually planned approach. In selected patients, the definitive repair may be safer as a staged operation with a covering loop-ileostomy. Rectal washouts with physiological saline are sufficient for bowel preparation in newborns. Older children and children with long-segment disease often require formal bowel preparation with polyethylene glycol or a similar laxative.

Anesthesia

Standard general anesthesia with endotracheal intubation is used. Antibiotic prophylaxis is recommended. The authors use intravenous kefuroxime and metronidazole.

OPERATIONS

In the following sections the two techniques that are most commonly used to treat HD are described, namely endorectal pull-through using a totally transanal approach and the Duhamel retrorectal pull-through.

Totally transanal endorectal pull-through

POSITION OF PATIENT

The patient is placed in a modified lithotomy position with thighs abducted and knees in flexion. An indwelling urinary catheter is placed and the operative field including the anal canal is prepared with an antiseptic solution. Sufficient anal retraction is achieved with a Lone Star™ retractor or with radial 5-0 monofilament stay sutures through the perianal skin to the anal canal at the dentate line. The stay sutures are brought through the edge of a stoma plate with a central round opening and the plate is fixed to the perineum around the anus (**Figure 6.17.2**). Use of a fiberoptic headlight and magnifying operative telescope facilitate the operation. The surgeon sits between the patient's legs and a first assistant stands on the right side of the patient.

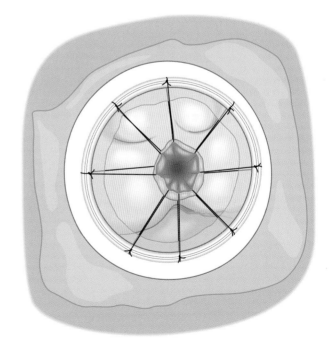

6.17.2

MUCOSECTOMY

The mucosectomy is started 5 mm proximal to the dentate line (**Figure 6.17.3**). Prior to the incision, adrenaline diluted with physiological saline (1:100 000) is injected into the submucosal layer of the anal canal. The needle should be parallel to the bowel wall just below the mucosa at the time of injection. Successful injection visibly separates the mucosa from underlying layers of the bowel wall facilitating the beginning of dissection. A circumferential mucosal

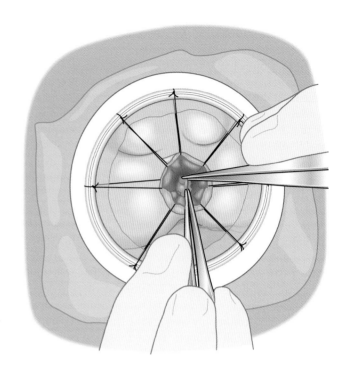

6.17.3

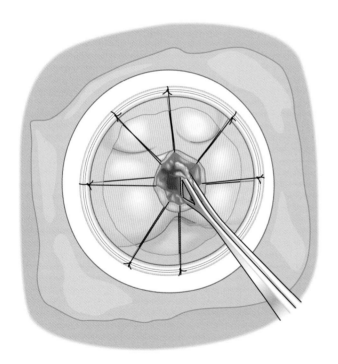

6.17.4

incision 5 mm proximal to the dentate line is made using a fine-tipped monopolar diathermy. Fine-tipped dissection scissors may be also used for mucosectomy. Next, the mucosa is separated from the underlying sphincter muscle by retracting the incised mucosal edge with fine dissecting forceps pushing the internal anal sphincter muscle layer laterally (**Figure 6.17.4**). Dissection proceeds systematically in a circumferential manner in order to avoid unnecessary handling of thin and friable mucosa.

After the mucosa is circumferentially mobilized for a distance of 3–5 mm, the developing mucosal tube is more easily controlled with triangular clamps or fine monofilament stay sutures (**Figure 6.17.5**). From this point onwards an assistant can facilitate exposure by proving gentle counter-traction at the site of dissection. At the site of previous rectal biopsy, the mucosa may be especially adherent due to submucosal scarring. It is very important to avoid forceful anal retraction and subsequent sphincter damage at any stage of the operation.

Mucosectomy is continued for about 3–4 cm. Sufficient length of mucosectomy is at the point where the muscle cuff starts to invaginate when downward traction is applied from the mobilized mucosal tube. This point represents the level of the rectum just above the levator muscles.

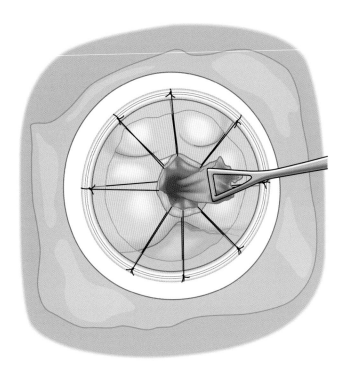

6.17.5

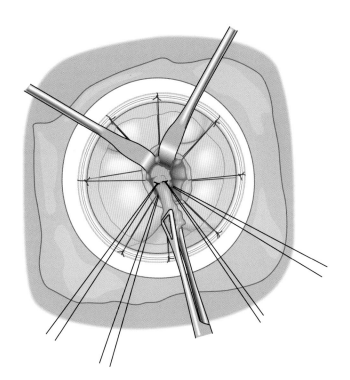

6.17.6

DIVISION OF THE MUSCLE CUFF

The next step of the operation involves exposure of the seromuscular surface of the rectum by division of the muscle cuff. This is facilitated by placing four 5-0 monofilament stay sutures at 11, 1, 5, and 7 o'clock through the muscle cuff and the most proximal part of the mobilized mucosal tube. The muscle cuff is divided just above each stay suture until the seromuscular surface of the rectum is identified. These four small incisions are then joined to complete the circumferential division of the muscle cuff. This can be safely performed with bipolar scissors or forceps (**Figure 6.17.6**). It is important to stay close to the bowel wall in order to avoid damage to prostate and urethra.

MOBILIZATION OF THE RECTOSIGMOID COLON

The rectosigmoid colon is mobilized by combining downward traction from the mucosal tube and sequential coagulation of blood vessels on the bowel wall using bipolar forceps (**Figure 6.17.7** and **6.17.8**).

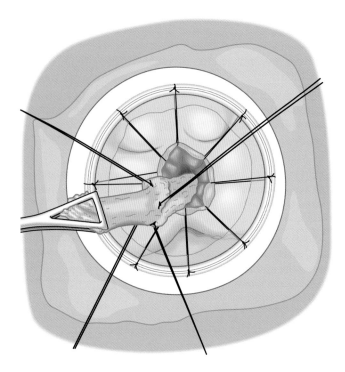

6.17.7

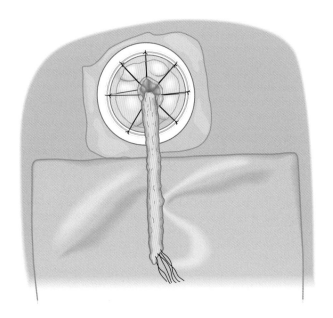

6.17.8

The surgeon can freely pull and manipulate the rectosigmoid colon with one hand and coagulate blood vessels with the other hand as they appear in the surgical field. An assistant helps by providing gentle counter-traction at the site of dissection. The blood vessels are often found in shallow clefts on the bowel wall which they cause when the bowel is pulled downwards. Rectosigmoid mobilization is continued until bowel with normal caliber and thickness is identified.

In infants, this involves mobilization of 20–25 cm of the rectosigmoid colon through the anus. In older children up to 55–60 cm of distal bowel can be mobilized transanally (**Figure 6.17.9**).

A seromuscular frozen section biopsy is then performed just distal to the level planned for coloanal anastomosis to confirm normal innervation with ganglion cells of the pulled-through colon.

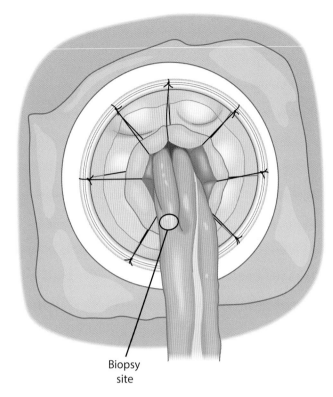

Biopsy site

6.17.9

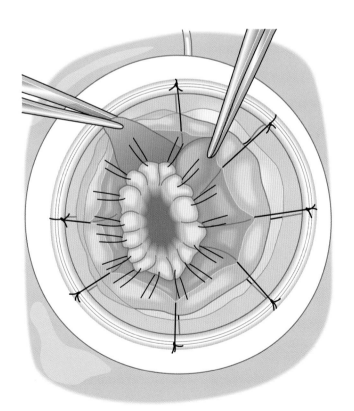

COLOANAL ANASTOMOSIS

It is important to ensure that the pulled-through colon is not rotated before it is divided. Once the colon is divided with monopolar diathermy, coloanal anastomosis is performed with between 10 and 12 5-0 colorless monofilament full-thickness stitches (**Figure 6.17.10**). The anal retractor is then removed and the anus is allowed to retract to its normal position.

6.17.10

POSTOPERATIVE CARE

Enteral feeds are started and the urinary catheter removed on the morning after transanal endorectal pull-through. Full enteral feeds are usually reached by the second postoperative day. Following the operation, bowel movements are usually frequent, especially in infants, often resulting in a perianal rash that requires local treatment with protective creams. The bowel frequency usually normalizes within three to six months of operation. Anal calibration is performed 2 weeks after the operation and dilatations are commenced if the anus does not accept a Hegar size 12 dilator. Edema of the muscle cuff occasionally causes temporary narrowing of the anal canal which may be treated with daily anal Hegar dilatations for 4–6 weeks.

Duhamel operation

POSITION OF THE PATIENT

As for the transanal endorectal pull-through, an infant patient is placed at the lower end of the operating table in a lithotomy position with thighs abducted and knees flexed. The lower limbs are placed on soft silicone cushions and taped to the operating table. Leg stirrups or cushioned supports can be used in older children. An indwelling urinary catheter is placed using aseptic technique after the skin preparation.

INCISION

A low transverse Pfannensteil or muscle cutting incision is most commonly used to enter the abdominal cavity. In infants and smaller children, the whole abdominal cavity can be explored through this approach. The surgeon stands on the right side of the patient and the assistant across on the left side. Self-retaining retractors are rarely needed.

EXPLORATION AND PEROPERATIVE FROZEN SECTION BIOPSIES

After entering the abdomen the colostomy (if present) is mobilized. If the colostomy is a leveling colostomy (colostomy made in the most distal section of the bowel with still normal ganglion cells) no frozen section biopsies are required. In a primary operation and in situations in which the colostomy is not at the level of distal extent of normally ganglionated bowel (non-leveling defunctioning colostomy), frozen section biopsies are obtained to determine the level of normally ganglionated bowel. A transition zone, a funnel-like narrowing of the dilated proximal bowel is usually well visible, especially in older children. The biopsies (one or two) are taken above the transitional zone. In patients with long segment disease or TCA the visual assessment of the transitional zone is not reliable. In these cases, multiple biopsies are often required. The biopsies can be full-thickness biopsies or, more practically, seromuscular biopsies that are obtained without opening the mucosa.

MOBILIZATION, RETRORECTAL PULL-THROUGH AND ANASTOMOSIS

After confirmation of the presence of ganglion cells, the proximal ganglionic bowel, usually the sigmoid colon, is mobilized to reach the perineum without tension. Usually, mobilization of the whole left colon and splenic flexure is required to gain sufficient length for the pull-through. The aganglionic rectum is mobilized below the peritoneal reflection and the rectum is stapled across and divided at this level. Stay sutures placed on both ends of the staple line facilitate further orientation. A space directly behind the rectum is developed by blunt finger dissection down to the level of the levator muscle (**Figure 6.17.11**).

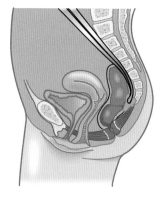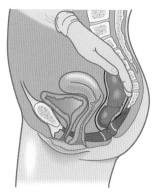

6.17.11

The abdominal phase of the operation can be performed laparoscopically. The blunt retrorectal dissection towards the anal canal is easily performed by a laparoscopic dissecting forceps or Babcock-grasping forceps.

The operation is continued from the perineum. The anal canal and rectum are cleaned with antiseptic solution. The anus is retracted by narrow retractors or preferably by Lone Star™ retractor. The posterior 180° of the rectal wall is exposed and a transverse full-thickness incision through the posterior half of the anal canal is made by monopolar diathermy 1–1.5 cm above the dentate line. The incision connects the anal canal with the previously developed retrorectal space. Stay sutures are inserted to both ends of the transverse incision and the passage connecting the retrorectal tunnel and anal canal is bluntly widened to allow bowel pull through (**Figure 6.17.12**).

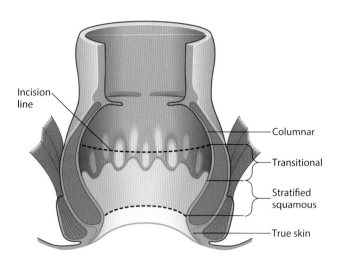

6.17.12

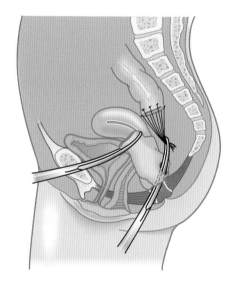

6.17.13

The mobilized proximal ganglionic bowel is pulled through the retrorectal space and through the opening in the posterior wall of the anal canal. It is important to ensure that the bowel is not twisted during pull-through. The pulled-through colon is opened and anastomosed with the opening in the posterior wall of the anal canal using absorbable sutures (**Figure 6.17.13**).

A GIA stapler (or endo-GIA stapler in small infants) is used to create a side-to-side anastomosis between posterior rectal wall and anterior wall of the pulled-through colon. Before firing the device, the correct orientation has to be ensured visually and by palpation from the abdominal side. A colotomy is made in the pulled-through colon at the level of the proximal staple line in the native rectum (**Figure 6.17.14**).

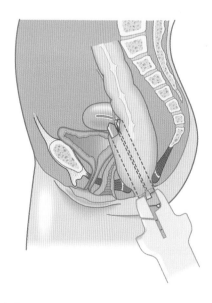

6.17.14

An opening is also made in the rectal staple line and a GIA stapler is inserted distally into each lumen. The position of the device in relation to the previous suture line is checked by finger palpation and the device is fired (**Figure 6.17.15**). Complete elimination of the common wall is confirmed by digital examination.

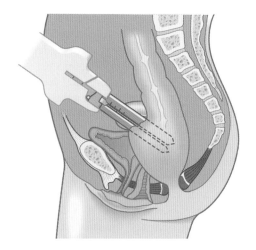

6.17.15

The colotomy and the opening in the rectal staple line are closed by interrupted absorbable sutures (**Figure 6.17.16**).

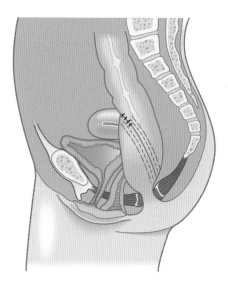

6.17.16

WOUND CLOSURE

After confirming hemostasis, the wound is closed in two layers. The fascial layers are closed with running absorbable sutures and the skin with running subcuticular sutures. No drains are required. Postoperative pain control is facilitated by epidural analgesia or infusion of long acting local anaesthetics to the fascial level of the wound using an automatic pump system (Pain Buster®).

POSTOPERATIVE CARE

There is usually no need to use nasogastric tubes postoperatively. Enteral feeding with liquids can be started when the patient has regained normal bowel sounds, usually on postoperative day 2 or 3. The patient can advance to normal food intake usually in 2-4 days. The urinary catheter can be taken out when the epidural anesthesia is discontinued, usually on day 3. The recovery from surgery is slower than after totally transanal procedure because

of the laparotomy or laparoscopy that is required to mobilize and prepare the proximal bowel. Severe diarrhea or perineal rash are uncommon after Duhamel operation. No anastomotic calibrations or dilatations are required. Some patients may have constipation postoperatively and may require early laxative treatment.

OUTCOME

Postoperative enterocolitis occurs in 10–25 percent of patients. This is usually mild and can be controlled by oral antibiotics. Enterocolitis is most common during the first two postoperative years.

A significant percentage of patients suffer from functional problems especially during the first postoperative year. Some degree of fecal soiling is common, on the other hand, frank incontinence is very uncommon. Constipation also occurs in some patients; constipation is most commonly caused by achalasia of the internal sphincter. The outlet obstruction caused by sphincter achalasia may also cause recurrent bouts of enterocolitis.

The overall functional outcome is very similar following all surgical techniques that are in common use. The experience of the operating surgeon is more important than the choice of surgical technique in terms of obtaining favorable functional results. The functional problems of early childhood tend to improve with growing age. At adolescence, the vast majority of patients have no soiling or constipation. As adults, most patients can lead a normal life with no social or occupational restrictions. The patients with the worst late functional outcome are those who have syndromic HD with mental retardation and those who have had significant anastomotic complications.

FURTHER READING

De La Torre L, Langer JC. Transanal endorectal pull-through for Hirschsrung's disease: technique, controversies, pearls, pitfalls and an organised approach to the management of postoperative obstructive symptoms. *Seminars in Pediatric Surgery* 2010; **19**: 96–106.

Georgeson KE, Robertson DJ. Laparoscopic-assisted approaches for the definitive surgery for Hirschsprung's disease. *Seminars in Pediatric Surgery* 2004; **13**: 256–62.

Hirschsprung H. Stuhltragheit Neugeborener in Folge von Dilatation und Hypertrophie des Colons. *Jahrbuch für Kinderheilkunde* 1887; **27**: 1–3.

Martin LW, Caudill DR. A method for elimination of the blind rectal pouch in the Duhamel operation for Hirschsprung's disease. *Surgery* 1967; **62**: 951–3.

The APPEAR procedure

NORMAN S WILLIAMS AND KHALID A EL-GENDY

HISTORY

The advent of circular stapling instruments and advanced surgical techniques has resulted in sphincter-saving rectal resections becoming common practice in the surgical management of both benign and malignant rectal pathology. Using abdominal approaches to rectal resection further improvements in the rates of anal sphincter preservation for distal rectal pathology are limited by anatomical considerations. A number of additional surgical techniques have been developed to be used in combination with an abdominal approach to effectively excise rectal pathology while preserving the anal sphincter complex. Historically, these include abdominoanal pull-through, parasacral and abdominotranssphincteric techniques. More recently, intersphincteric resection has been introduced. However, such techniques are often associated with significant morbidity and poor, even unacceptable functional outcome following inadvertent or intentional injury to the anal sphincter complex.

The Anterior Perineal PlanE for ultra-low Anterior Resection of the rectum (the APPEAR technique) is an extrasphincteric, anterior perineal approach used in combination with conventional open or laparoscopic abdominal procedures to restore gastrointestinal continuity.[1] The technique may be used once a trial dissection with the standard abdominal approach reveals that formation of a permanent stoma is necessary to safely and adequately remove the rectal pathology. The APPEAR approach permits the operator to determine whether sphincter preservation is feasible, and if not, then appropriately convert to an abdominoperineal excision of the rectum or panproctocolectomy.

PRINCIPLES AND JUSTIFICATION

The APPEAR technique negates challenging pelvic anatomy by permitting access to and visualization of the distal few centimeters of rectum within the pelvic floor, termed the 'rectal no-man's land' – defined above by the junction of the levator ani and rectum to below by the superior border of the external anal sphincter.[1] This allows accurate rectal transection at the desired level and construction of an anastomosis under direct vision while preserving the anal sphincter complex and its nerve supply in their entirety. This is of particular benefit when combined with a laparoscopic low anterior resection where distal rectal transection is often inaccurate and problematic with currently available stapling devices. Furthermore, this approach permits retrieval of the pathological specimen through the perineal wound avoiding the requirement for an abdominal wound when combined with a laparoscopic approach.

Operative indications include: **proven carcinoma of the lower third of rectum** where anatomical restrictions prevent satisfactory rectal dissection and/or transection with a potential inadequate distal clearance margin; ileal pouch anal anastomosis for **ulcerative colitis** or familial adenomatous polyposis (FAP) where retained rectal tissue is at risk of future malignancy or continuation in symptoms; difficult or previously failed restoration of gastrointestinal continuity in patients with a **short or strictured rectal stump including reversal of a Hartmann's procedure**. This chapter outlines the principles of this technique, highlighting various alterations in the technique dependent on the indications of the operation and potential difficulties encountered.

PREOPERATIVE

Patient status

The patient's fitness for treatment, irrespective of operative indication, must be assessed for safety to undergo a full laparotomy and optimized accordingly. Complete preoperative evaluation of the patient's pathology should be undertaken in each case. Furthermore, suitability to undergo a restorative procedure in each individual should be assessed prior to undertaking an ultra-low anastomosis accounting for preoperative bowel function, general health and mobility.

Patients not suitable to undergo the APPEAR procedure include those in whom anal sphincter preservation has already been deemed inappropriate for medical or surgical (particularly oncological) reasons by multidisciplinary team, or in whom surgery has been deemed inappropriate. These include patients with cancers that invade the anal sphincter mechanism, or those with T3 or T4 tumors identified by staging magnetic resonance imaging and which have not responded to preoperative chemoradiation.

Counseling

The APPEAR procedure aims to reduce the incidence of permanent stoma formation, however, all patients must be counselled by an appropriately trained surgical team member or colorectal nurse specialist regarding the possibility of permanent stoma formation in the event that the operation fails to restore gastrointestinal continuity.

Patients should be warned of the potential of poor postoperative bowel function, termed anterior resection syndrome, which includes increased frequency of defecation, urgency, and fecal incontinence.[2] Those counseling should reassure patients that postoperative bowel dysfunction gradually improves over 12–24 months. Should bowel function continue to be suboptimal after this time with conservative measures, options including neuromodulation or electrically stimulated gracilis neo-sphincter may be discussed (Chapters 9.2 and 9.3). As with all pelvic surgery, the sequelae of pelvic nerve damage including urinary and sexual dysfunction must be stressed, with reassurances that such adverse events can be improved by specialist consultation. A particular complication of the procedure may be a perineal fistula, and patients should be warned that this may require remedial surgery. The best way of preventing this complication is a prophylactic EUA before temporary ileostomy closure plus or minus revision of the colo/ileo anal anastomosis; patients should be counselled accordingly.

Anorectal physiology

Assessment of preoperative continence status and anorectal physiology (station pull-through anal manometry, pudendal nerve terminal motor latencies, and endoanal ultrasound) is advisable in all patients to determine the strength and function of the anal sphincter muscles. Furthermore, anorectal physiology should be repeated prior to the reversal of a defunctioning ileostomy as the APPEAR technique can theoretically result in sphincter damage. Those identified with poor function or weak anal sphincters that are at high risk of fecal incontinence or significant bowel dysfunction after surgery will be encouraged to undergo both a pre- and postoperative nurse-led program to strengthen the anal sphincter muscles.

Stoma planning

All patients undergoing the APPEAR procedure are recommended to have a temporary divided loop ileostomy constructed to mitigate the effects of a clinically detectable anastomotic leak including sepsis, poor functional outcome, and increased risk of local recurrence.[3] Stoma site marking should, if possible, always be carried out prior to the operation, preferably by a colorectal specialist nurse. As previously discussed, all patients must be warned of the risk of permanent stoma formation.

Bowel preparation

An empty colon and rectum is preferable for the APPEAR procedure, and is usually achieved with clear fluids in combination with purgatives and/or enemas 24–48 hours prior to surgery. On-table lavage can be undertaken if required in those found to have unsatisfactory bowel preparation during surgery.

Anesthesia

The operation is performed under full general anesthetic and muscle relaxant with those undergoing an open abdominal approach potentially benefiting from the insertion and infusion of anesthesia and analgesia via an epidural catheter. On induction, patients receive prophylactic antibiotics, a urethral catheter is inserted and the skin prepared and draped to allow simultaneous access to both the perineum and abdomen.

OPERATION

Position of patient

Patients are placed in the lithotomy-Trendelenburg position with pneumatic compression stockings to reduce the risk of thromboembolism. Good lighting is essential for this operation, and it is the authors' preference to use a headlight during the perineal phase to accurately identify and preserve relevant pelvic anatomical landmarks.

Abdominal phase (open/laparoscopic)

For rectal cancer and restoration of gastrointestinal continuity in those with a short or strictured rectal stump, the left colon and splenic flexure are fully mobilized to the mid-transverse colon and the inferior mesenteric vessels divided and ligated (described in Chapters 5.6 and 5.7). Rectal mobilization and total mesorectal excision is performed as low as possible in the pelvis, (described in Chapters 6.1 and 6.2).

For patients with ulcerative colitis or FAP a two- or three-stage restorative proctocolectomy is performed, with a stapled J ileal pouch fashioned after adequate small bowel mobilization as described in Chapters 6.6, 6.8, and 6.9. The APPEAR procedure is performed during the stage when the ileal pouch anal anastomosis is constructed.

Perineal phase

INCISION

Prior to incision, the rectovaginal/prostatic plane is infiltrated with a 1 in 300 000 adrenaline–saline solution. A convex cresenteric skin incision is then made in the perineum midway between the vagina or base of the scrotum and the anal verge (**Figure 6.18.1**). The skin and subcutaneous tissues are dissected from the underlying external anal sphincter and transverse perinei muscles, thus creating an extrasphincteric plane (**Figure 6.18.2**).

In the female, the plane between the posterior vaginal wall and anterior rectal wall is developed anterior to the perineal body using diathermy and sharp dissection. Infiltration with adrenaline–saline solution aids in development of this plane and prevention of sphincter injury or buttonholing of the rectum or vagina. The dissection is continued in a cephalad manner until contact is made with the abdominal operator.

In the male, this approach resembles that of a perineal prostatectomy entering the rectourethral/prostatic plane dividing the rectourethralis muscle close to the rectum. Hydrodissection with adrenaline–saline solution aids in the identification and preservation of the membranous urethra. The anterior rectal wall is then mobilized, using a combination of blunt and diathermy dissection, from the prostate in close proximity to the rectum to avoid damage to the neurovascular bundles located at the inferolateral aspect of the prostate. The perineal operator continues dissection in a cephalad direction until the abdominal operator is reached.

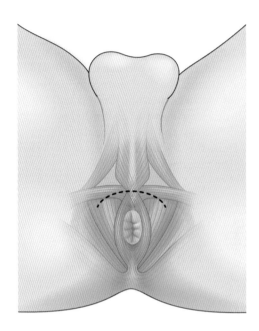

6.18.1

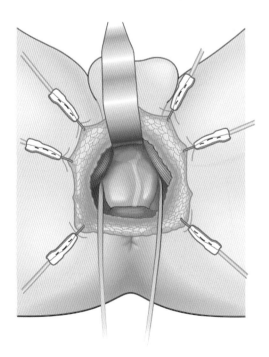

6.18.2

RECTAL EXCISION

The posterior and lateral rectal walls are mobilized by diathermy division of the attachments to the puborectalis muscle. The abdominal operator transects the rectosigmoid junction using a transverse stapling device and passes the transected stapled end of the upper rectum through the perineal wound, effectively everting it. Downward traction allows for visualization and diathermy division of the residual posterolateral attachments to completely free the rectum, if necessary down to and including the junction of the puborectalis and external anal sphincter (**Figure 6.18.3**). Thus, the anorectal stump can be exteriorized through the perineal wound.

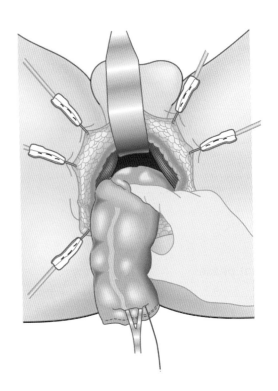

6.18.3

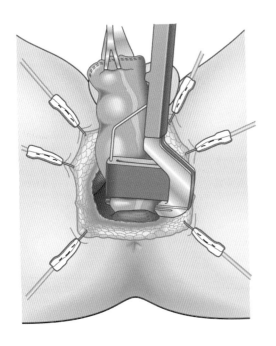

6.18.4

With an abdominal operator exerting upward traction, the rectum is transected at the desired level using a linear transverse stapler placed across the rectum. Once the stapling instrument is fired, the rectum can be removed after transection between the stapler and a proximally placed crushing bowel clamp (**Figure 6.18.4**). Alternatively, if deemed appropriate a Contour® circular stapling instrument can be used. Due to the nature of the pathology in some patients it may not be possible to apply a transverse stapler, and thus the upper anal canal is transected with a knife below a straight crushing bowel clamp.

CONSTRUCTION OF ANASTOMOSIS

In patients with cancer and those with a benign short or strictured rectal stump, the previously mobilized left colon is delivered through the perineal wound (**Figure 6.18.5**). Whenever possible a short colonic J pouch (5–6 cm limbs) is fashioned but otherwise a straight coloanal anastomosis is constructed, preferably in an end-to-side fashion. For patients with ulcerative colitis or FAP, an ileal J pouch is constructed primarily and then delivered through the perineal wound. An ileal pouch anal or colopouch anal anastomosis can then be constructed either manually or using a circular stapling instrument.

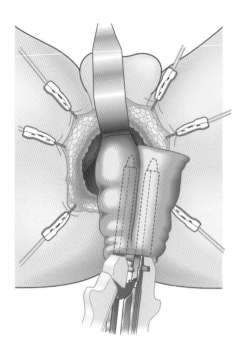

6.18.5

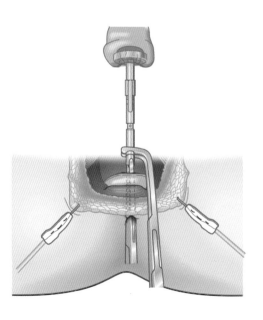

A stapled anastomosis is to be preferred as there is evidence to indicate a more favorable functional outcome compared to hand-sewn anastomosis.[4] The authors' favored stapling technique, known as the endoanal docking technique, negates the difficulty in docking the anvil and stapling device trocar within the narrow perineal wound. A Lone Star retractor™ is used to provide optimal views and access to both the perineal wound and anal canal during this technique (**Figure 6.18.6**). A straight Spencer Wells artery forceps is placed into the anal canal and advanced through an enterotomy made adjacent to the staple line in the distal anorectal stump using diathermy. The Spencer Wells artery forceps and a Chex anvil grasping forceps can then be used to grasp and draw the specially extended shaft of the anvil of a Compact™ circular stapling instrument, previously secured within the colopouch/ileal pouch with a purse string suture, down and through the enterotomy into the anal canal.

6.18.6

Once the shaft of the anvil has been sufficiently drawn through the anal canal, the trocar of the appropriate sized circular stapling device is fully extended and docked extracorporeally with the anvil while ensuring the bowel is not rotated (**Figure 6.18.7**).

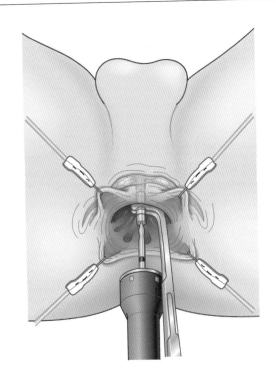

6.18.7

The trocar must be in the fully seated position with the anvil (confirmed both visually and audibly – as described by the manufacturer of the stapling device) prior to closing the instrument (**Figure 6.18.8a**). The position of the anvil and anorectal stump should be continuously checked during device closure by reapplication of the Lone Star™ retractor to fully view the anal canal or the perineal wound as required (**Figure 6.18.8b**).

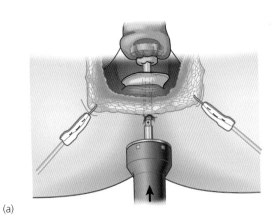

(a)

6.18.8

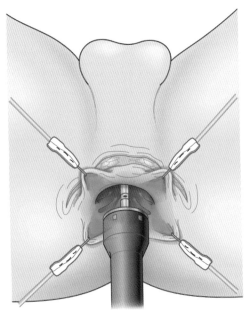

(b)

The stapling instrument is slowly closed, ensuring no extraneous tissue is involved, drawing the gun into the anal canal. The gun should only be fired after obtaining visual confirmation of adequate tissue compression, while directly visualizing the anastomosis in the perineal wound using a Lone Star™ retractor (**Figure 6.18.9**).

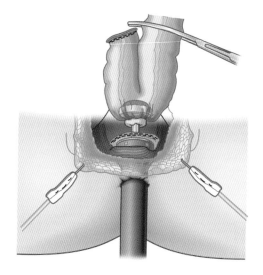

6.18.9

Alternatively, a standard double/triple stapling technique can be employed (described in Chapter 1.9), whereby the circular stapling device is placed within the anal canal and the trocar extended to perforate the anorectal stump, adjacent to the staple line, and docked with the anvil within the perineal wound. The authors have found this a difficult maneuver to perform in such a restricted space and would recommend the endoanal docking technique.

In those situations in which a transverse stapler cannot be applied across the anorectal stump, the proximal colon may be drawn through the anorectal stump and a transanal ileo/coloanal anastomosis is manually constructed with the aid of a Lone Star™ retractor (**Figure 6.18.10**).

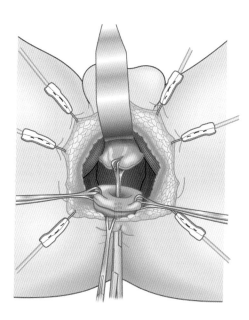

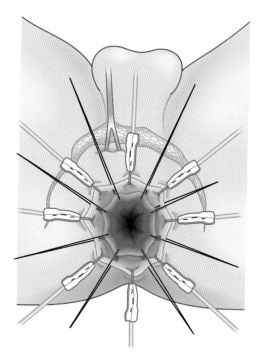

6.18.10

A covering ileostomy should be constructed in all cases by the abdominal operator once the anastomosis is successfully constructed. The authors' preference is to exteriorize a small bowel loop that is transected and a spout created from the proximal limb. The transected distal end is left in a subcutaneous position (**Figure 6.18.11**). This prevents overflow and reduces the risk of pelvic sepsis while allowing for a relatively easy closure in due course (described in Chapter 3.2).

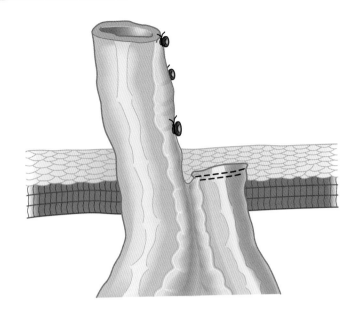

6.18.11

Wound closure

After hemostasis has been achieved, a levatorplasty is performed to reinforce the anastomosis and prevent perineal herniation. At least two negative pressure drains are placed within the wound, and both the subcutaneous tissues and the skin approximated with absorbable sutures (**Figure 6.18.12**).

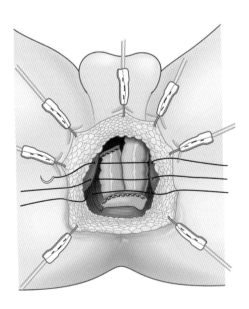
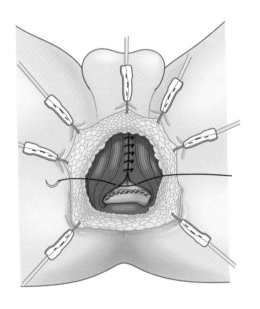

6.18.12

POSTOPERATIVE MANAGEMENT

Postoperative management is according to the patient's pathology (see Chapters 5.12, 6.1, 6.2, 6.6, 6.7, 6.8, and 6.9).

Reversal of ileostomy

Assessment of anastomotic integrity is performed at three to six months with a water-soluble enema and an examination under anesthesia with or without revision of anastomosis prior to consideration of reversal. Once these examinations have demonstrated an intact anastomosis and acceptable sphincter function has been noted on anorectal physiology, the patient can be counseled for reversal of ileostomy.

Complications

Potential complications include those described for the abdominal phase of the procedure, with bowel frequency and severity dependent on the primary pathology (Chapters 5.12, 6.1, 6.2, 6.6, and 6.7). Complications of the APPEAR procedure that are either specific to or occur with higher frequency compared to the conventional techniques are perineal herniation, anastomotic stricturing, and anastomotic-perineal fistulation.

ANASTOMOTIC STRICTURE

Symptomatic patients may be offered examination under anesthetic and stricture dilatation. If recurrent, patients can be taught the practice of self-dilatation using Hegar dilators and monitored appropriately.

ANASTOMOTIC LEAKAGE

The risk of anastomotic dehiscence and subsequent leakage increases the closer an anastomosis is constructed to the anal verge.[5] The APPEAR technique is an ultra-low anterior resection, and is therefore likely to have an increased incidence of pelvic sepsis and fistula formation compared to higher anterior resections.

The incidence of pelvic sepsis with abscess formation can be reduced with the introduction of negative pressure drains within the perineal wound during wound closure and is further reduced as surgeons progress the learning curve. Pelvic sepsis with abscess formation can be treated by computed tomography-guided drainage of a collection and infusion of empirical antibiotics in a similar fashion to those that occur after the abdominal phase of the operation only (see Chapter 6.1).

Fistula formation secondary to the APPEAR technique presents as perineal-anastomotic fistulae invariably emanating from the anterior aspect of the anastomosis. In the authors' experience, these are best prevented by routinely performing an examination under anesthetic two to three months postoperatively prior to ileostomy closure. The anastomosis is examined carefully and any defect or established fistula is repaired by revising the anastomosis transanally with the use of a Lone Star™ retractor. Revision is best done by mobilizing the anterior aspect of the anastomosis and advancing the mobilized colon or ileum forwards to cover the defect; this is akin to an advancement flap technique although lateral incisions are not made. Should the defect be significant, this may warrant laparotomy, redoing APPEAR, excision and refashioning of anastomosis after mobilization of the colonic or ileal pouch. Reversal of ileostomy should not, under any circumstance, be considered until all sepsis has settled with no evidence of an anastomotic dehiscence or fistula.

PERINEAL HERNIATION

Perineal herniation is rare following the APPEAR technique provided a levatorplasty is performed routinely, but may manifest as perineal bulging during defecation or symptoms of obstructed defecation and incomplete evacuation. This is best investigated with evacuation proctography that will demonstrate the perineal hernia and usually demonstrate retention of contrast. Should a hernia develop this is best treated with a levatorplasty reinforced with a biological mesh.

REFERENCES

1. Williams NS, Murphy J, Knowles CH. Anterior perineal plane for ultra-low anterior resection of the rectum (the APPEAR technique): a prospective clinical trial of a new procedure. *Annals of Surgery* 2008; **247**: 750–8.
2. McDonald PJ, Heald RJ. A survey of postoperative function after rectal anastomosis with circular stapling devices. *British Journal of Surgery* 1983; **70**: 727–9.
3. Laurent C, Nobili S, Rullier A *et al.* Efforts to improve local control in rectal cancer compromise survival by the potential morbidity of optimal mesorectal excision. *Journal of the American College of Surgeons* 2006; **203**: 684–91.
4. Kirat HT, Remzi FH, Kiran RP, Fazio VW. Comparison of outcomes after hand-sewn versus stapled ileal pouch-anal anastomosis in 3,109 patients. *Surgery* 2009; **146**: 723–9; discussion 729–30.
5. Rullier E, Laurent C, Garrelon JL *et al.* Risk factors for anastomotic leakage after resection of rectal cancer. *British Journal of Surgery* 1998; **85**: 355–8.

Vertical reduction rectoplasty for idiopathic megarectum

MARC A GLADMAN AND NORMAN S WILLIAMS

HISTORY

A subgroup of patients with functional constipation has persistent dilatation of the rectum, which in the absence of an organic cause, is termed 'idiopathic megarectum' (IMR).[1] Despite the etiology being unknown, certain pathophysiological features have been documented. As well as chronic dilatation, rectal compliance is increased (resulting in 'excessive laxity'), perception of rectal distension and evacuatory function are impaired, and colonic transit is often delayed.[2]

Several surgical procedures including rectal resection, restorative proctocolectomy, pelvic floor procedures, and fecal diversion have been attempted in such patients with variable results and often unacceptably high morbidity and mortality.[3] To specifically address the rectal pathophysiology, the operation of vertical reduction rectoplasty (VRR) was devised based on the premise that reducing rectal capacity and compliance would restore the perception of rectal fullness and improve rectal sensory and evacuatory function, and improve colonic transit.[4]

PRINCIPLES AND JUSTIFICATION

Indications

Operating on a grossly dilated rectum is technically challenging and potentially hazardous, since mobilization is difficult due to gross distortion of the normal anatomy within the confines of the bony pelvis, and due to the presence of the hugely dilated rectal blood vessels that are invariably encountered in this condition. Accordingly, surgery carries a significant risk of pelvic hemorrhage and sepsis (resulting in a mortality rate of 5 percent) in patients with IMR.[3] In the longer term, there is a risk of pelvic nerve injury and bowel obstruction.[3] VRR is a less radical procedure and has been shown to be safe and effective when performed in carefully selected patients.[5] However, patients should be warned about the potential risks of pelvic surgery. Accordingly, surgery is reserved for patients with confirmed idiopathic megarectum with sufficiently severe symptoms who wish to avoid a stoma. Specifically, each of the following criteria should be fulfilled:

1 Severe constipation (± fecal incontinence) with impaired quality of life.
2 Persistent dilatation limited to the rectum without organic cause (see below under Preoperative assessment and preparation).
3 Failure of non-surgical interventions (conservative, behavioral/biofeedback and medical treatments).
4 Satisfies detailed physiological assessment.
5 Satisfies detailed psychological assessment.

Due to the relative infrequency with which surgery is performed, patients should also understand that the outcome is unpredictable and carries a risk of permanent stoma formation.

Contraindications

Contraindications are as follows:

1 Rectal dilatation secondary to Hirschsprung's disease, anorectal obstruction, or disorders of the endocrine or central nervous system.
2 Coexisting (gross) dilatation of all the colon, i.e. extensive megacolon. In this setting, alternative options such as restorative proctocolectomy are more appropriate.
3 Inadequate assessment of rectal diameter and physiology prior to surgery (see below under Preoperative assessment and preparation).

PREOPERATIVE ASSESSMENT AND PREPARATION

Counseling

This is a crucial part of the preparation for surgery, during which the details of the procedure, the risks, and the outcomes are explained. In particular, it should be stressed that no form of surgical intervention offers certainty of cure. Counseling is best performed by a multidisciplinary team of professionals and thus surgery is most ideally performed in a specialist unit. It must be emphasized that embarking on surgical intervention requires detailed clinical, psychological, and physiological assessment prior to surgery and that the procedure involves two stages and the creation and subsequent closure of a diverting stoma. Ideally, prospective patients should be given the opportunity to meet other patients who have undergone the procedure. The patient must be allowed sufficient time to make a fully informed and considered decision and this may involve returning for further discussion.

Confirmation of diagnosis: clinical and physiological assessment

It is assumed that organic disease of the colon, rectum, and anus has been excluded by appropriate investigation. As patient selection is crucial for a successful outcome, the importance of a thorough and comprehensive clinical and physiological assessment cannot be overstressed. It is useful to obtain objective information about patient symptoms and their severity using validated constipation (± fecal incontinence) scoring systems (e.g. the Cleveland Clinic Constipation score). A detailed history also provides the opportunity for the clinician to exclude other causes of megarectum (e.g. psychiatric/endocrine diseases) and to ensure that all non-surgical interventions have been exhausted.

Many patients may be referred with a presumptive diagnosis of a megarectum, e.g. on plain radiography or during endoscopic examination. However, it is obligatory to obtain objective evidence of the diagnosis of megarectum using one of the following criteria:[2]

1. A rectal diameter at the pelvic brim of >6.5 cm on a lateral x-ray obtained during double-contrast barium enema.
2. Widest rectal diameter of >8.3 cm on lateral x-ray during evacuation proctography.[6]
3. A rectal diameter of >6.3 cm at the minimum distension pressure during controlled (pressure-based) distension using a barostat during anorectal physiology combined with fluoroscopic imaging.[6]

Of these three imaging methods, only a double-contrast barium enema study will enable exclusion of proximal bowel dilatation. However, it should be noted that this technique is not sensitive for diagnosing megarectum and can underestimate dilatation.[6] Therefore, if clinical suspicion is high the other techniques should be employed. By contrast, a diagnosis based on elevated sensory threshold volumes during anorectal manometry should not be used as it is not specific and overdiagnoses the condition.[6]

Patients should also undergo full and comprehensive physiological assessment of hindgut function using anorectal physiology that incorporates anorectal manometry including sensory testing, endoanal ultrasound, measurement of pudendal nerve terminal motor latencies, evacuation proctography, and studies of colonic transit as a minimum. It is increasingly the case that more detailed assessment of rectal compliance and sensation is performed in such patients.[2] Appropriate measures need to be taken to exclude a diagnosis of Hirschsprung's disease (including short and ultra-short segment). In the authors' experience, the absence of the rectoanal inhibitory reflex is insufficient to confirm the diagnosis of Hirschsprung's disease, as this may also be absent in patients with IMR. Therefore, full-thickness rectal biopsy and confirmation of aganglionosis may be necessary.

Stoma therapist assessment/education

It is the authors' recommendation that the colo-neorectal anastomosis is covered with a temporary diverting stoma. A defunctioning loop ileostomy is most suitable for this purpose. Consequently, it is imperative that the patient receives adequate education from the stoma therapist preoperatively. Such education may prove particularly useful as some patients may require or elect to have a permanent stoma following surgery. An appropriate site in the right iliac fossa for the covering ileostomy should be marked by the stoma therapist prior to surgery.

Bowel preparation and prophylactic antibiotics

A full bowel preparation is required for surgery. Due to the gross impaction observed in patients with IMR, this may require a staged approach requiring admission to hospital. The first stage should involve complete disimpaction of the rectum and distal colon, if at all possible, and frequently requires a manual evacuation under anesthesia in the days immediately prior to surgery. Repeated evacuations over successive days may be necessary. Only then can oral bowel cleansing safely begin without fear of bowel perforation proximal to the 'obstructing' impacted fecoloma. More aggressive and more prolonged administration of purgatives may be required than the surgeon is accustomed to. For this purpose, a clear fluid diet for 72 hours and two sachets of sodium picosulfate/magnesium citrate per 24-hour period over 2 days are given prior to surgery. Antibiotic prophylaxis is provided at induction of anesthesia by metronidazole and cefuroxime.

DVT prophylaxis

Patients should receive subcutaneous heparin or low-molecular weight heparin according to their weight and the unit's policy, prior to surgery and until fully ambulant postoperatively.

Anesthesia

The procedure is performed under general anesthesia, although an epidural catheter is often used to supplement the general anesthetic and to provide initial postoperative analgesia for 48–72 hours.

OPERATION

Position/preparation of the patient

The patient is positioned in the modified Lloyd-Davies position, ensuring full access to the anus for completion of the stapled colo-neorectal anastomosis. Once general anesthesia has been induced, a Foley urethral catheter is inserted into the bladder; pneumatic calf compressing stockings are applied routinely to minimize the risk of thromboembolism and peripheral neuropathy. The entire abdomen is prepared with povidone–iodine from above the xiphisternum to below the symphysis pubis.

Incision

A midline incision is made down to the level of the symphysis pubis. The greater curvature of the stomach should be visible in the upper aspect of the wound to allow adequate access to complete full mobilization of the splenic flexure.

Exploration, planning, and preparation

A laparotomy is performed. Specifically, the colon and rectum are inspected to identify the extent of the dilated megabowel. With appropriate preoperative selection, megacolon should have been excluded. The rectum is identified, inspected, and the degree of dilatation evaluated. It is preferable to avoid use of the sigmoid colon for the colo-neorectal anastomosis, as it is invariably dysfunctional in patients with megarectum. Accordingly, the sigmoid colon is resected and a site in the descending colon is chosen for anastomosis.

The patient is positioned in the exaggerated Trendelenburg position and the operative field is then set-up to begin the procedure. This involves packing of the small bowel away from the operative site and adequate retraction of the anterior abdominal wall. The bladder (which may also be grossly dilated, 'megacystis') may need to be mobilized and, in women, the fundus of uterus is sutured to the lower aspect of the wound to facilitate access to the rectum within the pelvis.

Mobilization of the left colon and splenic flexure

To ensure adequate colonic length for a tension-free pelvic anastomosis, the left colon and splenic flexure are routinely mobilized.

A large, moistened pack is placed over the sigmoid colon. Mobilization is performed using electrocautery and begins by dividing the congenital sigmoid adhesions. The left colon is retracted anteromedially out of the wound to expose the lateral peritoneal attachments. The full-thickness of the peritoneum is incised from sigmoid colon in a craniad direction towards the splenic flexure. Care is taken to incise the peritoneum alone without entering the fascia of the mesocolon. It is common for the peritoneum to be thickened and for the sigmoid mesocolon to be elongated (**Figure 6.19.1**).

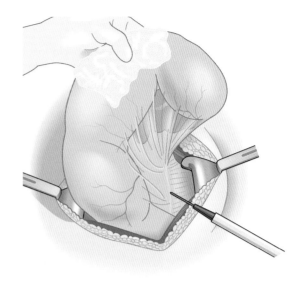

6.19.1

The extrafascial plane between the left mesocolon and Gerota's fascia is developed and the gonadal vessels and left ureter are identified. In cases of megarectum, their location is extremely variable and they are often pulled anteromedially by the elongated sigmoid mesocolon. Once identified, they are displaced posteriorly and mobilization continues under the left colon mesentery towards the midline. Mobilization continues in this plane in a craniad direction to approach the splenic flexure inferiorly (**Figure 6.19.2**).

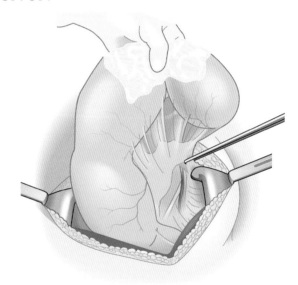

6.19.2

Further mobilization of the splenic flexure is performed along the transverse colon within the lesser sac. The transverse colon is delivered out of the wound, the gastrocolic omentum is reflected in a craniad direction, and its attachments with the traverse colon are divided, allowing entry into the lesser sac. Mobilization continues in the lesser sac laterally towards the splenic flexure. The splenocolic ligament is then incised at the superolateral margin of the colon to complete the mobilization (**Figure 6.19.3**).

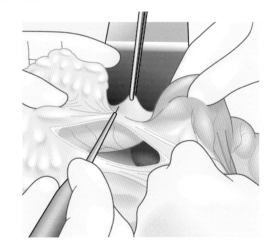

6.19.3

The colon is then retracted anterolaterally to complete the medial mobilization. The duodenal attachments to the mesocolon are divided and the inferior mesenteric vein (IMV) is identified at the inferior border of the pancreas (**Figure 6.19.4**). The peritoneum overlying the IMV at this point is incised and the vessel is skeletalized, clamped, divided, and ligated to provide further colonic mobility to perform a tension-free anastomosis.

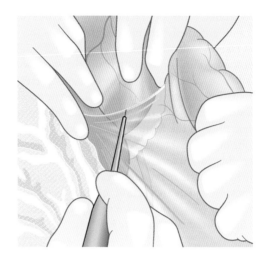

6.19.4

Division of the mesentery and resection of the sigmoid colon

The sites of resection in the descending colon and the rectosigmoid are identified, and windows are created in the mesentery close to the bowel wall. With the left colon and splenic flexure fully mobilized to the midline, the colon is suspended out of the midline wound on its mesentery to inspect the mesenteric vasculature by transillumination. In contrast to oncological resections, the inferior mesenteric and superior rectal vessels are identified and preserved. Further windows are created in the mesentery to allow skeletalization of the marginal artery and mesenteric vessels close to the colonic wall, which are then clamped, divided, and ligated. Solid fecal matter that invariably persists despite bowel preparation is 'milked' into the segment of colon to be resected.

A 75 mm linear stapling device (e.g. TLC™ 75; Ethicon, Cincinnati, OH, USA) is then applied to the descending colon and rectosigmoid to allow the sigmoid colon to be resected (**Figure 6.19.5**).

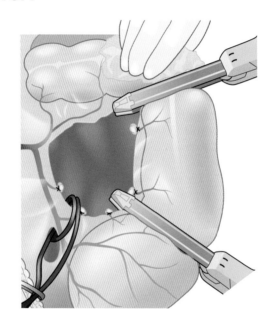

6.19.5

Mobilization and vertical reduction of the megarectum

Prior to mobilization of the rectum, the location and course of both ureters is again confirmed, bearing in mind that their usual anatomy is often disturbed due to distortion by the grossly dilated rectum. To ensure complete preservation of the superior rectal vessels, a vascular sling is applied. During mobilization, it is useful to use a large, moistened pack to protect the rectum while being retracted. Great care needs to be taken to prevent injury to the grossly dilated vessels that are present at the mesenteric border of the rectum and within the mesorectum. It should also be noted that the fascial planes within the pelvis are less obvious in patients with megarectum.

The rectum is retracted inferiorly towards the symphysis pubis, and anteriorly to elevate it out of the pelvis. Time is taken to identify and enter the extrafascial plane of the mesorectum posteriorly in the first instance. The hypogastric nerves are identified and preserved by careful dissection off the mesorectal fascia. Continued mobilization is then performed posteriorly down towards the pelvic floor in the familiar plane used for oncological resections involving total mesorectal excision. This ensures that the dilated mesorectal vessels are not injured and that the hypogastric nerves are preserved. As mobilization progresses, adequate retraction of the rectum can be achieved using a large moistened pack under one or two St Mark's lipped retractors (**Figure 6.19.6**).

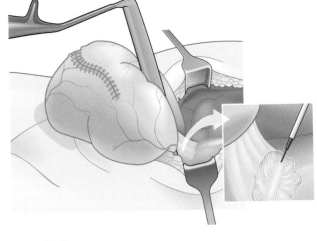

6.19.6

Additional mobilization of the rectum is performed anterolaterally. This involves incision of the peritoneum and continued mobilization in the extrafascial plane that has been developed posteriorly. The anterior plane, which may be difficult to identify in the presence of a grossly dilated bladder (megacystis) can be accentuated using hydrodissection. A Babcock's forceps applied to the bladder or vagina can help demonstrate the correct plane. Full mobilization of the extraperitoneal lower rectum anteriorly is crucial to protect the anterior viscera during reduction of rectal capacity with the stapling devices. The mobilization is complete when the fascia covering the levator muscles is reached (**Figure 6.19.7**).

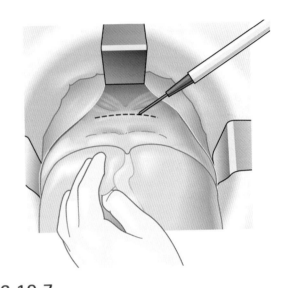

6.19.7

The grossly dilated rectum is washed out with copious volumes of povidone–iodine and then deflated in preparation for vertical reduction. A 100 mm linear stapling device (e.g. TLC 100; Ethicon) is then applied along the antimesenteric border of the rectum in a vertical direction to reduce its capacity, and bisecting it into anterior and posterior portions. In most instances (e.g. rectal diameter approximately 10 cm), reduction by approximately one-half (to 5 cm diameter) is usually sufficient. However, in cases of more extreme dilatation, disproportionately more rectum is excised than is retained. Several, usually two to three, fires of the stapling device are required, depending on the degree of elongation of the megarectum, until the anorectal junction is approached. Occasionally, it may be necessary to divide the rectum between clamps and suture manually if the rectum is exceptionally thickened.

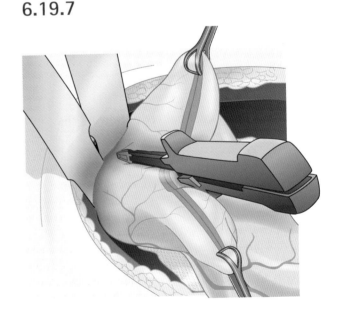

6.19.8

The anterior portion of the rectum is then excised. This is achieved by applying a 50 mm TLH™ instrument (Ethicon) at right angles to the vertical staple line at its lower limit. In a narrow male pelvis, it may be necessary to use a 30 mm stapler. A right-angled crushing bowel clamp is placed proximal to the TLH stapler and the anterior portion of the rectum is excised by cutting onto the stapling device using a 15 blade long-handle scalpel. The staple lines are oversewn with a continuous layer of 2-0 polygluconate sutures (**Figure 6.19.9**).

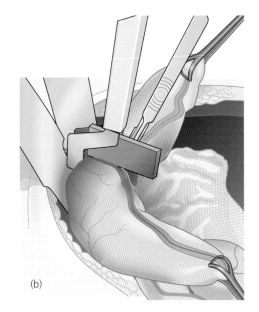

(b)

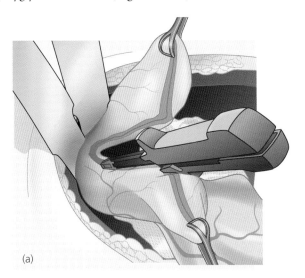

(a)

6.19.9

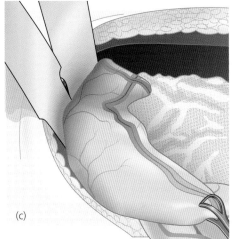

(c)

Construction of the coloneorectal anastomosis

A coloneorectal anastomosis is then constructed between the proximal stapled end of the neorectum and the proximal descending colon using a 31 or 33 mm circular stapling device. In view of the extended length of the anastomosis, it is often necessary to use an endoscopic curved intraluminal stapler (e.g. Endopath® ILS; Ethicon). The staple line is excised from the descending colon and a purse-string inserted using a 2-0 polygluconate suture. The anvil from the stapler is inserted and secured in place by tightening the purse-string suture. The circular stapling device is then gently inserted through the anal canal, into the neorectum. Great care must be taken to guide the circular stapler gently up the neorectum to the proximal staple line without disrupting the anterior staple line along its antimesenteric border. The spike of the stapling device is extended and the anvil is connected, retracted and fired to allow construction of the anastomosis. The integrity of the staple lines is checked by inflating the neorectum with air introduced via a large Foley catheter per anum, after filling the pelvis with saline (**Figure 6.19.10**).

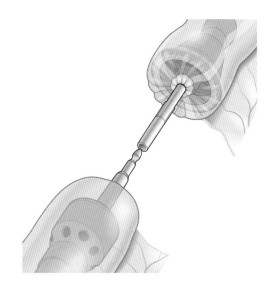

6.19.10

Construction of a loop ileostomy

The anastomosis is protected with a defunctioning loop ileostomy, details of which can be found in Chapter 3.1.

Wound closure

After achieving hemostasis, the abdomen is irrigated and fluid is suctioned. A closed-system drain (e.g. Robinson 20F) is inserted into the pelvis. The fascia is closed, the subcutaneous tissue is irrigated and the skin approximated.

POSTOPERATIVE CARE

Oral fluids are commenced immediately and the diet is gradually advanced to a normal intake. The pelvic drain is removed once the output is reduced. Patients are generally discharged 7–10 days after surgery. A water-soluble contrast enema is performed approximately 6 weeks after the procedure and the ileostomy is closed if leakage is excluded.

OUTCOME

Medium-term (five-year) follow-up of ten (six female) constipated patients with IMR undergoing VRR revealed that there were no deaths or late complications.[5] Specifically, there were no complications related to bowel obstruction or pelvic nerve dysfunction reported following traditional procedures for idiopathic megarectum. Patients were evaluated before and after surgery by independent assessment of symptoms using scoring systems and anorectal physiology, including detailed evaluation of rectal diameter, compliance, and sensory and evacuatory function. Recurrence of symptoms that necessitated permanent ileostomy formation occurred in two patients. However, constipation scores improved, bowel frequency increased, and laxative usage reduced postoperatively. Further, VRR was successful in achieving and maintaining correction of rectal diameter, compliance, and sensory function in seven of eight patients following surgery.[5]

REFERENCES

1. Todd IP. Discussion on megacolon and megarectum with the emphasis on conditions other than Hirschsprung's disease. *Proceedings of the Royal Society of Medicine* 1961; **54**: 1035–40.
2. Gladman MA, Knowles CH. Novel concepts in the diagnosis, pathophysiology and management of idiopathic megabowel. *Colorectal Disease* 2008; **10**: 531–8.
3. Gladman MA, Scott SM, Lunniss PJ, Williams NS. Systematic review of surgical options for idiopathic megarectum and megacolon. *Annals of Surgery* 2005; **241**: 562–74.
4. Williams NS, Fajobi OA, Lunniss PJ *et al*. Vertical reduction rectoplasty: a new treatment for idiopathic megarectum. *British Journal of Surgery* 2000; **87**: 1203–8.
5. Gladman MA, Williams NS, Ogunbiyi OA *et al*. Medium-term results of vertical reduction rectoplasty and sigmoid colectomy for idiopathic megarectum. *British Journal of Surgery* 2005; **92**: 624–30.
6. Gladman MA, Dvorkin LS, Scott SM *et al*. A novel technique to identify patients with megarectum. *Diseases of the Colon and Rectum* 2007; **50**: 621–9.

7

Perineal reconstruction

VRAM flap

JÉRÉMIE H LEFÈVRE AND EMMANUEL TIRET

PRINCIPLES AND JUSTIFICATION

Perineal wound complications occur frequently after abdominoperineal resection (APR), particularly if radiotherapy has been given preoperatively. These complications include abscess formation, wound dehiscence, and delayed wound healing,[1, 2, 3, 4, 5] and the incidence ranges from 25 to 60 percent. Two factors are responsible: impaired healing of the perineum secondary to radiation effects and tension at the site of wound closure. As tumor-free margins are required to minimize local recurrence, extensive resection is sometimes needed with a resulting perineal defect. The larger the perineal resection, the greater is the risk of postoperative perineal wound complications. Several techniques have been developed in an attempt to improve perineal healing. These include omentoplasty, gracilis flap, vertical rectus abdominis myocutaneous (VRAM) flap, and gluteus maximus flap. All these approaches facilitate closure of the perineal defect without undue tension by bringing in healthy and well-vascularized tissue.[6] This chapter describes the authors' technique in performing a VRAM flap for perineal reconstruction. The reader is also directed to Chapters 2.15 and 7.3 for other techniques.

The VRAM flap technique was first described by Taylor *et al.* in 1983.[7] The initial description of a long myocutaneous flap was initially designed to be mobilized from the contralateral side as an island flap to cover large groin and thigh defects.[7] The large paddle of skin and underlying rectus abdominis muscle were vascularized by the deep inferior epigastric vessels. In subsequent application following APR, the flap is passed into the pelvis and brought down to the perineum. Should a posterior colpectomy be required for tumor extension to the vagina, the VRAM flap can also be used to reconstruct a neovagina.

PREOPERATIVE EXPLORATION

No preoperative examination is required systematically for the VRAM flap. The patient should be seen by a plastic surgeon before the procedure. For patients with vascular risk factors, such as diabetes, arterial hypertension, obesity, or with previous surgical history (appendicectomy, inguinal hernia repair, laparotomy or laparoscopy, stoma formation), a Doppler ultrasound is required to assess patency of the deep inferior epigastric vessels. Usually in the case of APR, the flap is taken from the right side of the abdominal wall, because end colostomy is usually placed in the left iliac fossa. In case of previous damage to the right epigastric vessels, the flap can be taken from the left side as well, after having checked vessel patency.

SURGICAL TECHNIQUE

APR is performed through a midline incision. Caution must be taken at this stage to keep the umbilicus on the contralateral side of the future flap, in order to avoid further umbilical necrosis (**Figure 7.1.1**). The colostomy site should have been marked preoperatively by a specialized nurse.

VRAM reconstruction does not modify the technique used to perform the APR (see Chapter 6.10). After removal of the specimen, the width and the length of the perineal defect are measured with a ruler. The size of the required flap is then calculated and the dimensions transferred to the anterior abdominal skin. The shape of the flap is usually oblique, parallel to the rib along an axis starting from the umbilicus to the scapula (**Figure 7.1.1b**).[7] It can be alternatively vertical[4, 8] or horizontal (**Figure 7.1.1a, c**).

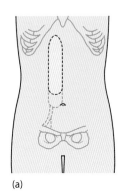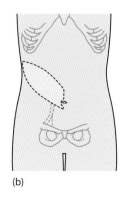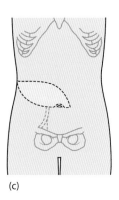

(a)   (b)   (c)

7.1.1 VRAM flaps: (a), vertical; (b), oblique; (c), horizontal.

In the authors' experience, VRAM flap with an oblique skin paddle[9] allows a larger area of skin to be harvested for reconstruction (**Figure 7.1.2a, b**). The main drawback of this oblique skin paddle is the additional wound incision to the midline incision. Conversely, a vertical skin paddle does not add another incision but may increase the risk of wound dehiscence, and in the case of a large paddle extending to the pubic skin, the inferior part of the flap may have been irradiated. The maximum width of the vertical flap should be 7–8 cm to allow a tension-free closure of the abdominal wall.[4] The four main steps of the flap dissection are shown in **Figure 7.1.3**.

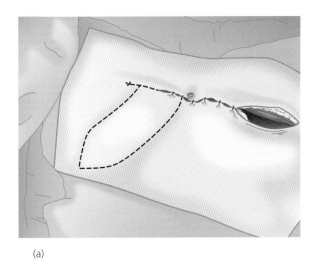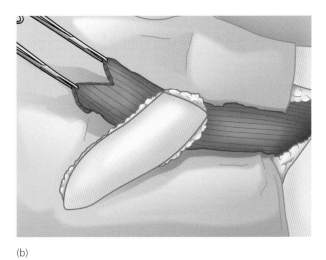

(a)   (b)

7.1.2 (a) Drawing of the oblique flap and (b) final aspect after complete dissection.

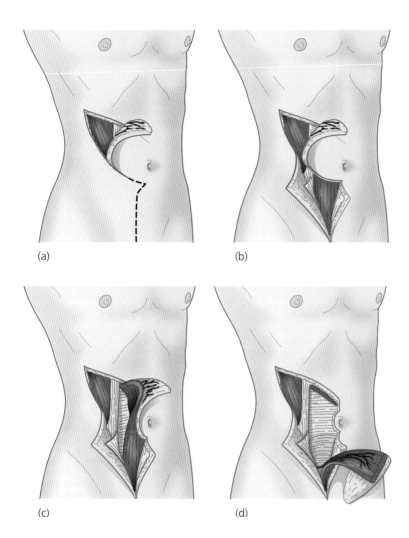

(a)

(b)

(c)

(d)

7.1.3 Schematic representation of the dissection of the VRAM flap.

The skin and subcutaneous tissues are incised down to the level of the anterior rectus sheath. The dissection of the skin flap begins on the lateral side and extends to the external border of the anterior rectus sheath. The anterior rectus sheath is then incised vertically along its external border. The VRAM dissection is continued with transverse division of the anterior rectus sheath just above (**Figure 7.1.4**) and below the skin paddle. Therefore, the anterior rectus sheath and the myocutaneous perforating vessels remain included within the flap.

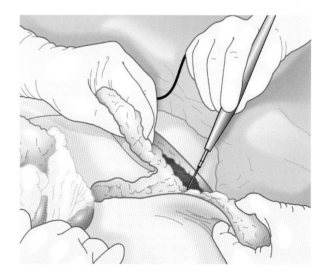

7.1.4 Beginning of the VRAM dissection at its lateral extremity over the anterior rectus sheath.

In the next step, the rectus muscle is divided transversally close to its cranial insertion (**Figure 7.1.5**a, b). The superior epigastric vessels are carefully ligated. After proximal division, the rectus abdominis muscle can be easily freed from its posterior sheath. (**Figure 7.1.5**c). At this point, the anterior rectus sheath below its caudal transverse incision must be dissected from subcutaneous tissue and skin to allow a tension-free closure of the abdominal wall at the end of the procedure. Therefore, the posterior sheath has been completely preserved all along the midline incision, with the anterior sheath below its caudal transverse incision.

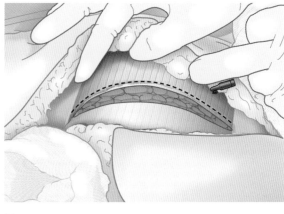

(b)

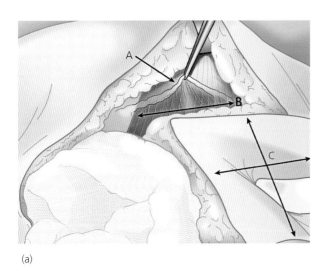

(a)

7.1.5 (a) Separation of the anterior rectus sheath (A), (B) rectus abdominis, (C) VRAM flap. (b) Division of the cranial insertion of the rectus abdominis. (c) Separation of the VRAM flap from the posterior rectus sheath.

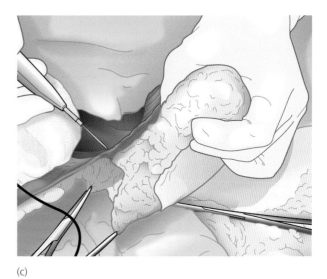

(c)

The rectus muscle is then freed from the lower part of the anterior sheath down to the pubic bone (**Figure 7.1.6**). At this point, particular care is taken to preserve the inferior epigastric vessel and the pedicle should not be skeletalized.[4]

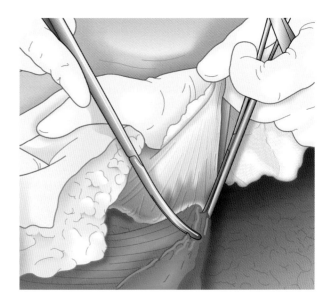

7.1.6 Separation of the anterior rectus sheath from the rectus muscle.

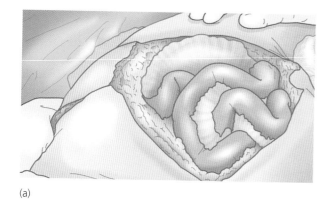

(a)

At the end of the dissection, the VRAM flap can be fully mobilized and brought down to the pelvis (**Figure 7.1.7**). The VRAM flap is then rotated to the perineal defect. At this stage, caution must be taken to avoid a twist of the muscle or its pedicle that could lead to flap ischemia. Perineal closure is started from the bottom of the defect with interrupted sutures and continued laterally. In the case of posterior colpectomy, the upper part of the flap can be flipped inside the perineal cavity to create a neo-vagina with absorbable interrupted stitches (**Figure 7.1.8**).

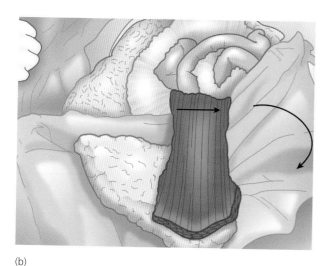

(b)

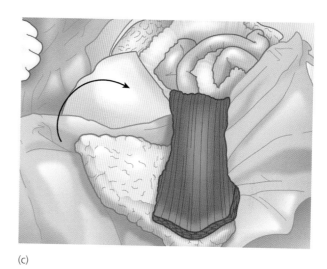

(c)

7.1.7 Aspect of the abdominal wall (a) after full dissection of the VRAM (b) and the mobilization of the subcutaneous tissue below the flap (c).

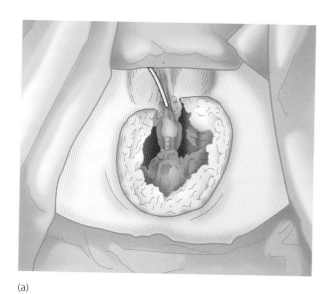

(a)

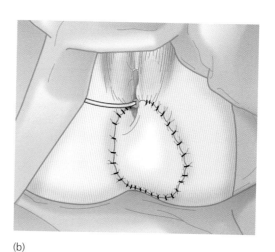

(b)

7.1.8 Perineal wound before and after fixation of the VRAM flap.

Abdominal closure

Two suction drains are placed in the pelvis and the end colonic stoma is created on the contralateral abdominal wall. The anterior abdominal wall is closed in separate layers. No prosthetic mesh is needed to prevent a wound hernia.[6,9] Above the umbilicus, the posterior sheath is closed with continuous suture to the contralateral side. Below the umbilicus, the two layers (anterior and posterior sheaths) are closed with continuous suture to the contralateral side. As the remaining subcutaneous tissues and skin have been freed, a tension-free skin closure can be performed (**Figure 7.1.9**). The final aspect is an L-shaped incision (**Figure 7.1.10**).

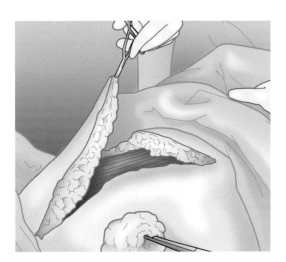

7.1.9 Abdominal wall closure.

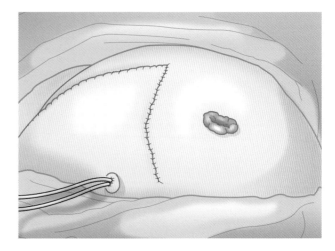

7.1.10 Final aspect of the wound incision after abdominal closure.

POSTOPERATIVE CARE

During the first 5 postoperative days, the patient should be nursed in the lateral decubitus position to avoid pressure on the perineal flap, which should be inspected daily by the surgeon. Patients are asked to avoid direct pressure on the flap and walking for 12 days. Otherwise, postoperative care is not different from that usually following APR.

RESULTS OF THE VRAM FLAP

The authors have published their experience with the VRAM flap,[9] and a recent meta-analysis has assessed the different flaps after APR.[10] The VRAM flap ($n = 43$) was compared with classical omentoplasty ($n = 41$) after APR for anal canal squamous cell carcinoma. Size of the skin paddle was recorded in 20 patients. The mean size was 15.3 ± 4.7 cm (6–22) $\times$ 7.6 ± 1.4 cm (6–11). The VRAM flap was harvested from the right side in 40/43 patients. VRAM flap confection was not associated with higher morbidity or mortality. All patients with a VRAM flap had successful perineal closure, while six patients (11.5 percent) in the other group did not ($p = 0.02$). The VRAM flap reduced perineal morbidity (26.8 versus 44.2 percent, $p = 0.10$) and time to wound healing (18.7 ± 34.9 versus 95.1 ± 113.2 days, $p < 0.01$). No differences were observed between the two groups in relation to wound hernia or evisceration (7 versus 9.6 percent). However, no perineal hernia was observed in the VRAM flap group while this complication occurred in eight patients in the omentoplasty group (15.4 percent, $p < 0.01$).

Nisar and Scott reported the results of 19 studies on VRAM flap reconstruction in a total of 385 patients.[10] The VRAM flap was performed mainly for rectal cancer ($n = 191$), anal cancer ($n = 91$), and gynecological cancer ($n = 89$). Most studies were retrospective and the largest included 73 patients.[4] The rate of perineal healing varied from 90 to 100 percent and the largest series reported immediate perineal healing for 85 percent of patients and 95 percent at follow-up.[4] The lowest rate of 54 percent was observed in one series with many obese patients who had received high doses of radiotherapy, but at the end of follow-up every patient achieved perineal healing. Several studies have confirmed the reduction of perineal complications after VRAM flap when compared with primary closure or omentoplasty.[5, 10] In the meta-analysis by Nisar and Scott,[10] no demonstrable increase in abdominal wall complications after VRAM flap was observed after a mean 3.8 years of follow-up. Moreover, no significant difference was observed in the mean hospital stay.

REFERENCES

1. Arnold PG, Lovich SF, Pairolero PC. Muscle flaps in irradiated wounds: an account of 100 consecutive cases. *Plastic and Reconstructive Surgery* 1994; **93**: 324–7; discussion 328–9.

2. Yeh KA, Hoffman JP, Kusiak JE *et al.* Reconstruction with myocutaneous flaps following resection of locally recurrent rectal cancer. *American Journal of Surgery* 1995; **61**: 581–9.

3. Shibata D, Hyland W, Busse P *et al.* Immediate reconstruction of the perineal wound with gracilis muscle flaps following abdominoperineal resection and intraoperative radiation therapy for recurrent carcinoma of the rectum. *Annals of Surgical Oncology* 1999; **6**: 33–7.

4. Buchel EW, Finical S, Johnson C. Pelvic reconstruction using vertical rectus abdominis musculocutaneous flaps. *Annals of Plastic Surgery* 2004; **52**: 22–6.

5. Chessin DB, Hartley J, Cohen AM *et al.* Rectus flap reconstruction decreases perineal wound complications after pelvic chemoradiation and surgery: a cohort study. *Annals of Surgical Oncology* 2005; **12**: 104–10.

6. Butler CE, Gundeslioglu AO, Rodriguez-Bigas MA. Outcomes of immediate vertical rectus abdominis myocutaneous flap reconstruction for irradiated abdominoperineal resection defects. *Journal of the American College of Surgeons* 2008; **206**: 694–703.

7. Taylor GI, Corlett R, Boyd JB. The extended deep inferior epigastric flap: a clinical technique. *Plastic and Reconstructive Surgery* 1983; **72**: 751–65.

8. Tei TM, Stolzenburg T, Buntzen S *et al.* Use of transpelvic rectus abdominis musculocutaneous flap for anal cancer salvage surgery. *British Journal of Surgery* 2003; **90**: 575–80.

9. Lefevre JH, Parc Y, Kerneis S *et al.* Abdomino-perineal resection for anal cancer: impact of a vertical rectus abdominis myocutaneus flap on survival, recurrence, morbidity, and wound healing. *Annals of Surgery* 2009; **250**: 707–11.

10. Nisar PJ, Scott HJ. Myocutaneous flap reconstruction of the pelvis after abdominoperineal excision. *Colorectal Disease* 2009; **11**: 806–16.

Martius flap

HUEYLAN CHERN AND MADHULIKA VARMA

HISTORY

The Martius flap was first described using bulbocavernosus fat and muscle to repair large, complex or postradiation rectovaginal or vesicovaginal fistulae. This procedure is credited to Dr Heinrick Martius. He described using the flap for repair of a large urethral defect in 1928 and subsequently used it for successful repair of vesicovaginal and/or rectovaginal fistulae. However, the idea of using the bulbocavernosus flap can be traced back as far as 1905 to Dr Sellheim.[1] Since the introduction of the Martius flap in the early 1900s, there have been many modifications to this procedure. Some are done with full skin harvest from the inner thigh or from the labia in conjunction with the bulbocavernosus flap to allow repair of large epithelial defects. Another modification is the use of the bulbocavernous fat pad alone, rather than including the bulbocavernosus muscle for the graft. As the most commonly performed technique for repairing rectovaginal and vaginovesical fistulae uses the bulbocavernosus fat, this chapter will describe harvest of the bulbocavernous fat flap.

PRINCIPLES AND JUSTIFICATION

While primary repairs of simple rectovaginal or vesicovaginal fistulae are feasible, repairing a large, complex, recurrent, or postradiation rectovaginal or vesicovaginal fistula is a challenge to surgeons and a daunting task. The devascularized tissues involved, as well as the dead space created from the dissection, make primary repair of these complex fistulae more prone to failure.

There have been many flap procedures described to protect the repair and obliterate dead space in these complex fistulae. The flaps enhance healing by bringing new blood supply, providing tissue support and creating a physical barrier between the sutured repairs of the walls of the fistula. Tissues proposed for use include bulbocavernosus, gracilis, omentum, rectus abdominis, sartorius, and gluteus maximus muscles, as well as biologic meshes. Martius flaps have been described and reported extensively for the repair of large and complex urethrovaginal or vesicovaginal fistulae in the urologic literature. They have also been used for complex rectovaginal fistula repair. The advantages of using a bulbocavernous flap include the ease of approach, one operative field involvement, low postoperative mobidity, minimal cosmetic defect, obliteration of dead space in the dissected region, and bringing a new blood supply to a devascularized area.

The labial area is well vascularized with perineal branches from the pudendal artery (**Figure 7.2.1**). The superior vascular supply to the Martius flap comes from the external pudendal artery branches and the inferior

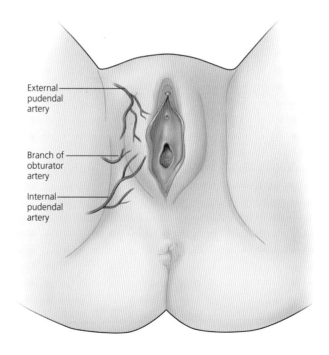

External pudendal artery

Branch of obturator artery

Internal pudendal artery

7.2.1

vascular supply to the Martius flap comes from the internal pudendal artery branches. The Martius flap is a pedicled bulbocavernous fat pad harvested from the labia majora while preserving the inferior vascular pedicle. The tissue harvested should be as thick as a thumb and as long as a finger. The Martius flap is an adjunct measure used to repair rectovaginal or vesicovaginal fistulae using a transanal, transvaginal, or transperineal approach. We will describe the transperineal approach for rectovaginal fistula repair here.

PREOPERATIVE ASSESSMENT AND PREPARATION

The patient should undergo routine work up for rectovaginal fistula. For patients with an obstetric history, endoanal ultrasound and manometry may be helpful to define associated sphincter defects and define baseline sphincter function. Colonoscopy should be performed if indicated for screening or in those where Crohn's disease is suspected. For patients with failed prior repairs, uncontrolled perineal sepsis, severe fecal incontinence, or large and irradiated complex fistulae, fecal diversion with a colostomy should be considered. Any inflammation or sepsis should be resolved, which can take four to six months, before any attempts at repair. Full mechanical bowel preparation is used and a standard one dose perioperative antibiotic covering the gastrointestinal tract flora should be given prior to incision.

OPERATION

The procedure is routinely performed under general anesthesia supplemented by local anesthesia. The operation is typically performed in the lithotomy position. A Foley catheter is usually placed. A Lone Star™ retractor may be helpful for exposure. A transverse perineal incision is made. The dissection is carried out cranially in between the rectum and the vagina. The posterior vaginal wall is dissected away from the anterior rectal wall outside the sphincter complex. The fistula is identified and divided (**Figure 7.2.2**). The dissection should extend to approximately 2 cm cranial to the fistula to allow tension-

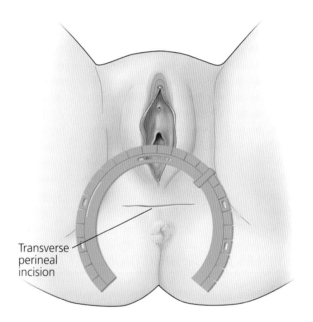

Transverse perineal incision

7.2.2

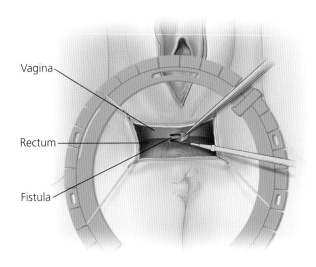

Vagina

Rectum

Fistula

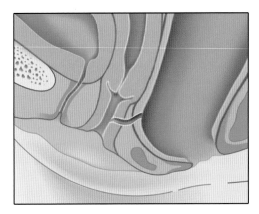

7.2.3

free closure of the vagina and rectum. The rectal defect is closed in one or two layers with interrupted 3-0 polyglactin transversely. The vaginal defect is closed with interrupted 3-0 polyglactin sutures (**Figure 7.2.3**).

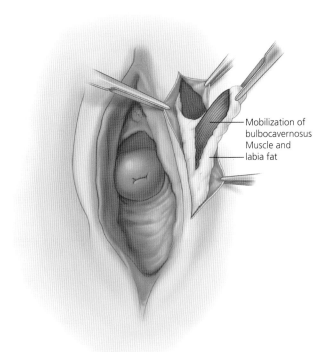

Mobilization of bulbocavernosus Muscle and labia fat

The Martius flap is harvested from the labia majora (**Figure 7.2.4**). It can be harvested from the right or left side depending on the location of the fistula and the ease of the flap to reach the fistula location. A vertical labial incision is made.

7.2.4

The bulbocavernosus fat flap is mobilized immediately underneath the skin. The borders of dissection are the labiocrural fold laterally, the fascia covering the inner aspect of the labial minor, bulbocavernosus muscle, and the vestibular bulb medially, and Colle's fascia as the deep border.[2] It is dissected out leaving it attached to the inferior or posterolateral vascular pedicle. A subcutaneous tunnel is created connecting the two incisions. The tunnel should be generous enough so as not to cause vascular compromise of the bulbocavernosus flap. The flap is tunneled in the correct orientation from the labial incision to the perineal incision and area of fistula repair (**Figure 7.2.5**). The flap is

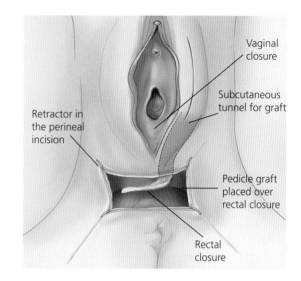

7.2.5

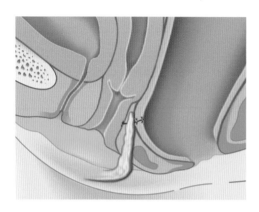

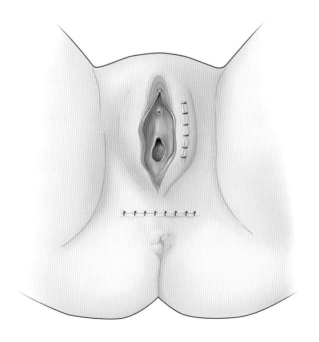

7.2.6

secured over the fistula repair with several interrupted 3-0 polyglactin sutures. Both the labial and perineal incisions are closed with 4-0 absorbable subcuticular sutures (**Figure 7.2.6**). Drains are not routinely used.

POSTOPERATIVE CARE

Postoperatively, diet is advanced as tolerated. Routine pain management and bowel regimen to prevent constipation are indicated. Bathing should be avoided. Normal activity can be resumed as tolerated, except sexual activity.

OUTCOME

Most studies on the use of Martius flap for the repair of rectovaginal fistula are limited to case series. The results are encouraging, both for non-irradiated rectovaginal fistulae and for irradiated rectovaginal fistulae.[3,4,5] The risk of wound complication is rare. One commonly reported complication is dyspareunia, reported in 13–31 percent of patients. However, the Martius flap procedure is not associated with a significant amount of perceived cosmetic disfigurement.[6] Sexual and bowel functions after Martius flap are not well studied and are only limited to small case series. Given the major morbidities associated with other types of flaps, the Martius flap serves as a good adjunct measure to repair complex rectovaginal fistulae.

REFERENCES

1. Given FT Jr, Acosta AA. The Martius procedure – bulbocavernosus fat flap: a review. *Obstetrical and Gynecological Survey* 1990; **45**: 34–40.
2. Elkins TE, DeLancey JO, McGuire EJ. The use of modified Martius graft as an adjunctive technique in vesicovaginal and rectovaginal fistula repair. *Obstetrics and Gynecology* 1990; **75**: 727–33.
3. White AJ, Buchsbaum HJ, Blythe JG, Lifshitz S. Use of the bulbocavernosus muscle (Martius procedure) for repair of radiation-induced rectovaginal fistulas. *Obstetrics and Gynecology* 1982; **60**: 114–18.
4. McNevin MS, Lee PY, Bax TW. Martius flap: an adjunct for repair of complex, low rectovaginal fistula. *American Journal of Surgery* 2007; **193**: 597–9; discussion 599.
5. Gosselink MP, Oom DM, Zimmerman DD, Schouten RW. Martius flap: an adjunct for repair of complex, low rectovaginal fistula. *American Journal of Surgery* 2009; **197**: 833–4.
6. Petrou SP, Jones J, Parra RO. Martius flap harvest site: patient self-perception. *Journal of Urology* 2002; **167**: 2098–9.

Local advancement flaps

MICHAEL J EARLEY

PRINCIPLES AND JUSTIFICATION

In order to understand what is required for reconstruction, one must consider the requirements for the perineum. It must be sufficiently padded to cover bony prominences, sufficiently elastic to allow the hips and symphysis pubis to move and stretch, and sufficiently taut and robust to support the abdominal contents. In addition, the reconstructed perineum must not lose its integrity while at the same time providing openings for micturition, defecation, intercourse, and childbirth.

Most reconstructions follow excisions for cancer which result in 'extirpative defects'. These may be small (e.g. posterior vaginal wall, anal canal, etc.) or large (e.g. pelvic exenteration with loss of bowel support leading to pelvic perineal herniation, or large, slowly healing cavities). Childbirth trauma or surgical trauma may result in vesicovaginal or rectovaginal fistulae which need closure and flap repair. Irradiated tissues are non-pliable, scarred, and may repeatedly break down leading to a need for excision of the affected area and subsequent reconstruction. Inflammatory diseases, such as Crohn's disease, and hidradenitis suppurativa may cause multiple abscesses in both groin and perineal areas. Surgical treatment of both conditions will create complex defects requiring reconstruction.

The key to success is the use of well-vascularized flaps from outside the zone of trauma whatever the cause. Immediate reconstruction is preferable to delayed as primary wound closure and primary healing is achieved thereby leading to easier postoperative management with less pain, less discharge, no dressing packs, and less risk of infection. Overall, primary healing causes less postoperative morbidity with little risk of fistula formation. The pressure of already displayed anatomy with open tissue planes in primary reconstruction gives a major advantage when compared to the difficulties met by the scarring and contracture seen typically in later or 'delayed' (secondary) reconstruction.

One must first consider 'the reconstructive ladder' which has as its first rung primary closure and next has skin grafting, with complex microvascular flaps at the highest rung. Between these options lie local, regional, and distant flaps (**Figure 7.3.1**).

Skin grafts are not relevant in this difficult area of folds, cavities, and ligamentous and bony prominences, and the vascularity brought with a flap is essential. It is beyond the scope of this chapter to consider decubitus ulcers of the ischial, trochanteric, and sacral areas, and vaginal or penile reconstruction. There is, however, considerable overlap between the flaps used in these instances and those used in large perineal defects, such as the vertical, transverse, and oblique rectus abdominus flaps.

The local flaps discussed below are those based on the pudendal arterial system and the gluteal arterial system,

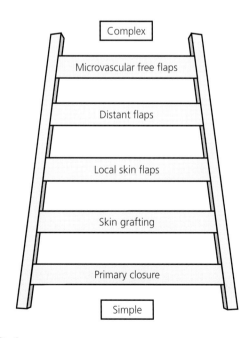

7.3.1 The reconstructive ladder.

both superior and inferior. Regional flaps considered below are gracilis, either myocutaneous or muscle alone, and the infragluteal posterior thigh flap.

PUDENDAL FLAPS

Arterial anatomy

Manchot in 1889 provided the first description of genital blood supply and appreciated that the cutaneous supply could be divided into anterior and posterior. The anterior supply consists of the superficial and deep external

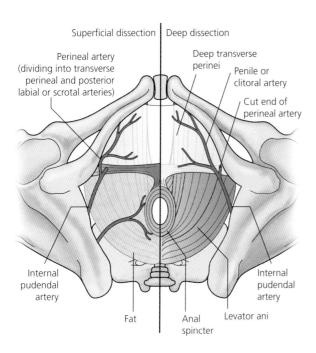

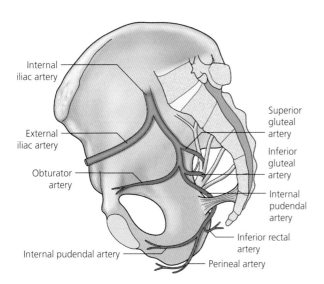

7.3.2

pudendal arteries which are branches of the femoral artery. These form a rich anastomosis with the anterior branch of the obturator artery. The posterior supply is mainly from the internal pudendal artery, a branch of the internal iliac artery. This gives rise to lateral and medial branches, the latter anastomosing with branches of the inferior gluteal artery, before the internal pudendal artery divides into its two terminal branches, the penile or clitoral branch and the perineal artery. The terminal branches of the perineal artery form the transverse perineal artery and the posterior labial (scrotal) arteries which anastomose with branches of the deep external pudendal, obturator, and medial circumflex femoral arteries (**Figure 7.3.2**).

Applications of the knowledge

Flaps designed around the genital area were first described in 1973, but were limited due to poor application of the anatomical knowledge described above. In practical terms, many of the surgical procedures resulting in defects of this area disrupt the anterior blood supply (e.g. vulvectomy and inguinal block dissection). The posterior blood supply provides viability to the pudendal thigh fasciocutaneous flap, also known as the Singapore flap, and the so-called lotus flap variations. The Martius flap (see Chapter 7.2) is supplied by branches of the perineal artery. The safest way in which to ensure viability of these flaps is to use a Doppler to identify the arterial perforators entering the base of the flap. As long as the relevant perforators are included in the raised flap, it can be islanded and mobilized to reach defects without tension, while simultaneously avoiding folds of tissue known as 'dog ears' as the flaps are turned.

Specific flap designs

The pudendal thigh fasciocutaneous flap, also known as the Singapore flap, must include the posterior perforators of the deep pudendal artery to ensure its viability. As with all of these flaps, it is helpful but not essential to identify perforators with preoperative Doppler mapping. It is described as including the deep fascia throughout its length but if perforators are preserved this is unnecessary.

It may be bilateral and closely resembles the 'inner petal flap' of the lotus flap design. It is, however, compromised in a radical vulvectomy (**Figure 7.3.3**a,b).

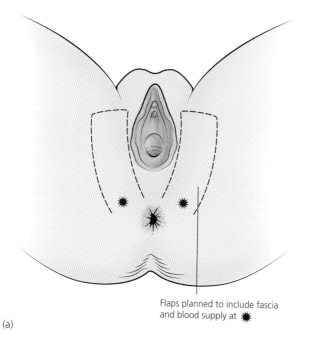

(a)

Flaps planned to include fascia and blood supply at ✳

(b)

One flap folded into neovagina and donor site closed

One flap raised

7.3.3 The Singapore flap.

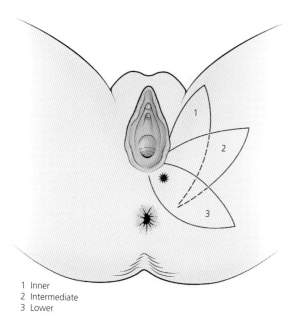

1 Inner
2 Intermediate
3 Lower

✳ The position of the arterial perforators of the deep pudendal artery

7.3.4 The lotus flaps. 1, inner; 2, intermediate; 3, lower; *, the position of the arterial perforators of the deep pudendal artery.

The lotus flap designs display versatility in filling several different defects based again on the posterior perineal blood supply. Inner, intermediate, and lower 'petals' are described (**Figure 7.3.4**). The lower lotus flap can be large, extending around the inferior gluteal fold, being useful therefore even if a radical vulvectomy has been performed. The flap base must always include the deep perforator branches of the posterior or proximal part of the perineal artery.

The V–Y fasciocutaneous pudendal thigh flap is essentially a variation on a lower petal lotus flap. It is also based on the cutaneous perforators of the deep pudendal artery but obviously includes part of the anastomosis with the inferior gluteal arterial system (**Figure 7.3.5**). A 'stepladder' V–Y advancement variation has been described in large flaps in order to avoid straight scar contracture. Their main application is in the treatment of perianal disease. Both flaps do not need undermining to allow movement but instead require 'islanding' with all margins of the flap being incised. Prior Doppler identification of perforators, although not absolutely necessary, is helpful.

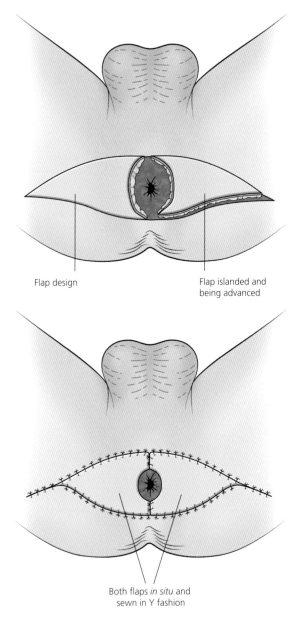

Flap design

Flap islanded and being advanced

Both flaps *in situ* and sewn in Y fashion

7.3.5 The V–Y fasciocutaneous pudendal thigh flap.

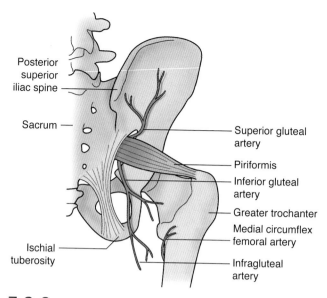

7.3.6 Posterior view of the pelvis.

Posterior superior iliac spine

Sacrum

Ischial tuberosity

Superior gluteal artery

Piriformis

Inferior gluteal artery

Greater trochanter

Medial circumflex femoral artery

Infragluteal artery

GLUTEAL FLAPS

Arterial anatomy

The superior and inferior gluteal arteries are branches of the internal iliac artery. As they leave the pelvis, they are separated by the piriformis muscle (**Figure 7.3.6**). The superior gluteal artery divides into deep, superior and inferior branches which supply the glutei and give arterial muscular perforators to the overlying skin. The inferior gluteal artery in a similar fashion supplies the glutei and the lower buttock skin becoming the infragluteal artery at the lower border of the gluteus maximus. This artery anastomises with branches of the medial femoral circumflex artery to form a subfascial plexus along the posterior thigh. This plexus is the basis of the posterior thigh fasciocutaneous flap which is described below.

Flaps based on the gluteal arterial system

CUTANEOUS

A gluteal rotation flap of skin and subcutaneous fat alone can be raised and rotated either inferiorly or superiorly (**Figure 7.3.7**). It has a limited arc and will not reach many defects. It also lacks the bulk of myocutaneous flaps.

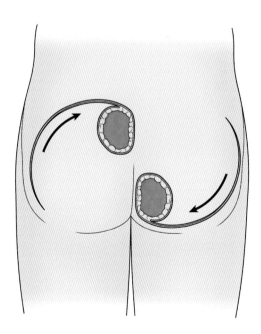

7.3.7 Gluteal rotation flaps. Alternative designs are shown for superior or inferior defects.

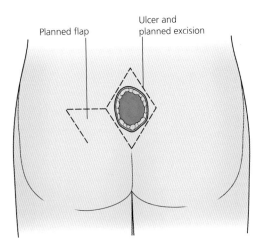

The same is true for rhomboid (Limberg) flaps (**Figure 7.3.8**).

Cutaneous flaps slowly have evolved into perforator flaps where Doppler-identified myocutaneous branches are included in the flap. Slow accurate dissection results in large flaps being raised on the perforators alone. These are called SGAP (superior gluteal arterial perforator) and IGAP (inferior gluteal arterial perforator) flaps and can be used as rotation, transposition, or even free microvascular transfer flaps.

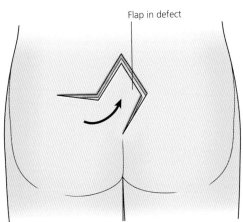

7.3.8 Limberg or rhomboid flap.

MYOCUTANEOUS

In order to increase the arc of rotation, the muscle attachments of the gluteus maximus to the iliac bone can be divided. This affects muscle function, increases blood loss, and increases operative time. Use of large gluteal myocutaneous flaps has, by and large, been superseded by perforator flap variations, such as the V–Y advancement and posterior thigh flaps, but they do have the advantage of introducing muscle bulk into a defect.

The common mistake is to plan V–Y advancement flaps too small. Used as bilateral advancement flaps with prior identification of perforators by Doppler, they are reliable and suitable for many midline perineal defects. If Doppler is unavailable they are still reliable if a wide subcutaneous base is included in these flaps and undermining is avoided (**Figure 7.3.9**). These flaps will advance further towards the midline if the gluteus maximus is divided from its iliac attachment peripherally.

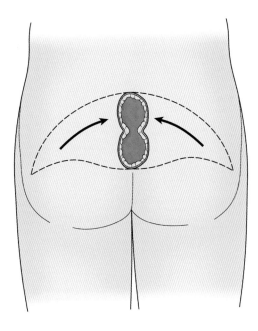

7.3.9 Large V–Y gluteal cutaneous or myocutaneous advancement flaps for midline defects.

The posterior thigh fasciocutaneous flap is a long posterior thigh flap based on the fascial plexus of the descending infragluteal artery. The fascia must be included and the flap base is bulky as it is turned to reach perineal defects. The infragluteal perforator flap overcomes this problem as it is islanded on a perforator. The main indication for the posterior thigh fasciocutaneous flap and its perforator variation is in the coverage of ischial and sacral pressure sores (**Figure 7.3.10**).

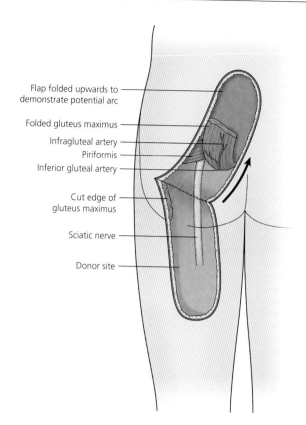

7.3.10 Posterior thigh fasciocutaneous flap.

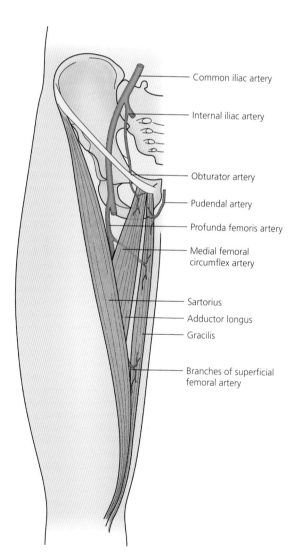

7.3.11 Arterial supply of gracilis.

GRACILIS FLAPS

Arterial anatomy

The gracilis is part of the adductor muscle group in the medial thigh. Its primary arterial supply, i.e. its dominant pedicle, arises from the medial femoral circumflex artery which is itself a branch of the profunda femoris. It enters the deep surface of the muscle at the junction of its proximal and middle thirds approximately 6–8 cm distal to the pubic tubercle, passing between adductor longus and brevis muscles. Accessory pedicles arise proximally from the terminal branches of the obturator and pudendal arteries and distally from the superficial femoral artery (**Figure 7.3.11**).

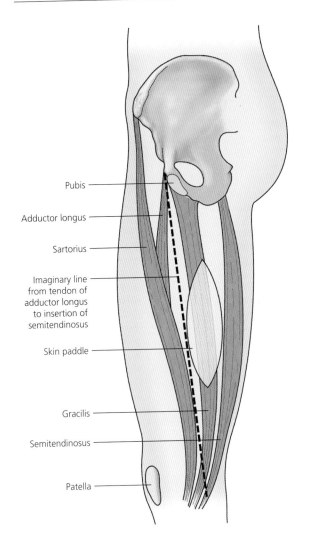

7.3.12 Medial view of the right thigh.

Pubis
Adductor longus
Sartorius
Imaginary line
from tendon of
adductor longus
to insertion of
semitendinosus
Skin paddle
Gracilis
Semitendinosus
Patella

Using the gracilis flap

It can be used bilaterally or unilaterally and can reach the groin, anterior vulva, vagina, posterior vulva, and perineum. As a myocutaneous flap, the skin paddle must be placed accurately over muscle perforators which can be identified using preoperative Doppler mapping. It must always be posterior to a line drawn from the adductor longus tendon at the pubic tubercle to the tendon of the semitendinosus (**Figure 7.3.12**) with the skin paddle directly over the muscle which may be difficult to achieve in the presence of fat or flabby thighs as in the elderly. Common causes of failure relate to a wrong location of the skin paddle, too big a skin paddle, and a twisted dominant pedicle. Safe raising of the flap should be from distal to proximal, constantly relating the skin position to the muscle, and a full dissection of the pedicle clearly identifying the medial femoral circumflex branches.

A 'short' gracilis flap has been described where the dominant vascular pedicle is divided and reliance for blood supply is placed on the proximal accessory pedicles which are branches of the obturator and pudendal arteries. It should be used with caution and a small skin paddle. It must not be used if the pelvis has been irradiated.

Gracilis advantages and disadvantages

Its main advantages lie in its ease of dissection, the absence of functional loss at the donor site, primary closure of the donor site, and its small size which allows its use in the closure of urethrocutaneous, vesicovaginal, rectovaginal, and rectocutaneous fistulae. It also usually lies outside the radiation fields if adjuvant radiotherapy has been used.

The main disadvantages are the flaps lack of bulk where defects are large, the occasionally unreliable skin paddle, and the upper inner thigh mound resulting where the transposed muscle is folded over on its proximal attachment to the pubis.

OTHER FLAPS

Rectus abdominus myocutaneous flaps

Although considered elsewhere (see Chapters 6.11 and 7.1), mention should be made of flaps based on the deep inferior epigastric arterial system. These are the workhorse flaps for large perineal and groin defects. There are three main variations, the transverse rectus abdominus myocutaneous flap (TRAM), the vertical rectus abdominus myocutaneous flap (VRAM), and the oblique rectus flap (**Figure 7.3.13**).

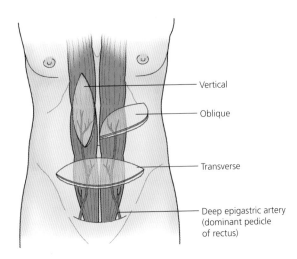

Vertical
Oblique
Transverse
Deep epigastric artery
(dominant pedicle
of rectus)

7.3.13 Varieties of rectus abdominus myocutaneous flap.

The VRAM flap is the most suitable for abdominoperineal resectional defects and may be used in conjunction with synthetic mesh pelvic floor reconstruction. The oblique rectus flap is particularly useful to cover groin defects and exposed femoral vessels or in resurfacing of the lower abdominal wall (**Figure 7.3.14**).

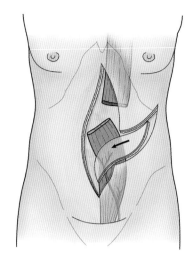

7.3.14 Oblique rectus flap (being used to fill a vertical abdominal defect).

Free microvascular transfer flaps

Finally, at the most complex and highest rung of the reconstructive ladder are 'free flaps'. These are flaps raised at a distant site, isolated on their vascular pedicle which is then divided, and then transferred to the surgical defect. The vessels, at least one artery and often two veins, are anastomosed using an operative microscope to recipient vessels. They are used in salvage situations where previous flaps have failed or in the presence of large defects where a more local or regional flaps cannot reach or fill the defect. The commonest flaps are the anterolateral thigh perforator flap or the latissimus dorsi myocutaneous flap.

FURTHER READING

Grant JCB. *An atlas of anatomy*, 6th edn. Baltimore: Williams & Wilkins, 1972.

Hurst RD, Gottlieb LJ, Crucitti P *et al.* Primary closure of complicated perineal wounds with myocutaneous and fasciocutaneous flaps after proctectomy for Crohn's disease. *Surgery* 2001; **130**: 767–72.

Saito A, Sawaizumi M, Matsumoto S, Takizawa K. Stepladder V–Y advancement medial thigh flap for the reconstruction of vulvoperineal region *Journal of Plastic, Reconstructive and Aesthetic Surgery* 2009; **62**: 196–9.

Standring S (ed.). *Gray's anatomy*, 39th edn. Philadelphia, PA: Churchill Livingstone, 2005.

Strauch B, Vasconez LO, Hall-Findlay EJ, Lee B (eds). *Grabb's encyclopedia of flaps*, 3rd edn. Torso, Pelvis, and Lower Extremities 3. Philadelphia: Lippincott, Williams and Wilkins, 2009.

Wee JT, Joseph VT. A new technique of vaginal reconstruction using neurovascular pudendal–thigh flaps: a preliminary report. *Plastic and Reconstructive Surgery* 1989; **83**: 701–9.

Yii NW, Niranjan NS. Lotus petal flap in vulvo-vaginal reconstruction. *British Journal of Plastic Surgery* 1996; **49**: 547–54.

8

Rectal prolapse

Delorme operation

DF ALTOMARE AND M RINALDI

HISTORY

Full-thickness rectal prolapse is a life-altering disability that commonly affects older people, while it is rare in childhood and younger adults. This condition is associated with a deep rectovaginal or rectovesical peritoneal pouch, laxity of the lateral ligaments, and loss of attachment of the rectum to the sacrum. Other associated conditions are perineal descent and a patulous anus. Fecal incontinence is present in 50–70 percent of patients, particularly the elderly. Surgical procedures for the treatment of rectal prolapse can be classified as plication, excision, rectopexy, and resection. All these operations may be performed via either an abdominal or a perineal approach, the latter being more suited to high-risk patients. Among perineal operations, encircling procedures (Thiersch ring and others) are not often performed in the modern era because they only offer a mechanical barrier to the prolapse and have high rates of infection and recurrence. On the other hand, perineal rectosigmoidectomy (Altemeier procedure) is a more major procedure with the potential risks of a pelvic anastomosis. The Delorme procedure was first described in 1900 by Edmond Delorme,[1] a French military surgeon. It is a relatively safe and simple perineal technique, that involves stripping the mucosa off the prolapsing segment and suture plication of the rectal muscular wall. The operation may be performed under spinal anesthesia, so it is particularly indicated in elderly or frail patients with coexisting morbidities or in patients otherwise deemed unfit for major surgery. Having initially fallen out of favor due to anecdotal reports of high recurrence and complication rates, the procedure has gained in popularity since the report by Uhlig and Sullivan.[2] The technique originally described has been modified by a number of authors to include anal sphincter repair or levatorplasty as treatment for associated fecal incontinence.

PRINCIPLES AND JUSTIFICATION

Indications and contraindications

The aim of the surgical treatment for rectal prolapse is to control (reduce or resolve) the prolapse and improve continence, as well as constipation that may result from associated obstructed defecation. Perineal procedures are particularly useful for elderly patients and for patients unsuitable for major abdominal surgery. The choice between the Delorme procedure and perineal rectosigmoidectomy is based on several elements; above all, the length of the prolapse: if the prolapsing rectal segment is shorter than 5 cm, perineal rectosigmoidectomy is difficult to perform, while the Delorme operation is indicated when the prolapse is not full thickness around the entire circumference. An internal Delorme operation may be suitable in patients with internal prolapse or rectal intussusception leading to obstructed defecation. Complete mucosectomy is difficult in patients with extensive diverticular disease, and the Delorme procedure may be contraindicated in such patients. The decision about which operation to perform in rectal prolapse must be individualized and based on provision of full and complete information on the available options to the patient, who can then make an informed decision in consultation with their surgeon. After all, the Delorme can always be repeated if a recurrence does later occur.

PREOPERATIVE

Patient evaluation

Preoperative assessment should include routine rectosigmoidoscopy to exclude coincident colorectal pathology. Anal manometry is recommended to evaluate anal sphincter function but may not always be possible in view of the prolapse. Dynamic enterocolpodefecography can provide further information about associated pelvic floor dysfunction (enterocele, rectocele, etc.) that may require simultaneous correction.

A cleansing enema (sometimes difficult because of anal incontinence) is administered on the day of the operation and prophylactic antibiotics are given (metronidazole and cephalosporin in the authors' institution). Deep venous thrombosis prophylaxis is also advisable.

Anesthesia

Delorme's procedure may be performed under general, spinal, caudal, or local anesthesia using a peripheral bilateral pudendal nerve block.

OPERATION

Patient position

Although the jackknife position is traditionally preferred in the US, most European surgeons, including the authors, favor the lithotomy position.[3] The lithotomy position facilitates exteriorization of the rectal prolapse, especially in the conscious patient, making the procedure easier for the surgeon. A Foley catheter is positioned in the bladder before surgery.

Mucosal dissection

Before starting the mucosal dissection, the rectum is exteriorized and grasped by two Babcock forceps, and the level of the mucosal incision is marked by diathermy (**Figure 8.1.1**). To facilitate the dissection and reduce bleeding a submucosal infiltration of an adrenalin solution (1/200 000) is performed. A Lone Star™ self-retaining retractor is positioned.

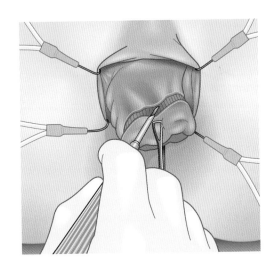

8.1.1

Starting about 1 cm proximal to the dentate line, the rectal mucosa is incised by diathermy until the muscular layer is exposed and the mucosa stripped off the underlying muscle, again by diathermy to minimize blood loss. This step of the operation is the only one that requires particular surgical skill to identify the correct plane of dissection (**Figure 8.1.2**).

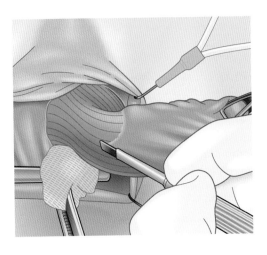

8.1.2

The mucosa is progressively dissected from the underlying muscular layer (which appears paler than the mucosa) by diathermy and using small swabs mounted on the forceps. Gentle traction of the mucosa will facilitate detachment from the underlying muscular layer. Progressive dissection of the rectal mucosa should be stopped when it cannot be pulled down any further. A mucosal cylinder several centimeters long (more than 10 cm) is usually removed. Careful hemostasis with diathermy must be achieved during this step of the procedure.

Muscle plication

The muscular layer of the rectum is then plicated using four absorbable polyglycolic sutures (3-0), one for each quadrant (**Figure 8.1.3**). Further sutures are often necessary to complete the plication between the main sutures. Each of the sutures starts from the apex of the mucosal dissection and extends down to the distal part of the dissection. When the sutures are tied the rectum will appear plicated like a concertina. Some surgeons skip this step of the procedure by directly performing coloanal mucosal anastomosis, but the authors prefer the original version of the procedure, since omission of the muscle sutures can leave a potentially contaminated dead space and increase the risk of subsequent hematoma or abscess formation.

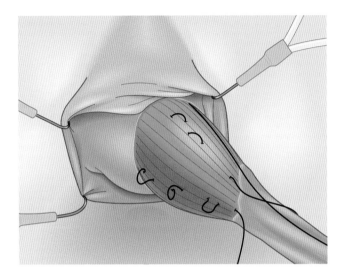

8.1.3

Coloanal anastomosis

After completion of the muscle plication, the mucosal cylinder is progressively divided, starting at the 12 o'clock position, and a mucosa-to-mucosa coloanal anastomosis suture is performed using 3-0 polyglycolic sutures (**Figure 8.1.4**). The authors suggest that it is better to partially include the underlying muscle in the mucosal suture. After the four cardinal sutures, one or two more intervening sutures can be placed to complete the coloanal anastomosis. Too many interrupted stitches or continuous suture may give rise to a postoperative stricture and should be avoided.

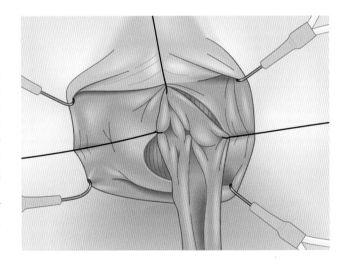

8.1.4

The final appearance of the coloanal anastomosis (**Figure 8.1.5**) shows the prolapsed reduced hemostasis has been achieved and the suture line is well above the dentate line. Endoanal placement of an absorbable hemostatic sponge may be advisable.

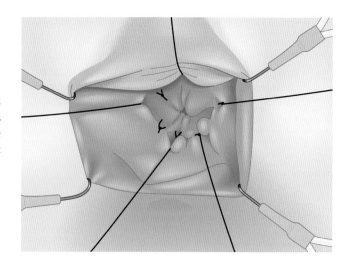

8.1.5

POSTOPERATIVE CARE

Postoperative care is usually easy because the patient has very little or no pain, and oral feeding can be resumed immediately. The urinary catheter can be removed as soon as the effect of the spinal anesthesia wears off. Antibiotic prophylaxis can usually be stopped within 24 hours in almost all cases. The patient's hospital stay is usally short and indeed the operation can be done in one-day surgery in many patients.

COMPLICATIONS

The operation is safe and serious complications are uncommon. The most frequent early complication is postoperative bleeding, which rarely requires reoperation (resuturing of the mucosa). Another described complication is immediate postoperative suture line dehiscence, with or without recurrent prolapse, often due to persistent coughing or vomiting postoperatively. This requires immediate resuturing. Perineal cellulitis may also arise and short-term oral antibiotics are generally used to resolve the problem. Urinary retention is another common postoperative problem, most often related to the spinal anesthesia.

Possible late complications include mucosal prolapse, successfully treated by rubber band ligation, and suture line stricture that can usually be resolved by mechanical dilation.

A rare complication is acute ischemic proctitis, described in a recent report one month after a Delorme operation, that required anterior rectal resection and a transverse colostomy diversion.[4]

OUTCOME

Data in the literature report mortality rates ranging from 0 to 4 percent and recurrence rates from 4 to 38 percent, but in many series the real incidence of recurrence or residual functional disorders is poorly documented. This is because long-term follow-up is rarely achievable due to the older age of patients. Good results in terms of improved continence (70 percent) are reported in patients treated with the Delorme operation and sphincteroplasty, but many other series have shown an improved continence even without sphincteroplasty.[5]

The largest randomized controlled trial to compare the Delorme operation with the Altmeier operation and abdominal rectopexy (the PROSPER trial) has recently reported no significant difference in recurrence between the Altemeier operation (24%) and the Delorme Operation (31%) (p=0.4).[6] These data confirm the conclusion of a recent Cochrane review[7] that there is no evidence to support preference for one operative approach over the other, thus the treatment should be decided on the basis of the patient's informed opinion and surgeon's preference.

REFERENCES

1. Delorme E. Sur le traitement des prolapsus du rectum totaux par l'excision de la muquese rectale ou rectal-colique. *Bulletin et Mémoires de la Société des Chirurgiens de Paris* 1900; **26**: 499–518.
2. Uhlig BE, Sullivan ES. The modified Delorme operation: its place in surgical treatment for massive rectal prolapse. *Diseases of the Colon and Rectum* 1979; **22**: 513–21.
3. Binda GA, Serventi A. Perineal approach to external rectal prolapse: the Delorme procedure. In: Altomare DF, Pucciani F (eds). *Rectal prolapse. Diagnosis and clinical management.* Berlin: Springer-Verlag, 2008: 89–95.
4. De Nardi P, Osman N, Viola M, Staudacher C. Ischemic proctitis following Delorme procedure for external ractal prolapse. *Techniques in Coloproctology* 2006; **10**: 253–5.
5. Wexner SD, Khanna AA. Surgery of rectal prolapse: functional outcome from the perineal approach. An overview. In: Altomare DF, Pucciani F (eds). *Rectal prolapse. Diagnosis and clinical management.* Berlin: Springer-Verlag, 2008: 103–6.
6. Senapti A, Gray RG, Middleton LJ *et al.* PROSPER: a randomised comparison of surgical treatments for rectal prolapse *Colorectal Disease* 2013 Jul; 15(7): 858–68.
7. Bachoo P, Brazelli M, Grant A. Surgery for complete rectal prolapse in adults. *Cochrane Database of Systematic Reviews* 2000; (**2**): CD001758; update in *Cochrane Database of Systematic Reviews* 2008; (**4**): CD001758.

Perineal rectosigmoidectomy

J GRAHAM WILLIAMS AND ROBERT D MADOFF

HISTORY

The first description of perineal rectosigmoidectomy was provided by Miculicz. The first operation he reported was for an incarcerated, gangrenous prolapse, but he also treated five other patients with uncomplicated prolapse by perineal amputation.[1] The operation was popular during the first half of the twentieth century, but a recurrence rate of over 50 percent reported from St Mark's Hospital lessened surgeons' enthusiasm for this procedure.[1] Altemeier published a large series of patients with rectal prolapse treated by perineal rectosigmoidectomy with few recurrences.[2] This revived interest in the procedure and earned him eponymous recognition. There have been a number of reported series of patients treated with this operation with variable recurrence rates and low morbidity.[3] The role of concomitant levatoroplasty has not been the subject of a randomized trial, although observational studies suggest a role in improving postoperative continence.[4]

PRINCIPLES AND JUSTIFICATION

The principle of the operation is to excise the prolapsing segment of rectum from below, thus avoiding the morbidity of a transabdominal approach. However, the operation should involve more than merely amputating the prolapsed rectum, and mobilization and excision of redundant pelvic large bowel is essential to avoid recurrence. Circumferential and full-thickness rectal prolapse is required for the operation to be technically feasible.

Perineal rectosigmoidectomy is associated with low morbidity and mortality rates and traditionally has been preferred for elderly or high-risk patients. While the 'minimally invasive' nature of the operation makes it an attractive alternative to transabdominal repair for fit patients with prolapse, the recurrence rate is higher and the long-term functional consequences of resection of the rectal reservoir and its replacement by less compliant proximal colon are poorly understood. Furthermore, younger patients may experience higher recurrence rates with time, simply as a consequence of their longer life expectancy.

Unlike most abdominal approaches, perineal rectosigmoidectomy avoids dissection at the pelvic brim and hence avoids the potential for hypogastric nerve damage and presacral hemorrhage. The operation lends itself to the treatment of incarcerated or gangrenous prolapse. Pelvic floor repair is easily performed during rectal excision, which is not the case with Delorme's operation (mucosectomy and rectal wall plication, see Chapter 8.1). Care should be exercised in patients who have undergone previous sigmoid or rectal excision as the proximal blood supply to the rectum may be compromised. Under these circumstances, perineal rectosigmoidectomy may lead to an ischemic segment of rectum when the distal rectal blood supply is divided.

PREOPERATIVE PREPARATION

The diagnosis of full-thickness rectal prolapse should be obvious from the history and clinical examination. Clues to the presence of a rectal prolapse include a patulous anus with mucus staining of the anal margin. It is often difficult to demonstrate a prolapse with the patient in the left lateral position or the prone position, but the prolapse can usually be demonstrated by asking the patient to strain seated on a commode. Full-thickness rectal prolapse is differentiated from mucosal prolapse by the presence of concentric rather than radial mucosal folds, and by the presence of a palpable sulcus between prolapse and the anal margin.

Preoperative assessment of the colon by barium enema, colonoscopy or computed tomography (CT) colonography is required to exclude an associated proximal lesion. Colonoscopy can be performed intraoperatively if required, but this approach requires a full bowel preparation.

Defecography is useful when the diagnosis is in doubt and to demonstrate associated abnormalities, such as enterocele or pelvic organ prolapse. Anal manometry provides an objective measure of sphincter function if resection rectopexy is being considered, and endoanal ultrasound can be used to identify sphincter injury. Colonic transit studies are mandatory if subtotal or total abdominal colectomy is being considered in constipated patients.

Full mechanical bowel preparation is unnecessary and especially likely to be detrimental to elderly or infirm patients. A phosphate enema can be administered to clear the rectum and make manipulation easier. Patients should be fitted with sequential compression stockings and commenced on low-molecular weight heparin prior to surgery to reduce the risk of venous thromboembolism. A single dose of antibiotics is given intravenously within 1 hour of surgery. The bladder is emptied with a Foley catheter, and the perineum is sterilely prepped and draped.

Anesthesia

Perineal rectosigmoidectomy can be performed under general or regional anesthesia. Regional neural block by spinal or epidural anesthesia is appropriate for elderly or frail, high-risk patients, who are the majority of patients suitable for this approach.

OPERATION

Position of the patient

The operation can be performed in the lithotomy or the prone jack-knife position. The prone jack-knife position has several major advantages over the lithotomy position. First, it is easier to position assistants around the operating table and train junior surgeons to perform the procedure as all the surgical team have an excellent view of the operative field. Second, bleeding is reduced because the perineum is uppermost and venous congestion less. Third, it is easier to achieve good illumination within the pelvis.

Our preference is for the prone position. The patient is turned onto a suitable large hip roll to flex the hips. The chest is supported to allow the abdomen to hang free. The knees are padded and slightly flexed with the feet supported on pillows. The arms are brought forward and placed on a padded arm board. The head is slightly flexed and turned to one side on a padded ring. The buttocks are taped apart with wide adhesive tape. The operating table is slightly broken at the hips and placed with a head-down tilt (**Figure 8.2.1**).

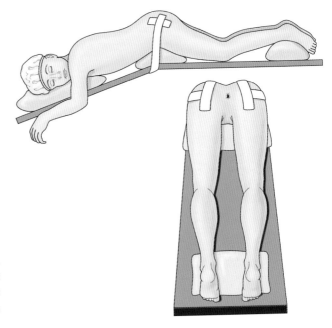

8.2.1

Incision

A Lone Star™ self-retaining ring retractor is useful to efface the anal canal and improve exposure and access. The ring is placed over the anus against the buttocks and eight hooks are inserted into the perianal skin radially, 1 cm from the anal margin and then inserted into the grooves on the ring on a degree of tension. The rectal prolapse is delivered from the pelvis by gentle traction on the rectal wall grasped by a Babcock forceps passed through the anus. Some surgeons prefer to infiltrate the lower rectal wall with 1:200 000 adrenaline solution in 0.25 percent bupivicaine prior to incision. Initial scoring of the mucosa with electrocautery 1.5 cm proximal to the dentate line is helpful in keeping the incision at the right level around the whole circumference of the rectum. An incision is made at this level through all the layers of the rectal wall using electrocautery. The wall can be thicker than anticipated and the incision is deepened until the bowel wall of the inner loop of the prolapse is identified. The incision is then continued circumferentially until the entire circumference of the outer bowel ring has been divided (**Figure 8.2.2**).

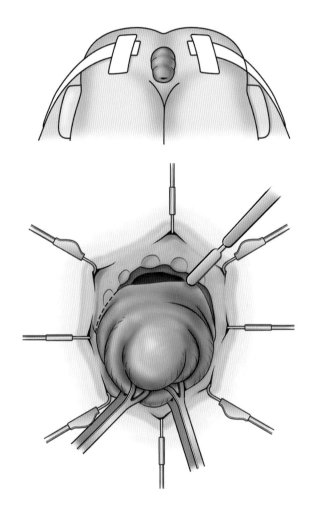

8.2.2

Mobilization of the rectum and sigmoid

Rectal mobilization is performed by dividing the tissues of the mesorectum, working round the full circumference of the prolapse. A small right-angle clamp such as a Lahey clamp is useful. Strands of mesorectal tissue are elevated and either divided with electrocautery (if thin) or clamped, divided and ligated with fine absorbable suture material (**Figure 8.2.3**). A vessel sealing device such as the small jaw Ligasure® is handy for dividing the mesentery and frequently saves time. Care must be taken to achieve accurate hemostasis as divided structures will quickly retract out of sight into the pelvis and produce troublesome bleeding. During the early stage of this dissection, the pouch of Douglas is usually encountered anteriorly. It is helpful to open the peritoneum at this stage as it improves access to the pelvis and aids mobilization of the rectum and distal sigmoid colon. Dissection continues cephalad, dividing the mesorectal tissues close to the rectal wall.

A surprising length of bowel may be mobilized as the dissection proceeds (30 cm or more). The mobilization is complete when more than gentle retraction is required to pull down more colon and it is possible to palpate a straight sigmoid colon through the opened peritoneum anteriorly.

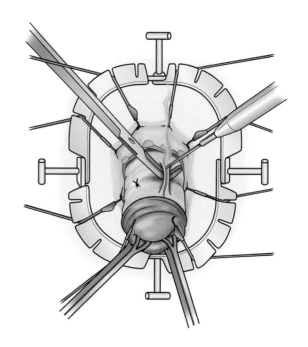

8.2.3

Levatoroplasty

Levatoroplasty is easily performed during perineal rectosigmoidectomy. While posterior levatoroplasty most replicates the normal anatomy, repair can be anterior, posterior or both. Levatoroplasty is thought to have a beneficial effect on postoperative continence and, by supporting the repair and narrowing the pelvic floor, may help prevent recurrence. The levator muscles can be directly visualized at the levator hiatus. Anterior levatoroplasty is performed with the aid of narrow retractors pulling the outer tube of the distal rectum and the perineal body anteriorly while simultaneously drawing the fully mobilized rectum and distal sigmoid posteriorly (**Figure 8.2.4**). Care should be taken not to confuse the external sphincter for levator muscle. A posterior levatoroplasty can be performed by drawing the mobilized bowel anteriorly and the distal rectal segment posteriorly. Levatoroplasty is performed by placing a series of interrupted 2-0 polypropylene or polydioxanone sutures through the levator ani muscle on each side and tying the sutures sequentially to create a hiatus that is snug but still allows a finger to be passed into the pelvis alongside the rectum without difficulty.

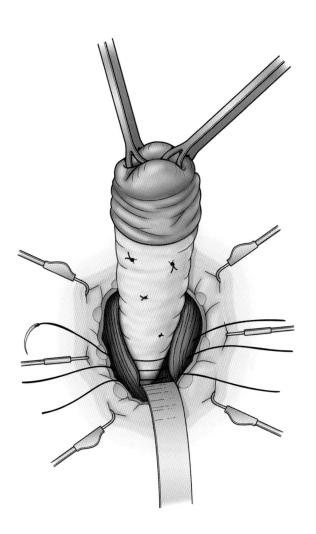 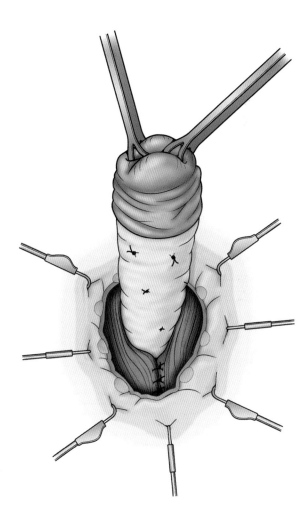

8.2.4

Anastomosis

The final phase of the operation is to resect the mobilized rectum and distal sigmoid and perform an anastomosis. The level of the proximal resection should be at the limit of mobilization to maintain a good blood supply and it is important that the remaining dissection of the mesorectum and mesocolon stops at the level of the anastomosis.

A small incision is made into the proximal intestine at the site of resection and a stay suture of 3-0 polyglactin is placed through the full thickness of the cut edge of the rectum and the proximal intestinal wall (**Figure 8.2.5**). This is tied and tagged and the incision in the proximal colon is extended to one side for one-quarter of the circumference.

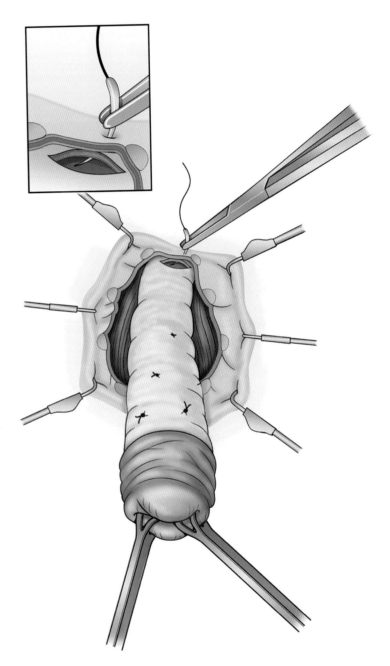

8.2.5

A further stay suture is placed at one end of this incision through both edges of the bowel and tied and tagged. A series of further full-thickness polyglactin sutures are inserted between the two sutures to complete the anastomosis in the first quadrant (**Figure 8.2.6**). There is usually a significant size discrepancy as the proximal colon is much narrower and the anastomosis has to be tailored appropriately such that there are no gaps. This is best done by splitting the difference between sutures to ensure even spacing.

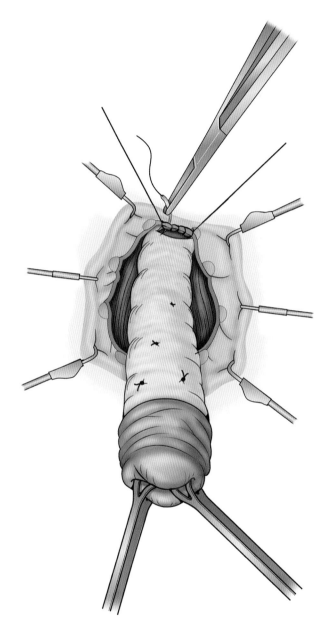

8.2.6

The next quadrant of proximal colon is incised, and a further stay suture is inserted. The anastomosis in this quadrant is completed as previously. The procedure is repeated for the remaining circumference of the colon. It is important to perform the anastomosis in segments, because the proximal intestine may retract into the pelvis if the colon is simply divided at the limit of dissection before stay sutures are inserted. When complete, the anastomosis can be inspected with a suitable anal retractor, to check for gaps or bleeding points. The anastomosis retracts into the pelvis once the Lone-Star™ retractor is removed (**Figure 8.2.7**).

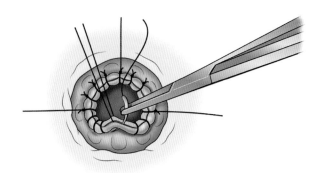

8.2.7

The anastomosis can be performed with a circular stapler. The anvil is passed into the proximal intestine and a purse-string suture is placed and tied round the shaft. A second purse-string suture is placed in the cut edge of the distal rectum and tied. The instrument is closed within the pelvis and fired. The stapled approach is often more difficult than a sutured anastomosis due to the size discrepancy between the proximal colon and distal rectum. In addition, it is difficult to perform a stapled anastomosis when a levatoroplasty has been performed.

POSTOPERATIVE CARE

The postoperative course after a perineal rectosigmoidectomy is usually very smooth. Patients experience minimal pain, which is usually easily controlled with a mild oral opiate. Oral intake can commence as soon as the patient has recovered from the anesthetic. Bowel function usually returns within a few days of the operation. Most patients will be ready for discharge home after 3–4 days. Potential complications include anastomotic bleeding, which is usually easily controlled by suture ligation of the bleeding point. Anastomotic breakdown and pelvic sepsis is unusual, which is surprising, given that the anastomosis is very low in the rectum. An anastomotic stricture is unusual and can be dealt with by gentle dilatation.

OUTCOME

The recurrence rate after perineal rectosigmoidectomy is dependent on the length of follow-up. Reported rates are variable, of the order of 5–25 percent, and this should be borne in mind when counseling younger patients as to the merits and drawbacks of this procedure.[3, 4, 5] Recurrence probably reflects inadequate mobilization and resection of the distal sigmoid. Care should be taken to ensure that all redundant pelvic colon has been dealt with during mobilization and resection should be performed such that the anastomosis is performed within the rectum and not at the surface of the perineum. Improvement in fecal incontinence is less likely following perineal rectosigmoidectomy than following an abdominal repair of rectal prolapse. Concomitant levatoroplasty can help improve anal control, with some patients regaining full continence.

REFERENCES

1. Madoff RD, Mellgren A. One hundred years of rectal prolapse surgery. *Diseases of the Colon and Rectum* 1999; **42**: 441–50.
2. Altemeier WA, Culbertson WR, Schowengerdt C, Hunt J. Nineteen years' experience with the one-stage perineal repair of rectal prolapse. *Annals of Surgery* 1971; **173**: 993–1006.
3. Kim DS, Tsang CB, Wong WD *et al*. Complete rectal prolapse: evolution of management and results. *Diseases of the Colon and Rectum* 1999; **42**: 460–6; discussion 466–9.
4. Chun SW, Pikarsky AJ, You SY *et al*. Perineal rectosigmoidectomy for rectal prolapse: role of levatoroplasty. *Techniques in Coloproctology* 2004; **8**: 3–9.
5. Altomare DF, Binda G, Ganio E *et al*. Long-term outcome of Altemeier's procedure for rectal prolapse. *Diseases of the Colon and Rectum* 2009; **52**: 698–703.

Abdominal rectopexy – open

J GRAHAM WILLIAMS AND ROBERT D MADOFF

HISTORY

Abdominal prolapse repairs were first described at the turn of the twentieth century.[1] Pemberton and Stalker advocated anterior sigmoid fixation following posterior rectal mobilization in 1939.[2] Direct suture fixation of the mobilized rectum to the sacrum was first described by Cutait in 1959.[3] Numerous rectal fixation procedures have since been described, with and without foreign material, all of which emphasize the importance of adequate rectal mobilization. In 1969, Frykman and Goldberg combined rectal mobilization with both suture rectopexy and sigmoid resection for the treatment of rectal prolapse.[4] This forms the basis of the operation described in this chapter.

PRINCIPLES AND JUSTIFICATION

Transabdominal fixation procedures for rectal prolapse are widely popular as they retain the rectum and return it to its rightful place in the pelvis. These techniques involve securing the mobilized rectum to the presacral fascia, with or without foreign material. Older versions of this approach included the anterior sling rectopexy (Ripstein's operation) and the posterior sling rectopexy (Wells' operation). These approaches fell out of favor because of concerns about troublesome constipation and infection of the foreign material. However, in more recent times there has been resurgence in interest in suspension/fixation operations with the description of the lateral mesh rectopexy originally popularized by Loygue et al.[5] and now advocated using a laparoscopic approach by d'Hoore (see Chapter 8.6). Suture fixation of the rectum can be combined with sigmoid resection. The avoidance of foreign material for fixation lessens the risks and consequences of postoperative infection, particularly if colonic resection is included in the procedure.

The original rationale for resection in addition to fixation was to prevent early recurrence by suspending the left colon from the splenocolic ligament. However, this is unlikely to be effective as the ligament is very variable and often nonexistent in patients with functional bowel disorders. Concomitant sigmoid resection does eliminate the risk of volvulus of the characteristically redundant sigmoid colon that becomes even longer following rectal mobilization. Furthermore, resection of redundant sigmoid colon combined with rectopexy should, in theory, alleviate postoperative constipation, although there are conflicting data in support of this assertion. The extent of rectal mobilization is controversial. Many surgeons advocate full mobilization of the rectum to the pelvic floor. However, there are data to indicate that while this is associated with a lower recurrence rate than when partial mobilization is performed (preserving the lateral support to the rectum), postoperative constipation is more of a problem, presumably as a consequence of denervation of the rectum during the mobilization.[6] Finally, the combination of subtotal colectomy with rectopexy has been successful in treating patients suffering from severe slow transit constipation and rectal prolapse. Such patients are unusual and great care must be taken in establishing slow colonic transit and excluding significant sphincter weakness.

PREOPERATIVE ASSESSMENT AND PREPARATION

Preoperative assessment and preparation are similar as for perineal rectosigmoidectomy (see Chapter 8.2).

OPERATION

Patient position

The patient is placed in the modified Lloyd-Davies position, using Yellowfin™ stirrups or a suitable alternative. These are easily adjustable and the foot rests relieve pressure on the calves and perineal nerve. Pneumatic compression boots are routinely used to further reduce the risk of venous thrombosis. The foot table is removed or dropped to facilitate access for an assistant (**Figure 8.3.1**).

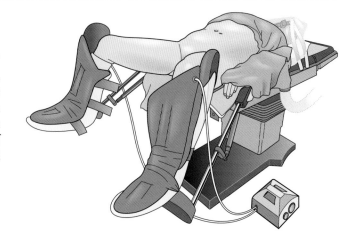

8.3.1

Incision

While both lower midline and Pfannenstiel incisions are acceptable, the latter should be avoided in obese patients where exposure may prove difficult (**Figure 8.3.2**).

A self-retaining retractor is inserted and the pelvis is explored. A steep head down tilt aids exposure and the small bowel and proximal colon are lifted out of the pelvis and packed away in the upper abdomen.

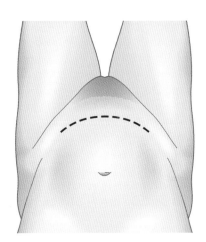

8.3.2

Rectosigmoid mobilization

Dissection commences by mobilizing the distal sigmoid colon along the line of Toldt with electrocautery or scissors. The rectosigmoid junction is mobilized to the right. The pelvic nerve plexus should be identified at the pelvic brim and the dissection kept anterior to these nerves. The incision is continued in the anatomic plane between the fascia propria of the mesorectum and the parietal endopelvic fascia. The correct plane is composed of loose areolar tissue and should be largely avascular. The rectosigmoid junction is then retracted to the left and the peritoneal reflection is incised to enter the presacral plane from the right, again taking care to identify and preserve the pelvic nerve plexus. Throughout the dissection, care should be taken to preserve the ureters on both sides and the gonadal vessels on the left (**Fig 8.3.3**).

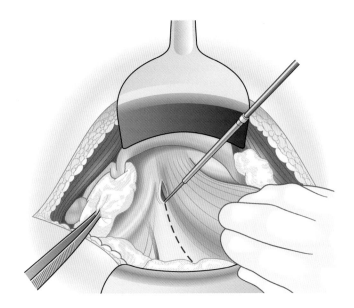

8.3.3

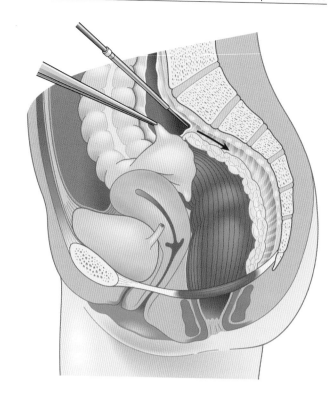

Once the presacral plane is entered at the sacral promontory, posterior mobilization in the avascular presacral (total mesorectal excision) plane is completed under direct vision, dividing the loose areolar tissue with scissors or electrocautery. The dissection is facilitated by insertion of a retractor, such as a Harrington or long St Mark's Lloyd-Davies, behind the mesorectum. Waldeyer's fascia is divided and posterior mobilization continues to the pelvic floor (**Fig 8.3.4**).

8.3.4

Anterior dissection is performed by retracting the uterus anteriorly with a suitable pelvic retractor and incising the pouch of Douglas. This peritoneal incision is carried laterally on either side to meet the previous posterior dissection. Our routine anterior dissection does not extend beyond the upper one-third of the rectovaginal septum in women or below the top of the seminal vesicles in men. Division of the 'lateral ligaments' can be associated with constipation, so we leave these intact. We specifically avoid anterolateral dissection in men to minimize the risk of parasympathetic nerve injury and erectile dysfunction (**Figure 8.3.5**).

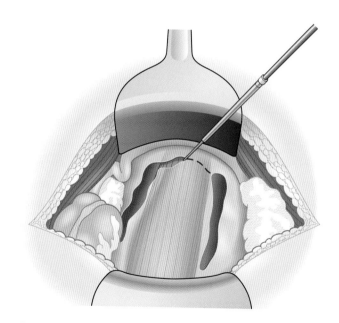

8.3.5

The mobilized rectum is then fixed to the presacral fascia with non-absorbable sutures. We prefer 0 polypropylene, on a 40 mm half-curved round body needle. Horizontal mattress sutures are used, taking a generous bite of the mesorectum immediately adjacent to but strictly avoiding the rectum. The second bite is taken through the presacral fascia in the upper sacral hollow of S2 or S3. This should be just off the midline to avoid the presacral artery, and not too far laterally to avoid the venous plexus around the sacral foramina. The needle then passes back through the mesorectum roughly 1 cm from the original point of insertion (**Figure 8.3.6**).

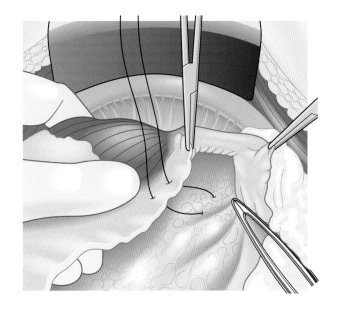

8.3.6

We utilize two sutures for fixation, both on the same side of the rectum, the second placed cephalad to the first. The sutures are tagged as they are inserted and are tied only after the final position of the rectum has been confirmed to be satisfactory. The rectum should be on gentle stretch, without laxity caudad to the fixation sutures (**Figure 8.3.7**).

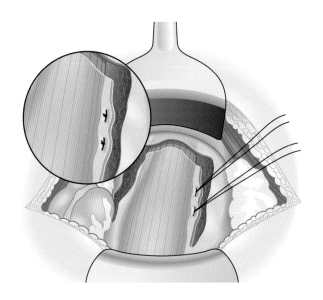

8.3.7

SIGMOID RESECTION

Where required, a sigmoid resection is performed to remove the redundant sigmoid colon. We preserve the inferior mesenteric and superior rectal vessels to maintain good blood supply to the rectum and lessen the risk of anastomotic breakdown. A hand-sewn anastomosis performed at a comfortable level using peritonealized upper rectum (for technique, see Chapter 1.8). Similarly, if total or subtotal colectomy is performed, the whole of the rectum should be retained with an ileorectal or ileosigmoid anastomosis. A stapled anastomosis can also be performed, but care must be taken not to tear the rectal wall as the instrument is passed up the mobilized rectum. When performing a resection, we do not tie the rectopexy sutures until the anastomosis is complete. Tying the rectopexy sutures first can hamper access to the rectal side of the anastomosis and make anastomotic suture placement difficult.

POSTOPERATIVE CARE

The orogastric tube is removed after extubation. The patient is mobilized as soon as possible and certainly by postoperative day 1. Either patient-controlled analgesia or an epidural catheter is acceptable. Oral fluids and diet are introduced early as tolerated by the patient and the intravenous infusion removed as soon as the patient has an adequate oral fluid intake. No postoperative antibiotics are used.

OUTCOME

The recurrence rate for abdominal rectopexy is accepted to be lower than for perineal procedures and is usually less than 10 percent.[7, 8] The recurrence rate is influenced by the adequacy and the length of follow-up. Concomitant sigmoid resection does not appear to influence the recurrence rate but may influence incidence of postoperative constipation. In a University of Minnesota series, 70 percent of severely constipated patients with rectal prolapse improved following rectopexy and subtotal colectomy,[9] but there is a significant risk of incontinence when sphincter function is poor.

Restoration of continence is reported in 50–90 percent of incontinent patients who undergo rectopexy. These widely variable results reflect both the degree of underlying sphincter dysfunction and the stringency of patient follow-up.

REFERENCES

1. Madoff RD, Mellgren A. One hundred years of rectal prolapse surgery. *Diseases of the Colon and Rectum* 1999; **42**: 441–50.
2. Pemberton J, Stalker L. Surgical treatment of complete rectal prolapse. *Annals of Surgery* 1939; **109**: 799–808.
3. Cutait D. Sacro-promontory fixation of the rectum for complete rectal prolapse. *Proceedings of the Royal Society of Medicine* 1951; **52** (Suppl.): 105.
4. Frykman HM, Goldberg SM. The surgical treatment of rectal procidentia. *Surgery, Gynecology and Obstetrics* 1969; **129**: 1225–30.
5. Loygue J, Nordlinger B, Cunci O *et al*. Rectopexy to the promontory for the treatment of rectal prolapse. Report of 257 cases. *Diseases of the Colon and Rectum* 1984; **27**: 356–9.
6. Speakman CT, Madden MV, Nicholls RJ, Kamm MA. Lateral ligament division during rectopexy causes constipation but prevents recurrence: results of a prospective randomized study. *British Journal of Surgery* 1991; **78**: 1431–3.
7. Kim DS, Tsang CB, Wong WD *et al*. Complete rectal prolapse: evolution of management and results. *Diseases of the Colon and Rectum* 1999; **42**: 460–6; discussion 466–9.
8. Raftopoulos Y, Senagore AJ, Di Giuro G, Bergamaschi R. Recurrence rates after abdominal surgery from complete rectal prolapse: a multicentre pooled analysis of 643 individual patient data. *Diseases of the Colon and Rectum* 2005; **48**: 1200–6.
9. Madoff RD, Williams JG, Wong WD *et al*. Long-term functional results of colon resection and rectopexy for overt rectal prolapse. *American Journal of Gastroenterology* 1992; **87**: 101–4.

Abdominal rectopexy – laparoscopic

ANDREW RL STEVENSON

PRINCIPLES AND JUSTIFICATION

While multiple approaches and operations have been devised over the years for the treatment of rectal prolapse, it is generally accepted that the abdominal approach has a lower recurrence and improved function when compared with the perineal repairs. However, as the abdominal approach is more physiologically demanding for the patient, this requires careful selection of patient suitability for a major abdominal procedure. Laparoscopy is less invasive than traditional open abdominal repair and so may extend the suitability of abdominal approach to the more elderly and debilitated patients that would otherwise have been deemed only suitable for a perineal approach.

When considering the appropriate operation for your patient with rectal prolapse, one needs to consider the expected recurrence as well as the functional outcome. This includes consideration for whether or not the patient has constipation or fecal incontinence, or both. This may provide some guidance as to whether or not a sigmoid resection (high anterior resection) is combined with the rectopexy. This obviously increases the potential risks and morbidity associated with any colonic or rectal anastomosis. Although uncommon, the risk of anastomotic complications needs to be weighed up against the potential for improved function with lower levels of constipation and improved continence when compared with less extensive rectal prolapse repairs, such as mesh or suture rectopexy. The resection rectopexy may be generally regarded as the benchmark in terms of rectal prolapse recurrence, as well as offering good functional outcome with low rate of constipation and improved levels of continence. This chapter outlines the general principles and highlights some of the techniques to perform a laparoscopic resection rectopexy. The steps for resection can be omitted in patients in whom a suture rectopexy alone is desired. In this case, set-up and port positions are identical, apart from the 12 mm hypogastric port which is no longer needed.

PREOPERATIVE

Patient status

Laparoscopic surgery has become widely applied to almost all aspects of colorectal surgery. Careful patient selection for laparoscopy is particularly important when still on the learning curve for any new procedure or skill. The patient should be generally fit to undergo general anesthesia and without prohibitive intra-abdominal adhesions. However, even though a patient may have had multiple laparotomies in the past, it is generally found that those patients that present with full-thickness rectal prolapse often have very few adhesions. As such, it may still be worth an initial inspection or laparoscopy before deciding the patient is not suitable because of expected adhesions.

Specific risks

Detailed preoperative discussion with the patient should include the risks associated with general anesthesia and laparoscopy. Specific complications, such as anastomotic leakage (0–5 percent), hemorrhage (2 percent), and infection should also be discussed along with expected change in bowel function. Invariably, bowel function is more frequent and may initially have impairment of continence, but should be expected to improve with time. Particularly in male patients, careful discussion is required regarding the risks of pelvic nerve injury, retrograde ejaculation, impotence, or bladder dysfunction. These complications should be uncommon but rates vary according to surgeon experience.

Investigations

As the majority of patients with rectal prolapse present with some form of bowel dysfunction or fecal incontinence, preoperative assessment including anorectal physiology, pudendal nerve studies, and endoanal ultrasound can be useful. This may demonstrate concomitant sphincter defect that may require future repair. Similarly, profound neuropathy, multiple defects in the internal sphincter, or profoundly low resting pressure may indicate the need for further procedures after prolapse repair, such as sacral nerve stimulation. Having such information preoperatively can allow the surgeon to discuss the expected functional outcome with the patient and so prepare the patient for the possibility of other procedures further down the track.

Defecating proctogram can be useful for patients with early full-thickness prolapse, suspected rectal intussusception, or solitary rectal ulcer syndrome. These patients can also benefit from resection rectopexy if their symptoms warrant intervention and are not improved with conservative measures. Nuclear colonic transit studies may be indicated if there is a history of severe constipation. Pan-colonic dysmotility may indicate a more extensive subtotal colectomy is warranted in patients that otherwise have normal sensation and normal continence.

General patient considerations and investigations may depend on comorbidities, such as diabetes, hypertension, and cardiopulmonary problems. A detailed history of any previous bowel resection or pelvic surgery must be obtained as such information may alter the decision to perform the resection in combination with the rectopexy.

Bowel preparation

There is currently much debate regarding the type and extent of mechanical bowel preparation that may be required prior to colorectal surgery. If a resection is not planned with the rectopexy, an enema on the morning of the operation is usually sufficient. This may be combined with a diet of clear fluids for 24 hours prior to the operation. This may be considered sufficient for many surgeons, even with a resection. However, it is still quite widely accepted to perform routine complete bowel preparation in a routine manner.

Prophylactic antibiotics are routinely given 1 hour prior, or on induction, such as a second generation cephalosporin (assuming no allergies).

An orogastric tube may be placed at the time of surgery if there is a distended stomach noted at laparoscopy. Decompression may help to keep the omentum and small bowel out of the field of view when performing the laparoscopic mobilization. The orogastric tube can then be removed at the end of the procedure.

ANESTHESIA

A general anesthetic is required to perform laparoscopy. An epidural catheter is not required to supplement general anesthesia nor to provide postoperative analgesia.

As this is a minimally invasive procedure, simple analgesics or patient-controlled analgesia is generally all that is required. A Foley urethral catheter is inserted into the bladder to facilitate the view in the pelvis.

OPERATION

Position of patient

For laparoscopic resection rectopexy, the patient is placed in the modified lithotomy position with the legs supported by Allen stirrups (**Figure 8.4.1**). A non-slip 'jelly' mattress can be used to reduce any patient movement when the table is tilted or rolled to one side. Alternatively, a beanbag can be wrapped around the patient's shoulders and sides before applying vacuum suction.

The right arm needs to be held in by the side, either with a pillowcase or towel, or using the beanbag. The left arm may remain out for intravenous access by the anesthetist. However, careful attention needs to be observed of any pressure areas, such as the brachial plexus, elbow, and wrist.

Both the surgeon (S) and the assistant (A) stand on the patient's right side. The scrub nurse (N), or second assistant (if available – but not necessary), can be positioned between the patient's legs. Only one monitor is required, positioned on the patient's left side. Ideally, this should now be a flat screen monitor, on a separate arm to allow easy movement from the patient's left shoulder and then down towards the

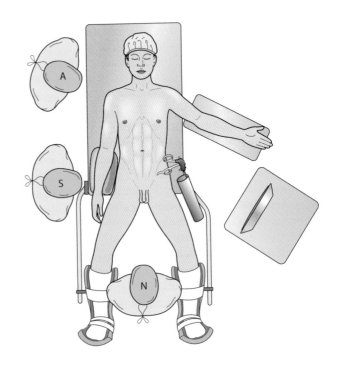

8.4.1

pelvis. In order to improve access and movement around the operating table, care should be taken to have all of the laparoscopic leads, electrocautery and energy source leads all leading off in one direction.

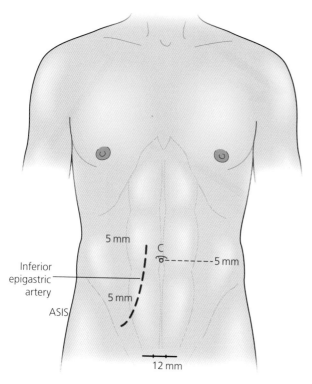

8.4.2

Mobilize left colon

A lateral to medial approach to mobilizing the left colon is the preferred method of left colon mobilization in our hospital. This is a similar approach as to open surgery, which usually allows surgeons to be familiar with the planes of dissection. With the operating table and patient rolled towards the surgeon (left side up), the sigmoid colon is mobilized by freeing any congenital or inflammatory attachments to the left pelvic and abdominal side wall. This is achieved by grasping the colon or appendix epiploica with the surgeon's graspers (S_{LEFT}) through the right upper quadrant port. Countertraction is then provided by another 5 mm grasper through the left flank port, held by the assistant's left hand (A). This then exposes the line of dissection along the left peritoneal reflection. The rectosigmoid junction is retracted to the right and mobilized sufficiently to the right to visualize the gonadal vessels and left ureter. Great care must be taken during this time to minimize the chance of inadvertent injury to these structures, either by direct contact or lateral thermal spread from the energy source. The left ureter should be found in a horizontal position as a reference to establish the correct 'horizon' and camera orientation (**Figure 8.4.3**).

Position of ports

Wherever possible, it is the preference of the author to use 5 mm ports, including the camera port. This requires a good quality 5 mm laparoscope (0° and 30°) to be available. A 5 mm port can then be placed at the umbilicus, at the very base of the cicatrix which further improves cosmesis, with less pain and less chance of port site hernia.

A 5 mm optical port is inserted in the right upper quadrant in the anterior auxiliary line, using low insufflation of CO_2 (3 liters/minute). This should be away from any previous incisions and just above the level of the midabdomen (in the anterior axiliary line). After pneumoperitoneum has been achieved, the 5 mm port can be inserted at the base of the umbilicus, which will then serve as the main camera port. The main operating port for the right-handed surgeon (S_{RIGHT}) will be the right iliac fossa, level with the anterior superior iliac spine (ASIS) and just lateral to the inferior epigastric vessels. The main port for the assistant surgeon (A) will be in the left flank, level with the umbilicus but right out laterally at the anterior auxiliary line. Once the operating table is rolled towards the surgeon, this port on the left side is easily reached (even by the shortest surgeon, in the largest patient). Finally, a 12 mm port can be placed where a small low Pfannenstiel incision can be planned for specimen extraction. Often, this can be below the hairline and so provide excellent cosmesis (**Figure 8.4.2**).

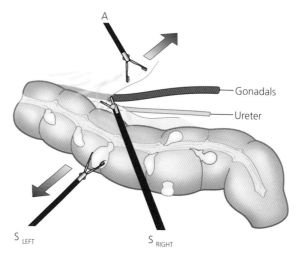

8.4.3

There will soon come a point where the surgeon has difficulty reaching any further up the left colon from the right iliac fossa port. At this point, the harmonic scalpel is then placed in through the left flank port. The assistant's grasper is taken out from the left flank port and then placed through the right iliac fossa port (i.e. both graspers from the right, pulling the left colon and splenic flexure across to the right). This grasper in the right iliac fossa can be placed via the surgeon, then held by the nurse (or second assistant) who is standing between the legs (N). The other grasper is still through the right upper quadrant and held by the operating surgeon (S_{LEFT}) to allow fine manipulation of the tissues and more rapid exposure as the dissection progresses. With the harmonic scalpel now through the left flank port (S_{RIGHT}), this provides a better angle of approach to mobilize the attachments from the spleen, omentum, left kidney, and perinephric fat. A complete mobilization of the splenic flexure from the tail and body of the pancreas is not typically required for this operation. However, the same technique can be extended to provide greater mobility as is required for an ultra-low anterior resection (**Figure 8.4.4**).

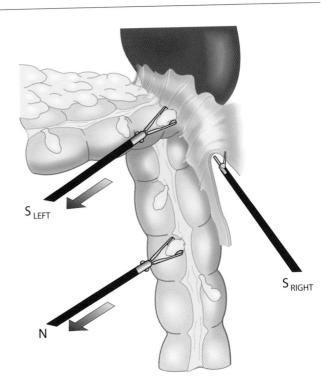

8.4.4

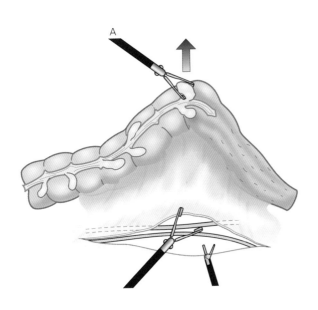

8.4.5

The rectosigmoid junction is then retracted to the left and held anteriorly by the assistant's grasper which is now again through the left flank port (A). The light source for the 30° 5 mm laparoscope is then turned 90° clockwise. This provides a better angle to visualize across towards the left ureter. The peritoneum is then scored just dorsal to the inferior mesenteric vessels over the sacral promontory. A window is then made through to the ureter which has previously been exposed from the lateral aspect. Care must be taken to identify the hypogastric nerves, which should be gently pushed backwards. The window is then extended in a cephalad direction, hence isolating the inferior mesenteric vessels. Through this window, the left ureter must be identified. Correct orientation is important and, again, the ureter should be in a horizontal position (**Figure 8.4.5**).

The assistant's grasper now lifting the mesocolon just cephalad to the inferior mesenteric vessels (A), a window is made above the left colic artery. The surgeon's left grasper can then be placed through this window (S_{LEFT}). The harmonic scalpel can be placed through the more distal window just beyond the inferior mesenteric vessels (S_{RIGHT}). The surgeon's grasper and harmonic scalpel act like a pair of 'chopsticks' which then lift up and expose the inferior mesenteric vein and inferior mesenteric artery. Using this 'chopsticks maneuver', a 12 mm endoscopic stapler can be placed through the hypogastric port to secure the vessels. Alternative methods for securing the vessels can be employed, such as clips or other thermal devices. However, it is convenient to use the stapler as it will be later used for division of the upper rectum (**Fig 8.4.6**).

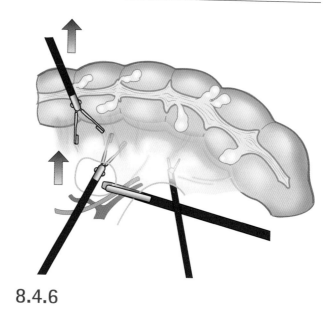

8.4.6

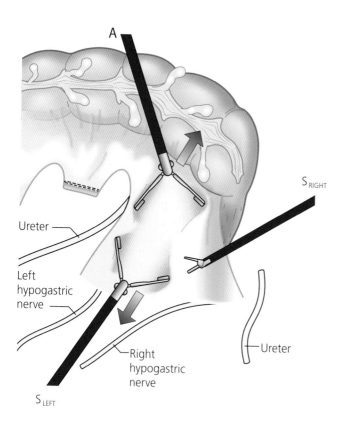

8.4.7

Attention is now towards the pelvis and the beginning of the mesorectal mobilization. The rectosigmoid junction is lifted forward by the surgeon to allow the assistant to place their opened grasper between the cut edges of the peritoneum of the mesorectum (A). The grasper ends are opened wide and the mesorectum lifted up and pushed forward. This exposes the plane of dissection behind the mesorectum. The presacral space is entered at the level of the sacral promontory. Fine grasping of the posterior tissues can be performed with the surgeon's left-hand grasper (S_{LEFT}) as the posterior mobilization in the avascular plane continues. Further traction can also be applied forward in the mesorectum by careful placement of the surgeon's grasper. Once again, care must be taken of the hypogastric nerves which should be pushed backwards as the dissection continues. If the assistant's grasper has been placed correctly, it is often possible to continue the dissection under direct vision down to the pelvic floor without the assistant having to make any adjustments to their grasping. Mobilization is complete when Waldeyer's fascia has been divided and the levator ani muscles have been reached. The dissection can then be carried around laterally from the posterior aspect (**Figure 8.4.7**).

With the rectosigmoid now pulled taut by the assistant's grasper from the left flank (A), this then exposes the right peritoneal reflection in the mesorectum. Lateral tension from the tissues can be gained by either a suction irrigator or grasper placed through the 12 mm hypogastric port, held by the scrub nurse (or second assistant standing between the legs, N). This then exposes the line of lateral dissection, which continues down to the front of the rectum at the pouch of Douglas. The left side can then be dissected, with the rectosigmoid being pulled across by the surgeon's left-hand grasper (**Figure 8.4.8**).

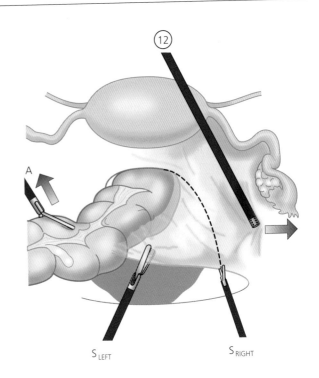

8.4.8

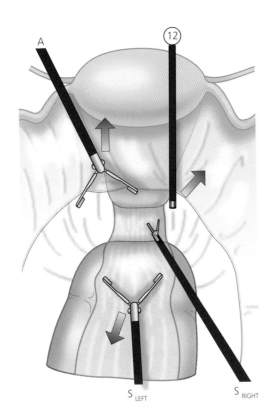

8.4.9

Anterior dissection is continued to at least 5 cm beyond the peritoneal reflection. Exposure is achieved with the assistant's open grasper lifting the vagina up and forward (A). This can be also aided by a grasper or suction irrigator via the 12 mm port held by the scrub nurse (N). The exposed rectum can then be gently pulled cephalad using the open grasper in the surgeon's left hand (S_{LEFT}). In males, the dissection is carried down to the level of the seminal vesicles. The lateral stalks are preserved (**Figure 8.4.9**).

Now that the mesorectal mobilization is complete, the level of division of the upper rectum is then chosen if a resection is to be combined with the rectopexy. This is best assessed by having the assistant (A) grasp the rectosigmoid and pull the rectum straight and out of the pelvis. The level of suture rectopexy is then chosen adjacent to the upper part of the sacral promontory. The level of division of the rectum should be just a few centimeters proximal to this point. The mesorectum can then be divided using the harmonic shears or stapler. The rectum can then be divided using an appropriate sized stapler reload via the 12 mm hypogastric port. The specimen is then delivered via a small 40 mm Pfannenstiel incision, utilizing the previously made 12 mm port incision (**Figure 8.4.10**).

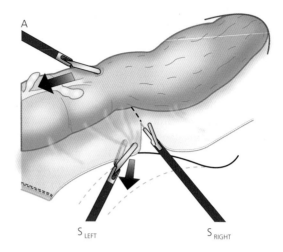

8.4.10

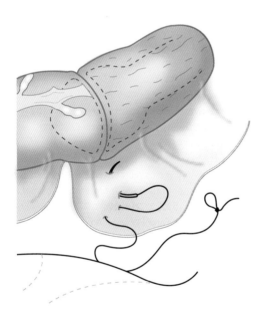

Rectal fixation

Once the sigmoid specimen has been resected via the Pfannenstiel incision and the anvil inserted securely, this is then returned to the abdominal cavity. An end-to-end colorectal anastomosis is then effected, typically with a 29 mm circular stapler. This part can be performed either through the open Pfannenstiel wound or laparoscopically. Either way, care must be taken to ensure the proximal colon is not twisted (**Figure 8.4.11**).

8.4.11

Before firing the stapler, a suture rectopexy is performed using a 2-0 Novafil™ suture. We have found that only one suture is required and placed just in front of the sacral promontory. A secure placement of the suture through the periosteum is important, away from the hypogastric nerves or presacral vein. The suture is then passed through the fascia of the mesorectum just distal to the level of the anastomosis. The position of the anastomosis can be controlled by the assistant holding the stapler per rectum. When the knot is about to be tied, the stapler can be fired and gently removed. The anastomosis can then be checked for integrity with air sufflation via the rectum and saline in the pelvis. Any small bubbles can be a potential source of anastomotic leak and so should be secured with a 3-0 polydioxanone suture. A closed suction drain is then inserted into the pelvis and brought out through the left flank port.

POSTOPERATIVE CARE

Nasogastric or orogastric tubes used during the operation for gastric decompression can be removed at the end of the operation. Patients can then commence oral intake as tolerated. Mobilization should be encouraged on day 1 with removal of intravenous cannula. Indwelling catheter and rectal tube can typically be removed over the following 24–48 hours.

OUTCOME

Most patients should expect an excellent and rapid recovery after a laparoscopically performed resection rectopexy. Typically, the length of stay is between 3 and 5 days, often dependent upon other comorbidities. Recurrence rate after suture rectopexy, with or without resection ranges from 0 to 9 percent.[1]

The recurrence rate in our unit is under 3 percent with a median follow-up of 62 months.[2] The same technique has also been used for symptomatic rectal intussusception in patients who have otherwise failed medical treatment, as well as patients with solitary rectal ulcer syndrome.[3] No patients in these series have had worsening of preoperative constipation, or obstructed defecation. There has been significant improvement with constipation between 63 and 70 percent. Similarly, problems with fecal continence also have significant improvement in over 60 percent of patients without further intervention.

There are limited data available from randomized trials comparing the different approaches for the treatment of rectal prolapse. Two smaller trials had been performed in the 'open' era comparing mesh or suture with resection and suture-rectopexy.[4, 5] In both of these trials, the rate of constipation was significantly lower in the patients who also had resection. While there is a potential disadvantage for anastomotic leakage to occur, this should be uncommon and is less that 1 percent in our series with only one minor leak occurring. We have now performed over 550 laparoscopic resection rectopexies in our unit with very low morbidity. In addition to the 550 resection rectopexies, the author has also performed over 250 laparoscopic ventral rectopexies for treatment of patients with both full-thickness rectal prolapse, as well as rectal intussusception and rectocele. The early results of this technique also seem promising, and it has become the procedure of choice in many parts of Europe, UK and Australia. Recurrence rates and function after VR are similar to those achieved with resection rectopexy, but can be achieved with potentially lower risk/morbidity and even performed as a day-case procedure[6]. Ideally, a randomized trial comparing the two techniques would seem appropriate. However, it seems historically difficult to enroll sufficient patients for such trials although there is now good evidence that at least the laparoscopic approach has significant advantages over traditional laparotomy with similar long-term outcomes.[7, 8]

REFERENCES

1. Stevenson ARL, Stitz RW, Lumley JW. Laparoscopic-assisted resection-rectopexy for rectal prolapse: early and medium follow-up. *Diseases of the Colon and Rectum* 1998; **41**: 46–54.
2. Ashari LHS, Lumley JW, Stevenson ARL, Stitz RW. Laparoscopically-assisted resection rectopexy for rectal prolapse: ten years' experience. *Diseases of the Colon and Rectum* 2005; **48**: 982–7.
3. Von Papen M, Ashari LHS, Lumley JW *et al.* Functional results of laparoscopic resection rectopexy for symptomatic rectal intussusception. *Diseases of the Colon and Rectum* 2006; **50**: 50–5.
4. Luukkonen P, Mikkonen U, Jarvinen H. Abdominal rectopexy with sigmoidectomy versus rectopexy alone for rectal prolapse: a prospective, randomized study. *International Journal of Colorectal Disease* 1992; **7**: 219–22.
5. McKee RF, Lauder JC, Poon FW *et al.* A prospective randomized study of abdominal rectopexy with and without sigmoidectomy in rectal prolapse. *Surgery, Gynecology and Obstetrics* 1992; **174**: 145–8.
6. Powar M, Ogilvie J, Stevenson ARL. Day-case laparoscopic ventral rectopexy: An achievable reality. *Colorectal Diseases* 2013; **15(6)**: 700–6.
7. Solomon MJ, Young CJ, Eyers AA, Roberts RA. Randomised clinical trial of laparoscopic versus open abdominal rectopexy for rectal prolapse. *British Journal of Surgery* 2002; **89**: 35–9.
8. Senapati AI, Gray RG, Middleton LJ *et al.* PROSPER: a randomised comparison of surgical treatments for rectal prolapse. *Colorectal Disease* 2013 July 15(7): 858–68.

Laparoscopic ventral rectopexy

ANDRÉ D'HOORE

PRINCIPLES AND JUSTIFICATION

Background

Rectal prolapse is a full-thickness intussusception of the rectum that can be retained within the anal canal (internal rectal prolapse) or can protrude through the anal ring (overt total or complete rectal prolapse). Untreated, it will lead to structural damage to the anal sphincter complex and ultimately fecal incontinence.

Rectal prolapse is often associated with varying degrees of prolapse of the middle pelvic compartment consequent on structural damage to the different levels of vaginal support. Insufficiency of the sacrouterine ligament (level I) may lead to vaginal vault prolapse and enterocele formation. Damage to the rectovaginal septum will lead to a high rectocele (level II). Damage to the perineal body (level III), often in combination with rupture of the anterior quadrant of the anterior sphincters, may result in a low rectocele (perineocele).

Surgery for rectal prolapse is intended to restore the anatomy and to improve function (preservation of anal continence, and improved rectal voiding) while avoiding surgery-related morbidity and functional sequelae (constipation).

Laparoscopic ventral rectopexy is a relatively new technique that uses a polypropylene mesh to suspend the middle compartment of the pelvic floor and in doing so not only corrects rectal intussusception but also suspends the middle pelvic compartment (levels I and II) (**Figure 8.5.1**). It has been shown to be a reproducible and safe technique which, as it is 'nerve-sparing' also reduces the incidence of postoperative constipation.

PREOPERATIVE INVESTIGATION

In most patients with external prolapse, the clinical picture will be evident; however, it can be important to visualize the other pelvic compartments. Therefore

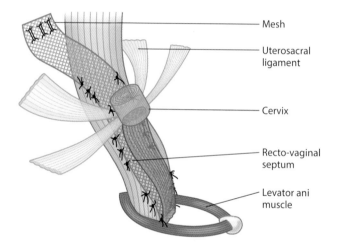

8.5.1 Position of the mesh in the rectovaginal septum. Level I and II suspension of the middle pelvic compartment.

Labels: Mesh, Uterosacral ligament, Cervix, Recto-vaginal septum, Levator ani muscle

colpocystodefecography or dynamic magnetic resonance imaging (MRI) of the pelvis is often indicated. Anal manometry is indicated to document residual anal sphincter function.

Preoperative anesthetic consultation is important, particularly in the elderly, to determine whether the patient is fit for general anesthetic and a laparoscopic approach. In an elderly or unfit patient, a perineal approach such as a Delorme operation (see Chapter 8.1) or an Altemeier operation (see Chapter 8.2) may be indicated.

PREOPERATIVE PREPARATION

The patient is given a preoperative enema to empty the rectum. Standard thromboprophylaxis using low molecular weight heparin is started before surgery. Antibiotic prophylaxis is indicated (the author routinely uses a single perioperative dose of cefazolin).

OPERATION

Patient positioning

The patient is positioned in a modified Lloyd-Davis position on a moldable beanbag and arms along the body. Fixation should allow a steep Trendelenburg position.

Trocar placement

An optical trocar is placed at the umbilical site. A 30° optic is preferable to facilitate deep pelvic visualization. An open Hassan technique is preferable in the case of previous surgery. A blind Veress needle technique can be used in other circumstances.

Under direct vision the other three trocars are placed: a 10 mm trocar in the right iliac fossa and 5 mm trocars in the left and right flanks. Special care must be taken not to injure the inferior epigastric artery. Too low a placement of the 10 mm port could injure the ilioinguinal nerve (**Figure 8.5.2**).

The vagina is cleaned with a povidone iodine solution as an obturator will be used during the operation to identify the position of the vaginal vault.

A urinary catheter is inserted.

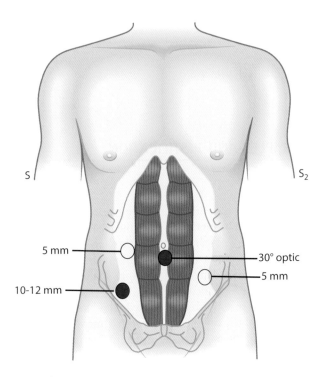

8.5.2 Trocar positioning: red dot, 10 mm trocar; S, surgeon; open dot, 5 mm trocar.

Anatomic landmarks

The first step is to perform adhesiolysis as required to visualize the pelvic organs. Care must be exercised as the small bowel is particularly at risk of inadvertent injury. The sigmoid colon is only partially mobilized from adhesions within the pelvis to allow straightening of the rectum.

Landmarks of interest are the right ureter, the right iliac artery, and the impression of the sacral promontory. The left iliac vein can be very close to the sacral promontory. The small bowel is kept out of the operative field by using a steep Trendelenburg position. Temporary suspension of the uterus with transcutaneous sutures through the lateral ligament is useful to optimize the operator's view of the pelvis (**Figure 8.5.3**).

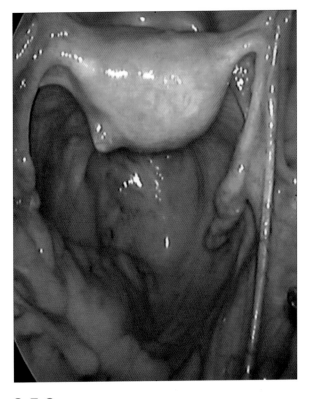

8.5.3 Pelvic view after temporary uterosuspension.

Dissection at the sacral promontory

Dissection is started (either using monopolar energy or an ultrasonic dissection tool) along the rectum at the site of the sacral promontory. The assistant surgeon gently retracts the sigmoid colon to the left.

Sharp incision of the peritoneum allows some pneumodisection. Special care is taken to avoid injury to the right hypogastric nerve which crosses the pelvic brim at this level.

Care should be taken not to injure the left iliac vein as bleeding at that site can be very troublesome. If it occurs, localized compression is advisable and in most instances a conversion to open laparotomy will be indicated.

Some smaller veins can run over the sacral promontory. They are easily controlled by coagulation. A zone of about 2–3 cm should be freed to allow safe mesh fixation.

Mesh fixation to the sacral promontory is safer in comparison to presacral fascia fixation (as in more conventional rectopexy techniques) to avoid cumbersome presacral bleeding.

Opening of the pelvic peritoneum

An inverted 'J' incision (**Figure 8.5.4**) is extended along the right side of the rectum over the deepest part of the pouch of Douglas. Special care is taken not to damage the autonomic nerve supply to the rectum.

Firm retraction should be exerted on the rectum to reduce the prolapse and to visualize the place for the anterior incision at the apex of the pouch of Douglas.

A lateral peritoneal flap is created to allow closure over the mesh at the end of the procedure.

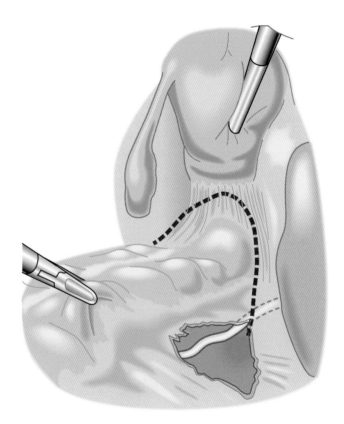

8.5.4 Inverted 'J' incision to open the peritoneum. Note the close relationship with the right hypogastric nerve.

Dissection of the rectovaginal septum

The rectovaginal septum is opened by incision of Denonvilliers' fascia 1 cm distance from the vaginal vault. Dissection is performed on the anterior aspect of the rectal wall leaving all areolar and fibrous tissue on the posterior side of the vagina. This is important to minimize later mesh erosion into the vagina (**Figure 8.5.5**). In women who have had a hysterectomy, inserting an obdurator into the vagina can facilitate this maneuver. Depending upon the individual patient, deeper dissection along the rectovaginal septum may be needed, especially to correct a concomitant rectocele. When a low rectocele is present, the dissection should be continued until the pelvic floor is reached. In certain situations, it may be necessary to fix the mesh at the top of the anal sphincter complex, in which case the laparoscopic dissection can be completed by a transperineal dissection.* Occasionally, there is a very thick, fatty pouch of Douglas that will inhibit good mesh fixation. The author has, on occasions, excised 'fatty pad' taking special care not to damage the rectal wall and to ensure meticulous hemostasis.

*Transperineal dissection may increase the incidence of mesh erosion.

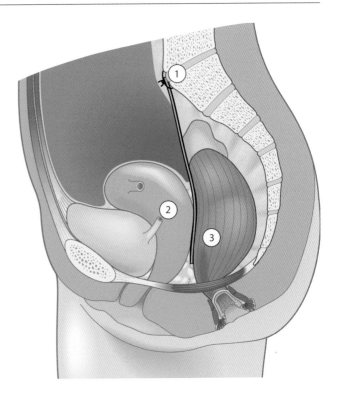

8.5.5 Sagittal view on the position of the mesh in the rectovaginal septum. The mesh is fixed upon the anterior aspect of the rectum [3] and to the sacral promontory [1]. A colpopexy [2] is performed upon the same mesh.

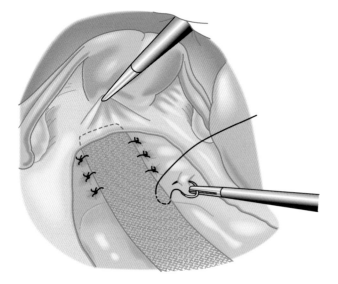

8.5.6 Fixation of mesh to the anterior side of the rectum.

Fixation of the mesh to the anterior side of the rectum

A non-absorbable strip of mesh polypropylene (4 × 18 cm) is used (**Figure 8.5.6**). The author finds this easy to handle and its texture ensures good tissue incorporation. There has been recent interest in the use of biological meshes. The mesh is sutured (absorbable and non-absorbable sutures can be used) to the ventral aspect of the rectum. An extracorporeal knot tying technique with a knot pusher is used. The sutures are passed through the right iliac fossa cannula. Further suturing will fix the mesh to the lateral border of the rectum proximal and distal to the pouch of Douglas. This will inhibit further intussusception of the rectum. The deep position of the mesh will reinforce the rectovaginal septum.

Fixation of the mesh to the sacral promontory

The mesh is then fixed to the sacral promontory (**Figure 8.5.7**) using an endofascial stapler or endo tacker. This fixation is the Achilles heel of the intervention and therefore it is advisable to use another two deep Ethibond 0 sutures to secure the fixation. No traction should be exerted to the rectum (which should remain in the sacrococcygeal hollow) but the prolapse should be reduced.

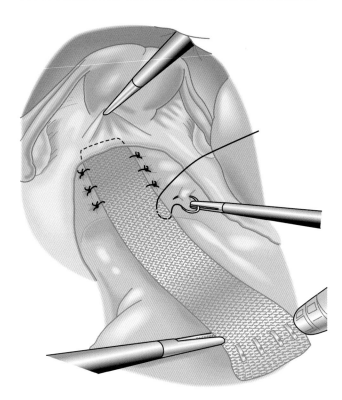

8.5.7 Rectopexy: fixation of the mesh to the anterior aspect of the rectum and fixation to the sacral promontory.

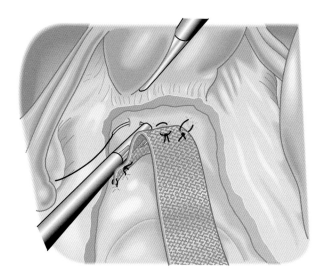

8.5.8 Colpopexy to the same mesh.

Colpopexy

In most patients, an additional colpopexy will be performed (**Figure 8.5.8**), especially in the presence of an enterocele or sacrouterine ligament insufficiency. The vaginal fornix or posterior vaginal vault will be fixed on the same mesh.

Two lateral sutures will incorporate the fibrous part of the cardinal ligament.

In the case of vaginal vault prolapse, additional sutures will be used to allow suspension of the middle compartment.

Peritoneal closure

The peritoneum is now closed over the mesh (**Figure 8.5.9**). This elevates the 'neo-pouch' of Douglas over the colpopexy. The peritoneal closure is also of importance to avoid later small bowel fixation (erosion) to the mesh.

The laparoscopic ports are then removed. The fascia at the 12 and 10 mm ports is closed.

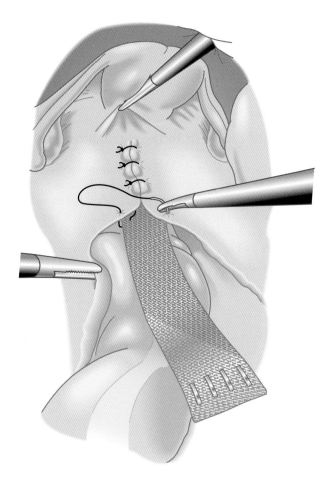

8.5.9 Closure of the peritoneum over the mesh ('neo-pouch' of Douglas).

POSTOPERATIVE MANAGEMENT

The urinary catheter is removed after surgery and early ambulation is advised. A normal diet is resumed as soon as possible. A fiber-enriched diet is prescribed and straining effort in the absence of any urge is discouraged. Patients are usually discharged from hospital 1–2 days postoperatively.

OUTCOME

Perioperative complications

Conversion is seldomly required (<5 percent) despite the proportion of patients who have had previous pelvic surgery. Dense pelvic adhesions can necessitate a conversion to laparotomy.

Inadvertent trauma to the left iliac vein will indicate an emergent laparotomy to provide hemostasis.

Postoperative morbidity and mortality

The laparoscopic approach is safe even in the aged population. Cardiac events are the most common reason of major morbidity (eventual mortality).

Care should be taken not to damage the rectum or vagina in order to avoid septic mesh complications. Some cases of septic spondylodiscitis have been described.

Mesh infections and erosions should be <1 percent.

The incidence of dyspareunia is less if the mesh is fixed to the rectum rather than a denuded posterior vaginal wall. Mesh erosion is uncommon following LVMR (<1% in our series), but the consequences can be severe and the risk of erosion should be fully discussed with the patient prior to the procedure.

Recurrence

Recurrence rate is in the range of other more classical mesh repairs and is in the order of 5 percent after five years of follow-up. The most common site of recurrence is the detachment of the mesh at the fixation site of the sacral promontory.

Relaparoscopy with refixation of the mesh should therefore be the approach of choice in the case of recurrence.

In patients with an important enterocele, the colpofixation can be insufficient and result in a recurrent prolapse of the middle pelvic compartment.

FUNCTIONAL OUTCOME

Most patients (up to 90 percent) will experience a significant improvement in fecal incontinence. Recovery of sphincter function can take time and no further incontinence surgery (sacral nerve stimulation, gracilis neosphincter) should be proposed within 6–12 months of prolapse surgery.

Laparoscopic ventral rectopexy results in an improved rectal emptying in about 70–80 percent of patients. These results have been reproduced in other series. The development of new-onset constipation is rare (about 5 percent) and most often is mild.

The location of the mesh in the rectovaginal septum leads less to dyspareunia the more that the mesh is fixed upon the rectum rather than against a denuded posterior vaginal wall.

FURTHER READING

Boons P, Collinson R, Cunningham C, Lindsey I. Laparoscopic ventral rectopexy for external rectal prolapsed improves constipation and avoids de novo constipation. *Colorectal Disease* 2010; **12**: 526–32.

D'Hoore A, Cadoni R, Penninckx F. Long-term outcome of laparoscopic ventral rectopexy for total rectal prolapse. *British Journal of Surgery* 2004; **91**: 1500–5.

D'Hoore A, Penninckx F. Laparoscopic ventral recto(colpo)pexy for rectal prolapse: surgical technique and outcome for 109 patients. *Surgical Endoscopy* 2006; **20**: 1919–23.

D'Hoore A, Vanbeckevoort D, Penninckx F. Clinical, physiological and radiological assessment of rectovaginal septum reinforcement with mesh for compex rectocele. *British Journal of Surgery* 2008; **95**: 1264–72.

STARR

LUKAS MARTI AND DAVID JAYNE

HISTORY

Stapled transanal rectal resection (STARR) is a relatively new procedure for the treatment of obstructed defecation syndrome (ODS). It aims to achieve a full-thickness, circumferential resection of the distal rectum, together with accompanying internal prolapse (intussusception) and/or rectocele, resulting in a neorectum, which is devoid of any mechanical impediment to evacuation. In the absence of a dedicated device to perform STARR, the original technique employed separate firings of two 33 mm circular staplers (PPH-01™; Ethicon Endo-surgery, Cincinnati, OH, USA); one stapler to perform each of the anterior and posterior semi-circumferential resections. Subsequently, the Contour Transtar™ (STR5G; Ethicon Endo-surgery) stapler was developed specifically for STARR, with the ability to perform a continuous circumferential transanal rectal resection. For the purpose of this chapter, the PPH-STARR procedure will be considered, as it is the simpler of the two techniques and, as yet, no clinical advantage has been demonstrated for the Transtar procedure, although it is accepted that this may only become apparent on long-term follow-up. It should be noted that both techniques, PPH-STARR and Transtar, produce the same anatomical outcome, namely a full-thickness distal rectal resection. The difference between the two techniques is the device and method used to achieve the full-thickness resection. For further information on Transtar the reader is referred to Jayne and Stuto.[1]

PRINCIPLES AND JUSTIFICATION

STARR is indicated for the treatment of obstructed defecation associated with internal rectal prolapse with or without rectocele. There is no proven value for STARR in functional outlet obstruction, such as anismus/spastic pelvic floor syndrome. The patient should present a good history of rectal evacuatory difficulty, which may include some of the following symptoms: prolonged straining to defecate, excessive time spent on the toilet, a sense of incomplete evacuation, frequent calls to defecate, use of digital manipulation or perineal support to initiate evacuation, a dependency on laxatives and enemas, and a feeling of pelvic pressure or rectal discomfort. Attention should be paid to symptoms of other pelvic organ prolapse, which exist in some 30–40 percent of patients with ODS. Appropriate investigation is of paramount importance in defining the anatomical defects (internal prolapse, rectocele, perineal descent) which may be amenable to surgical correction and thus to guide patient selection.

Coexistent rectal pathology is an absolute contraindication to STARR and includes anorectal sepsis, proctitis, anal stenosis, and chronic diarrheal states, and underlines the need for prior evaluation of at least the left colon and rectum. Relative contraindications to STARR, which must be treated according to their individual merits, include the presence of foreign material adjacent to the rectum (e.g. mesh from a previous rectocele repair), significant anal sphincter injury with fecal incontinence, a fixed, low enterocele, and concurrent psychiatric disorders.

Patients should be appropriately counseled about expected outcomes and associated risks. Current evidence suggests that with good patient selection some 70–80 percent of patients will achieve a good outcome, with improvement in ODS symptoms and quality of life.[2] Complications have been reported in 15–30 percent of cases, with the most frequently encountered being transient defecatory urgency (20 percent), anorectal pain (7.1 percent), urinary retention (6.9 percent), bleeding (5 percent), localized sepsis (4.4 percent), and anastomotic stricture (0.6 percent).[3] Despite the proximity of the vagina to the area of resection, the incidence of rectovaginal fistula and dyspareunia is very low.

PREOPERATIVE ASSESSMENT AND PREPARATION

Thorough investigation remains the cornerstone of good patient selection for STARR. The following investigations are mandatory: imaging of the colon and rectum, with flexible sigmoidoscopy as a minimum; and dynamic assessment of rectal evacuation, either by defecating proctography or dynamic MRI. It is the authors' preference to always perform anorectal manometry and endoanal ultrasound to characterize sphincter function, and this is mandatory if there is a history of fecal incontinence or evidence of sphincter weakness on clinical examination. Colonic transit studies may be helpful in differentiating slow transit constipation from rectal evacuatory dysfunction, which may have an influence on postoperative outcome. Symptoms of other pelvic organ prolapse should be sought and, if present, investigated by a gynecologist. The information from these investigations, combined with the history and clinical examination, should enable the clinician to select those patients most likely to benefit from STARR and to advise on probable outcome. If desired, the STARR procedure may be safely performed in combination with other gynecological procedures.

The lower colon and rectum is prepared by means of an enema administered prior to surgery; there is no need for full bowel preparation. A single dose of broad-spectrum antibiotics is administered at induction of anesthesia, which may take the form of either a general or regional anesthetic.

OPERATION

Patient position

The operation is performed with the patient in the 'forced' lithotomy position, with the hips flexed greater than 90°. This helps to expose the perineum and provides the best operative view for the surgeon. Head-down tilt of around 30° is employed to optimize views into the anorectum and to displace any small bowel from the pouch of Douglas. There is no place for operating in the prone position, which precludes adequate access to the vagina.

Initial assessment and preparation

Bimanual examination is performed to determine the degree of rectocele, the presence of coexistent enterocele, and to assess sphincter integrity. Assessment of internal rectal prolapse may be performed by insertion of a proctoscope or Eisenhammer retractor, but is best judged following insertion of the PPH circular anal dilator (CAD).

Four silk retaining sutures are placed at the anoderm in the 12, 3, 6, and 9 o'clock positions and used to apply traction and aid insertion of the lubricated anal dilator and obturator (CAD). The sutures are then tied around the flanges of the CAD to hold it securely in position.

A swab on a sponge holder is inserted into the anorectum and gradually withdrawn to determine the extent and apex of the internal rectal prolapse; the apex of the prolapse marks the midpoint of the resection (**Figure 8.6.1**).

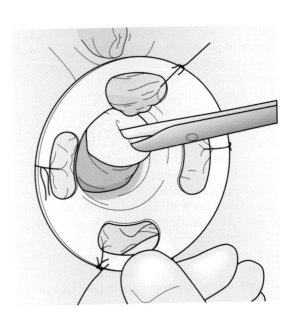

8.6.1 The circular anal dilator is held securely to the anoderm with four retaining sutures. A swab is inserted into the distal rectum to reveal the apex of the internal rectal prolapse.

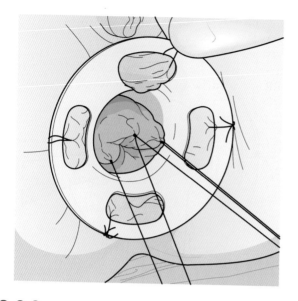

8.6.2 Three traction sutures are placed at the apex of the prolapse in the 10, 12, and 2 o'clock positions. The two strands of the middle 12 o'clock suture are separated and one of each tied to the 10 o'clock and 2 o'clock traction sutures.

Anterior semi-circumferential resection

Three 2-0 prolene traction sutures are placed in the apex of the prolapse at the 10, 12, and 2 o'clock positions, taking full-thickness bits of the rectal wall. The traction sutures are loosely tied. The two strands of the middle 12 o'clock suture are separated and the individual strands tied separately to the 10 o'clock and 2 o'clock sutures, to make a total of two traction sutures (each comprising three suture strands; **Figure 8.6.2**).

A malleable retractor is inserted through the posterior flange of the CAD to protect the posterior anorectum during the anterior semi-circumferential resection.

The first PPH-01 stapler is fully opened, lubricated, and inserted into the anorectum, such that the anvil is beyond the area of prolapse. The two traction sutures are threaded through the holes in the sides of the stapler and held together with a clamp. Tension is applied to the traction sutures while the stapler is closed, incorporating the prolapse within the stapler housing. Care is taken to ensure that all maneuvers are performed in line with the anorectal axis and that on closure the stapler is well within the distal rectum. A digital vaginal examination is performed to ensure that the vaginal mucosa has not been inadvertently incorporated into the stapler; the vaginal mucosa should move freely over the surface of the stapler (**Figure 8.6.3**). The stapler is held closed for 30 seconds to facilitate tissue compression and hemostasis and then fired. To remove the stapler, the opening mechanism is rotated one half turn anti-clockwise and the stapler withdrawn. The resection specimen should be retrieved from the stapler housing and the extent and integrity of resection assessed.

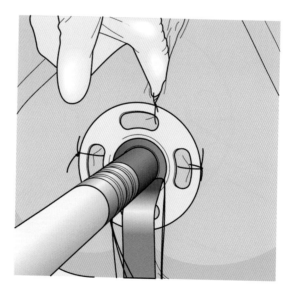

8.6.3 A malleable retractor is inserted beneath the posterior flange of the circular anal dilator. The first PPH-01 stapler is inserted into the anorectum incorporating the prolapse. A digital vaginal examination is performed.

It is usual for a 'mucosal bridge' to be encountered posteriorly. This should be looked for and if present divided with scissors (**Figure 8.6.4**).

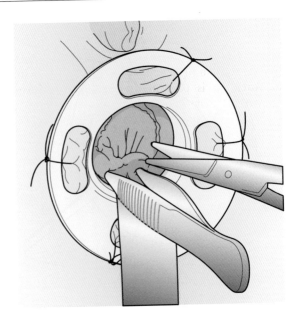

8.6.4 A posterior mucosal bridge is often present following the anterior resection and is divided with scissors.

Posterior semi-circumferential resection

Resection of the posterior rectum proceeds in much the same manner as the anterior semi-circumferential resection. Three 2-0 prolene traction sutures are placed; one at each 'dog-ear', which mark the lateral extent of the anterior semi-circumferential resection, and one at the 6 o'clock position. The two strands of the middle 6 o'clock suture are separated and one strand tied to each of the lateral sutures, such that two traction sutures remain. A malleable retractor is inserted through the anterior flange of the CAD to protect the anterior anorectum (**Figure 8.6.5**). The second PPH-01 stapler is inserted, lubricated and fully opened, into the anorectum such that the anvil is beyond the area of prolapse to be resected. The two traction sutures are threaded through the holes in the sides of the stapler and held together with a clamp. Traction is applied to the traction sutures and the stapler closed, incorporating the prolapse into the stapler housing. The stapler is held closed for 30 seconds and then fired. The stapler is withdrawn and the specimen inspected.

An anterior mucosal bridge may or may not be present; if so, this is divided. The lateral dog-ears, which mark the crossing of the anterior and posterior staple lines, are buried with a 3-0 dissolvable suture.

Hemostasis is checked with the aid of the anoscope and any bleeding points arrested with interrupted dissolvable sutures. The retaining sutures on the CAD are cut and the CAD removed. If necessary, a hemostatic sponge can be inserted into the anorectum and local anesthetic infiltrated as a pudendal nerve block.

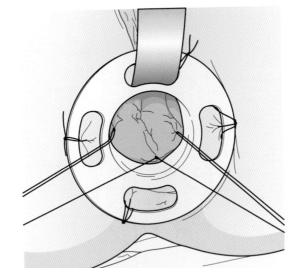

8.6.5 Three traction sutures are placed for the posterior semi-circumferential resection: one at each lateral extent of the anterior resection (the dog-ears), and one in the 6 o'clock position. The anterior rectum is protected with a malleable retractor.

POSTOPERATIVE CARE

Postoperatively, the patient is provided with adequate analgesia, which may include an opioid for the first 24 hours. Attention is paid to the possibility of urinary retention, which, if it occurs, is managed with an indwelling catheter. A stool bulking agent and softener is prescribed for 5 days. Patients are fit for discharge as soon as they are mobile, comfortable on oral analgesia, have passed urine, and are tolerating a normal diet. About half of patients will be discharged the day following surgery; the remainder a day later.

OUTCOME

Several personal series, multicenter studies, one randomized trial, and a large European Registry have assessed the short-term safety and efficacy of STARR. The randomized trial compared STARR with biofeedback therapy and demonstrated an efficacy of 81.5 percent for STARR as compared to 33.3 percent for biofeedback therapy.[4] In this study, the morbidity following STARR was 15 percent, with one serious adverse event (bleeding), but minimal risk of impaired continence. These results were reflected in the European STARR Registry, which collected data on almost 3000 patients and showed a significant improvement in symptom scores and quality of life, which was maintained throughout the 12 months of follow-up.[3] The issue that remains controversial and incompletely explained is the observation of post-STARR defecatory urgency, which may be problematic in some 20 percent of patients. Although urgency is usually transient, with resolution seen by three months postoperatively, a small proportion of patients will experience protracted symptoms. It is likely that these patients had sphincter dysfunction preoperatively, which may not have been apparent due to the predominant effect of the rectal obstruction; removal of the obstructing element subsequently uncovers the sphincter weakness and precipitates urgency. For this reason, the authors advocate formal evaluation of sphincter function as part of routine preoperative assessment and, in the presence of severely weakened sphincters, caution prior to undertaking STARR.

REFERENCES

1. Jayne D, Stuto A (eds). *Transanal stapling techniques for anorectal prolapse.* London: Springer-Verlag, 2009.
2. Boccasanta P, Venturi M, Stuto A *et al.* Stapled transanal rectal resection for outlet obstruction: a prospective, multicenter trial. *Diseases of the Colon and Rectum* 2004; **47**: 1285–96.
3. Jayne D, Schwandner O, Stuto A. Stapled transanal rectal resection for obstructed defecation syndrome: one-year results of the European STARR Registry. *Diseases of the Colon and Rectum* 2009; **52**: 1205–12.
4. Lehur PA, Stuto A, Fantoli M *et al.* Outcomes of stapled transanal rectal resection vs. biofeedback for the treatment of outlet obstruction associated with rectal intussusception and rectocele: a multicenter, randomized, controlled trial. *Diseases of the Colon and Rectum* 2008; **51**: 1611–18.

The EXPRESS procedure

NORMAN S WILLIAMS AND CHETAN BHAN

HISTORY

Rectal intussusception is a full-thickness invagination of the rectal wall occurring during evacuation and may result in symptoms of rectal evacuatory dysfunction (**Figure 8.7.1**). The presence of a rectocele, anterior bulging of the rectum into the posterior vaginal wall, is commonly associated with this finding and may also contribute to symptomatology (**Figure 8.7.2**). Diagnosis of both these rectal wall morphological 'abnormalities' is traditionally made during evacuation proctography and, more recently, using magnetic resonance proctography.[1]

Traditional surgical approaches for rectal intussusception have tended to be modifications of operative procedures to correct overt rectal prolapse, such as the intrarectal Delormes, or the various forms of abdominal rectopexy (suture, resection, etc.). More recently, stapled transanal rectal resection (STARR)[2] and laparoscopic ventral mesh rectopexy have been introduced.[3]

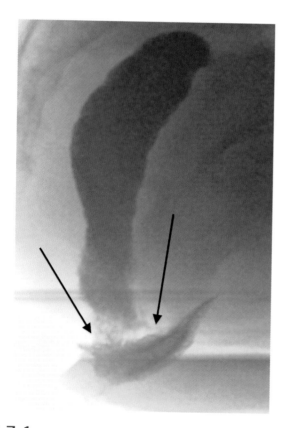

8.7.1 Evacuation proctogram demonstrating a circumferential full-thickness rectal intussusception. The arrows demonstrate the point and direction of the intussuscepting rectal wall.

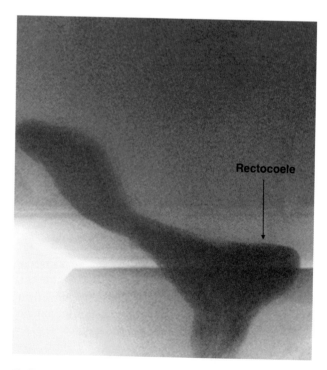

8.7.2 Evacuation proctogram demonstrating a rectocele formation. The rectal wall can be clearly seen bulging anteriorly.

PRINCIPLES AND JUSTIFICATION

The external pelvic rectal suspension (EXPRESS) is an anterior perineal rectopexy, which involves fixation of the rectum to the periosteum of the superior pubic ramus. The advantage of this technique, over abdominal procedures, is that any concomitant rectocele can be repaired simultaneously by reinforcement of the rectovaginal septum with a Permacol™ patch.[4]

Permacol is utilized as it is an acellular biological implant that has low immunogenicity, thus provoking a minimal inflammatory reaction when implanted. Furthermore, its cross-linked structure means host tissue collagenases are unable to degrade it as rapidly as with other biological implants.

The primary indication for the procedure is severe rectal evacuatory dysfunction, associated with the presence of an obstructing rectal intussusception, with or without a concomitant rectocele of greater than 2 cm that traps neo-stool on proctography. Patients with symptoms including tenesmus or the sensation of a lump within the rectum after defecation (in association with an intussusception) and/or an uncomfortable swelling within the vagina, or the need for vaginal digitation (in association with a rectocele) may also be considered for surgery.

Full anorectal physiological assessment is undertaken prior to consideration for surgery. This includes station pull-through anal manometry, to assess anal sphincter function, rectal sensory thresholds and endoanal ultrasound. In addition, evacuation proctography or magnetic resonance proctography is performed to confirm the presence of an obstructing rectal intussusception and whether or not a significant rectocele is also present. A radiopaque marker study should exclude a primary colonic dysmotility that could be contributing to the patient's symptoms.

All prospective patients must undergo conservative management. In the authors' institution, this service is delivered by a team of specialist nurses and includes dietary modification, toilet retraining to improve defecatory dynamics, biofeedback, and the use of rectal medication or irrigation to aid evacuation.

Patients keen to undergo surgery after failure of conservative management are counseled fully prior to surgery. During this consultation, they are warned that surgery may not result in symptom resolution and can be associated with rare but significant complications, including the requirement for stoma formation.

PREOPERATIVE

An empty colon and rectum is preferable prior to the EXPRESS procedure because of the risk of rectal perforation during the procedure, and is usually achieved with clear fluids in combination with purgatives and/or enemas 24–48 hours prior to surgery. The operation is performed under full general anesthetic with antibiotic prophylaxis at induction.

OPERATION

Position of patient

The patient is placed in a modified Lloyd-Davies position, on the operating table, with pneumatic compression stockings to reduce the risk of thromboembolism. A urethral catheter is inserted to empty the bladder and the skin is prepared and draped to allow access to the perineum as well as the suprapubic region.

Incision

A convex crescenteric incision is made between the rectum and the vagina/scrotum (**Figure 8.7.3**). The skin and subcutaneous tissue are dissected from the underlying anterior sphincter complex so as not to damage the anterior aspect thus enabling entry into the extra sphincteric plane.

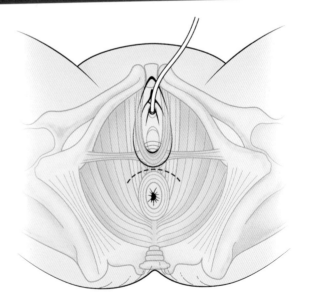

8.7.3

Perineal dissection

FEMALE

Using a combination of sharp, with diathermy, and blunt dissection, the plane between the posterior wall of the vagina and the anterior wall of the rectum is entered taking care not to injure the sphincter complex or buttonhole the rectum or vagina (**Figure 8.7.4**). Infiltration with saline solution aids in development of this plane. Another useful technique to aid dissection is to use an overglove to grip the rectum between the index finger within the rectum and thumb thus enabling the rectal wall to be placed under gentle traction aiding dissection and clarification of the anatomy within this region. These techniques are especially useful during dissection of the lower third of the rectovaginal plane particularly in the presence of a large rectocele, which produces an inflammatory reaction within the tissues resulting in almost complete obliteration of this plane.

The dissection is continued cephalad as far as the posterior fornix of the vagina to the level of Denonvilliers' fascia. Troublesome bleeding may be encountered from the perivaginal venous plexus, which invariably needs to be controlled by under-running of the vessels. Once the anterior plane has been dissected satisfactorily, the lateral wall of the rectum can be mobilized using blunt dissection.

MALE

Although the operation is much more commonly performed in women, the procedure can be applied to male patients. The dissection in the male resembles that of a perineal prostatectomy in which the rectourethral/prostatic plane is entered by dividing the rectourethralis muscle close to the rectum. Hydrodissection with adrenaline–saline solution aids in the identification and preservation of the membraneous urethra. The anterior rectal wall is then mobilized, using a combination of blunt and diathermy dissection, from the prostate in close proximity to the rectum to avoid damage to the neurovascular bundles located at the inferolateral aspect of the prostate.

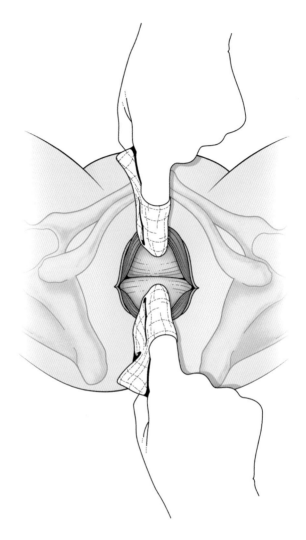

8.7.4

Suprapubic dissection

The assistant makes two transverse incisions over the lateral aspects of the superior pubic rami 2–3 cm long. The dissection is deepened to gain access to the retropubic space bilaterally. Two 1 polydiaxone (PDS) sutures are placed through the periosteum of the superior pubic ramus using a J needle through both suprapubic incisions with the needles preserved. A custom-made tunneler (a long artery forceps can be used instead) is advanced through the perineal incision retropubically – care is taken not to damage the vagina at this point – and delivered through the suprapubic incisions (**Figure 8.7.5**).

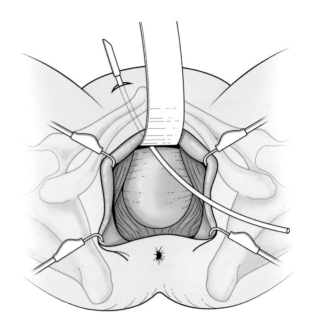

8.7.5

Rectal suspension

Two T-shaped strips of Permacol measuring 5 × 20 cm are utilized for the rectal suspension. The corner of the transverse portion of the T piece is sutured to a specially designed olive which can be secured to the end of the tunneling device (if a long artery forceps is used, this can be clipped directly to the corner of the transverse portion of the T piece) and then delivered through the retropubic tunnel back into the perineal wound (**Figure 8.7.6**). Care is taken to maintain axial alignment of the T piece during this maneuver.

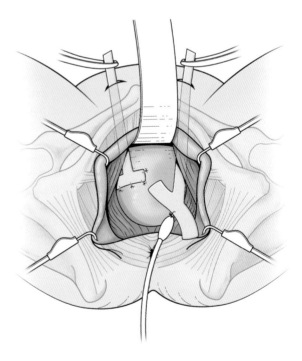

8.7.6

The transverse portion of the T piece should be sutured to the anterolateral rectal wall with its upper margin at approximately 8 cm from the upper margin of the external anal sphincter using 3-0 PDS interrupted sutures and involving the rectal serosa and muscle but not the mucosa. Once the transverse portions are secured to the anterolateral wall, the assistant applies upward traction on the longitudinal portion of the T strips through the suprapubic wounds (**Figure 8.7.7**). The previously placed pubic rami sutures are then attached to the longitudinal aspect of the T strip and tied, resulting in suspension of the rectum to the superior pubic ramus. At this stage, any redundant Permacol is excised.

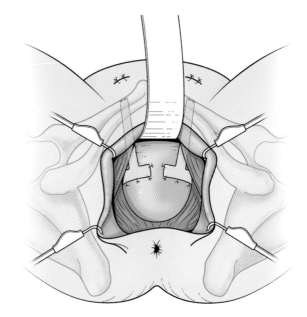

8.7.7

Rectocele repair

Any coexistent rectocele can now be repaired. Initially, the redundant bulging anterior rectal wall is plicated with a 2-0 polyglactin suture. Inserting a custom-designed square 5 × 5 cm Permacol patch with 5 × 2 cm wings then reinforces the rectovaginal septum (**Figure 8.7.8**).

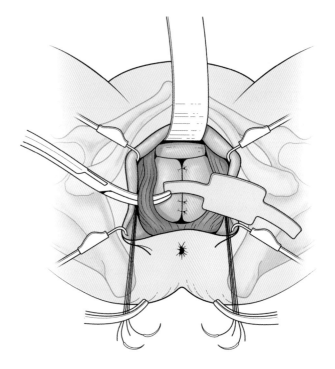

8.7.8

The square portion of the patch is fixed to the anterior rectal wall with interrupted 2-0 PDS sutures and the winged portion is fixed to the periosteum of the ischial tuberosities, again with 2-0 PDS (**Figure 8.7.9**).

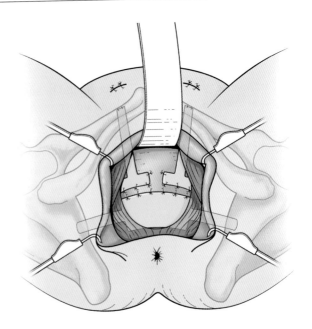

8.7.9

Closure

After hemostasis is secured two suction drains are left *in situ*. The subcutaneous tissues are closed and the skin approximated with interrupted absorbable sutures.

POSTOPERATIVE

Patients are allowed to eat and drink on the first postoperative day as tolerated, during which time full mobilization is encouraged. After 48 hours, the urethral catheter and suction drains (if output is less than 30 mL) are removed.

Patients are discharged after the first bowel movement and are reviewed in the surgical outpatient clinic after two months.

Most complications are related to minor wound infections or erosions through the posterior vaginal wall. The latter can usually be treated conservatively; however, sometimes they require surgical drainage or, rarely, removal of the Permacol patch.

The Permacol implant is well tolerated on the whole but initially may result in some vaginal discharge, which typically settles after 6–8 weeks. This is more common if a rectocele repair has been performed, and may result in dyspareunia, normally transient, that patients should be warned about preoperatively.

The most significant complication is associated with inadvertent rectal perforation particularly if unnoticed at the time of surgery, as this is likely to result in sepsis within the rectovaginal plane with subsequent rectovaginal/perineal fistulation. The management of such a complication would be surgical drainage of the sepsis and temporary defunctioning stoma formation.

REFERENCES

1. Shorvon PJ, McHugh S, Diamant NE *et al.* Defecography in normal volunteers: results and implications. *Gut* 1989; **30**: 1737–49.
2. Naldini G. Serious unconventional complications of surgery with stapler for haemorrhoidal prolapse and obstructed defecation due to rectocele and rectal intussusception. *Colorectal Disease* 2011; **13**: 323–7.
3. Wijffels N, Cunningham C, Lindsey I. Laparoscopic ventral rectopexy for obstructed defecation syndrome. *Surgical Endoscopy* 2009; **23**: 452; author reply 53.
4. Williams NS, Dvorkin LS, Giordano P *et al.* EXternal Pelvic REctal SuSpension (Express procedure) for rectal intussusception, with and without rectocele repair. *British Journal of Surgery* 2005; **92**: 598–604.

9

Surgery for incontinence

Surgical repair of the anal sphincters following injury

DANIEL SHIBRU AND ANN C LOWRY

HISTORY

Direct surgical repair of anal sphincters following injury may be approached in several ways: completely divided muscle ends may be overlapped or brought together by direct apposition; partially injured sphincter muscle may be plicated.

The theoretic advantages of an 'overlapping' sphincter repair include utilization of fibrous scar, which provides substantial tissue to hold sutures, and increased contact areas of muscle tissue decreasing the chance of suture disruption. However, both a retrospective study and a randomized trial found no difference in functional outcome between an overlapping repair and direct apposition.[1, 2] In situations where residual intact muscle is identified at the time of surgery, plication is an acceptable option to avoid division of intact muscle. Proponents argue that if the repair disrupts, the patient will not be clinically worse than preoperatively.

PRINCIPLES AND JUSTIFICATION

Sphincter repair is most commonly performed for an obstetrical injury of the anterior anal sphincter muscle resulting in fecal incontinence and/or a rectovaginal fistula.[1, 3, 4] Other indications are sphincter injuries secondary to previous anorectal surgery, trauma, or congenital abnormality.

The best results from sphincter repair are obtained in those patients who have an anatomical injury. Physical examination is sufficient to confirm a sphincter defect when a cloaca is present but imaging is important in most circumstances. Either endoanal ultrasound or magnetic resonance imaging will detect the presence of a sphincter defect more accurately than clinical examination. Evaluation of the colon by radiographic contrast studies or endoscopy should also be performed to exclude underlying disorders such as inflammatory bowel disease in patients with suggestive symptoms. Clinical history and perhaps other testing (such as anal manometry) are necessary to determine the estimated contribution of a sphincter defect to a patient's fecal incontinence.

A patient with a sphincter defect and fecal incontinence that developed soon after the injury is most likely to benefit from repair. If incontinence develops later in life and testing identifies a sphincter defect, repair offers less certain benefit. Patients with acute sphincter injuries should wait at least three months before repair to allow local edema and inflammation to resolve.

PREOPERATIVE

Preoperative preparation includes a complete mechanical bowel preparation and intravenous antibiotics with broad-spectrum coverage. Oral antibiotics are not necessary. Diverting stomas are not necessary in most circumstances since they offer no benefit in terms of wound healing or functional outcome and can be a source of morbidity.[5] Stomas may be considered in the presence of extensive perineal damage.

OPERATION

Anesthesia

Complete relaxation of the perineum is critical, therefore general or regional anesthesia is necessary. Supplemental local anesthetic aids immediate postoperative pain relief.

Patient position

The patient is placed in the prone jack-knife position with a roll placed under the hips to elevate the hips. The buttocks are taped apart for maximum exposure (**Figure 9.1.1**). A urinary catheter is inserted. A headlight worn by the operating surgeon is recommended.

The critical anatomy includes the location of the innervation and blood supply of the external sphincter. Because of the abundance of collateral circulation, blood supply is not as critical an issue as the innervation. Branches of the pudendal nerve which innervate the sphincter muscle approach the sphincter bilaterally from the posteriolateral position.

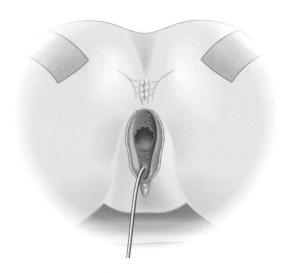

9.1.1

Incision

A curvilinear incision is made in the perineum. In most patients with anterior sphincter injury, the perineum is very thin or nonexistent. In these situations, the incision is made through the thin skin between the vagina and anus. Laterally, the incision is made 1.5–2 cm lateral to the anal verge and parallel to the outer edges of the external sphincter muscle (**Figure 9.1.2a**). The incision is extended into subcutaneous tissue of the ischiorectal fossa. Further extension posteriorly is not advised because of the risk of injury to the branches of the pudendal nerve.

In the presence of a cloaca, the incision is made at the fusion of the anterior rectal wall and posterior vaginal walls in the midline (**Figure 9.1.2b**). Laterally, the incision extends parallel to the curve of the external sphincter muscle in the subcutaneous fat.

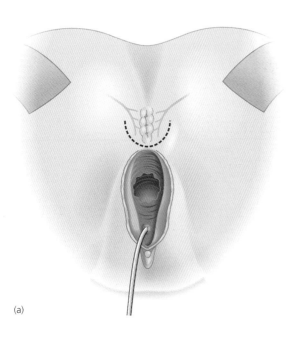

(a)

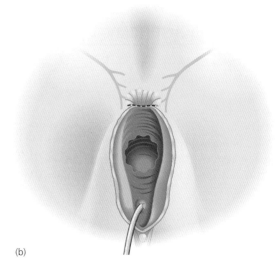

(b)

9.1.2

Mobilizing the muscle

A Lone Star retractor™ is placed to maximize exposure before starting to develop flaps (**Figure 9.1.3**). As the incision is deepened into the ischiorectal fat, the dissection is carried lateral to all identifiable fibers of the subcutaneous sphincter. Inclusion of all external sphincter muscle fibers is achieved if the dissection remains in the ischiorectal fat plane. In the midline the vaginal wall is dissected carefully off the residual scar. In some cases, the vaginal and rectal walls may be fused with little intervening tissue. Alternately applying traction by placing a finger in the vagina and anus will help identify the appropriate planes for separation and avoid injury to the rectum or vagina.

If a true cloaca exists, the first step in developing flaps is to dissect the rectal wall off the underlying vagina. The dissection proceeds cephalad until a normal appearing rectovaginal septum is reached. During this dissection venous sinuses may be encountered on the vaginal wall; suture ligation is required to stop bleeding from these sinuses.

Once the lateral borders of the external sphincter are clearly identified, the anoderm and distal rectal wall are elevated off the internal sphincter muscle laterally and off scar in the midline. It is easiest to start this dissection laterally and work medially, because in that manner planes of dissection can be developed in tissues that have not been previously injured. Early in the course of this dissection, the fibrous scar connecting the two functional limbs of the sphincter mechanism should be identifiable. The use of a Pratt bivalve anal speculum or a Fansler operative anoscope may be helpful when initiating the dissection. It is important to avoid stretching the sphincter any more than is necessary. Once the muscle is defined, the Lone Star retractor can be deepened for better exposure.

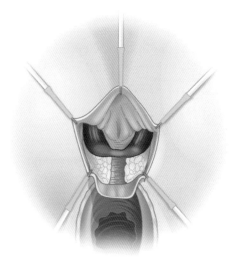

9.1.3

The dissection is complete when soft pliable tissue is reached in the midline and the external sphincter is well mobilized bilaterally. At this time the fibrotic scar joining the ends of the sphincter can be sharply divided. An attempt should be made to leave equal parts of fibrous tissue on each of the ends of the sphincter. In some situations, the divided ends of sphincter muscle will be adherent to the posterior vaginal wall and require separation from the vagina. Finally, a mixture of fibrotic scar and intact sphincter muscle may be identified in the midline. In that case a decision needs to be made whether to divide the muscle in the midline or leave it intact.

Identifying the levator ani

For deep injuries or a true cloaca, the plane between the vagina and rectum is further developed until normal planes of dissection cephalad to the injury are entered. At that point, separation of the rectovaginal septum should occur with ease. In this instance, the levator ani muscles will be identified laterally on either side of the rectum (**Figure 9.1.4**).

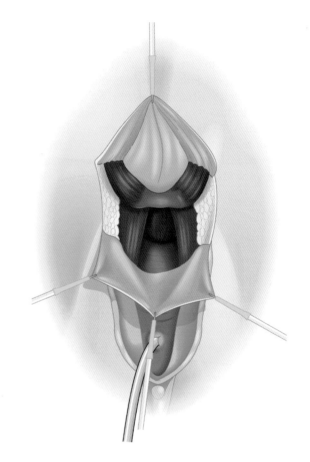

9.1.4

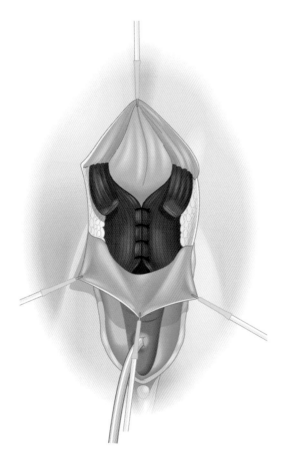

9.1.5

Levatoroplasty

A levatoroplasty can now be performed by placing several interrupted sutures of 2-0 polydioxanone or 2-0 polypropylene (**Figure 9.1.5**). The sutures will plicate the levator muscles to the midline, with the goal of lengthening the anal canal. This is most useful in true cloacal defects. Traditional teaching is that the downside of levatoroplasty is a higher incidence of dyspareunia. While there is some supportive evidence in the literature about rectocele repair, the one study in sphincteroplasty patients found no difference in sexual function between patients undergoing anal sphincteroplasty with and without levatorplasty.[3]

Sphincteroplasty

The sphincteroplasty may now be performed. Before proceeding any tears in either the vaginal or the rectal walls should be meticulously repaired with absorbable sutures (**Figure 9.1.6**).

OPTIONAL INTERNAL SPHINCTER REPAIR

In many cases, the ends of internal sphincter muscle have retracted further posteriorly than the ends of the external sphincter muscle. A standard overlapping repair may not eliminate the defect in the internal sphincter. Although controversial, a separate internal sphincter repair may improve the functional outcome. This procedure should only be done if it is easy to identify and separate the internal and external sphincters; if the tissue is too scarred attempts to separate the two muscles may lead to additional injury. Once separated, the internal sphincter muscle can either be approximated with simple stitches or overlapped with mattress stitches using 4-0 polydioxanone suture.

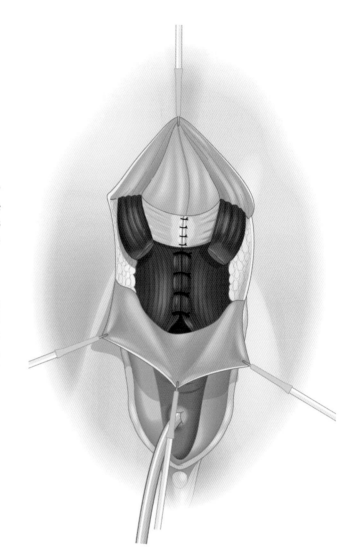

9.1.6

OVERLAPPING SPHINCTEROPLASTY

Regardless of the approach to the internal sphincter, the key portion of the procedure is the repair of the external sphincter. An overlapping sphincteroplasty is the most commonly utilized repair (**Figures 9.1.7** and **9.1.8**). Six mattress stitches of 2-0 polydioxanone sutures are placed to bring each fibrous end as far as possible to the opposite side. Three sutures are placed in each end of the sphincter. The sutures should be placed so that the sphincter can be tightened to allow the entrance of just the tip of the index finger into the anal canal. The sutures are then tied, completing the wrap.

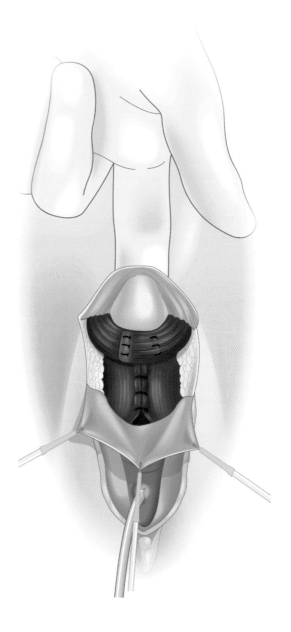

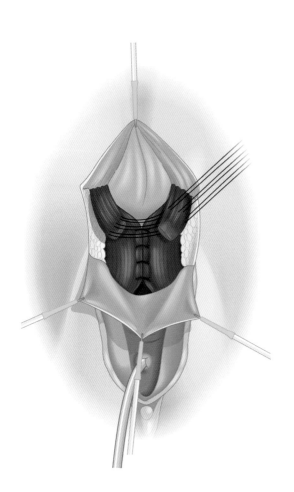

9.1.7

9.1.8

PLICATION

For partial sphincter injuries an option is to plicate the muscle (**Figure 9.1.9**). Lembert stitches of 2-0 polydioxanone suture invert the scarred portion of the muscle in the midline and imbricate the healthy muscle. Often a second layer of imbricating stitches is necessary to achieve the appropriate anal canal diameter.

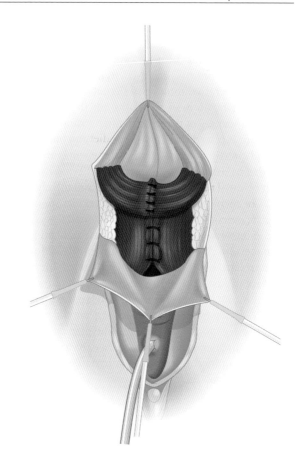

9.1.9

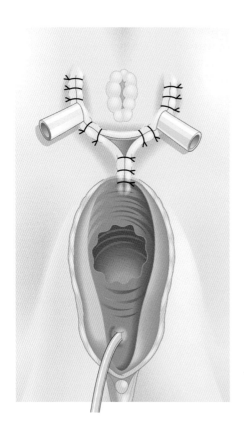

9.1.10

WOUND CLOSURE

If the transverse perineal muscles can be identified, they should be brought together in the midline to reconstruct the perineal body. The wound is closed with interrupted simple 3-0 absorbable sutures. The curvilinear incision is converted into a T-like incision or V–Y plasty to allow closure over the broadened perineum without undue tension (**Figure 9.1.10**). The wound is not closed tightly in the midline so it can drain. A 0.25-inch Penrose drain may be placed through the wound to prevent accumulation of blood or serous fluid. Well-lubricated vaginal packing is utilized for 24 hours to ensure hemostasis. The wounds are dressed lightly with a gauze sponge.

POSTOPERATIVE CARE

After operation, the urinary catheter is removed when adequate pain control is achieved, usually on postoperative day 2. Postoperative antibiotics are not necessary. Patients may shower or do brief sitz baths but they should avoid prolonged soaking of the wound. After postoperative day 2, the patient is placed on a high-fiber diet and bulk laxatives. To avoid constipation, daily tap water enemas are initiated after the patient begins to pass flatus. Typically, a small well-lubricated red rubber catheter and 200 mL tap water is used. The enemas are continued until regular spontaneous complete evacuation is occurring. Although less common, it is also imperative to avoid diarrhea so stimulant laxatives are not recommended. Loperamide hydrochloride or diphenoxylate hydrochloride are prescribed for patients who have persistent diarrhea or loose bowel movements.

It is not uncommon for the loosely approximated skin incision to separate. This separation should not cause undue concern to the patient or to the physician provided that the muscular sutures stay in place. Barrier ointments are useful to prevent perianal skin irritation secondary to wound drainage.

OUTCOME

Sphincteroplasty is highly successful for correction of rectovaginal fistulas.[6] In the short term, satisfactory functional results are obtained in 75–85 percent of patients after sphincteroplasty.[3] However, there is a growing body of evidence documenting deterioration of functional outcome after sphincteroplasty over time.[7] Predictive factors are difficult to determine. Recently, sacral nerve stimulation has been suggested as a treatment option following failed sphincteroplasty.[8]

REFERENCES

1. Oberwalder M, Dinnewitzer A, Nogueras J et al. Imbrication of the external anal sphincter may yield similar results as overlapping repair in selected patients. Colorectal Disease 2008; 10: 800–4.
2. Tjandra J, Han WR, Goh J et al. Direct repair vs. overlapping repair: a randomized, controlled trial. Diseases of the Colon and Rectum 2003; 47: 937–42.
3. Fang DT, Nivatvongs S, Vermeulen FD et al. Overlapping sphincteroplasty for acquired anal incontinence. Diseases of the Colon and Rectum 1984; 27: 720–2.
4. Dudding TC, Vaizey CJ, Kamm MA. Obstetric anal sphincter injury: incidence, risk factors, and management. Annals of Surgery 2008; 247: 224–37.
5. Hasegawa H, Yoshioka K, Keighley MR. Randomized trial of fecal diversion for sphincter repair. Diseases of the Colon and Rectum 2000; 43: 961–4; discussion 964–5.
6. Riss S, Stift A, Teleky B et al. Long-term anorectal and sexual function after overlapping anterior anal sphincter repair: a case-match study. Diseases of the Colon and Rectum 2009; 52: 1095–100.
7. Goetz LH, Lowry AC. Overlapping sphincteroplasty: is it the standard of care? Clinics in Colon and Rectal Surgery 2005; 18: 22–31.
8. Ratto C, Litta F, Parello A et al. Sacral nerve stimulation is a valid approach in fecal incontinence due to sphincter lesions when compared to sphincter repair. Diseases of the Colon and Rectum 2010; 53: 264–72.

Sacral nerve stimulation

KLAUS E MATZEL

HISTORY

Electrical stimulation of the pelvic floor was proposed as far back as early in the last century. However, once the concept of moving the stimulation from the target organs of the pelvic floor to its peripheral nerve supply was introduced, this therapeutic approach gained broader acceptance and clinical application. The aim of sacral nerve stimulation (SNS) is to recruit residual function and to re-establish lost function.

The technique used today was adapted in the early 1990s from the field of urology. The rationale for applying SNS to fecal incontinence arose from the observation of improved bowel habits and anorectal continence, increased anorectal angulation, and greater anal canal closure pressure in urologic patients. Also, anatomic dissection demonstrated a dual peripheral nerve supply of the striated pelvic floor muscles. It was reasoned that because the sacral spinal nerve site is the most distal common location of this dual nerve supply, stimulating there would enhance physiologic function (the observed increases in anorectal angulation and anal canal closure) through an easily accessible (dorsal, transforaminal) approach.

Subsequently, in 1994, SNS was first applied for the treatment of fecal incontinence in a distinct group: patients with functional deficits of the anal sphincter but no morphologic defect in whom conservative treatment had failed; traditional surgical options (e.g. sphincter repair) were conceptually questionable; and the high morbidity of sphincter-replacement procedures would outweigh the potential benefit.

Based on the positive outcome of SNS in this distinct population and the finding that a clinically efficient, minimally invasive trial stimulation could predict the outcome of permanent stimulation, selection criteria were expanded and a pragmatic 'trial-and-error' approach evolved.

PRINCIPLES

The procedure of SNS consists of three steps: the first two diagnostic, the third therapeutic. In the diagnostic stage, the accessibility of the nerve through the sacral foramen and the feasibility of electrode placement are determined; then the clinical effect of a trial period of stimulation is evaluated. Each step follows specific principles and has specific goals:

- **Acute percutaneous nerve evaluation (PNE)** tests the relevance of each sacral spinal nerve to anal sphincteric contraction (anal canal closure) and pelvic floor contraction. This diagnostic information can help to distinguish between the true functional capability of the striated anal sphincteric muscles and the patient's ability to make full voluntary use of them. By testing the functional relevance of each sacral spinal nerve (or multiple nerves) to anal sphincteric function, the individual pattern of peripheral innervation can be determined and the site of a possible lesion of the peripheral anal sphincteric nerve supply can be diagnosed. Individual differences of the somatomotor/somatosensory innervation pattern of the external anal sphincter and pelvic floor can be evaluated, and the dominance of the various levels of the sacral spinal nerves can be demonstrated to identify the optimal site for future stimulation.
- **Subchronic PNE** assesses therapeutic potential by temporarily stimulating the sacral nerve deemed most efficient functionally at acute testing (acute PNE). As a therapeutic trial it serves to select patients who may benefit from permanent neurostimulation. To confirm a beneficial response, a standardized questionnaire covers the phases before, during, and after subchronic PNE. The trial is considered effective if the frequency of incontinent episodes or days with incontinence is reduced by at least 50 percent and if the improvement is reversed after discontinuation. The trial should be long enough to confirm the 50 percent reduction.

- **Continuous low-frequency stimulation** with a permanently implanted neurostimulator (INS) aims to achieve the effect of temporary test stimulation and to improve symptoms permanently.

PREOPERATIVE ASSESSMENT AND PREPARATION

Indications

As no reliable clinical or physiologic predictor for a positive outcome of chronic SNS with a permanent neurostimulation device exists, the clinically efficient, minimally invasive, test stimulation is used on a pragmatic trial-and-error basis. Patients are appropriate for test stimulation with PNE if they have existing, even if residual, voluntary anal sphincteric function or existing reflex sphincteric activity, indicating a nerve–muscle connection (confirmed by intact anocutaneous reflex activity, reflex contraction during sneezing or coughing, or a muscle response to pudendal stimulation with a St Mark's electrode).

Contraindications

In addition to general contraindications (unfitness for surgery or prone placement), contraindications to SNS include: bony abnormalities of the sacrum preventing electrode placement in the sacral canal (e.g. severe sacral trauma distorting the anatomy); skin disorders, especially sepsis, in the areas of implantation of the electrode and pulse generator; pregnancy; bleeding diathesis; mental instability or retardation that would impede understanding and handling the device programmer; the presence of a cardiac pacemaker or implantable defibrillator; and any condition in which the risk of infection is unacceptable. Further, as the current generation of stimulation systems is not magnetic resonance imaging (MRI) safe, the need for full body MRI in diagnosing or treating any other medical condition must be excluded before offering SNS to the patient.

ANESTHESIA

Percutaneous nerve evaluation and permanent implantation can be performed under local or general anesthesia. If general anesthesia is used, muscle relaxants should be avoided; they will suppress the motor reaction when the sacral nerves are stimulated and complicate identification of the optimal position for the electrode. If local anesthesia is used, accidental blockade of the relevant sacral spinal nerves must be avoided, as the technique of electrode placement depends on a conducting nerve.

OPERATION

Anatomy

During each stage – acute testing, subchronic test stimulation, implantation of the permanent device – appropriate placement of the electrode is of upmost importance to the outcome. It should be placed close to the site where the sacral spinal nerves enter the pelvic cavity through the ventral opening of the sacral foramen and proximal to the sacral plexus (**Figure 9.2.1**).

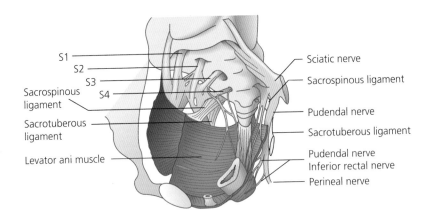

9.2.1 Anatomy: sacral spinal nerves.

Palpable anatomic landmarks are helpful in identifying the sacral foramina. Most commonly S3 is used for stimulation; it is also used as a reference location for orientation to place electrodes on S4. The S3 foramen level is located medial to the upper edge of the greater sciatic notch and a finger breadth from the sacral spine (**Figure 9.2.2**).

The foramina are located 1–2 cm from the midline, which is marked by the spinal processes (median sacral crest) and is easily palpable. The arrangement of the foramina relative to the midline may vary from parallel to a more V-shaped pattern. The distance between the levels of the sacral foramina is approximately 1.5 cm.

Preoperative or intraoperative imaging in two planes is helpful to identify individual variances in bony anatomy of the sacrum and the arrangement of the sacral foramina.

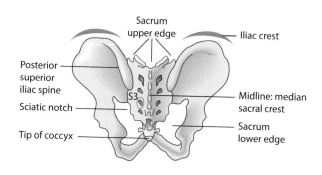

9.2.2 Anatomical landmarks.

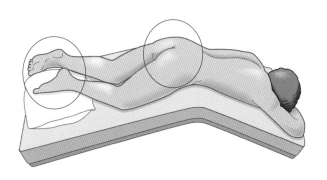

9.2.3 Patient positioning.

Procedures

The patient is positioned prone (on an x-ray-capable operating table if fluoroscopy with lateral imaging of the sacrum is required). The pelvis is supported; the legs and feet are fixed, but should be movable, as concomitant movements of the ipsilateral lower extremity during stimulation may aid electrode placement (**Figure 9.2.3**).

The operative field (sacrum and buttock) is draped and sterile. However, visualization of a motor response of the anus and perineal area, as well as the feet, must be ensured. Perioperative antibiotic prophylaxis is advisable.

Acute PNE

For acute PNE, needle electrodes (Medtronic model 041828 or 041829 foramen needles; Medtronic, Minneapolis, MN, USA) are inserted into the dorsal sacral foramina of the potentially relevant nerves S2, S3 and S4 (**Figure 9.2.4**). This positioning is mainly guided by anatomical landmarks of the sacrum and can be confirmed by fluoroscopy.

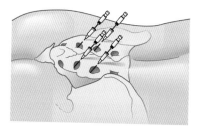

9.2.4 Acute percutaneous nerve evaluation: stimulation needle insertion.

Once the sacral foramina are identified (a distinct sensation of entering the dorsal opening of the foramen, perforating ligamentous structures as compared to hitting the periosteum of the sacrum), the needle electrode should be inserted at an acute angle to minimize the risk of nerve or vascular damage and then moved in a ventral direction (or back) with intermittent stimulation of graduated amplitudes.

The acute angle of insertion corresponds to a 60° angle at the level of the skin (**Figure 9.2.5**).

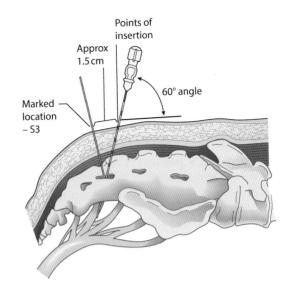

9.2.5 Acute percutaneous nerve evaluation: set-up.

A motor response of the pelvic floor and anus (if done under general anesthesia) or a sensory response (if local anesthesia) will optimize the positioning of the needle electrode. Although the effect of stimulation on pelvic floor and lower extremity activity may vary among individuals, the following responses are generally typical:

- S2 stimulation results in a clamp-like contraction of the perineal muscles and an outward rotation of the leg.
- S3 stimulation leads to contraction of the levator ani and external anal sphincter, resulting in a bellows-like movement, along with plantar flexion of the first and second toes.
- S4 stimulation produces a bellows-like contraction of the levator ani without movement of leg, foot, or toe.

If a sensory response is used to guide the placement of the electrode, it can range from a tingling 'pins-and-needles' sensation to the perception of a contracting muscle in the vaginal, perineal, perianal, or anal area.

Slow movements of the electrode into the foramen and back in millimeter steps with intermittent stimulation will help to optimize positioning, and markers on the needle electrode help to determine the depth of placement. The position is optimal when the motor/sensory response is most pronounced and the applied current is lowest. If acute PNE successfully elicits the required reaction, an electrode is inserted for subchronic PNE.

Subchronic PNE

To assess the clinical effect of temporary stimulation before permanent implantation, two technical options are available: (1) a temporary, percutaneously placed, test stimulation lead (or multiple leads) (Medtronic temporary screening lead (test electrode, 30571SC)) that will be removed at the end of this phase; or (2) a quadripolar electrode, the so-called 'tined lead', operatively, but minimally invasively, placed with the aid of fluoroscopy through a trochar (Medtronic model 3886) in a Seldinger technique. This electrode will remain in place for permanent stimulation. This procedure is termed stage 1 of a two-stage implant.

After acute PNE is performed the needle is removed, leaving the sheath in place. If a temporary electrode is used it will be inserted through the sheath and maneuvered to the appropriate sacral nerve. Intermittent stimulation is used to confirm positioning. The sheath is then withdrawn and the electrode is secured in place by adhesive dressing and its position again confirmed by stimulation and radiography (either intraoperatively with fluoroscopy or postoperatively with a two-plane sacral x-ray or fluoroscopy).

If the two-stage option is used, the needle is removed and, through the remaining sheath, an introducer guide is placed to direct the introducer for placement of the quadripolar tined lead electrode (see under Permanent implant).

For screening, both types of leads are connected to an external pulse generator (Medtronic screener 3625) (**Figure 9.2.6**); this has an extension cable connected to the electrode at the location of the future placement of the INS and tunneled percutaneously, usually to the contralateral side. Sterile dressing is used to decrease the risk of infection at the skin perforation of the extension cable during the course of the test stimulation.

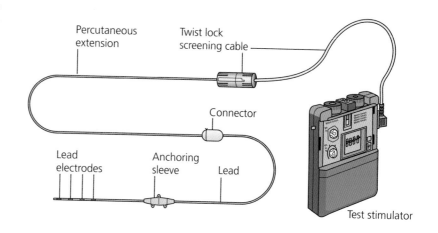

9.2.6 Set-up for timed lead electrode connected with extension to an external pulse generator.

For test stimulation with the external stimulator and the temporary electrodes, options are limited to unipolar stimulation. The parameters used are the same as for permanent stimulation (see under Permanent implant). If multiple temporary electrodes are in place, the one with the most pronounced sensory/motor response and the lowest threshold is chosen. If a tined lead has been placed as the first stage in the two-stage procedure, bipolar stimulation can be applied by setting the external pulse generator accordingly. Patients are instructed to interrupt stimulation only for defecation and micturition.

At the end of the screening phase, the percutaneously placed temporary test stimulation lead is removed and a permanent system consisting of an electrode and INS is implanted, usually some weeks after the screening to ensure intact skin conditions.

If the operatively placed quadripolar foramen electrode has been used, the percutaneous extension is removed and only the INS is added (the second stage of the two-stage implant).

Pros and cons of temporary and tined leads for PNE

Percutaneous placement of temporary test stimulation leads can be done on just one sacral spinal nerve or on multiple spinal nerves to offer the option of testing the effect of stimulation of different sides and levels or of synchronous stimulation of multiple nerves. With temporary test stimulation leads, only unipolar stimulation is possible. The fixation of the electrode is external with dressing.

The operative placement of tined lead electrodes is usually limited to one site, as it is costly and more invasive than the temporary lead. Tined lead test stimulation offers internal fixation by tines and the advantage of bipolar stimulation during testing. As there is no need for electrode removal after successful testing, the location of the electrode is retained for therapeutic chronic stimulation.

Permanent implant

The electrode is inserted with a minimally invasive technique with intraoperative fluoroscopy and neurostimulation with a Seldinger technique. After positioning the needle electrode close to the site where the target nerve enters the pelvic cavity the needle is removed, leaving the sheath in place; through this an introducer guide is placed to accept the introducer with a radiopaque depth marker through which the tined lead quadipolar electrode is pushed (if it has not already been placed as stage 1 during subchronic PNE).

The electrode consists of four contacts (Medtronic tined lead, 3889 or 3093), each of which can be stimulated separately. With intermittent stimulation and imaging, the position of the electrode is optimized; ideally, the electrode should be parallel to the nerve in a caudolateral position with all four contacts resulting in an adequate motor/sensory response at low-amplitude stimulation (**Figure 9.2.7**).

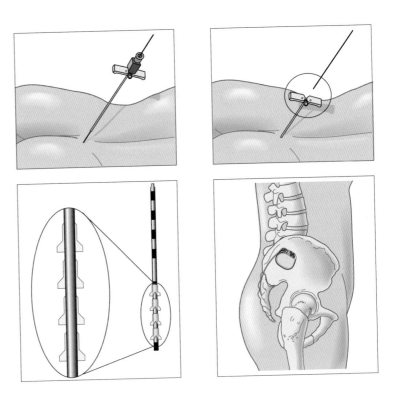

9.2.7 Tined lead electrode placement with pulse generator (four steps).

Once the position has been optimized, the introducer is pulled back and the plastic tines of the lead unfold and anchor the electrode in the surrounding tissue (**Figure 9.2.8a, b**).

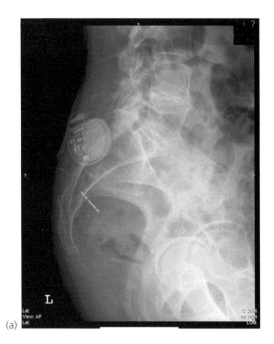

(a)

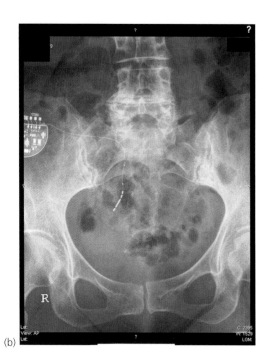

(b)

9.2.8 Electrode placement in caudolateral direction parallel to the nerve. (a) Lateral view; (b) anteroposterior view.

Depending on the type of pulse generator used, either the electrode is connected directly to the INS or an extension cable is needed. Either way, the electrode or connecting cable is tunneled subcutaneously to the position of the INS. Care should be taken to avoid proximity of the electrode/connecting cable track to bony structures, such as the iliac crest.

Currently, two INS models are available: a smaller one with a direct connector to the electrode (Medtronic model 3058) and a larger one (Medtronic model 3023) with longer battery life, requiring the use of an additional connecting cable to the electrode.

The INS is most commonly placed in a subcutaneous pocket in the buttock, medial to the dorsal axillary line (**Figure 9.2.9**).

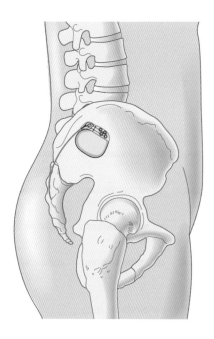

9.2.9 Tined lead electrode positioning.

The position should be discussed with the patient and marked preoperatively; it should avoid interference with clothing or habits and allow the patient to reach it with the programmer to activate and deactivate it or to change stimulation amplitude in a preset range. The skin incision for the subcutaneous pocket should be large enough to cover the INS, but not too wide (to avoid device rotation). In patients unable to reach around to the buttocks, the pocket can be placed in the abdominal wall.

During operative placement any manipulation can potentially result in a change of the electrode's position and stimulation is advised to ensure that this has not occurred and that the response is the same.

Bilateral use of foramen electrodes is uncommon, but may be chosen on the basis of an improved outcome of bilateral stimulation during the screening phase. The electrodes can be connected to two single INS devices or to a dual-channel INS (Medtronic model 7427T) that allows separate programming.

Open insertion of the electrode via an incision over the sacrum and operative exposure of the dorsal opening of the foramen is now largely reserved for patients in whom there is difficulty locating the sacral foramen with the Seldinger technique, such as those with bony abnormalities.

POSTOPERATIVE CARE

The pulse generator is activated by telemetry (Medtronic model 7432 console programmer) (**Figure 9.2.10**) early in the postoperative course. Patient cooperation is essential as programming is largely based on the patient's perception of the stimulation effect.

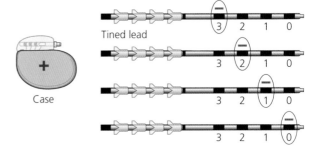

9.2.10 Postoperative electrode setting: unipolar stimulation.

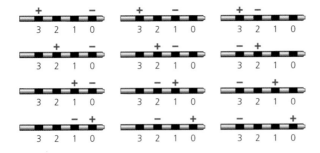

9.2.11 Postoperative electrode setting: Examples of bipolar stimulation.

Each of the four contact electrodes can be programmed as anode, cathode, or neutral (switched off). In combination with the pulse generator, which can be programmed as anode or neutral, multiple settings for stimulation are possible (**Figure 9.2.11**).

It is advisable to do the programming in a structured way and to follow an algorithm in the selection of the best parameters. The electrode combination most effective with regard to required voltage and the patient's perception of sensation or muscle contraction of the perineum and anal sphincter is commonly chosen for permanent stimulation: pulse width, 210 μsec; frequency, 15 Hz; on:off, 5 seconds:1 second or continuous stimulation. The level of stimulation is usually adapted to be above the individual patient's perception of muscular contraction or perianal sensation and adjusted if necessary. In principle, bipolar stimulation is preferable to unipolar stimulation.

Patients are instructed to interrupt stimulation with a hand-held programmer (iCon) (Medtronic model 3037) for defecation and micturition only, and to decrease or increase the intensity/amplitude of stimulation in a preset range.

COMPLICATIONS AND LIMITATIONS OF SNS

Serious complications are uncommon and require device removal in fewer than 5 percent, and are mostly prompted by infection or device malfunction. There are no reports of an infection of the spinal cord. Even if the electrode is removed, reimplantation has been successful. The most common complication is pain at the site of the INS, especially in thinner patients; however, the need for replacement is rare.

Electrode migration can occur, mostly in a ventral direction. Perforation of the rectum has not been reported. If reprogramming is ineffective, repositioning of the electrode is unavoidable.

The longevity of the INS is limited, depending on battery size, ranging between four and seven years. Current amplitude and stimulation usage mainly determine lifespan. A cycled program (alternating on and off for a set duration) or switching off the generator at regular intervals (such as during sleep) helps to prolong it. When the battery is drained the INS is exchanged in a minor intervention with disconnection and replacement.

The INS is sensitive to magnetic fields. If a need for MRI arises, the INS and electrode should be removed and can be reimplanted when the medical condition is controlled. The device is also sensitive to unipolar cautery, and bipolar cautery is advised for surgical interventions.

OUTCOME AND RECOMMENDATIONS

Published reports on SNS are heterogeneous with regard to patient selection, representing an evolution of the clinical indications. Early studies included patients with physiologic deficits in external anal sphincter and levator function, but who were otherwise morphologically intact. With the increasing experience that a positive test stimulation is highly predictive of the outcome of the permanent SNS and the expanding use of PNE as a screening tool for patient selection, it became clear that SNS improves not only external anal sphincter and levator ani muscle function, but also benefits patients with other conditions resulting in fecal incontinence, such as neuropathic fecal incontinence, cauda equina syndrome, internal anal sphincter (autonomic innervation) dysfunction, and incontinence following surgery for rectal prolapse and rectal resection. SNS also has the potential to benefit patients with concurrent fecal and urinary incontinence. Even patients with structural defects of internal or external anal sphincters have been treated successfully with SNS.

The clinical efficacy of SNS has been proven with reproducible results in multiple studies since 1994. The extent of improvement varies among the studies, but it is significant in all. Primary outcome measures, most commonly frequency of involuntary loss of bowel content but also the Cleveland Clinic Incontinence Score and the ability to postpone the call to stool, show a significant improvement. The clinical benefit is not confined to amelioration of symptoms; quality of life has been shown to be enhanced with successful SNS. The number of reports on long-term use of SNS are increasing and they uniformly demonstrate a sustained clinical benefit – for up to 18 years. Based on its limited invasiveness, the possibility to select patients for permanent therapeutic stimulation with a test trial, the reproducible clinical efficacy, and its low morbidity, SNS has become a crucial tool in the armamentarium of surgical treatment of fecal incontinence.

A systematic comparison with other surgical techniques – based on the existing level of evidence – led to the 2013 guidelines of the International Consultation on Incontinence (ICI). Surgical treatment is advised if conservative means do not result in adequate symptom relief. When conditions that secondarily result in fecal incontinence are excluded, the choice of treatment is based mainly on the findings of endoanal ultrasound. The role of SNS is central; it is recommended in patients presenting without a sphincteric lesion and is a therapeutic alternative to surgical repair in those with a sphincteric gap of up to 180°. In 2007, the UK National Institute of Clinical Excellence (NICE) considered the trial period the main advantage of SNS. Test stimulation should be considered for people with fecal incontinence in whom sphincteric surgery is deemed inappropriate. This is not limited to patients with an intact sphincter, but may include patients with sphincteric disruption. Permanent stimulation should be offered on the basis of the response to temporary stimulation.

FURTHER READING

Madoff R, Laurberg S, Lehur PA, et al. Surgery for fecal incontinence. In Abrams P, Cardozo L, Khoury S, Wein AJ (Eds): Incontinence. 5th International Consultation on Incontinence, ICUD-EAU, 2013.

Matzel KE, Kamm MA, Stösser M et al. MDT 301 Study Group. Sacral nerve stimulation for fecal incontinence: a multicenter study. Lancet 2004; **363**: 1270–6.

Matzel KE, Stadelmaier U, Hohenfellner M, Gall FP. Electrical stimulation of sacral spinal nerves for treatment of faecal incontinence. Lancet 1995; **346**: 1124–7.

Melenhorst J, Koch SM, Uludag O et al. Sacral neuromodulation in patients with faecal incontinence: results of the first 100 permanent implantations. Colorectal Disease 2007; **9**: 725–30.

National Institute for Health and Clinical Excellence Guidelines. Available from: www.nice.org.uk/guidance/IPG099.

Tan JJ, Chan M, Tjandra JJ. Evolving therapy for fecal incontinence. *Diseases of the Colon and Rectrum* 2007; **50**: 1950–6.

Tjandra JJ, Lim JF, Matzel K. Sacral nerve stimulation: an emerging treatment for faecal incontinence. *ANZ Journal of Surgery* 2004; **74**: 1098–106.

Wexner SD, Coller JA, Devroede G *et al*. Sacral nerve stimulation for fecal incontinence: results of a 120-patient prospective multicenter study. *Annals of Surgery* 2010; **251**: 441–9.

Construction of an electrically stimulated gracilis neoanal sphincter

NORMAN S WILLIAMS AND CHRISTOPHER LH CHAN

HISTORY

Efforts to create a neoanal sphincter have relied principally on the transposition of skeletal muscle, usually the gracilis, around the anal canal. Pickrell et al.[1] were the first to use this technique in man, and although satisfactory results were reported, other investigators have found the technique unreliable.[2] To improve the procedure, Cavina et al.[3] stimulated the gracilis muscle intermittently for several weeks after operation to prevent atrophy.

The original technique and subsequent modifications were poor as the gracilis, a fast-twitch muscle, was incapable of prolonged contraction without fatigue. Salmons and Henriksson[4] demonstrated in animals that long-term low-frequency electrical stimulation to a fast-twitch, fatiguable muscle could be converted to a slow-twitch, fatigue-resistant organ. Using this principle, further studies showed that, although the technique was practicable, the results were inconsistent. The technique has since been modified and is now an acceptable treatment for highly motivated patients with end stage fecal incontinence who wish to avoid a permanent stoma.[5]

PRINCIPLES AND JUSTIFICATION

Indications

The neosphincter can be used for several types of patients:

1 Incontinent patients with a deficient anal sphincter mechanism as a result of trauma or neurogenic damage with an intact rectum and anal canal. Construction of a neosphincter is indicated when other methods, such as sacral nerve stimulation or overlapping sphincteroplasty, have failed or are contraindicated.[6, 7]
2 Select patients with anorectal agenesis who have had an unsuccessful pull-through procedure and in whom endoscopic ultrasound (EUS) and ARP (anorectal physiology) indicate the absence of any functioning anal sphincter (thus ruling out a rerouting procedure).
3 Select patients who have undergone an abdomino-perineal excision of the rectum for cancer are suitable provided they have no evidence of local recurrence or distant metastases and are highly motivated to avoid a permanent stoma. The colon must be brought down to the perineum and sutured to the perineal skin several months before considering neosphincter construction.[8] Similarly, patients who have low rectal cancer and are about to undergo abdominoperineal excision of the rectum may be considered for the procedure. In such individuals, the colon is sutured to the perineal skin at the time of the resection.

We would also now recommend that in patients undergoing total ano-rectal reconstruction with a gracilis neosphincter following rectal excision a concomitant ACE procedure should be considered as a means of dealing with subsequent neorectal evacuation problems.

Contraindications

1 Damaged gracilis muscle: in practice, this includes patients with spina bifida and those with generalized neurological diseases, such as multiple sclerosis. Similarly, patients with myopathic disease affecting the limb muscles are unsuitable for the procedure. If there is any doubt about gracilis muscle function, it should be tested by electromyography.
2 Disseminated malignant disease or local pelvic recurrence.
3 Lack of sufficient manual dexterity to use the magnetic controls of the electrical stimulator.
4 Persistent perineal sepsis or Crohn's disease.
5 A cardiac pacemaker in situ.

PREOPERATIVE ASSESSMENT AND PREPARATION

Counseling

This is a most important part of the preparation in which the procedure must be fully explained. It must be stressed that there are usually three stages to the procedure and that a leg wound will result. The latter is an important consideration, particularly for women. The pros and cons of the procedure compared with a permanent colostomy must be discussed, and it must be made clear that success cannot be guaranteed. The prospective patient should meet a patient of similar age and same sex who has had the procedure for a similar indication. The patient should be shown the stimulator and programmer and provided with appropriate literature. He/she must be given sufficient time to make a decision and encouraged to return for further discussion.

Marking the site of the stimulator and covering stoma

Having made the decision to undergo the operation, a site is chosen where the stimulator is to be implanted. This is usually in a subcutaneous pocket overlying the lower ribs anteriorly. This will be on the left side if the covering stoma is to be on the right. In women, the site must be chosen so as to avoid rubbing by the brassiere. Once chosen, the site must be marked with indelible ink. Similarly, the stoma care nurse must site the position for the covering stoma. In those patients in whom a colonic pull-through procedure

is not to be performed, a loop ileostomy in the right iliac fossa is used. In those who are to have a colonic pull-through, a loop ileostomy is essential. If an ACE procedure is to be constructed simultaneously its site also needs to be marked.

Bowel preparation and prophylactic antibiotics

A full bowel preparation is required for all operative stages, unless it is to include a colonic pull-through. It is usually sufficient to give a low residue diet for 48 hours and two sachets of sodium picosulfate/magnesium citrate (Picolax®) during the 24 hours before the procedure. Antibiotic prophylaxis is provided by metronidazole and cefuroxime sodium. For stages 1 and 3, one dose is given with the premedication and two more are given at 6 and 12 hours after the procedure. For stage 2, the same antibiotics are continued for 5 days after the operation.

Deep vein thrombosis prophylaxis

Patients should be given subcutaneous low molecular weight heparin once a day, depending on their body weight.

Anesthesia

It is imperative that the anesthetist uses no muscle relaxants when the gracilis muscle is transposed and the neurostimulator implanted. If muscle relaxants are used, they will make it impossible to observe muscle contraction during nerve stimulation.

OPERATIONS

Mobilization of gracilis muscle

The patient is placed in the modified Lloyd-Davies position (as described in Chapter 1.3, Safety and positioning in the operating room). The skin of the perineum, groin, and inner aspect of the thigh on the side chosen for mobilization of the gracilis is prepared with povidone-iodine. If the covering stoma is to be eventually sited on the right side of the patient's abdomen, the left gracilis muscle is chosen for mobilization.

A longitudinal incision is made along the length of the innermost aspect of the thigh along a line from the medial femoral condyle towards the inferior pubic ramus, commencing approximately 2 cm proximal to the femoral condyle (**Figure 9.3.1**).

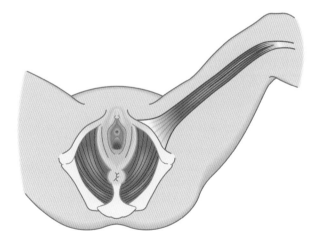

9.3.1

The skin incision is deepened through the superficial and deep fascia, and the gracilis muscle is identified. The gracilis is the most superficial muscle on the medial side of the thigh. Its tendon is easily identified in the lower part of the incision by the fact that its upper edge is overlapped by the tendon of the sartorius muscle as the latter arches over it to be inserted into the upper part of the medial surface of the shaft of the tibia below the tibial condyle. The tendon of the gracilis muscle is inserted into the tibia just behind the insertion of the sartorius tendon.

The gracilis muscle is mobilized in its distal half by division and ligation of the two or three distal vessels that supply it on its lateral surface (**Figure 9.3.2**). The intervening and overlying areolar tissue is also cleared from the muscle.

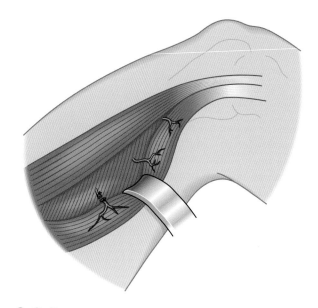

9.3.2

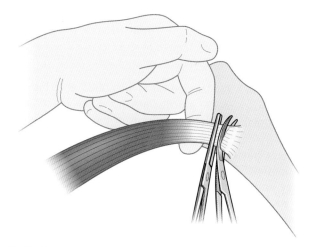

9.3.3

Transposition of gracilis muscle, implantation of electrode and neurostimulator and construction of covering stoma

The tendon of the gracilis muscle is traced down to its insertion on the tibia. The tendon is divided with strong scissors as close to its insertion as possible. It is also necessary to separate the gracilis tendon from the sartorius tendon by dividing the tissue that binds the two tendons together (**Figure 9.3.3**).

Once the tendon has been divided, it is clamped using a small artery forceps, which is then used as a retractor. By exerting traction in a proximal direction, the muscle can be mobilized upwards towards the main vascular pedicle. All areolar tissue overlying the muscle and binding it to the deeper muscles is divided (**Figure 9.3.4**).

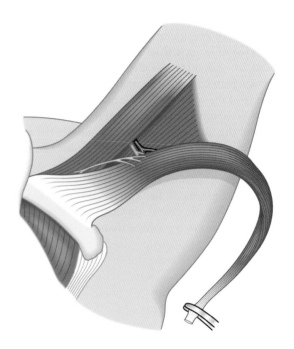

9.3.4

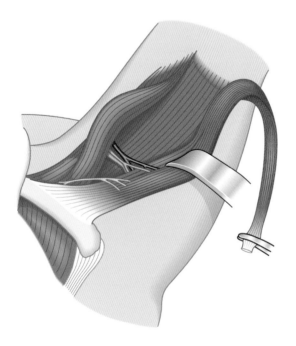

9.3.5

The main vascular pedicle is identified entering the lateral border of the gracilis, usually at the junction of the proximal and distal two-thirds of the muscle (**Figure 9.3.5**).

The pedicle consists of an artery and two venae comitantes. The artery is a branch of the obturator artery and emerges from beneath the medial border of the adductor longus to supply the gracilis muscle. Once identified, the vascular pedicle is carefully cleared of areolar tissue and freed to its point of exit beneath the adductor longus. The peripheral branches of the nerve to the gracilis lying above the main vascular pedicle can be identified using a nerve stimulator to ensure their preservation.

Mobilization of the muscle continues proximally by dividing the areolar tissue overlying its medial surface on the upper third to its origin from the lower half of the body of the pubic symphysis and the inferior pubic ramus.

The main nerve to the gracilis is sought by entering the plane between the adductor longus and adductor brevis muscles approximately 3 cm proximal to the main vascular bundle.

The main nerve is a continuation of the anterior branch of the obturator nerve. It traverses the superior surface of the adductor brevis muscle in a lateral to medial direction. In its upper part, it gives off a branch to the adductor brevis and then emerges from beneath the medial border of the overlying adductor longus to split into several branches, which enter the upper part of the lateral border of the gracilis muscle. By exerting downward traction on the upper part of the gracilis muscle, the main nerve is stretched. Identification of the nerve is confirmed by stimulation with a disposable nerve stimulator (set at 0.5 V), observing an en masse contraction of the gracilis muscle.

The areolar tissue on either side of the nerve binding it to the adductor brevis muscle is cleared. The tissue overlying the nerve is left undisturbed, and the site for electrode implantation is selected distal to the branch to the adductor brevis, but proximal to the main nerve division into its peripheral branches.

A 2 cm incision is made approximately 5 cm above the mid-inguinal point on the side on which the muscle has been mobilized. A pair of long artery forceps (Lloyd-Davies type) is passed under the adductor longus muscle in the plane between it and the adductor brevis muscle, and is tunneled subcutaneously until its tip emerges through the skin incision above the inguinal ligament. The track that has been created is enlarged by opening and closing the artery forceps several times. The tip of the electrode is grasped in the jaws of the artery forceps and gently brought through the subcutaneous tunnel, so that it emerges parallel to the main nerve (**Figure 9.3.6**).

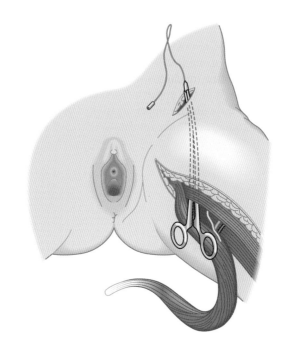

9.3.6

A transverse incision approximately 5 cm in length is made over the left anterior abdominal wall in the midclavicular line just above and lateral to the umbilicus. This incision is deepened to create a subcutaneous pocket large enough to take the simulator.

The tunneler with the trocar *in situ* is then introduced through the lower incision above the groin and advanced in the subcutaneous plane to emerge through the upper incision (**Figure 9.3.7**).

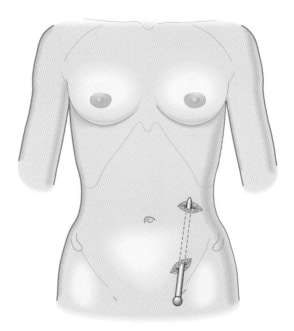

9.3.7

The trocar is removed from the plastic tube, and the proximal end of the lead with its connector destined for connection to the implant is threaded through the plastic tube to emerge in the upper incision. The plastic tube is withdrawn through the upper incision, leaving the lead ready for connecting to the implant (**Figure 9.3.8**).

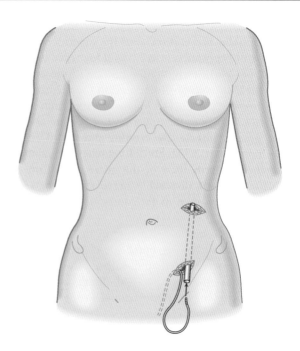

9.3.8

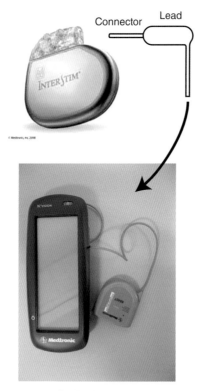

Radiotelemetry
programming unit

The connector part of the lead is passed through the silicone boot (**Figure 9.3.9**). The connector is inserted into the port on the superior surface of the implant after first releasing the screws at each connector point. It is essential to ensure that the connector part of the lead is fully pushed into the port of the implant. Only then is it fixed in place by screwing the screws down so they abut firmly against the connector part of the lead. The implant is programmed at 1 V and 10 Hz (pulse width 210 μs) using the radiotelemetry programming unit.

9.3.9

The electrode plate is sutured over the main nerve in its long axis. The non-absorbable sutures should all be placed before they are tied. Six interrupted 3-0 non-absorbable Goretex™ sutures on a round-bodied needle are used. Each suture passes through the periphery of the electrode plate, through the underlying adductor brevis muscle, taking care not to damage the nerve, and back through the plate, so that when tied the knot lies on the superior surface of the plate (**Figure 9.3.10**). From time to time, the implant is turned on by using the programmer so as to ensure that the electrode lies on the main nerve and that an en masse contraction of the gracilis muscle is achieved. Once the position of the electrode is correct, all the sutures are tied.

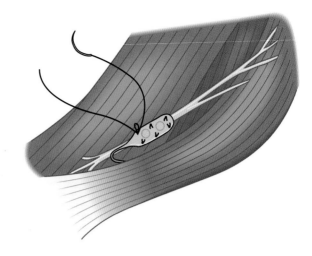

9.3.10

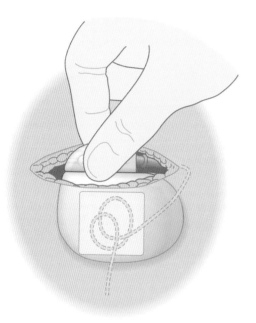

The simulator is turned off with the programmer and is placed in the subcutaneous pocket, ensuring that any redundant lead is placed behind the simulator (**Figure 9.3.11**). The transverse skin wound is closed with subcuticular 3-0 Monocryl.

The small wound above the groin is closed after first ensuring that a loop of excess lead no less than 1.5 cm in length is left in a small subcutaneous pocket at this point. This will relieve strain on the system and provide for patient growth and mobility.

9.3.11

Transposition of the gracilis muscle around the anal canal is started by two curvilinear incisions approximately 2 cm from the right and left margins of the anal verge. A circumferential subcutaneous tunnel around the anal canal, external to any remaining external anal sphincter, is created (**Figure 9.3.12**). This is deepened to ensure that it can easily accommodate the gracilis muscle when it is transposed. The skin bridges anteriorly and posteriorly are preserved. Care must be exercised in creating the space anteriorly between the anterior wall of the anorectum and the posterior vaginal wall in women. In many of these patients, there is considerable scarring in this region, and the vaginal and rectal walls are closely applied to each other. This dissection is aided by infiltration of the plane with a weak solution of adrenaline in saline (1:300 000).

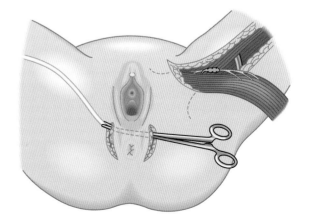

9.3.12

By gentle dissection with scissors, the plane is opened sufficiently to allow the insertion of a Jacques catheter, which can then be used to retract the anorectum downwards and allow the plane to be further dissected under direct vision. A headlight is particularly useful for this part of the procedure (**Figure 9.3.13**).

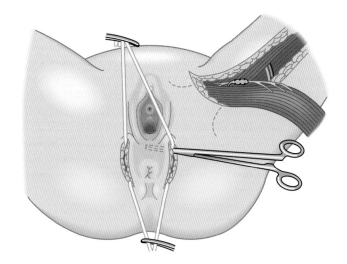

9.3.13

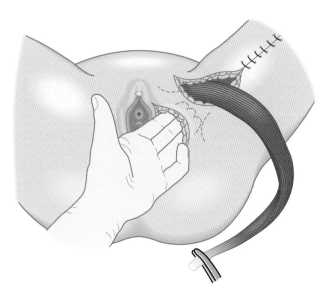

9.3.14

An incision is made in the skin crease between the thigh and the buttock on the side of the muscle to be transposed. Through this incision, a tunnel is created into the thigh to emerge close to the upper part of the mobilized gracilis muscle. It is necessary in creating this tunnel to divide Scarpa's fascia with scissors. The tunnel must be at least three finger-breadths wide. A similar tunnel is created from this incision to that on the lateral side of the anal verge (**Figure 9.3.14**).

Using a pair of long artery forceps attached to the free tendon of the gracilis, the muscle is brought into the perineum through the tunnel that has been created, ensuring that the muscle is not twisted (**Figure 9.3.15**).

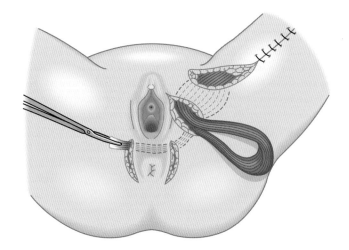

9.3.15

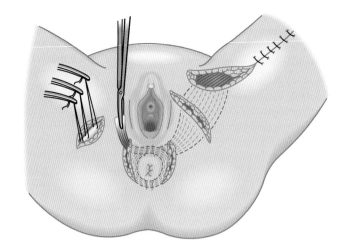

9.3.16

The muscle is brought round the anal canal in a gamma configuration. A small incision is made over the contralateral ischial tuberosity. The incision is deepened down to bone, and three interrupted 0-Ethibond sutures are attached to the underlying periosteum. The sutures are left long and clipped with the needles attached (**Figure 9.3.16**).

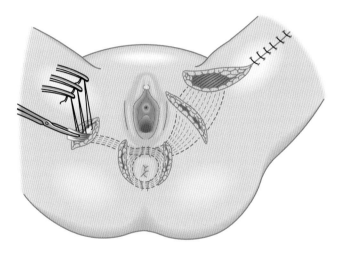

9.3.17

The gracilis muscle is transposed in an anticlockwise or clockwise direction depending on the side used, and its tendon is brought out through the incision overlying the ischial tuberosity (**Figure 9.3.17**).

The ipsilateral leg is then adducted to the midline, and the muscle is pulled through its tunnels so that it fits snugly around the anal canal, which should allow insertion of the tip of the index finger. The tendon of the gracilis muscle is then sutured to the ischial tuberosity using the previously placed interrupted Ethibond sutures (**Figure 9.3.18**).

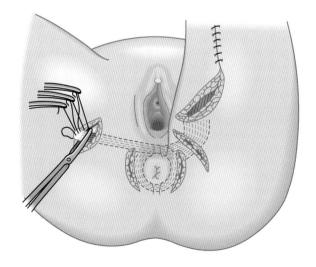

9.3.18

Once positioned, the stimulator is turned on with the programmer to ensure that contraction of the gracilis muscle occurs and occlusion of the anal orifice is achieved. The hand-held programmer is then used to check that it is able to turn the stimulator off (**Figure 9.3.19**).

The leg is closed with 3-0 Monocryl. Subcuticular polypropylene (Prolene) is used for the leg wound and interrupted 2-0 polyglactin (Vicryl) for the perineal skin wounds.

A covering loop stoma is then constructed. The authors usually use a loop ileostomy sited in the right iliac fossa and performs the operation laparoscopically (as described in Chapter 3.1).

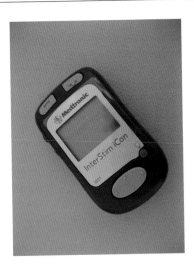

9.3.19

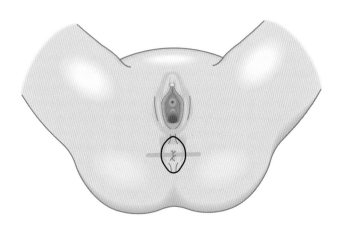

9.3.20

Total reconstruction of the perineum after rectal excision

This part of the operation differs from that previously described, in that stage 1 consists of a colonic pull-through operation with a coloperineal anastomosis.

Rectal excision is performed by an abdominoperineal approach (as described in Chapter 6.10). Before the perineal dissection is commenced, however, the position of the anal verge is marked with indelible ink, so that the neoanal canal can be positioned correctly. The perineal incision is elliptical in shape and commences anteriorly midway between the anus and the bulb of the urethra in the male or the posterior vaginal fourchette in the female, extending backwards to a point midway between the coccyx and posterior anal verge. Laterally, the incision lies approximately 1–2 cm from the anal verge. See **Figure 9.3.20**.

The incision is deepened through the para-anal tissue and ischiorectal fossa up to the plane of the pelvic floor muscles. The extent of radial dissection is not usually as wide as previously advocated, provided that this is compatible with lateral clearance of the tumor and the coccyx is not routinely removed. The dissection continues cranially, and the muscles of the pelvic floor and the lateral ligaments of the rectum are divided closer to the rectum than described previously, although it is essential to remove all the mesorectum. Therefore reconstruction as detailed below is not suitable for patients in whom a cylindrical excision of the rectum and levator muscle is being undertaken.

After the rectum and sigmoid colon have been fully mobilized, the descending colon is transected with a linear stapler at a convenient point, ensuring that the proximal side has an adequate blood supply. The rectum and sigmoid colon are removed. The descending colon is mobilized proximally around the splenic flexure to the mid-transverse colon. Care is taken to preserve the left branch of the middle colic artery which supplies the distal colon.

Stay sutures are secured to each end of the stapled line of the transected distal colon. The perineal operator then passes two pairs of long artery forceps via the perineal wound into the pelvis. The abdominal operator attaches the ends of the stay sutures into the jaws of the artery forceps in such a way that when the colon is brought down to the perineum it is not twisted. The perineal operator then gently pulls the colon down through the perineal wound; the abdominal operator assists in this process by gently guiding its passage (**Figure 9.3.21**).

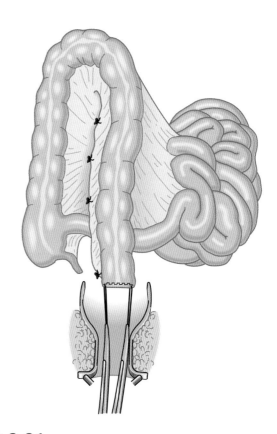

9.3.21

The abdominal operator tacks the colon to the sacrum with three or four non-absorbable sutures, which pass from the promontory of the sacrum through the serosa. Care must be taken not to damage the blood supply to the colon during this maneuver.

The perineal operator repairs any muscle that remains in the perineum and tacks the cut levator ani muscles to the serosa of the colon. The stapled end of the colon is cut off. Redundant colon is excised to prevent prolapse and the mucosa is sutured circumferentially to the perineal skin at the previous site of the anal verge (**Figure 9.3.22**). Interrupted polyglactin sutures on a taper cut needle are used for this anastomosis in the same manner as for a colostomy construction. The remainder of the perineal wound is then closed with interrupted polyglactin sutures (**Figure 9.3.23**).

A loop ileostomy is constructed in the right iliac fossa (as described in Chapter 3.1). If an ACE procedure is to be performed simultaneously (which we would now recommend) this is carried out using either the appendix or terminal ileum. The abdomen is closed in the usual manner, leaving two suction drains positioned in the pelvis emerging through the abdominal wall.

About two months, after all wounds have healed, the electrically stimulated gracilis neosphincter is constructed around the neoanal canal, as previously described.

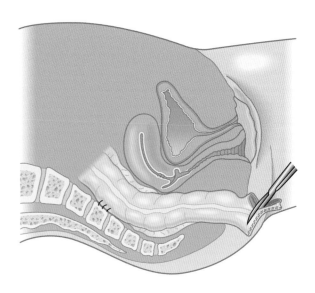

9.3.22

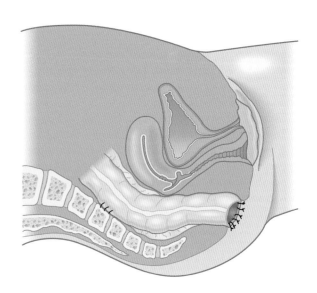

9.3.23

POSTOPERATIVE CARE

The patient is nursed with the legs together for the first 3 days and is then encouraged to become mobile. Oral fluids are commenced on the first postoperative day. Long-term electrical stimulation commences once all wounds have healed at the first outpatient visit. The stimulator is programmed using the programming unit. The 'training' protocol at present is as shown in **Table 9.3.1**.

Table 9.3.1 Training protocol for electrical stimulation of gracilis neoanal sphincter.

	Weeks 1 and 2	Weeks 3 and 4	Weeks 5 and 6	Weeks 7 and 8	After week 8
Pulse width (μs)	210	210	210	210	210
Frequency (Hz)	12	12	12	12	12
Time on (s)	2	2	2	2	4
Time off (s)	6	4	2	1	1

After 8 weeks, some conversion of 'fast-twitch' to 'slow-twitch' muscle should have occurred, which can be demonstrated by anorectal manometry using a microtransducer. With the probe positioned in the anal canal at the site of the neosphincter, the frequency of stimulation can gradually be increased until a smooth (fused) contraction takes place. The minimum frequency that produces such a tetanic contraction is known as the tetanic fusion frequency (TFF). Immediately after the operation, TFF is usually 25 pulses per second; after 8 weeks, it invariably decreases to about 10–15 pulses per second. When this reduction has occurred, the 'off' time can be reduced to zero, so the stimulator is working in continuous mode and the neosphincter is also contracting continuously, thus occluding the anal canal.

The authors' current practice is to perform a digital rectal examination rather than performing formal anorectal physiologic investigations. The patient is admitted for stage 3, i.e. closure of the covering stoma (as described in Chapter 3.1).

After closure of the stoma, the patient should be instructed on how to turn the stimulator off or on using the hand-held programmer.

Initially, there may be problems in rectal evacuation. Evacuatory problems seem to be due to the bulk of the muscle and difficulty pushing stool past this. Thus dietary manipulation with or without stool softening agents, so that stool is formed but soft may be used afterwards if necessary. Suppositories or enemas may also be used as necessary. In patients with no anal sensation, a regular daily regimen is used or if unsuccessful an ACE procedure (see Chapter 3.5) may be considered. If total anorectal reconstruction has been performed simultaneously with an ACE the patient is also taught how to irrigate distally via the ACE orifice using a catheter.

REFERENCES

1. Pickrell KL, Broadbent TR, Masters FW, Metzger JL. Construction of a rectal sphincter and restoration of anal continence by transplanting the gracilis muscle: a report of four cases in children. *Annals of Surgery* 1952; **139**: 853–62.

2. Yoshioka K, Keighley MRB. Clinical and manometric assessment of gracilis muscle transplant for faecal incontinence. *Diseases of the Colon and Rectum* 1988; **31**: 767–9.

3. Cavina E, Seccia M, Evangelista G *et al*. Construction of a continent perineal colostomy by using electrostimulated gracilis muscles after abdominoperineal resection: personal technique and experience with 32 cases. *Italian Journal of Surgical Sciences* 1987; **17**: 305–14.

4. Salmons S, Henriksson J. The adaptive response of skeletal muscle to increased use. *Muscle and Nerve* 1981; **4**: 94–105.

5. Hallan RI, Williams NS, Hutton MRE *et al*. Electrically stimulated sartorius neosphincter: canine model of activation and skeletal muscle transformation. *British Journal of Surgery* 1990; **77**: 208–13.

6. Williams NS, Hallan RI, Koeze TH, Watkins ES. Construction of the neorectum and neoanal sphincter following previous proctocolectomy. *British Journal of Surgery* 1989; **76**: 1191–4.

7. Williams NS, Hallan RI, Koeze TH *et al*. Construction of a neoanal sphincter by transposition of the gracilis muscle and prolonged neuromuscular stimulation for the treatment of faecal incontinence. *Annals of the Royal College of Surgeons of England* 1990; **72**: 108–13.

8. Williams NS, Hallan RI, Koeze TH, Watkins ES. Restoration of gastrointestinal continuity and continence after abdominoperineal excision of the rectum using an electrically stimulated neoanal sphincter. *Diseases of the Colon and Rectum* 1990; **33**: 561–5.

9. Saunders JR, Williams NS, Eccersley AJ. The combination of electrically stimulated gracilis neoanal sphincter and continent colonic conduit: a step forward for total anorectal reconstruction. *Diseases of the Colon and Rectum 2004*; **47**: 354–66.

Artificial bowel sphincter

PAUL-ANTOINE LEHUR AND MARK TC WONG

HISTORY

Fecal incontinence is a potentially debilitating condition that can have devastating consequences on both the physical and psychosocial well-being of afflicted individuals. Cross-sectional surveys of adult subjects from the general community have reported a prevalence of between 0.9 and 15 percent, with increasing prevalence with age, female sex, and obstetric injury. Most patients are treated by conservative measures, but selected individuals can benefit from traditional surgical procedures, such as sphincteroplasty, postanal repair, or transposition myoplasty. However, results have not always been favorable or consistent, and patients failing such interventions are often relegated to suffering lifelong fecal incontinence or to live with the morbidity of a permanent colostomy. In 1987, Jon Christiansen from Denmark first described the use of an artificial perianal sphincter (AMS 800™; American Medical Systems, Minnetonka, MN, USA), which was adapted from the artificial urological sphinter (AUS). Subsequent design modifications led to the development of the Acticon™ Neosphincter (by AMS), designed specifically for anal incontinence. The first implantation was performed in Nantes, France in May 1996. Since then, more than 60 cases have been performed in our center, with more than 500 cases already performed worldwide.

PRINCIPLES

Currently, the primary indication for the artificial anal sphincter is a well-motivated patient, suffering from severe anal incontinence for more than one year, who has failed or is not suitable for conventional treatments. This technique should be offered to patients as an alternative to a permanent colostomy. The patients must have sufficient mental capacity and manual dexterity to operate the device, so as to ensure regular bowel movements. The artificial anal sphincter attempts to correct the loss of resting anal pressure by restoring the high-pressure zone in the anal canal. However, this is static without the capacity to increase the pressure in imminent incontinence, and fecal continence is often never completely restored, particularly to liquid and gas.

Indications and contraindications

Paramount to the success of this procedure is careful patient selection and thorough counseling regarding the associated risks and expectations. Patients should be made aware that this device primarily serves to restore the loss of resting anal pressures and thus best provides continence to solid stools. Furthermore, being a foreign body implanted into an easily contaminated region of the body, particular attention must be paid to patients' ability to heal from surgery. The consequence of infection must be made known as this may require implant removal if antibiotics are not effective. As such, patients with active pelvic or perineal sepsis will not be candidates for this device. The ideal indication would be a young patient with sphincter injury not amenable to anal sphincter repair. The indications and contraindications are summarized in **Table 9.4.1**.

Components and function

The artificial bowel sphincter (ABS) is a semi-automated device, constructed of solid silicone rubber and consists of three fluid-filled components linked by kink-resistant tubing (**Figure 9.4.1**). The components include an inflatable cuff implanted circumferentially around the anal canal, a pressure-regulating balloon placed in the preperitoneal space of Retzius and a control pump placed in the subcutaneous tissue of the labia in women and the scrotum in men (**Figure 9.4.2**). The cuff is available in different sizes, varying from 9 to 14 cm in length and 2.0 to 2.9 cm

Table 9.4.1 Indications and contraindictions for implantation of the Acticon™ Neosphincter (artificial bowel sphincter).

Indications	Traumatic sphincter injury
	Neurological incontinence
	Neurogenic (idiopathic) incontinence
Relative indications	Agenesis of the anus
	Extensive perianal scar formation
	Thinned rectovaginal space
	Advanced age
	Diabetes mellitus
	Hand deformities
Contraindications	Extensive perineal descent
	Severe obstipation
	Radiation to the perineum
	Perineal sepsis
	Crohn's disease
	Anoreceptive sexual intercourse

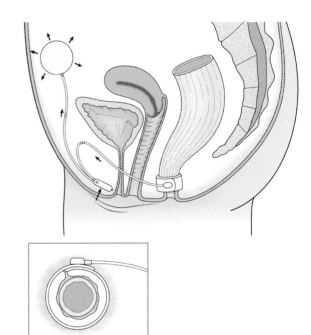

(a)

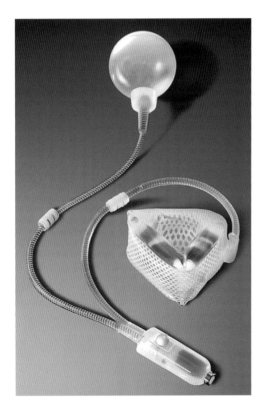

9.4.1 The Acticon™ Neosphincter.

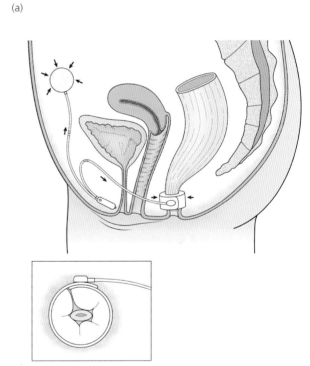

(b)

9.4.2 The Acticon™ Neosphincter device (a) deactivated with the control pump and (b) activated by passive refilling.

in width. The pressure-regulating balloon also comes with pressures ranging from 80 to 120 cmH$_2$O, in 10 cmH$_2$O steps. The control pump transfers fluid between the cuff and balloon, during activation and deactivation. When the

device is activated, the cuff is filled with fluid with pressure maintained by the regulating balloon, thus providing the necessary continence. Defecation is initiated by the patient, during which the control pump is compressed several times to displace fluid from the cuff to the balloon, thereby emptying the cuff and allowing evacuation to occur. Over the ensuing 5–8 minutes, the pressure stored in the balloon automatically repressurizes the cuff through passive fluid transfer, gradually restoring continence once defecation is complete. This returns the balloon to its original volume, thereby restoring equal pressure throughout the system, and the device is activated once again.

PREOPERATIVE

The patient should be counseled extensively regarding the risks and complications of this procedure, as well as expectations of outcome. Preoperative care comprises both meticulous cutaneous and bowel preparation over

a 48-hour period. Two douches of the operative field are performed daily with an iodinated solution and colonic preparation is performed using enteral preparations (e.g. X-prep®) and enemas, until the effluent becomes clear. There is no need for a routine colostomy, except in patients with severe preoperative diarrhea, which may contaminate the perineal wound postoperatively. Antibiotic prophylaxis using a third-generation cephalosporin and an aminoglycoside is administered in a single dose at the induction of anesthesia. In a multivariate analysis of 51 ABS implantations, Wexner *et al.* identified the early return of bowel movements (before day 2) and a history of perianal infections as independent risk factors for early postoperative infections, further reinforcing the need for conscientious bowel preparation.

OPERATION

The patient is placed in a modified lithotomy position, to allow for a combined perineal and abdominal approach for the implantation of the ABS. The first phase of the operation involves the placement of the perianal occlusive cuff (**Figure 9.4.3**).

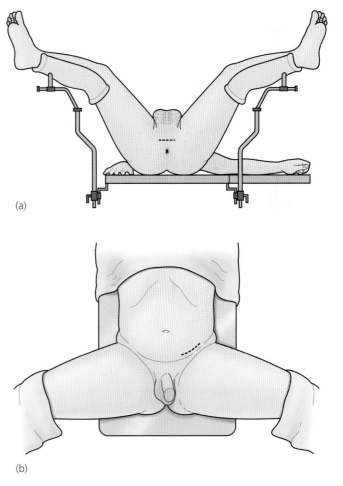

(a)

(b)

9.4.3 Patient positioning for (a) the perineal part and (b) the abdominal part of the procedure.

Perineal procedure

INCISION

A single preanal incision is made, from which a perianal tunnel can be created around the anal canal by blunt finger dissection, approximately 5–6 cm deep. This is to provide for a distance of at least 2–3 cm from the skin to the inferior edge of the implanted cuff, so as to comfortably close the perineum in layers, over the cuff without tension (**Figure 9.4.4**).

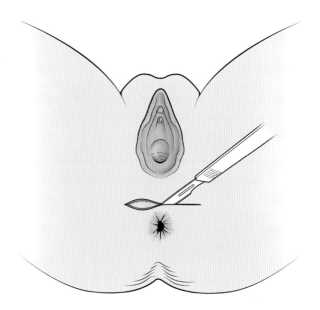

9.4.4 Perineal (preanal) incision.

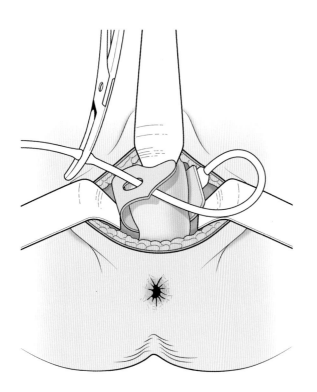

9.4.5 Placement of cuff around dissected anal canal.

SIZING THE CUFF

The length of the occlusive cuff is determined using a specially designed sizer with centimeter markings, which is wrapped around the mobilized anus and distal rectum. The cuff should be snug and not narrow the anal canal excessively, guided by digital rectal examination. The circumference is noted, to which 1 cm is added, and this length represents the final length of cuff to be used. In the event of perforation of the rectum at any point in the dissection, implantation of the ABS should be deferred or possibly abandoned. Once the perianal tunnel has been made, the preparation of the ABS device can begin on a separate sterile table. The device components are filled with sterile radio-opaque fluid, ensuring the entire system is free of air bubbles, and then occluding the ends of the tubing with silastic-shod mosquito clamps, in preparation for placement.

CUFF PLACEMENT

The perianal cuff is the first component put in place. With the cuff length determined, the space is inspected to decide between a 2.0 or 2.9 cm wide cuff. The selected cuff is then wrapped around the anus and this is secured in place by locking the silastic-holed tab over a corresponding knob. The tubing from the cuff is directed superiorly to either the right or left side depending on the planned placement of the control pump (**Figure 9.4.5**).

Abdominal procedure

Using a left iliac fossa incision, the rectus abdominis is split longitudinally to provide access to the preperitoneal space of Retzius, creating necessary space lateral to the bladder to accommodate the pressure-regulating balloon (**Figure 9.4.6**). The balloon is then filled with 55 mL of radio-opaque fluid and the tubing is similarly occluded using a silastic-shod mosquito clamp. The cuff tubing is secured to the superior end of a tunneling trocar, which is then used to create the subcutaneous tunnel, by advancing upwards above the superior pubic ramus lateral to the pubic tubercle, to emerge from the abdominal incision above.

The cuff tubing is then connected via a temporary plastic connector to the tubing of the balloon, and the pressure within the system is allowed to equilibrate for approximately 1 minute, after which the silastic-shod mosquito clamps are replaced on the cuff tubing. The balloon is emptied and the new volume of fluid now in the syringe is subtracted from the original 55 mL, giving the volume within the cuff after pressurization; this is usually between 4 and 8 mL. This volume of fluid allows the surgeon to advise the patient on the approximate number of pumps required for deactivation (each pump withdraws 0.5 mL of fluid from the cuff). Next the balloon is implanted empty and then filled with 40 mL of radio-opaque fluid, as recommended by the manufacturer, for sufficient pressurization of the system.

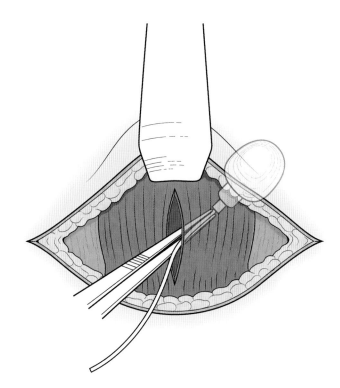

9.4.6 Placement of pressure-regulating balloon.

Control pump placement

The control pump is then positioned in a predetermined accessible position, allowing for ease of manipulation by the patient. In males, a subcutaneous tunnel is created from the abdominal wound to the scrotum by blunt dissection facilitated using a Hagar dilator (**Figure 9.4.7**); in females, a similar maneuver is performed to reach the labia majora. The control pump is placed within the subcutaneous pocket created. The pump should be secured such that the activation and deactivation buttons face anteriorly or laterally for convenient usage. The tubing is then trimmed to an appropriate length and the occlusive cuff and pressure-regulating balloon are connected to the pump, using the color-coded kink-resistant quick-connectors (black from the balloon and clear from the cuff).

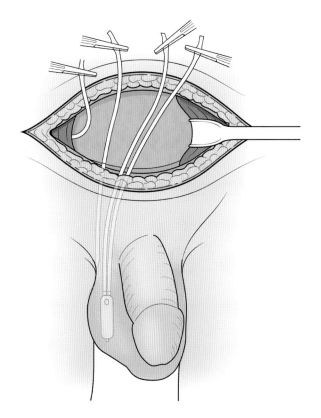

9.4.7 Placement of control pump in a male patient.

After assessing that cycling is correct, the incisions are closed in layers using absorbable sutures, with the tubing in the subcutaneous layer. No drains are used. The device is deactivated at the end of the procedure by pressing firmly on the deactivation button. In our experience, the entire procedure lasts around 90–120 minutes (**Figure 9.4.8**).

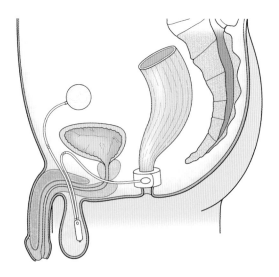

9.4.8 Final position of Acticon™ Neosphincter in a male patient.

POSTOPERATIVE CARE

Immediately after the operation, the patient is placed on a strict fluid-only diet for 3 days to avoid a resumption of bowel movements too early. The anal wound is cleaned regularly. The mean length of hospital stay is 7–10 days if there are no complications. The patient is discharged once defecation has become normal and the incisions are healed. The patient is readmitted 8 weeks later for 1 day during which the artificial sphincter is activated. A firm pressure on the control pump unblocks the deactivation button, allowing the filling of the cuff, which can then play its occlusive role. The patient is given the necessary instructions for opening the sphincter, allowing regular defecation, possibly initiated with small enemas in case of difficulty.

Follow-up of patients

Regular follow-up for patients is necessary, not only for research purposes but more importantly to check on the proper use of the device, its efficacy in restoring satisfactory anorectal function and the possible development of complications. Postoperative evaluation is based on annual examinations (clinical, plain x-rays, and anorectal manometry), as well as specific questionnaires relating to fecal incontinence and quality of life. It is important during the first postoperative months to detect any signs of cuff migration, assessing for signs of skin damage and erosion, which could lead to contamination of the material and explantation. Pressurization of the ABS with a radio-opaque fluid allows very simple radiological monitoring (**Figure 9.4.9**). These images can also be used for reference purposes in the event of subsequent dysfunction of the device. Endoanal ultrasonography can also be performed as a means of assessing the thickness of tissues encircled by the cuff and detecting any possible atrophy, which would be suggestive of ulceration of the device in the anal canal. Anal manometry, an important aspect of post-implantation monitoring, precisely and objectively estimates the efficiency of the ABS.

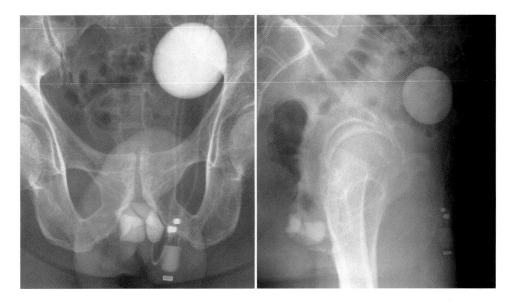

9.4.9 X-ray showing Acticon™ Neosphincter. Perianal cuff should be filled with radio-opaque fluid.

OUTCOME

In the 1990s, several centers in Europe, the United States, and Australia developed expertise in using the ABS to treat severe fecal incontinence not amenable to local repair. The emergence of less invasive treatment options, namely sacral nerve stimulation (SNS), has decreased the need for ABS implantation. However, there is still a place for this device in cases of non-response to conservative treatment, failure of local repair as well as unsatisfactory outcome following SNS. In this situation, the ABS is an effective solution for motivated patients and experienced surgeons. This is also echoed in the Standards Practice Task Force of the American Society of Colon and Rectal Surgeons and the National Institute for Clinical Excellence (UK), which stated in recent recommendations:

- Practice Parameters for the Treatment of Fecal Incontinence of the ASCRS (2007): 'The artificial bowel sphincter has a role in the treatment of severe fecal incontinence, especially in patients with significant sphincter disruption. Level of Evidence: III; Grade of Recommendation: B'.
- NICE (2008): '…If a trial of sacral nerve stimulation is unsuccessful, an individual can be considered for a neosphincter, for which the two options are a stimulated graciloplasty or an artificial bowel sphincter. People should be informed of the potential benefits and limitations of both procedures. Those offered these procedures should be informed that they may experience evacuatory disorders and/or serious infection, either of which may necessitate removal of the device. … People being considered for either procedure should be assessed and managed at a specialist centre with experience of performing these procedures'.

The authors' experience in more than 60 patients is that fecal continence can be restored for solid stool in more than 90 percent of cases, when ABS implantation has been successful, with the risk of early failure being 5–8 percent. Liquid stool and gas continence is less often achieved, estimated at 70 and 50 percent of cases, respectively. In 20–30 percent of reported series, evacuation difficulties impair daily life, with the need for regular enemas and/or laxatives, most often in the first year after implantation. We and others have shown that quality of life measured with the FIQoL instrument, improved significantly after ABS implantation.

Satisfactory results are usually sustained for five to seven years, after which late mechanical failure due to microperforation (usually inside the inflatable cuff) and loss of pressure in the system can begin to occur. ABS reimplantation after mechanical failure is a valid option for those patients who have had a good result previously. Patients usually accept the need for reimplantation, as in general they greatly appreciate the benefits obtained with the ABS.

CONCLUSIONS

With the advent of new, less invasive treatments for fecal incontinence, the role of the ABS must be put into perspective. Although morbidity and the need for revision surgery is high following implantation of the ABS, outcomes in terms of continence and improvement in quality of life are significantly improved in up to two-thirds of patients. Careful patient selection is the key to best results.

FURTHER READING

Christiansen J, Lorentzen M. Implantation of artificial sphincter for anal incontinence. *Lancet* 1987; **1**: 244–5.

Meurette G, La Torre M, Regenet N *et al*. Value of sacral nerve stimulation in the treatment of severe faecal incontinence: a comparison to the artificial bowel sphincter. *Colorectal Disease* 2008; **11**: 631–5.

Wexner SD, Jin HY, Weiss EG *et al*. Factors associated with failure of the artificial bowel sphincter: a study of over 50 cases from Cleveland Clinic Florida. *Diseases of the Colon and Rectum* 2009; **52**: 1550–7.

Wong WD, Congilosi S, Spencer M *et al*. The safety and efficacy of the artificial bowel sphincter for fecal incontinence: results from a multicenter cohort study. *Diseases of the Colon and Rectum* 2002; **45**: 1139–53.

Wong MT, Meurette G, Wyart V, *et al*. The artificial bowel sphincter - a single institution experience over a decade. *Annals of Surgery* 2011; **254**: 951-6.

Index

Note: Page numbers followed by f indicate figures; those followed by t indicate tables.